DISORDERS OF THE PANCREAS

NOTICE

Medicine is an ever-changing science. As new research and clinical experience broaden our knowledge, changes in treatment and drug therapy are required. The editors and the publisher of this work have checked with sources believed to be reliable in their efforts to provide information that is complete and generally in accord with the standards accepted at the time of publication. However, in view of the possibility of human error or changes in medical sciences, neither the editor, nor the publisher, nor any other party who has been involved in the preparation or publication of this work warrants that the information contained herein is in every respect accurate or complete, and they are not responsible for any errors or omissions or for the results obtained from use of such information. Readers are encouraged to confirm the information contained herein with other sources. For example and in particular, readers are advised to check the product information sheet included in the package of each drug they plan to administer to be certain that the information contained in this book is accurate and that changes have not been made in the recommended dose or in the contraindications for administration. This recommendation is of particular importance in connection with new or infrequently used drugs.

DISORDERS OF THE PANCREAS

Current Issues in Diagnosis and Management

Editors

Gerard P. Burns, M.Ch., F.R.C.S. (Eng. & Edin.), F.A.C.S.
Professor of Surgery
Albert Einstein College of Medicine
Bronx, New York
Chief of General Surgery
Long Island Jewish Medical Center
New Hyde Park, New York

Simmy Bank, M.D., F.R.C.P.
Professor of Medicine
Albert Einstein College of Medicine
Bronx, New York
Chief of Gastroenterology
Long Island Jewish Medical Center
New Hyde Park, New York

McGRAW-HILL, INC.
HEALTH PROFESSIONS DIVISION
New York St. Louis San Francisco Auckland Bogotá Caracas
Lisbon London Madrid Mexico Milan Montreal New Delhi
Paris San Juan Singapore Sydney Tokyo Toronto

DISORDERS OF THE PANCREAS

12345678910 HALHAL 98765432

ISBN 0-07-105402-2

This book was set in Times Roman by Bi-Comp, Incorporated.
The editors were Michael J. Houston and Muza Navrozov;
the production supervisor was Clare B. Stanley.
Project supervision was by Bermedica Production, Ltd.
Arcata Graphics/Halliday was printer and binder.

Library of Congress Cataloging-in-Publication Data

Disorders of the pancreas/edited by Gerard P. Burns, Simmy Bank.
p. cm.
Includes bibliographical references.
Includes index.
ISBN 0-07-105402-2
1. Pancreatitis. 2. Pancreatitis—Surgery. 3. Pancreas—Cancer.
I. Burns, Gerard P., date II. Bank, S.
[DNLM: 1. Pancreatic Diseases—diagnosis. 2. Pancreatic Diseases--therapy. 3. Pancreatitis—diagnosis. 4. Pancreatitis—therapy.
WI 805 D612]
RC858.P35D57 1992
616.3′7—dc20
DNLM/DLC
for Library of Congress 90-14244
CIP

Contents

Contributors*

Ira Agatstein, M.D. [11]
Fellow in Gastroenterology
University of Miami
School of Medicine
Miami, Florida

Rudolf W. Ammann, M.D. [16]
Professor of Medicine
Department of Medicine—
Gastroenterology Service
University Hospital
Zurich, Switzerland

Dana K. Andersen, M.D. [26]
Professor of Surgery and Medicine
Chief, Section of General Surgery
Department of Surgery
The University of Chicago
Chicago, Illinois

Emil J. Balthazar, M.D. [13]
Professor of Radiology
Department of Radiology
New York University Medical Center
New York, New York

Simmy Bank, M.D., F.R.C.P. [3,4,14]
Professor of Medicine
Albert Einstein College of Medicine
Bronx, New York
Chief of Gastroenterology
Long Island Jewish Medical Center
New Hyde Park, New York

Jamie S. Barkin, M.D., F.A.C.P. [11]
Professor of Medicine
University of Miami
School of Medicine
Chief of Gastroenterology
Mount Sinai Medical Center
Miami Beach, Florida

Les H. Blumgart, M.D. [22]
Enid A Haupt Professor of Surgery
Department of Surgery
Memorial Sloan-Kettering Cancer Center
New York, New York

Eric J. S. Boyd, M.D., M.R.C.P. [18]
Research Fellow
Ninewells Hospital and Medical School
Dundee, Scotland

Gerard P. Burns, M.Ch., F.R.C.S. (Eng. & Edin.), F.A.C.S. [4]
Professor of Surgery
Albert Einstein College of Medicine
Bronx, New York
Chief of General Surgery
Long Island Jewish Medical Center
New Hyde Park, New York

* The numbers in brackets following the contributor name refer to chapter(s) authored or co-authored by the contributor.

Donald R. Campbell, M.D. [19]
Assistant Professor of Medicine
Department of Medicine
University of Kansas School of Medicine
Kansas City, Kansas

Marc L. Citron, M.D. [27]
Associate Professor of Medicine
Albert Einstein College of Medicine
Bronx, New York
Head, Section of Medical Oncology
Long Island Jewish Medical Center
New Hyde Park, New York

Meinhard Classen, M.D. [8]
Professor of Medicine
Direktor der II medizinischen Klinik und Poliklinik
Der Technischen Universitat München
Munich, Germany

David A. Dreiling, M.D.* [15]
Alfred and Florence Gross Professor of Surgery
Vice Chairman
Department of Surgery
The Mount Sinai School of Medicine
New York, New York

Mary E. Estakhri, M.D. [12]
Resident in Surgery
Department of Surgery
University of California, Davis
Sacramento, California

Jack Farman, M.B., Ch.B., M.Med., F.A.C.R. [5]
Professor of Clinical Radiology
Columbia-Presbyterian Medical Center
New York, New York

Charles F. Frey, M.D. [12]
Professor and Vice Chairman
Department of Surgery
University of California, Davis
Sacramento, California

Philippe Gertsch, M.D. [22]
Professor of Surgery
Department of Visceral and Transplant Surgery
Universitat Bern
Klinik fur Viszerale Chirurgie
Bern, Switzerland

Pierce A. Grace, M.Ch., F.R.C.S.I. [24]
Senior Registrar
Royal College of Surgeons in Ireland
Dublin, Ireland

Ronald Greenberg, M.D. [3,14]
Assistant Professor of Medicine
Albert Einstein College of Medicine
Bronx, New York
Attending Physician
Long Island Jewish Medical Center
New Hyde Park, New York

Norton J. Greenberger, M.D. [19]
Chairman and Peter T. Bohan Professor of Medicine
Department of Medicine
University of Kansas School of Medicine
Kansas City, Kansas

Friedrich Hagenmueller, M.D. [8]
Professor of Medicine
Head of Gastroenterology
Altona Hospital
Hamburg, Germany

* Deceased.

Michael H. Harvey, M.B., F.R.C.S. [1]
Registrar in Surgery
Norfolk and Norwich Hospitals
Norwich, England

Martin Hirsch, M.D. [13]
Assistant Professor of Radiology
New York University Medical Center
New York, New York

Klaus Knyrim, M.D., Ph.D. [8]
Assistant Attending Kassel Hospital
Kassel, Germany

I. N. Marks, M.B., Ch.B., F.R.C.P. [2]
Professor of Gastroenterology
University of Cape Town
Head
Department of Gastroenterology
Groote Schuur Hospital
Cape Town, South Africa

Robert McGovern, M.D. [11]
Senior Fellow in Gastroenterology
University of Miami
School of Medicine
Miami Beach, Florida

Charles J. Mitchell, M.B., F.R.C.P. [9]
Consultant Physician and Gastroenterologist
Scarborough Hospital
Honorary Consultant Physician
St. James' University Hospital
Leeds, North Yorkshire United Kingdom

A. R. Moosa, M.D. [21]
Professor and Chairman
Department of Surgery
University of California
San Diego Medical Center
San Diego, California

Ali Reza Moattari, M.D. [25]
Assistant Professor of Internal Medicine
Northeastern University
Chicago, Illinois

Horst Neuhaus, M.D. [8]
Assistant Professor of Medicine
11 Medizinschen Klinik und Poliklinik
Der Technischen Universitat München
Munich, Germany

Benjamin W. Pace, M.D. [6]
Assistant Professor of Surgery
Albert Einstein College of Medicine
Bronx, New York
Associate Attending Department of Surgery
Long Island Jewish Medical Center
New Hyde Park, New York

Ivana Pavlic-Renar [25]
Research Fellow
Department of Internal Medicine
East Virginia Medical School
Norfolk, Virginia

Henry A. Pitt, M.D. [24]
Professor and Vice Chairman
Department of Surgery
Johns Hopkins Medical Institutions
Baltimore, Maryland

John H. C. Ranson, M.B., F.A.C.S. [7]
Professor of Surgery
New York University Medical Center
New York, New York

Howard A. Reber, M.D. [1]
Professor and Vice Chairman
Department of Surgery
U.C.L.A. School of Medicine
Los Angeles, California
Chief, Surgical service
Sepulveda Veterans Administration Hospital
Sepulveda, California

John Robert, M.D. [15]
Fellow in Research
Department of Surgery
The Mount Sinai School of Medicine
New York, New York

Henri Sarles, M.D. [17]
Director
Unite de Recherches de Pathologie Digestive
INSERM
Marseilles, France

Richard M. Schaffer, M.D. [5]
Assistant Professor of Clinical Radiology
Columbia-Presbyterian Medical Center
New York, New York
Attending Radiologist
St. Luke's-Roosevelt Hospital Center
New York, New York

Neal E. Seymour, M.D. [26]
Assistant Professor of Surgery
University of Texas
Southwestern Medical School in Dallas
Dallas, Texas

Frederick P. Smith, M.D. [27]
Clinical Professor of Medicine
Georgetown University
Washington, D.C.

Bernard Stark, M.D. [14]
Assistant Professor of Medicine
Albert Einstein College of Medicine
Bronx, New York
Attending Physician
Long Island Jewish Medical Center
New Hyde Park, New York

Norman W. Thompson, M.D. [25]
Henry King Ransom Professor of Surgery
University of Michigan, Ann Arbor
Ann Arbor, Michigan

Aholeab E. Toleldano, M.D. [15]
Research Fellow
Department of Surgery
The Mount Sinai School of Medicine
New York, New York

Philip Vigneri, D.O. [27]
Assistant Professor of Radiation Oncology
Albert Einstein College of Medicine
Bronx, New York
Attending Radiation Oncologist
Long Island Jewish Medical Center
New Hyde Park, New York

Aaron I. Vinik, M.D. [25]
Professor of Internal Medicine
Anatomy and Neuroanatomy
East Virginia Medical School
Norfolk, Virginia

Andrew L. Warshaw, M.D. [10]
Harold and Ellen Danset Professor of Surgery
Harvard Medical School
Associate Chief of Surgery
Massachusetts General Hospital
Boston, Massachusetts

Thomas Taylor White, M.D.* [20]
Clinical Professor of Surgery
University of Washington
Seattle, Washington

---

* Deceased.

Leslie Wise, M.D. [6]
Professor of Surgery
Albert Einstein College of Medicine
Bronx, New York
Chairman, Department of Surgery
Long Island Jewish Medical Center
New Hyde Park, New York

Kenneth G. Wormsley, M.D., D.Sc., F.R.C.P. [18]
Consultant Physician and Gastroenterologist
Ninewells Hospital and Medical School
Dundee, Scotland

David S. Zimmon, M.D. [23]
Professor of Clinical Medicine
New York University School of Medicine
St. Vincent's Hospital
New York, New York

Preface

Recent advances in the investigation and treatment of pancreatic disorders have greatly increased the choices in clinical management available to the physician. The purpose of this book is to explore selected areas in which there are often lack of agreement and sometimes contention regarding the most efficacious modality of diagnosis or therapy. It does not purport to cover the gamut of pancreatic diseases, as several comprehensive texts on the pancreas have appeared in recent years.

The selected topics have been discussed in most instances by two authors from whom diverging viewpoints might be expected. The authors were allowed considerable leeway in their discussions, which served both to highlight the controversial aspects and to reveal a considerable degree of unexpected unanimity of opinion. Individual topics have been preceded by an editorial statement of the controversies involved and comment on the views expressed by the authors.

All the contributors to this issue are pancreatologists who have spent most of their careers investigating and managing patients with pancreatic diseases. Each has taken up the challenge to present a forthright view on a controversial topic, and we are deeply appreciative of their efforts.

DISORDERS OF THE PANCREAS

CHAPTER

1

LESSONS FROM EXPERIMENTAL PANCREATITIS

Howard A. Reber and Michael H. Harvey

EDITORIAL COMMENT

It seems likely from the experimental models used to study pancreatitis that multiple factors are involved even when a single agent is responsible. These factors may include pancreatic duct permeability, capillary permeability, pancreatic secretion, intraductal pressure, bacterial contamination, decrease in blood flow, and activation of pancreatic enzymes.

It is clearly oversimplistic to emphasize a single etiologic factor such as pancreatic ductal obstruction, as this alone will not produce disease. Similarly, emphasis on single factors in treatment, such as inhibiting pancreatic secretion or removing peritoneal toxic fluid, leads to therapeutic disappointment. These experimental studies have been helpful in demonstrating the complexity of acute pancreatitis both in its etiology and pathophysiology, but therapeutic advances resulting from the studies have not been forthcoming. Nevertheless, continued studies are beginning to look promising. The pathophysiology is now being examined at the cellular level, and definition of the roles of prostaglandins, oxygen-free radicals, and changes in capillary permeability may eventually lead to new therapeutic approaches.

CONTROVERSY

Pancreatitis is impossible to study directly in humans because of the inaccessibility of the organ. The stages of evolution of human pancreatitis from mild disease to diffuse necrosis are poorly understood. Some would question whether such an evolution indeed occurs. Hence there has been widespread use of animal experimental models. But what is the best animal to use? What etiologic agent should be employed? Should normal animals be studied or rather those suffering from induced alcoholism, malnutrition, or a metabolic disorder? Is the isolated perfused pancreas from an animal a suitable model to study or does it represent a dying organ? This chapter addresses many of these issues.

Claude Bernard in 1856 created the first experimental model of acute pancreatitis when he injected bile and olive oil into the dog pancreas.[14] Despite considerable research, 130 years later there are still significant gaps in our understanding of the pathogenesis and pathophysiology of the disease. Advances in treatment have been made, but the search for a specific therapy continues to frustrate investigators. Today the management of these patients is still largely supportive.

In this chapter we review the various models of experimental pancreatitis and evaluate the contribution that each has made to our understanding of the human disease.

AN "IDEAL" MODEL OF ACUTE PANCREATITIS

Direct investigation of the human pancreas is difficult and potentially dangerous. Thus, clinical studies of acute pancreatitis have focused mainly on the epidemiology of the disease and its response to a variety of treatments. In order to study the etiology and pathophysiology of the disease, investigators have turned to animal models. A great number of experimental models of acute pancreatitis have been devised, each of which resembles the human condition to a greater or lesser extent. The "ideal" experimental model has yet to be described. The requisites for such a model include the following. The anatomy and physiology of the animal pancreas should be similar to that found in humans. Acute pancreatitis should occur spontaneously in the normal population, and the pathologic features of the disease should resemble those found in human acute pancreatitis. It should be possible to produce the disease with all known etiologic agents. The disease should run a similar course to that in human pancreatitis in terms of both its local and its distant manifestations. Morbidity and mortality rates should be similar. The system should not depend on circumstances or substances not found under physiologic conditions. Finally, the ideal model should be inexpensive, readily available, noninvasive, and easily reproducible.

Unfortunately such a model has been unattainable, and compromises have had to be made. Thus, some models produce a rapidly evolving lethal hemorrhagic pancreatitis. They are better suited to studies of pathophysiology and less well suited to studies involving treatment. Others are slow to evolve and produce a nonlethal form of the disease. Therefore, they may be useful for therapeutic studies. It is important for investigators to be aware of the strengths and weaknesses of each experimental model so that they can select the one that is best suited to answer their questions.

EARLIER MODELS

Much of our knowledge of human acute pancreatitis has come from the study of the three experimental models described below.

Duct Injection Models

The duct injection model has been widely used in attempts to test the *common channel* theory of acute pancreatitis described by Opie in 1901.[85] Opie suggested that a gallstone might produce obstruction of the ampulla of Vater, permitting bile to reflux from the common bile duct into the pancreatic duct. Since that time numerous investigators have produced acute pancreatitis by injecting gastric juice, hydrochloric and nitric acids, and sodium hydroxide, as well as bile or bile salts, into the main pancreatic duct. The model is adaptable to most animal species, but rats and dogs have been used most commonly. The substance (usually bile with or without activated pancreatic enzymes) is injected via a cannula placed in the main pancreatic duct in the head of the gland. The severity of the pancreatitis depends on the substance infused and the infusion pressure.

Flexner showed in 1906 that the deleterious effects of bile salt injection depend on the salt used and its concentration.[42] Unconjugated bile salts produce the most severe damage. A combination of bile and trypsin or pancreatic juice has been shown to increase the severity of pancreatitis.[33,117] Bacterial infection of the injected bile also increases the degree of pancreatic damage. Aho and Nevelainen studied the early histologic changes in the rat pancreas following bile injection.[2] They demonstrated severe ductal disruption within 5 minutes of manual injection of homologous bile, allowing bile and pancreatic enzymes to enter the pancreatic interstitium. Other experiments from the same laboratory showed that the rat pancreatic duct ruptures at a pressure of 82 mm Hg.[4] These observations suggested that injection pressure is an important determinant of pancreatic damage in this model. It is important to remember that even in the presence of pancreatic duct obstruction, such high pressure within the pancreatic duct does not occur in humans. Hence, the results of experiments using high-pressure injection techniques must be interpreted with caution.

Evidence against the common channel theory has come from experiments in which the entire output of bile has been diverted through the pancreatic duct of dogs[130] and goats[103] without producing acute pancreatitis. Other workers have shown in humans that the pressure within the pancreatic duct is consistently higher than that in the common bile duct under a variety of conditions,[7,18] Thus pancreatic juice would be expected to flow into the common bile duct when a common channel exists rather than the reverse. However, animal experiments suggest that under certain circumstances this pressure relationship may be reversed.[33,53,80] Recently Senninger et al. tested the common channel theory in a model of acute pancreatitis using the opossum.[113] This animal has a long common channel (2–3 cm) between the bile and pancreatic ducts. The unusual anatomic configuration allowed investigation of the effects of ligation of the common duct well below the junction of the bile and pancreatic ducts. They found that obstruction of the common duct, allowing biliary–pancreatic reflux, resulted in severe necrotizing pancreatitis. However, when the bile duct and the pancreatic duct were ligated above their confluence, thus preventing reflux, pancreatitis also developed. Ligation of the bile duct or pancreatic duct alone did not result in pancreatitis. They concluded that biliary obstruction rather than bile reflux is the prerequisite for the development of acute pancreatitis in this model, although the mechanism is obscure. Other observations indicate that only 18% of individuals have a common channel long enough to allow fluid to pass from one duct to another when the ampulla is blocked by a gallstone.[26]

The duct injection model has also been used to examine the effects of pancreatic enzymes on the development of acute pancreatitis. Polya[92] was the first to inject trypsin into the pancreatic duct and produce pancreatitis. Heat-inactivated trypsin had no effect. Anderson et al. infused specific pancreatic enzymes into the canine pancreatic duct.[9] They found that trypsin and chymotrypsin, but not amylase or carboxypeptidase, produced acute pancreatitis when infused at pressures of less than 140 mm Hg. Recently, however, the role of trypsin in producing pancreatic necrosis has come into question since it has been shown that the enzyme is incapable of digesting healthy cells or native protein.[99,41] The importance of trypsin in acute pancreatitis is perhaps more likely to be related to its role as an activator of other proteolytic enzymes such as elastase and phospholipase A. Geokas[45] produced acute hemorrhagic pancreatitis by injecting elastase into the canine pancreatic duct. He also demonstrated injury to elastic fibers of small vessels and ducts when pancreatic slices were incubated in vitro with elastase. Attention has focused recently on the possible role of phospholipase A in the pathogenesis of acute pancreatitis. The principal substrates of this enzyme are lecithin and cephalin, which are major components of cell membranes. Lecithin is an essential component of bile, and bile acids are known to activate phospholipase A.[73] In rats, intraductal phospholipase A_2 failed to produce necrotizing pancreatitis.[109] However, when a mixture of phospholipase A_2 and bile were injected, severe pancreatitis resulted. Lysolecithin (produced by the action of phospholipase on lecithin) injected into the pancreatic duct of rats also produced pancreatic necrosis. These authors also reported finding large amounts of lysolecithin in the pancreas of three patients who died of acute pancreatitis.

Pancreatic Duct Obstruction Models

Obstruction to the flow of pancreatic juice may result from a variety of causes including biliary calculi, tumor, stricture of the pancreatic duct, and ampullary edema, stenosis, and spasm. Simple ductal ligation does not produce acute pancreatitis but rather pancreatic atrophy.[126] However, when ductal ligation is combined with a stimulus to pancreatic secretion, edematous pancreatitis results.[71,93] These changes are thought to occur as a result of ductal hypertension and the escape of ductal contents into the interstitial tissues. The ability of the pancreatic duct to withstand elevated pressure has been studied. Bockman demonstrated disruption of duct and acinar plasma membranes by electron microscopy after injecting ferritin under pressure (150 mm Hg) into the pancreatic duct of dogs.[16] Pirola and Davis[91] elevated duct pressure in cats to within a range they had measured during active secretion of the pancreas (20–40 mm Hg) and observed extravasation of India ink particles from the ducts. The greatest degree of extravasation was seen in those animals with the highest pressures.

Vascular factors in the presence of pancreatic duct obstruction may be important in the pathogenesis of hemorrhagic pancreatitis. Popper et al. produced edematous pancreatitis in dogs by ductal ligation and intravenous secretin administration.[94] They were able to convert this to hemorrhagic pancreatitis by ligating the gastroduodenal artery for 15 minutes. Ligation of the artery alone had no effect. Menguy et al. reported similar results.[79]

Other investigators, using different models, have also stressed the importance of vascular factors. Pfeffer et al. interrupted the arterial supply of the dog pancreas by injecting microspheres of various sizes into the pancreaticoduodenal artery and observed the development of hemorrhagic pancreatitis.[89] The most severe lesions occurred with the smallest microspheres, suggesting that ischemia caused by occlusion of end arteries was the cause. Goodhead produced acute edematous pancreatitis by intraductal injection of autologous bile at a pressure of 140 mm Hg.[49] He showed that although total pancreatic blood flow increased, pancreatic perfusion decreased. When he injected a bile-trypsin mixture producing hemorrhagic pancreatitis, both flow and perfusion decreased. Furthermore he showed that hemorrhagic pancreatitis could be prevented by sympathectomy and heparin and low-molecular-weight dextran administration (all of which increased pancreatic blood flow). Other investigators, using duct injection models, have demonstrated a fall in pancreatic blood flow during the course of acute pancreatitis.[8,87] In contrast Berry et al., using a modification of the closed duodenal loop model (described below) in rats, demonstrated an increase in pancreatic blood flow and perfusion early in the course of hemorrhagic pancreatitis.[15] This suggested a primary inflammatory response.

Duodenal Reflux Models

Enterokinase, the enzyme responsible for the activation of trypsinogen, is synthesized by the enterocytes of the proximal small intestine.[57] The concept that reflux of duodenal contents into the pancreatic duct might be responsible for the activation of trypsinogen within the pancreas, and the subsequent development of acute pancreatitis, was first put forward by Williams and Busch in 1907.[131] However, the theory gained little acceptance until 1962, when McCutcheon and Race[78] performed a series of experiments in dogs using a model described by Pfeffer et al.[90] In this model the common bile duct was ligated and bile flow diverted by cannula to the duodenum. Then the duodenum was closed at the pylorus and at a point distal to the entry of the pancreatic duct. This created a blind duodenal loop. Gastrointestinal continuity was restored by a gastroduodenostomy distal to the loop. The model produces a rapidly evolving hemorrhagic pancreatitis with a high mortality rate. Using this model McCutcheon and Race showed that the pancreatitis that developed could be prevented by ligating the pancreatic duct. This suggested that duodenal reflux was the initiating event. However, there are a number of serious objections to this theory. Robinson and Dunphy[103] perfused duodenal secretions through the pancreatic duct of goats and found that despite the presence of activated pancreatic enzymes within the ductal lumen, pancreatitis did not occur. Strack et al. added barium to the duodenal contents in a Pfeffer loop preparation and found that duodenopancreatic reflux only occurred after pancreatitis had already developed.[116] These findings appear to substantiate those of Archibald, who, using postmortem specimens, was unable to demonstrate reflux of duodenal contents with an intraduodenal pressure of 1000 mm H_2O sustained for 1 hour.[10] Cavallari et al. were unable to confirm that pancreatitis could be prevented in the Pfeffer preparation by ligating the pancreatic duct.[19] Rosato et al. showed that duodenal obstruction in dogs, at pressures that were controlled to avoid vascular compromise of the duodenal mucosa, did not result in pancreatitis.[104] Thus the evidence implicating duodenal reflux as a pathogenic factor in acute pancreatitis is not strong. However experiments by Hammond and Mann[52] in which acute pancreatitis was produced by the intraductal injection of enterokinase, and observations by Grant et al.[50] and Talbot et al.[118] suggest that this enzyme may indeed play a role in the pathogenesis of the disease. Grant and associates demonstrated the presence of active enterokinase in human bile and excluded duodenobiliary reflux as the mechanism. They concluded that the enzyme must have been "absorbed" from the gut and carried to the liver, where it was excreted into bile. They suggested that biliary–pancreatic reflux might be the initiating event in acute pancreatitis. Indeed Talbot et al. showed that enterokinase can be readily displaced into the circulation following perfusion of the small bowel with saline. They suggested that this might occur normally as a response to a meal.

The three experimental models described above all have certain strengths and weaknesses. The *duct injection models* are simple to set up, inexpensive, and adaptable to many species. They produce rapidly evolving lesions and are readily reproducible. These histologic lesions bear some resemblance to the human disease. However, they require invasive techniques and in most cases involve the use of higher injection pressures than are likely to be found clinically. Models involving *pancreatic duct obstruction* are also simple and adaptable to a variety of species. Edematous pancreatitis can be produced by duct ligation and stimulation of pancreatic secretion, but the production of hemorrhagic pancreatitis requires additional invasive vascular maneuvers. An attractive feature of this model is its apparent high clinical relevance (e.g., duct obstruction by a gallstone with continued pancreatic secretion). The *duodenal reflux model* is highly invasive, is complex to prepare, and produces a rapidly evolving hemorrhagic pancreatitis. Another disadvantage of this model is its doubtful clinical relevance, except perhaps in the rare instance of pancreatitis associated with obstruction of an afferent loop.

RECENTLY DESCRIBED MODELS

In recent years several new models of acute pancreatitis have been described. Experiments using some of these models have provided important new information regarding the disease, and about the physiology of pancreatic secretion.

Diet-induced Pancreatitis

Lombardi et al. described a new model of acute pancreatitis that involved feeding young female mice a choline-deficient diet supplemented with 0.5% DL-ethionine (CDE diet).[72] The lesion was 100% fatal within 5 days, and death was due to massive hemorrhagic necrosis of the pancreas with extensive fat necrosis throughout the peritoneal cavity. Male mice treated with estradiol were also affected, suggesting that estrogens were important.[96] Gilliland and Steer modified the protocol by feeding the mice for only 24 hours preceded and followed by a 24-hour fast.[47] This reduced the mortality to 55% to 60% and allowed study of the alterations in acinar cell function induced by the diet. They found that digestive-enzyme secretion was blocked and zymogen granules accumulated within the cell. When the pancreas was removed 24 to 72 hours after starting the diet, large vacuoles were seen within the cytoplasm. These were subsequently shown to contain both digestive enzymes and lysosomal hydrolases. This suggested that one effect of the diet was to produce fusion of zymogen granules with lysosomes (a process known as *crinophagy*). This may be of importance in the development of pancreatitis, since the lysosomal hydrolase cathepsin B is capable of activating trypsinogen to trypsin.[51] However, the significance of this in the development of pancreatitis has been questioned since the reaction only occurs between pH 2.5 and pH 4 and trypsin is inactive within this range. Further experiments in the same laboratory using dispersed pancreatic acini revealed that the accumulation of zymogen granules within the cytoplasm was due to a block in stimulus–secretion coupling.[95] Despite these reservations, data using the model have suggested the intriguing possibility that activation of pancreatic enzymes could take place within the pancreatic acinar cell rather than in the interstitium. This is a new concept and may be a fruitful line of investigation.

The CDE-diet model is noninvasive, simple, and inexpensive, and the severity of pancreatitis is highly reproducible. The lesion is slow to evolve; thus the model is suitable for studies of potential new therapies. The major drawback is that there is no evidence that choline deficiency or ethionine plays any role in human acute pancreatitis. Thus the clinical relevance appears to be low. Moreover, only hemorrhagic pancreatitis has been produced.

Hypersecretion Model

Lampel and Kern described a new model of acute interstitial pancreatitis in rats characterized by marked edema of the pancreas and hyperamylasemia.[62] The lesion was produced by a supramaximal dose of the cholecystokinin analog caerulein (5 μg/kg per hour), and it developed within 3 hours of starting the infusion. Certain similarities have been noted with this model and the CDE-diet model. Vacuoles are seen within the cytoplasm of the acinar cells, which by immunocytochemical techniques have been shown to contain both proteolytic enzymes and lysosomal hydrolases.[105] The origin of these vacuoles is probably different from that of the crinophagic vacuoles seen in the diet-induced model; moreover, there is no excessive accumulation of zymogen granules following caerulein administration. As in the diet model, these findings suggest that intracellular activation of pancreatic enzymes might be important in the development of acute pancreatitis.

The hypersecretion model is simple, inexpensive, slow to evolve, and reversible. It has been extended to other species including the dog[101] and mouse.[82] However, the relevance of this model to the human situation is questionable, and the morphologic similarity to human pancreatitis is low. Moreover, only edematous pancreatitis has been produced.

Duct Perfusion Model

Reber et al. showed that the main pancreatic duct of cats could be made more permeable by perfusing the duct with ethanol or various bile acids at low pressures within the physiologic range (<20 mm Hg).[98] Farmer et al. showed that oral administration of ethanol to cats resulted also in an increase in pancreatic duct permeability to large dextran molecules.[38] The same group showed that perfusion of the duct with bile salts, at physiologic pressures, also increased permeability to macromolecules the size of pancreatic enzymes.[40] In all these experiments, when the permeable pancreatic duct was subsequently perfused with activated pancreatic enzymes, acute edematous pancreatitis resulted.[39] The characteristics of these models of acute alcoholic and biliary pancreatitis have been fully described.[128,129] The intravenous administration of 16-16 dimethylprostaglandin E_2 or histamine during the period of ductal perfusion resulted in acute *hemorrhagic* pancreatitis. Recent work suggests that the development of hemorrhage is a result of the increase in microvascular permeability caused by these vasoactive substances.[55] It is of interest that prostaglandins and other related agents that also increase vascular permeability have been detected in pancreatic exudate and the systemic circulation following both experimental and human pancreatitis.[6,37,48,83,120,124]

Permeability changes similar to those obtained by bile salt perfusion and oral alcohol have been described following both partial pancreatic duct obstruction with an actively secreting pancreas[12] and acute systemic hypercalcemia. Subsequent perfusion of the permeable duct with activated pancreatic enzymes also results in acute pancreatitis.[11]

The duct perfusion model of acute pancreatitis is expensive, complex, and invasive. However, one major attraction of this model is its high clinical relevance. Depending on the method used to induce pancreatic duct permeability, a model of either biliary or alcoholic pancreatitis can be produced with histologic features closely resembling those seen in the human disease.[43] The manipulations are performed using physiologic concentrations of ethanol and bile salts, and at physiologic pressures. Furthermore, the model is unique in that it can be manipulated to produce acute hemorrhagic or edematous pancreatitis. Exogenous activated pancreatic enzymes are needed to produce pancreatitis, and the experiments described do not address the question of how endogenous enzymes might become activated within the duct. However, the observation that enterokinase given intravenously can activate pancreatic enzymes within the pancreas[97] may be relevant in this regard, as may the experiments of Grant et al. and Talbot et al. described previously. Activated enzymes have also been found in the pancreatic juice of patients with acute pancreatitis.[46,100,125]

Other Models

Several other models of experimental pancreatitis have been described. Some of these involve the intraductal injection of bacteria or bacterial toxins[121,122] or the administration of immune serum to isolated components of the pancreas.[81] Others require the systemic injection of scorpion venom[86] or organophosphate insecticides.[30] The clinical relevance of these models is highly doubtful, except for acute pancreatitis caused by scorpion venom, which occurs in humans.

Isolated Perfused Pancreas

In recent years some interesting information has come from experiments involving the use of an ex vivo model of acute pancreatitis.[56] In this model the dog pancreas is removed with a short segment of duodenum to include the cannulated pancreatic duct. The preparation is perfused via the splenic and superior mesenteric arteries with oxygenated blood (or, as recently described, the blood substitute fluosol[84]) collected from the portal vein and recirculated through an oxygenator. Using this preparation Sanfey et al. have produced acute pancreatitis by a 2-hour period of ischemia, by the infusion of oleic acid, and by partial pancreatic duct obstruction and stimulation of pancreatic secretion.[108] These three manipulations were felt to mimic the clinical situations of ischemic, alcoholic (hyperlipidemic), and biliary pancreatitis, respectively. Studies of the effect of osmotically active agents on the development of pancreatitis suggested that an increase in capillary permeability may be an important early feature of the lesion.[107] Since endothelial injury in other organs has been shown to be mediated by the generation of oxygen-derived free radicals, they postulated that a similar mechanism might be operative in the pancreas. In a series of experiments (reviewed by Sanfey et al.[108]) they showed that the free-radical scavengers superoxide dismutase and catalase significantly reduced the edema and weight gain of the pancreas, as well as the hyperamylasemia produced in this model. This suggested that oxygen-free radicals played a significant part in this form of pancreatic injury. Furthermore, pretreatment of the preparation with allopurinol (a xanthine oxidase inhibitor) prevented the development of acute pancreatitis.

TREATMENT OF ACUTE PANCREATITIS

Efforts to find a specific therapy for acute pancreatitis have been hampered by a lack of understanding of the pathophysiology of the disease. They have been directed to several areas, based on certain assumptions. First, attempts have been made to inhibit pancreatic secretion because of the notion that continued production and/or leakage of digestive enzymes might be harmful. Second, because of the frequent presence of toxic peritoneal fluid associated with the disease, efforts have been made either to remove it from the body or to counteract its effects with specific antidotes.

Inhibition of Pancreatic Secretion

Putting the inflamed pancreas "to rest" has long been advocated as an essential part of treatment. A number of substances are known to inhibit pancreatic secretion directly or indirectly. These include glucagon, calcitonin, somatostatin, and cimetidine. Waterworth et al., in a pig model, demonstrated increased survival with glucagon given 18 hours after induction of pancreatitis.[127] However, other studies in dogs,[21] rats,[32,69,88] and mice,[74] in which the drug was given after the onset of pancreatitis, showed no benefit. In a number of double-blind clinical trials this agent has also been disappointing.[23,24,31]

Somatostatin, which directly inhibits pancreatic secretion, improved survival from bile-induced pancreatitis in dogs[112] and rats.[13] In contrast, Lankisch et al. were unable to demonstrate any benefit in rats.[65] Sporadic reports of a beneficial effect of somatostatin in human acute pancreatitis have appeared in the literature, but to date there are no reported double-blind clinical trials.

Cimetidine inhibits gastric acid secretion and hence indirectly inhibits pancreatic secretion stimulated by secretin. However, experimental and clinical studies suggest that this drug is of no benefit in the treatment of acute pancreatitis.[17,35,66,114]

Other studies have demonstrated that pancreatic secretion is suppressed spontaneously in the early stages of acute pancreatitis. This may explain why therapies aimed at inhibiting secretion have proved disappointing.[29,34] Furthermore, two recent reports indicate that stimulation of the pancreas with secretin does not influence the course of acute experimental pancreatitis.[36,63]

Removal of Toxic Substances

Peritoneal lavage has been advocated as a therapy for acute pancreatitis in the belief that some of the local and systemic effects of the disease are due to the presence of biologically active substances within the peritoneal cavity. Studies by Amundsen et al.[5] and Frey et al.[44] demonstrating the presence of hypotensive substances in the ascitic fluid of animals with acute pancreatitis lend support to this form of management. However, despite encouraging experimental work,[67,68] recent controlled clinical trials have failed to show any benefit of peritoneal lavage in patients with acute pancreatitis.[22,77]

Antiprotease Therapy

Proteolytic pancreatic enzymes are normally secreted in an inactive form, and mechanisms exist to prevent their intrapancreatic activation. However, during the course of acute pancreatitis, the trypsin inhibitory capacity of patients' sera has been shown to be reduced. This suggests that these defense mechanisms can be overwhelmed.[1] The hypothesis that decreased levels of trypsin inhibitor may be important in the pathogenesis of acute pancreatitis has led to the study of antiprotease agents as a therapy for the disease. Experimental work suggested that treatment with aprotinin was beneficial when the agent was given before or immediately after the onset of the disease.[59,123] Several reports of uncontrolled clinical studies also suggested that aprotinin was effective. However, the results of two double-blind controlled trials showed no benefit.[23,24,58] More recently the effect of the low-molecular-weight protease inhibitor leupeptin on experimental pancreatitis has been studied. Increased survival was demonstrated in a rat model when compared with either control animals or animals treated with aprotinin.[60]

As discussed earlier, the importance of trypsin in the pathogenesis of acute pancreatitis may be related to its role in activating other proteolytic enzymes such as phospholipase A. Aho et al. demonstrated a reduction in mortality with the phospholipase inhibitor procaine hydrochloride.[3] Schroder et al. reported increased survival in a pig model using another phospholipase inhibitor, xylocaine.[110] The same group demonstrated a reduction in phospholipase A levels and mortality rate using the potent phospholipase inhibitor chlorpromazine.[111] To date there are no reported clinical trials of the use of phospholipase inhibitors.

Other Therapeutic Studies

A number of other agents have been studied as potential treatments in acute pancreatitis. As discussed earlier there is some experimental evidence to suggest that a reduction in pancreatic blood flow and perfusion may play a role in the pathogenesis of the disease. Wright and Goodhead[132] and Donaldson et al.[28] showed that the fall in pancreatic blood flow that occurred in acute pancreatitis could be reversed by treatment with dextran 40. Plasma infusion also increased cardiac output and pancreatic blood flow, but only transiently. The latter group also showed that dextran 40 reversed the hypoxia of the pancreas that occurs early in the course of the disease.[27] Dextran 70 appears to have the same effect.[70] Sanfey et al. found that albumin prevented the development of acute pancreatitis in an ex vivo preparation and suggested that the protective effect was due to its action as an osmotically active agent rather than to any effect on blood flow.[106] They concluded from this and other studies that an increase in capillary permeability is an important early feature of acute pancreatitis.[107] It should be emphasized that despite these encouraging reports, there is at present no clinical evidence to support the use of these agents in the treatment of acute pancreatitis. It is possible that adequate fluid replacement to correct hypovolemia may in itself be as effective.

A new approach to therapy was suggested as a result of the observation that prostaglandins act as cytoprotective agents on the gastric mucosa.[102] Several groups have investigated the effect of prostaglandins in acute pancreatitis. Manabe and Steer[75], Coelle et al.[20] and Standfield and Kakkar[115] all demonstrated a protective effect of prostaglandin E_2 in the CDE-diet model of acute pancreatitis in mice. In contrast to these studies, Martin et al.,[76] Lankisch et al.,[64] and Crockett et al.,[25] using three different experimental models, were unable to demonstrate any protective effect of prostaglandins. Wedgwood et al. have shown that 16-16 dimethylprostaglandin E_2, far from being protective, converts edematous to hemorrhagic pancreatitis in the duct perfusion model of pancreatitis in cats.[129] Taylor et al., using the diet model, concluded that the ability to show a protective effect of prostaglandins is dependent on the exact experimental protocol used.[119] To date there are no reported clinical trials of the use of prostaglandins in acute pancreatitis.

Recent work suggests that oxygen free radicals may play a role in the pathogenesis of acute pancreatitis. These studies also suggest that treatment with free-radical scavengers and the xanthine oxidase inhibitor allopurinol may be effective. Harvey et al., using the duct perfusion model of pancreatitis in the cat, have also suggested that an increase in microvascular permeability is an important early feature in the pathogenesis of acute pancreatitis.[54] They hypothesized that this increase in permeability is brought about by the release of histamine, prostaglandins, and other vasoactive substances during the course of the disease. Because β-agonist drugs are physiologic antagonists to a variety of these vasoactive agents, they studied the effect of isoproterenol and terbutaline on their model of acute pancreatitis. Both drugs significantly reduced the degree of pancreatic edema and inflammation even when given up to 12 hours *after* the onset of pancreatitis. These studies complement those of Sanfey et al.[108] and suggest novel approaches to therapy that deserve further study, in both the experimental and clinical setting.

One important caution emerges from the results of these studies of therapy in experimental pancreatitis. Initial enthusiasm for new experimental treatments has turned to disappointment when the agents have been applied clinically. Well-controlled double-blind clinical trials with large numbers of patients are necessary before any new agent can become established therapy for acute pancreatitis.

CONCLUSIONS

We have learned a great deal about the evolution and physiology of acute pancreatitis from the experimental study of the disease. However, it is clear that many studies have produced conflicting results and that we still have much to learn. Advances in treatment can come only from a better understanding of the underlying pathophysiology. To gain such an understanding we must, wherever possible, employ models of pancreatitis that closely resemble the human situation. In assessing possible therapeutic agents we must remember that for any modality to be of use in humans, it must be effective when given *after* the onset of the disease. Agents that only prevent pancreatitis when given before or at the time of injury probably will be of no benefit in the clinical setting.

REFERENCES

1. Adham NF, Dyce B, Haverback BJ. Trypsin-binding α-2-macroglobin in patients with acute pancreatitis. Gastroenterology 61:365–372, 1972.

2. Aho, HJ, Nevelainen TJ. Experimental pancreatitis in the rat. Ultrastructure of sodium taurocholate-induced pancreatic lesions. Scand J Gastroenterol 15:417–424, 1980.
3. Aho HJ, Nevalainen TJ, Lindberg RLP, Aho AJ. Experimental pancreatitis in the rat. The role of phospholipase A in sodium taurocholate-induced acute haemorrhagic pancreatitis. Scand J Gastroenterol 15:1027–1031, 1980.
4. Aho HJ, Suonpaa K, Ahola RA, Nevalainen TJ. Experimental pancreatitis in the rat-ductal factors in sodium taurocholate induced acute pancreatitis. Exp Pathol 25:73–79, 1984.
5. Amundsen E, Ofstad E, Hagen P-O. Experimental acute pancreatitis in dogs, I: Hypotensive effect induced by pancreatic exudate. Scand J Gastroenterol 3:659–664, 1968.
6. Amundsen E, Ofstad E, Hagen P-O. Experimental acute pancreatitis in dogs: Histamine release induced by pancreatic exudate. Scand J Gastroenterol 4:73–79, 1969.
7. Anderson MC, Hagstrom WJ. A comparison of pancreatic and biliary pressures recorded simultaneously in man. Can J Surg 5:461–470, 1962.
8. Anderson MC, Needleman SB, Gramatica L, Toronto IR, Briggs DR. Further enquiry into the pathogenesis of acute pancreatitis. Arch Surg 99:185–192, 1969.
9. Anderson MC, Schiller WR, Gramatica L. Alterations of portal venous and systemic arterial pressure during experimental acute pancreatitis. Am J Surg 117:715–720, 1969.
10. Archibald, E. The experimental production of pancreatitis in animals as a result of the resistance of the common duct sphincter. Surg Gynecol Obstet 28:529–545, 1919.
11. Austin JL, Harvey MH, Sieckman G, Reber, HA. Pancreatitis and pancreatic duct obstruction. Surg Forum 37:172–174, 1986.
12. Austin JL, Wipfler J, Sieckman G: Pancreatic duct obstruction and permeability to macromolecules. Gastroenterology 90:1332, 1986.
13. Baxter JN, Jenkins SA, Day DW, et al. Effects of somatostatin and a long acting somatostatin analogue on the prevention and treatment of experimentally induced acute pancreatitis in the rat. Br J Surg 72:382–385, 1985.
14. Bernard C. Mémoire sur la pancreas. C R Searces Acad Sci 1(suppl), 1856.
15. Berry AR, Millar AM, Taylor TV. Pancreatic blood flow in experimental acute pancreatitis. Dig Dis Sci 27:444–448, 1982.
16. Bockman DE. Route of retrograde flow in the exocrine pancreas during ductal hypertension. Arch Surg 103:321–329, 1971.
17. Broe PJ, Zinner MJ, Cameron JL: A clinical trial of cimetidine in acute pancreatitis. Surg Gynecol Obstet 154:13–15, 1982.
18. Carr-Locke DCL, Gregg JA. Endoscopic manometery of pancreatic and biliary sphincter zones in man. Dig Dis Sci 26:7–15, 1981.
19. Cavallari A, Galleti G, Battisti C, et al. The vascular morphology of the pancreas in acute experimental pancreatitis due to creation of a closed duodenal loop in the dog. Bull Soc Ital Biol Sper 44:773–778, 1968.
20. Coelle EF, Adham N, Elashoff J, Lewin K, Taylor IL: Effects of prostaglandin and indomethacin on diet-induced acute pancreatitis in mice. Gastroenterology 85:1307–1312, 1983.
21. Condon RE, Woods JH, Poulin TL, Wagner WG, Pisiotis CA. Experimental pancreatitis treated with glucagon or lactated Ringers solution. Arch Surg 109:154–158, 1974.
22. Cooper MJ, Williamson RCN, Pollock AV. The role of peritoneal lavage in the prediction and treatment of severe acute pancreatitis. Ann R Coll Surg Engl 64:422–427, 1982.
23. Cox AG, Armitage P, Hogg R. Death from acute pancreatitis: MRC multicentre trial of glucagon and aprotinin. Lancet 2:632–635, 1977.
24. Cox AG, Armitage P, Hogg R. Morbidity of acute pancreatitis: The effect of aprotinin and glucagon. Gut 21:334–339, 1980.
25. Crocket KV, Brackett K, Crocket A, et al. Prostaglandin E_1 treatment in experimental acute pancreatitis in the rat. Eur Surg Res 16:265–273, 1984.

26. DiMagno EP, Shorter RG, Taylor WF. Relationships between pancreaticobiliary ductal anatomy and pancreatic ductal parenchymal histology. Cancer 49:361–368, 1982.
27. Donaldson LA, Schenk WG. Experimental acute pancreatitis. The changes in pancreatic oxygen consumption and the effect of dextran 40. Ann Surg 190:728–731, 1979.
28. Donaldson LA, Williams RW, Schenk WG. Experimental pancreatitis: Effect of plasma and dextran on pancreatic blood flow. Surgery 84:313–321, 1978.
29. Dreiling DA. Pancreatic function in acute pancreatitis. JAMA 175:183, 1961.
30. Dressel TD, Goodale RL, Arneson MA, Borner JW. Pancreatitis as a complication of anticholinesterase insecticide intoxication. Ann Surg 189:199–204, 1979.
31. Durr HK, Maroske D, Zelder O, Bode JC. Glucagon therapy in acute pancreatitis. Report of a double blind trial. Gut 19:175–179, 1978.
32. Durr HK, Weihe W, Bode C, Bode JC. A controlled trial of glucagon in acute experimental pancreatitis in rats. Z Gastroenterol 15:728–733, 1977.
33. Elliot, DW, Williams RD, Zollinger RM. Alterations in the pancreatic resistance to bile in the pathogenesis of acute pancreatitis. Ann Surg 146:669–682, 1957.
34. Evander A, Hederstrom E, Hultberg B, Ihse I. Exocrine pancreatic secretion in acute experimental pancreatitis. Digestion 24:159–167, 1982.
35. Evander A, Ihse I. Cimetidine treatment in acute experimental pancreatitis. Eur Surg Res 12:301–309, 1980.
36. Evander A, Lundquist I, Ihse I. Influence of gastrointestinal hormones on the course of acute experimental pancreatitis. Hepatogastroenterology 29:161–166, 1982.
37. Farias LR, Frey CF, Holcroft JW, Gunther R. Effect of prostaglandin blockers on ascites fluid in pancreatitis. Surgery 98:571–578, 1985.
38. Farmer RC, Maslin S, Reber HA. Effects of acute ethanol and aspirin ingestion on pancreatic duct permeability to macromolecules. Gastroenterology 82:1053, 1982.
39. Farmer RC, Maslin SC, Reber HA. Acute pancreatitis–Role of duct permeability. Surg Forum 34:224–227, 1983.
40. Farmer RC, Tweedie J, Maslin S, et al. Effects of bile salts on permeability and morphology of main pancreatic duct in cats. Dig Dis Sci 29:740–751, 1984.
41. Ferrini, U, Zito R. Action of trypsin on Bence Jones protein derivatives. Nature 189:485, 1961.
42. Flexner S. The constituent of the bile causing pancreatitis and the effect of colloids upon its action. J Exp Med 8:167–177, 1906.
43. Foulis AK. Histological evidence of initiating factors in acute necrotizing pancreatitis in man. J Clin Pathol 33:1125–1131, 1980.
44. Frey CF, Wong HN, Hickman D, Pullos T. Toxicity of hemorrhagic ascitic fluid associated with hemorrhagic pancreatitis. Arch Surg 117:401–404, 1982.
45. Geokas MC. The role of elastase in acute pancreatitis, III: The destructive capacity of elastase on pancreatic tissue in vivo and in vitro. Arch Pathol 86:135–141, 1968.
46. Geokas MC, Rinderknecht H. Free proteolytic enzymes in pancreatic juice of patients with acute pancreatitis. Dig Dis 19:591–598, 1974.
47. Gilliland L, Steer ML. Effects of ethionine on digestive enzyme synthesis and discharge by mouse pancreas. Am J Physiol 239:G418–G426, 1980.
48. Glazer G, Bennett A. Prostaglandin release in canine acute hemorrhagic pancreatitis. Gut 17:22–26, 1976.
49. Goodhead B. Vascular factors in the pathogenesis of acute pancreatitis. Ann R Coll Surg Engl 45:80–97, 1969.
50. Grant DAW, Talbot RW, Hermon-Taylor JH. Catalytically active enterokinase in human bile. Clin Chim Acta 142:39–45, 1984.
51. Greenbaum LM, Hirshkowitz A. Endogenous cathepsin activates trypsinogen in extracts of dog pancreas. Proc Soc Exp Biol Med 107:74–76, 1961.
52. Hammond JB, Mann NS. Pancreatitis following the intraductal injection of partially purified enterokinase in dogs. Dig Dis 22:182–188, 1977.
53. Hansson K. Experimental and clinical studies in aetiologic role of bile reflux in acute pancreatitis. Acta Chir Scand 375(suppl):1–102, 1967.
54. Harvey MH, Wedgwood KR, Reber HA. Treatment of acute pancreatitis with β-adrenergic agonist drugs. Surgery 102:229–234, 1987.

55. Harvey MH, Wedgwood KR, Reber HA. Vasoactive drugs, microvascular permeability and hemorrhagic pancreatitis in cats. Gastroenterology 93:1296–1300, 1987.
56. Hermon-Taylor J. A technique for perfusion of isolated canine pancreas. Gastroenterology 55:488–501, 1968.
57. Hermon-Taylor J, Perrin J, Grant DAW, et al. Immunofluorescent localization of enterokinase in human small intestine. Gut 18:259–265, 1977.
58. Imrie CW, Benjamin IS, Ferguson JC, et al. A single centre double blind trial of trasylol therapy in primary acute pancreatitis. Br J Surg 65:337–341, 1978.
59. Imrie CW, MacKenzie M. Effective aprotinin therapy in bile-trypsin canine experimental acute pancreatitis. Digestion 22:32–38, 1981.
60. Jones PA, Hermon-Taylor J, Grant DAW. Anti-protease chemotherapy of acute experimental pancreatitis using the low molecular weight oligopeptide aldehyde leupeptin. Gut 23:939–943, 1982.
61. Kioke H, Steer ML, Meldolesi J. Pancreatic effects of ethionine: Blockade of exocytosis and appearance of crinophagy and autophagy precede cellular necrosis. Am J Physiol 242:G297–G307, 1982.
62. Lampel M, Kern HF. Acute interstitial pancreatitis in the rat induced by excessive doses of a pancreatic secretagogue. Virchows Arch Pathol Anat 373:97–117, 1977.
63. Lankisch PG, Goke B, Folsch UR, et al. Influence of secretin on the course of acute experimental pancreatitis in rats. Digestion 26:187–191, 1983.
64. Lankisch PG, Goke B, Kunze H, Otto J, Winckler K. Does PGE_2 have a beneficial effect on acute experimental pancreatitis in the rat. Hepatogastroenterology 30:148–150, 1983.
65. Lankisch PG, Koop H, Winkler K, Folsch UR, Creutzfeldt W. Somatostatin therapy of acute experimental pancreatitis. Gut 18:713–716, 1977.
66. Lankisch PG, Koop H, Winckler K, Otto J. Cimetidine. Harmful in acute experimental pancreatitis? Hepatogastroenterology 29:195–197, 1982.
67. Lankisch PG, Koop H, Winckler K, Schmidt H. Continuous peritoneal dialysis as treatment of acute experimental pancreatitis in the rat. I: Effect on length and rate of survival. Dig Dis Sci 24:111–116, 1979.
68. Lankisch PG, Koop H, Winckler K, Schmidt H: Continuous peritoneal dialysis as treatment of acute experimental pancreatitis in the rat, II: Analysis of its beneficial effect. Dig Dis Sci 24:117–122, 1979.
69. Lankisch PG, Winkler K, Bokermann M, Schmidt H, Creutzfeldt W. The influence of glucagon on acute experimental pancreatitis in the rat. Scand J Gastroenterol 9:725–729, 1974.
70. Lehtola A, Kivilaakso E, Puolakkainen P, et al. Effects of dextran 70 versus crystalloids in the microcirculation of porcine hemorrhagic pancreatitis. Surg Gynecol Obstet 162:556–562, 1986.
71. Lium R, Portsmouth NH, Maddock S. Etiology of acute pancreatitis. Surgery 24:593–604, 1948.
72. Lombardi B, Estes, LW, Longnecker DS. Acute hemorrhagic pancreatitis (massive necrosis) with fat necrosis induced in mice by DL-ethionine fed with a choline deficient diet. Am J Pathol 79:465–480, 1975.
73. Magee LW, Gallai-Hatchard J, Sanders H, Thompson RHS. The purification and properties of phospholipase A from human pancreas. Biochem J 83:17–25, 1962.
74. Manabe T, Steer ML: Experimental acute pancreatitis in mice. Protective effects of glucagon. Gastroenterology 76:529–534, 1979.
75. Manabe T, Steer ML. Protective effects of PGE_2 on diet-induced acute pancreatitis in mice. Gastroenterology 78:777–781, 1980.
76. Martin DM, Someron AO, Nasrallah SM. The effect of prostaglandin E_2 on ethionine-induced pancreatitis in the rat. Gastroenterology 81:736–741, 1981.
77. Mayer AD, McMahon MJ, Corfield AP, et al. Controlled trial of peritoneal lavage for the treatment of severe acute pancreatitis. N Engl J Med 312:399–404, 1985.
78. McCutcheon AD, Race D. Experimental pancreatitis: A possible aetiology of postoperative pancreatitis. Ann Surg 155:523–531, 1962.

79. Menguy RB, Hallenbeck GA, Bollman JL, Grindley JH. Ductal and vascular factors in etiology of experimentally induced acute pancreatitis. Arch Surg 74:881–889, 1957.
80. Menguy RB, Hallenbeck GA, Bollman JL, Grindley JH. Intraductal pressures and sphincteric resistance in canine pancreatic and biliary ducts after various stimuli. Surg Gynecol Obstet 106:306–320, 1958.
81. Murray MJ, Thal A. The clinical significance of circulating pancreatic antibodies. Ann Intern Med 53:548, 1960.
82. Niederau, C, Ferell LD, Grendell JH. Onset, course and regression of caerulein-induced acute necrotizing pancreatitis in mice. Dig Dis Sci 29:962, 1984.
83. Ofstad E. Formation and destruction of plasma kinins during experimental acute hemorrhagic pancreatitis in dogs. Scand J Gastroenterol 5:1–44, 1970.
84. O'Malley VP, Keyes DM, Postier RG. The fluosol-perfused isolated canine pancreas: A model for the study of blood component effects in acute pancreatitis. J Surg Res 40:210–215, 1986.
85. Opie EL. The etiology of acute hemorrhagic pancreatitis. Bull Johns Hopkins Hosp 12:182–190, 1901.
86. Pantoja JL, Renner IG, Abramson SB, Edmondson HA. Production of acute hemorrhagic pancreatitis in the dog using venom of the scorpion, *Buthus quinquestriatus*. Dig Dis Sci 28:429–439, 1983.
87. Papp M, Makara GB, Hajtman B, Csaki L. A quantitative study of pancreatic blood flow in experimental pancreatitis. Gastroenterology 51:524–528, 1966.
88. Papp M, Ribet A, Fodor I, et al. Glucagon treatment of experimental acute pancreatitis. Acta Med Acad Sci Hung 32:105–116, 1975.
89. Pfeffer RB, Robertson AL, Safadi D et al. Gradations of pancreatitis, edematous through hemorrhagic, experimentally produced by controlled injection of microspheres into blood vessels in dogs. Surgery 51:764–769, 1962.
90. Pfeffer RB, Stasior O, Hinton JW. The clinical picture of the sequential development of acute hemorrhagic pancreatitis in the dog. Surg Forum 8:248–251, 1957.
91. Pirola RC, Davis AE. Effect of pressure on the integrity of the ductacinar system of the pancreas. Gut 11:69–73, 1970.
92. Polya E. Die Wirkung des Trypsins auf das lebende Pankreas. Pflugers Arch 121:483–493, 1908.
93. Popper HL, Necheles H. Edema of the pancreas. Surg Gynecol Obstet 74:123–124, 1942.
94. Popper HL, Necheles H, Russell KC. Transition of pancreatic edema into pancreatic necrosis. Surg Gynecol Obstet 87:79–82, 1948.
95. Powers RE, Saluja AK, Houlihan MJ, Steer ML. Diminished agonist-stimulated inisotol triphosphate generation blocks stimulus-secretion coupling in pancreatic acini during diet-induced experimental pancreatitis. J Clin Invest 77:1668–1674, 1986.
96. Rao KN, Eagon PK, Okamura K. Acute hemorrhagic pancreatic necrosis in mice: Induction in male mice treated with estradiol. Am J Pathol 109:8–13, 1982.
97. Reber HA. Pancreatic duct and microvascular permeability to macromolecules. Scand J Gastroenterol 20 (suppl 112):96–100, 1985.
98. Reber HA, Roberts C, Way LW. The pancreatic duct mucosal barrier, Am J Surg 137:128–134, 1979.
99. Reid LC, Paulette RE, Challis TW, Hinton JW. The mechanism of the pathogenesis of pancreatic necrosis and the therapeutic effect of propylthic acid. Surgery 43:538–549.
100. Renner IG, Rinderknecht H, Doublas AP. Profiles of pure pancreatic secretions in patients with acute pancreatitis: The possible role of proteolytic enzymes in pathogenesis. Gastroenterology 75:1020–1028, 1978.
101. Renner IG, Wisner J. Exogenous secretin ameliorates ceruletide induced acute pancreatitis in the dog. Dig Dis Sci 28:946, 1983.
102. Robert A. Prostaglandins and digestive diseases. In: Samuelsson B, Ramwell PW, Paoletti R eds. Advances in Prostaglandin and Thromboxane Research. New York, Raven Press, 1980.

103. Robinson TM, Dunphy JE. Continuous perfusion of bile and protease activators through the pancreas. JAMA 183:530–533, 1963.
104. Rosato EF, Cowan RP, Rosato FE. Duodenal pressure as a factor in the cause of pancreatitis. Surgery 68:837–841, 1970.
105. Saluja A, Saito I, Saluja M, et al. In vivo rat pancreatic acinar cell function during supramaximal stimulation with caerulein. Am J Physiol 249:G702–G710, 1985.
106. Sanfey H, Broe PJ, Cameron JL. Experimental ischemic pancreatitis: Treatment with albumin. Am J Surg 150:297–300, 1985.
107. Sanfey H, Cameron JL: Increased capillary permeability: An early lesion in acute pancreatitis. Surgery 96:485–491, 1984.
108. Sanfey H, Sarr MG, Bulkley GB, Cameron JL. Oxygen-derived free radicals and acute pancreatitis: A review. Acta Physiol Scand 548(suppl):109–118, 1986.
109. Schmidt H, Creutzfeldt W. The possible role of phospholipase A_2 in the pathogenesis of acute pancreatitis. Scand J Gastroenterol 4:39–48, 1969.
110. Schroder T, Kinnunen PKJ, Lempinen M. Xylocaine treatment in experimental pancreatitis in pigs. Scand J Gastroenterol 13:863–865, 1978.
111. Schroder T, Lempinen M, Nordling S, Kinnunen PK. Chlorpromazine treatment of experimental acute fulminant pancreatitis in pigs. Eur Surg Res 13:143–151, 1981.
112. Schwedes U, Althoff PH, Klempa I, et al. Effect of somatostatin on bile-induced acute hemorrhagic pancreatitis in the dog. Horm Metab Res 11:655–661, 1979.
113. Senninger N, Moody FG, Coelho JCU, Van Buren DH. The role of biliary obstruction in the pathogenesis of acute pancreatitis in the opossum. Surgery 99:688–693, 1986.
114. Sillero C, Perez-Mateo M, Vasquez N, Martin A. Controlled trial of cimetidine in acute pancreatitis. Eur J Clin Pharmacol 21:17–21, 1981.
115. Standfield NJ, Kakkar VV. Prostaglandins and acute pancreatitis—Experimental and clinical studies. Br J Surg 70:573–576, 1983.
116. Strack AA, Dreizin DH, Ketyer S, Lazaro EJ. Duodenal reflux in the genesis of acute pancreatitis. Can J Surg 10:68–74, 1967.
117. Summ PT, Bencomse SA, Beck JT. Pathogenesis of bile-induced acute pancreatitis in the dog. Experiments with detergents. Am J Dig Dis 15:637–646, 1970.
118. Talbot RW, Grant DAW, Hermon-Taylor J. Displacement of endogenous enterokinase into portal venous blood and bile following luminal perfusion of proximal small intestine in guinea pigs. Dig Dis Sci 29:1009–1014, 1984.
119. Taylor IL, Coelle EF, Adham NF. Factors that modify the effects of prostaglandin on diet-induced acute pancreatitis in mice. Scand J Gastroenterol 112(suppl):101–105, 1985.
120. Thal AP, Kobold EE, Hollenberg MJ. The release of vasoactive substances in acute pancreatitis. Am J Surg 105:708–713, 1963.
121. Thal A, Molestina JE. Studies on pancreatitis, III: Fulminating hemorrhagic pancreatic necrosis produced by means of staphylococcal toxin. AMA Arch Pathol 60:212, 1955.
122. Thal A, Tansathiahaya P, Egner W. An experimental study of bacterial pancreatitis. Surg Gynecol Obstet 103:459–468, 1956.
123. Thompson AG. Proteinase inhibitors in experimental and clinical pancreatitis. Ann NY Acad Sci 146:540–547, 1968.
124. Traverso LW, Pullos TG, Frey CF. Hemodynamic characteristics of porcine hemorrhagic pancreatitis ascites fluid. J Surg Res 34:254–262, 1983.
125. Troll W, Doubilet H. The determination of proteolytic enzymes and proenzymes in human pancreatic juice. Gastroenterology 19:326–330, 1951.
126. Wang CC, Wang KJ, Grossman MJ. Effects of ligation of the pancreatic duct upon the action of secretin and pancreozymin in rabbits with a correlated histological study. Am J Physiol 160:115–121, 1950.
127. Waterworth MW, Barbezat GO, Hickman R, Terblanche, J. A controlled trial of glucagon in experimental pancreatitis. Br J Surg 63:617–620, 1976.
128. Wedgwood KR, Adler G, Kern H, Reber HA. Effects of oral agents on pancreatic

duct permeability: A model of acute alcoholic pancreatitis. Dig Dis Sci 31:1081–1088, 1986.
129. Wedgwood KR, Farmer RC, Reber HA. A model of hemorrhagic pancreatitis in cats—Role of 16-16 dimethyl prostaglandin E_2. Gastroenterology 90:32–39, 1986.
130. White TT, Magee DF. Perfusion of the dog pancreas with bile without production of pancreatitis. Ann Surg 151:245–250, 1960.
131. Williams HU, Busch FC. The etiology and pathogenesis of acute pancreatitis. Trans Assoc Am Physicians 22:304–314, 1907.
132. Wright PW, Goodhead B. The value of dextrans in the treatment of experimental pancreatitis. Surgery 67:807–815, 1970.

CHAPTER

2

CLASSIFICATION OF PANCREATITIS

I. N. Marks

EDITORIAL COMMENT

Dr. Marks's review has demonstrated the evolution of the classification of pancreatitis from a purely clinical one in the 1940s and 1950s to an etiologic classification in the early 1960s and a clinicopathologic classification following the Marseilles Symposium in 1963. More recently, a classification combining clinical, pathologic, and radiologic criteria including endoscopic retrograde cholangiopancreatography (ERCP) has been suggested. Still more recently there has been an even simpler classification, that is, acute and chronic pancreatitis. Even the latter was short-lived, as the French group reclassified *chronic* into *chronic* and *chronic obstructive*. Even the clinical classification has become more specific with the introduction of more specific signs of severity of the attack. The fact that there has been such an evolution and progression in classification over the last 40 years implies that other classifications will undoubtedly emerge.

One area that seems likely to change is the probability that alcohol-induced pancreatitis, currently considered almost always chronic, may consist of at least two varieties, namely, the well-recognized chronic group and a second, namely, acute alcohol-induced pancreatitis occurring de novo. One awaits with interest further refinements to the classifications as MRI, skinny needle aspiration, and understanding of genetic factors with regard to fibrosis (vis-à-vis cirrhosis) become increasingly sophisticated.

CONTROVERSY

There have been three major international meetings on the classification of pancreatitis—two in Marseilles that bear this name, and one in England. The Marseilles classifications rely largely on pathologic findings that are rarely available in clinical practice, while the English classification attempts to be more comprehensive. Some workers feel that a simple etiologic classification is the most clinically appropriate, while reports of the Swiss group have taken the view that only time can tell to which group the patient will eventually conform. Hence, it seems timely to review the various classifications that prevail at the moment.

The wide spectrum of clinical, etiologic, and pathologic variants of pancreatitis virtually precludes an entirely satisfactory classification of the disease. Relatively simple classifications based on clinical, etiologic, or pathologic criteria have been suggested, but shortcomings inherent in most of them led to the use of combinations of two or more of these criteria. Advances in the understanding of the pathogenesis of various forms of the disease gave fresh impetus to the search for a perfect classification, and a degree of consensus was achieved at two recent international conferences convened for this purpose.

HISTORICAL OBSERVATIONS

Cawley's description in 1788 of a "free-living young man" who died of diabetes and emaciation and showed a pancreas full of calculi at necropsy is one of the earliest records of chronic pancreatitis.[5] Subsequent reports linked advanced chronic pancreatitis with inveterate alcoholics, and Friedreich, in 1878, suggested the term *drunkard's pancreas*.[9] Early reports, however, also linked alcohol with acute and, indeed, fulminating pancreatitis.[8,31] Alcohol, it seemed, was not only a major cause of chronic pancreatitis but also an important cause of clinically acute forms of the disease.

The landmark observations of Opie, in 1901, drew attention to the association between acute pancreatitis and a stone impacted in the lower end of the common bile duct or the ampulla of Vater.[23,24] These reports, however, tended to detract from the etiologic significance of cholelithiasis unassociated with demonstrable choledocholithiasis. The finding of dilatation, thickening, edema, and inflammation of the gallbladder in patients with chronic pancreatitis, led the Mayo workers to the view that disease of the biliary tract may be secondary to pancreatic disease, a view that detracted further from the etiologic significance of gallstones in pancreatitis.[11] Small wonder that Cattell and Warren, in 1953, were hesitant about accepting gallstones as a cause of pancreatitis.[4]

CONVENTIONAL CLINICAL CLASSIFICATION

Early workers classified pancreatitis into acute and chronic forms of the disease based largely on clinical criteria. Chronic relapsing pancreatitis, a third variety, was popularized by the Mayo group in 1946,[6] and other clinical variants were added. The classification was broadened to cover a large number of clinical syndromes ranging from acute fulminating to painless varieties (Table 2-1). The conventional classification of pancreatitis into acute, relapsing, and chronic varieties, while simple and descriptive, tended to the institution of a standard medical and surgical attack on the disease irrespective of the specific cause in the individual patient.[20] Little attempt was made to identify and eradicate the etiologic factor in each patient.

TABLE 2-1. CONVENTIONAL CLINICAL CLASSIFICATION

Acute
Fulminating
Severe
Mild
Relapsing
Chronic
Painless

ETIOLOGIC CLASSIFICATION

Classifications based on etiologic factors were presented in the mid 1950s,[3,16,17] but it was not until a few years later that the crucial prognostic value of an etiologic classification became apparent. The Philadelphia[13,14] and Cape Town groups,[20] in particular, showed that alcohol-induced and gallstone pancreatitis were essentially different entities, each having a distinct natural history and characteristic diagnostic and therapeutic aspects. Alcohol-induced pancreatitis repre-

TABLE 2-2. ETIOLOGIC CLASSIFICATION OF PANCREATITIS

Painful	Painless
Gallstone	Tropical or -nutritional
Alcohol-induced	Idiopathic
Tropical or nutritional	Alcohol-induced
Idiopathic	Miscellaneous
Miscellaneous	Fibrocystic disease
Congenital	Pancreatopathy
Pancreas divisum	Hemochromatosis
Duct anomalies	Cirrhosis
Hereditary	Small bowel disease
Metabolic	Diabetes mellitus
Hyperparathyroidism	Porphyria
Hyperlipemia	Infiltrations
Infective	Myeloma
Viral	Sarcoid
Contiguous	Chronic inflammatory
Penetrating peptic ulcer	Schistosomiasis
Obstructive	Syphilis
Carcinoma	Tuberculosis
Roundworm	Toxocariasis
Duodenal obstruction	Lipomatous atrophy
Vaterian stenosis	Juvenile forms
Perivaterian diverticulum	Adult varieties
Traumatic	Metabolic
External trauma	Uremia
Postsurgical	Hypoalbuminemia
Primary inflammatory	Duct obstruction
Vascular	Carcinoma
Drug-induced	

TABLE 2-3. ETIOLOGY OF CHRONIC PANCREATITIS (circa 1960)*

Howat	Chronic (40 Cases)	Dreiling	Chronic (100 Cases)	Calcific (24 Cases)
Gallstones (1 typhoid)	20	Gallbladder disease	42	2
Vaterian stenosis	2	Gallbladder disease	8	
Perivaterian diverticulum	2	Alcohol	22	11
Papilloma of ampulla of Vater	1	Alcohol	3	2
Hyperparathyroidism	1	Alcohol and gallbladder disease		4
Chronic alcoholism	1	Duodenal obstruction (cancer duodenum)	1	
Thrombosis of IVC	1	DLE (steroid therapy)	1	
Unknown	12	Unknown	23	5

* From Dreiling,[7] and Howat.[15]

sents about 60% of cases of pancreatitis in most western countries, and biliary disease, miscellaneous, and unknown causes account for the remainder. The etiologic classification may be considered under the headings of painful and painless forms of the disease (Table 2-2).

It is of interest that both the clinical and the etiologic classifications were broadened to include other criteria. Lagerlöf,[18] in 1942, classified pancreatitis as acute and chronic based on clinical, functional, and pathologic criteria, and the Mayo group in 1946 considered the tendency to relapse with eventual destruction of the pancreas as the predominant feature in chronic relapsing pancreatitis.[6] Pathologic features were thus closely interwoven into the clinical classifications of the disease, but the clinical presentation remained of paramount importance. The etiologic classification, on the other hand, was extended to make provision for clinical, radiologic, and functional aspects, but little allowance was made for the pathologic status of the pancreas.[21] The picture in the early 1960s was further complicated by a lack of consensus as to the causes of chronic pancreatitis. While the Philadelphia,[13] Marseilles,[27] and Cape Town[20] groups recognized alcohol as the major etiologic factor in chronic pancreatitis, both Howat[15] and Dreiling,[7] in 1962, regarded gallstones or gallbladder disease as the dominant cause (Table 2-3).

THE CLINICOPATHOLOGIC CLASSIFICATION

The Marseilles Symposium, in 1963, favored a clinicopathologic classification comprising acute, relapsing acute, chronic relapsing, and chronic pancreatitis.[26] The acute varieties were characterized by clinical and pathologic resolution after an attack and the chronic by permanent residual pancreatic damage (Table 2-4). This classification gained widespread acceptance since it had the virtue of seeming simplicity and carried with it the authority of most leading pancreatologists of the day. The delayed publication of the Marseilles report and the pathologic bias of the classification, however, created a certain amount of confusion in its appli-

TABLE 2-4. CLINICOPATHOLOGIC CLASSIFICATION (Marseilles, 1963)

1. Acute pancreatitis
2. Relapsing acute pancreatitis
3. Chronic relapsing pancreatitis
4. Chronic pancreatitis

cation. First, it may be difficult to distinguish the acute varieties from clinically acute attacks of chronic pancreatitis in the relatively early stage of the disease. Second, the use of the clinically descriptive word *acute* in the pathologic context created a semantic problem. The latter could, perhaps, be overcome by using the term *clinically acute pancreatitis* to refer to acute pancreatitis in the clinical sense.[19] However, most authors were, and are still, tethered to the usage of acute pancreatitis in the clinical rather than the clinicopathologic context. A third problem related to the stringency of the diagnostic criteria. The Marseilles group[28] was reluctant to accept anything other than radiologic evidence of calcific pancreatitis or histologic changes as evidence of chronic pancreatitis. The Marseilles definition of the latter allowed for residual loss of pancreatic function, but, despite this, little cognizance was taken of abnormal tests of pancreatic function. On the other hand, a serum amylase level >1000 units was considered diagnostic of acute pancreatitis, in the Marseilles context, provided that it was not due to alcohol! The Marseilles classification became more meaningful when considered in conjunction with etiologic criteria. Gallstone pancreatitis, with its tendency to pathologic and functional restitution between attacks, is predominantly an acute or relapsing acute disease, whereas alcohol-induced pancreatitis, associated usually with persistent pathologic and functional changes, is essentially a relapsing chronic or chronic one.

THE NEWER CLASSIFICATIONS

Advances in the understanding of the structural and functional changes of pancreatitis, facilitated by the advent of newer technologies such as ERCP, ultrasound, and CT scan, prompted a reevaluation of the Marseilles classification of 1963. This was clearly warranted since the new techniques, in conjunction with function data, provided some measure of organ damage and hence chronic change. Two further international symposia were convened, the first in Cambridge in 1983 and the second in Marseilles in 1984.

The Cambridge Workshop[29] saw no need for a radical revision of the Marseilles classification of 1963, but favored expansion to include clinical criteria to provide an index of severity, etiologic factors to help define prognosis, and fairly precise statements of functional and morphologic damage (Tables 2-5 and 2-6). They favored retention of the terms *acute pancreatitis* and *chronic pancreatitis* despite the confusion that had arisen from their use in the past.

The second Marseilles Symposium[12] also recommended that the classification consist simply of acute and chronic pancreatitis, and that the terms *relapsing acute pancreatitis* and *chronic relapsing pancreatitis* be omitted. Their modifica-

TABLE 2-5. CAMBRIDGE CLASSIFICATION, 1983

Acute pancreatitis
Chronic pancreatitis

tion involved further subdivision of the chronic form into classic chronic pancreatitis and chronic obstructive pancreatitis associated with duct obstruction due to scarring or tumor (Table 2-7). Apart from the latter, the Marseilles conferees were reluctant to include etiologic factors in their revised classification.

Omission of the relapsing forms of the disease by the delegates attending both the Cambridge Symposium and second Marseille Symposium, while simplifying the classification, left unanswered the problem of categorizing a patient having an initial attack of pancreatitis. The requirement that morphologic functional criteria be included in the Marseilles definitions of acute and chronic pancreatitis recreated one of the major dilemmas of the Marseilles classification of 1963. The Cambridge definition of acute pancreatitis, based on clinical criteria, allowed categorization into the acute group pending the availability of evidence of permanent structural damage—the delegates recognized that a single attack of acute pancreatitis may be associated with transient functional or anatomic change and, on the other hand, that a patient with silent underlying disease may present with an acute attack. Frey's masterly critique of the Cambridge and Marseilles classifications[10] and the views expressed by 12 signatories of a letter on the subject[2] warrant close attention. The latter stressed the need for an "operational classification" to provide as much pertinent and measurable information as possi-

TABLE 2-6. CHRONIC PANCREATITIS—IMAGE GRADING (Cambridge, 1983)

	ERCP	Ultrasound and CT Scanning
1. Normal	Quality study visualizing whole gland without abnormal signs.	
2. Equivocal	<3 abnormal branches	1 abnormal sign only
3. Mild	>3 abnormal branches	≥2 abnormal signs
4. Moderate	Above and main pancreatic duct changes	MPD 2–4 mm Gland up to 2 × normal Cavities <10 mm Irregular ducts Focal acute pancreatitis Parenchymal heterogeneity Duct wall echoes increased Irregular head or body contour
5. Marked	All of the above plus one or more of the following: Cavity >10 mm Intraduct filling defects Calculi Duct obstruction or stricture Severe duct irregularity Contiguous organ invasion	

TABLE 2-7. REVISED MARSEILLES CLASSIFICATION, 1984

Acute pancreatitis
Chronic pancreatitis
Obstructive chronic pancreatitis

ble to facilitate comparison of data from one institution with that from another. It is probable that their rather cumbersome classification will supplement the deceptively simple Cambridge and Marseilles classifications, and that a number of broad-based, mutually related classifications will be used in the future.[1]

Many problems remain unresolved, particularly the thorny issue of whether alcohol-induced disease, although not infrequently clinically acute, is invariably associated with chronic change. While most patients presenting with a clinically acute attack have preexistent chronic changes, a certain proportion of them are indeed acute in the clinicopathologic context.[22,30] Renner et al., in a recently published autopsy series of 247 patients with fatal alcohol-induced clinically acute pancreatitis, found that no fewer than 53% of them had histologic evidence of acute pancreatitis unassociated with chronic change—an incidence comparable to that found in lethal pancreatitis due to choledocholithiasis or miscellaneous causes.[25] This high incidence is probably considerably greater than that found in the usual clinical setting, but the study leaves no doubt as to the existence of alcohol-induced acute pancreatitis. The findings in the study of Renner et al. may also be reconciled with the suggestion by Scuro et al. that acute alcoholic pancreatitis "quite probably follows a pathophysiological pathway different from that of chronic alcoholic pancreatitis."[30]

REFERENCES

1. Bank S. Acute and chronic pancreatitis. In: Dent TL, ed. Pancreatic Disease. New York, Grune & Stratton, 1981, pp 167–188.
2. Banks PA, Bradley EL, Dreiling DA, et al. Classification of pancreatitis—Cambridge & Marseille. Gastroenterology, 89:928–930, 1985. Letter.
3. Blumenthal HT, Probstein JG. Pancreatitis: A Clinical-Pathological Correlation. Charles C Thomas, Springfield, Ill., 1959.
4. Cattell RB, Warren KW. Surgery of the Pancreas. Philadelphia, WB Saunders, 1953, p 58.
5. Cawley, T. A singular case of diabetes, consisting entirely in the quantity of urine: With an enquiry into the different theories of that disease. Lond Med J 9:286, 1788.
6. Comfort MW, Gambill EE, Baggenstoss, AH. Chronic relapsing pancreatitis: A study of twenty-nine cases without associated disease of the biliary or gastrointestinal tract. Gastroenterology 6:239–285, 1946.
7. Dreiling DA. Panel discussion: Chronic relapsing pancreatitis. In: Proceedings of the 2nd World Congress of Gastroenterology, Munich 1962. Vol 4, Topical Problems in Pancreatitis. Bartelheimer H, Lagerlöf H, eds. Basel, Karger, 1963, p 9.
8. Fitz RH. Acute pancreatitis: A consideration of pancreatic hemorrhage, hemmorrhagic, suppuration and gangrenous pancreatitis and of disseminated fat necrosis. Boston Med Surg J 120:181–235, 1889.
9. Friedreich N. Diseases of the pancreas. In: Cyclopedia of the Practice of Medicine. New York, Wood, 1878, Vol 8, p 599.

10. Frey CF. Classification of pancreatitis: State-of-the-art, 1986. Pancreas 1:62–68, 1986.
11. Gambill EE, Comfort MW, Baggenstoss AH. Chronic relapsing pancreatitis: An analysis of 27 cases associated with disease of the biliary tract. Gastroenterology 11:1–33, 1948.
12. Gyr KE, Singer MV, Sarles H. Pancreatitis: Concepts and Classifications. Proceedings of the Second International Symposium on the Classification of Pancreatitis, Marseille, France, 28–30; March, 1984. Amsterdam, Excerpta Medica, 1984.
13. Howard JM, Ehrlich EW. The etiology of pancreatitis—a review of clinical experience. Ann Surg 152:135–146, 1960.
14. Howard JM, Ehrlich EW. Gallstone pancreatitis: A clinical entity. Surgery 51:177–184, 1962.
15. Howat HT. Panel discussion: Chronic relapsing pancreatitis. In: Proceedings of the 2nd World Congress of Gastroenterology, Munich 1962. Vol 4, Topical Problems in Pancreatitis. Bartelheimen H, Lagerlöf H, eds. Basel, Karger, 1963, p 10.
16. Janowitz HD. The variety of pancreatic disease. Am J Dig Dis 2:41–42, 1957.
17. Joske RA. Etiologic factors in the pancreatitis syndrome. Br Med J 2:1477–1481, 1955.
18. Lagerlöf HO. Pancreatic function and pancreatic disease studied by means of secretin. Acta Med Scand 128 (suppl): 1942.
19. Marks IN. Alcohol-induced pancreatitis. In: Truelove SC, Willoughby CP, eds. Topics of Gastroenterology 7. Oxford, Blackwell, 1980, pp 303–322.
20. Marks IN, Bank S. The aetiology, clinical features and diagnosis of pancreatitis in the South Western Cape. S Afr Med J 37:1039–1053, 1963.
21. Marks IN, Bank S, Louw JH. The diagnosis and management of pancreatitis. In: Glass GBJ, ed. Progress in Gastroenterology. New York, Grune & Stratton, 1966, Vol 1, pp 412–472.
22. Marks IN, Girdwood AH, Bornman PC, Feretis C. The prevalence and etiology of pancreatitis in Cape Town. In: Gyr KE, Singer MV, Sarles H, eds. Pancreatitis: Concepts and Classification. Amsterdam, Excerpta Medica, 1984, pp 345–346.
23. Opie EL. The relation of cholelithiasis to disease of the pancreas and fat necrosis. Bull Johns Hopkins Hosp 121:19–20, 1901.
24. Opie EL. The etiology of acute haemorrhagic pancreatitis. Bull Johns Hopkins Hosp 121:182–188, 1901.
25. Renner IG, Savage WT, Pantoja JL, Renner VJ. Death due to acute pancreatitis: A retrospective analysis of 405 autopsy cases. Dig Dis Sci 30:1005–1018, 1985.
26. Sarles H. "Pancreatitis" Symposium, Marseille, April 25 & 26, 1963. S. Karger; Basel, NY 1965.
27. Sarles H, Muratore R, Sarles JC. Étude anatomique des pancréatites chroniques de l'adulte. Semin Hôp Paris 37:1507–1522, 1961.
28. Sarles H, Sarles JC, Camatte R, et al. Observations on 205 confirmed cases of acute pancreatitis, recurring pancreatitis and chronic pancreatitis. Gut 6:545–559, 1965.
29. Sarner M, Cotton PB. Classification of pancreatitis. Gut 25:756–759, 1984.
30. Scuro LA, Cavallini G, Vantini I. Etiology and pathogenesis of acute pancreatitis. In: Banks PA, Bianchi Porro G, eds. Acute Pancreatitis: Advances in Pathogenesis, Diagnosis and Treatment. Milano, Masson, 1984, p 13.
31. Symners WSTC. Acute alcoholic pancreatitis. Dublin J Med Sci 143:244, 1917.

CHAPTER

3

VALUE OF ASSESSING "RISK FACTORS" IN ACUTE PANCREATITIS

Simmy Bank and Ronald Greenberg

EDITORIAL COMMENT

The authors have thoroughly reviewed the many approaches to developing prognostic assessments of acute pancreatitis. No single system has universal application because of the variations in etiology, geography, and therapeutic approaches. The pragmatic conclusion is to recommend that each institution use the criteria that work best for its patient population and environment. The negative side to this is the accumulation of irreconcilable data for publication and studies that defy comparison. A plea is therefore made for an assessment to be made on Ranson's criteria as well as any other index that may be more acceptable at the local institutional level, so that reports of clinical studies will be comparable.

Early prognostic assessment is not an intellectual exercise for house staff but a valuable technic for selecting those 20% to 30% of patients who will develop severe disease. These patients should be treated in the intensive care unit and carefully monitored. As Dr. Bank points out, the mortality in this group already shows signs of decreasing. Intensive diagnostic scrutiny in these patients should lead to prompt detection of infected pancreatic necrosis, sterile necrosis abscess, or hemorrhage effusion with the potential for early intervention to prevent death from these complications.

CONTROVERSY

The prognostic signs for patients with acute pancreatitis formulated by Ranson in New York in 1974 have proved valuable in assessing severity and in planning treatment but have not been universally accepted. Modifications of the Ranson criteria have been established and used in other centers, particularly in Europe. Severity indices based on clinical features including shock, ileus, characteristics of the peritoneal fluid, and extrapancreatic involvement have their advocates. Even clinical assessment by the examining physician has been shown to be extremely accurate. These prognostic assessments and their role in therapy are discussed.

RISK FACTORS IN PANCREATITIS

The last 10 years has witnessed important advances in the understanding of the pathophysiology of acute pancreatitis and the use of physical and biochemical data to identify better the severity, prognosis, and treatment of the acute attack. This is not to say that symptoms and signs of imminent disaster, previously referred to as fulminating pancreatitis, have not been recognized since the 1940s.[55] Shock, ileus, or evidence of hemorrhagic pancreatitis and many single biochemical abnormalities have long been known to be associated with a downward course. However, Ranson and his group identified a group of biochemical criteria that assessed severity, and they popularized these criteria to assess the therapeutic value of peritoneal lavage for the acute attack. Since the evolution of Ranson's prognostic signs, which became widely used, there has been a veritable race to modify, improve, simplify, enhance—and even detract from—the original 11 early objective signs of severity. These have included attempts to resurrect single signs; propose clinical criteria to reassess severity; supercede biochemical criteria by radiologic findings; and even employ combinations of clinical, biochemical, and radiologic data. These attempts to categorize the clinical course better are, of course, highly commendable and should be pursued. However, lest we expend too much energy in this direction, it might be worth pausing to reflect on a few salient questions.

1. Has definition of the prognostic indicators made any material difference to the mortality of the disease?

2. Has definition of the prognostic factors made an impact on the intensity and type of treatment?

3. Has the definition of the prognostic factors led to the elaboration or discovery of new or alternate therapeutic measures directed at the pancreatic necrosis itself?

4. Has the definition of the prognostic factors really helped to group the disease into categories so that better stratified evidence of therapeutic successes can be ascertained?

5. Has it in fact helped to predict abdominal complications that could not have been ascertained by other means?

6. And in short, has it been an intellectual or statistical exercise rather than a therapeutic advance?

DEFINITION OF RISK FACTORS

Attempts to assess the severity of the attack before multiple criteria were popularized may best be considered under the clinical classification of the disease and the use of single criteria.

Clinical Classification (Table 3-1)

Clinical classification was one of the earliest methods of assessing severity. There are of course a group of patients in whom recognition of a fulminating

TABLE 3-1. SINGLE SIGNS OF SEVERITY

Clinical	Biochemical	Radiologic
Peritoneal aspiration	Hypocalcemia	Marked ileus
Shock	Fibrinogen*	CT scan
Ileus	Methemalbuminemia*	Ultrasound†
Hemorrhagic pancreatitis	Hypophosphatemia*	ERCP†
Fluid sequestration	AST*	
Ascites	BUN*	
Pa_{O_2}	Phospholipase A_2 activity†	
Nystagmus*	Endotoxemia†	
Encephalopathy*	α_1-Antitrypsin†	
	α_2-Macroglobulin*	
Diabetic or hyperosmolar coma*	Complement†	
Fever*	C-Reactive protein†	
Skinny needle aspiration†	Granulocyte elastase†	
	Urine trypsinogen-activating peptide†	
	Serum pancreatitis associated peptide (PAP)†	

* Rarely considered today because of obsolescence.
† Still under investigation or rarely available at present.

attack is so obvious that all other definitions of severity are really an exercise in futility. These patients usually present in a morbidly ill fashion with marked abdominal distension; ileus; ascites; shock; evidence of toxemia; and acidotic breathing and seem close to death and requiring extensive resuscitative measures. No prognostic signs or clinical criteria are needed to realize that these patients are likely to die or run a stormy course or develop serious complications. This group probably accounts for some 2% of all cases of acute pancreatitis, and the mortality in this group approximates 90%. Similarly, it was rarely a major prognostic problem when the patient presented with tetany, confusion, irritability, or stupor with localizing neurologic signs or combination of these. However, this clinical presentation accounts for a relatively small proportion of patients during their initial examination. Because of the relative rarity of this momentous onset, more refined attempts were made to classify the clinical aspects of the disease. One of the standard clinical classifications dating back to 1959 was that proposed by Marks, Louw, and Bank and encompassed four groups: (1) *fulminating*, with shock, ileus, or evidence of hemorrhagic disease, (2) *severe,* illness severe enough to require admission into hospital for intravenous fluids and nasogastric suction, (3) *mild,* in which abdominal pain and the raised amylase levels were the significant feature, and recovery was usually rapid in 3 to 7 days, and finally (4) *painless pancreatitis*.[7,55,56] How do these early criteria measure up to the present-day risk factors?

1. *Shock.* Louw, Marks, and Bank recorded a >50% mortality in patients with blood pressures below 100 mm Hg on admission and not rapidly corrected by fluid replacement.[55] Since then, conflicting mortality rates have been reported, using shock as a prognostic sign. The general evidence is that although shock has high specificity as an indicator, its sensitivity is low. There can be little doubt that shock either at the onset or any time during the course of an attack is a serious sign carrying a mortality of some 30% to 50%, especially as it is rarely a single sign and is often associated with evidence of either cardiopulmonary or renal insufficiency or other organ abnormality.

2. *Ileus*. Admission with or continuance of prolonged abdominal distension and a silent belly indicates either severe chemical peritonitis or severe inflammatory neuropraxia of the celiac plexus resulting in adynamic ileus. Temporary ileus is a relatively frequent manifestation in the early stages and thus only predicts severity in a small number of cases. However, if prolonged it indicates a poor prognosis (± 50%–60% mortality), and the return of bowel sounds can be of great reassurance that the severity of attack is subsiding.

3. *Hemorrhagic pancreatitis*. This was once considered a virtual sign of impending death. The presence or overt evidence of hemorrhagic or necrotic disease still denotes a mortality ranging from 40% to 90% in the literature and in our own study 50%, or equal to Ranson's or Bank's poor prognostic criteria. The usual indicators are Grey Turner's or Cullen's sign, the presence of hemorrhagic fluid if aspiration or operation is undertaken, and the rarely used test for methemalbuminemia. In our own studies, despite the high mortality of hemorrhagic disease, Ranson's and Bank's signs were still better indicators of prognosis than evidence of hemorrhagic disease alone.

Miscellaneous Individual Signs

Most of these are obviously indicative of severe metabolic or hemorrhagic phenomena and have limited value because of their relative infrequency as sole signs, for example, hypocalcemia, hypokalemia, hypomagnesemia, stupor, confusion associated with cephalomalacia and cerebral edema, or perivascular hemorrhagic phenomena.[4,27,79]

Other clinical manifestations such as age, ethnic group, fever, renal failure, respiratory rate, nystagmus, and abdominal mass have all been proposed but have since been found to have poor predictive value of outcome or complications on their own.[30,43,48]

Table 3-1 shows some of the many signs either clinical, biochemical, or radiologic that have been proposed as an indication of severe or necrotizing disease. In regard to the latter, it should be stressed that although necrotizing disease clearly tends to be severe, the edematous form may also be severe. One recent study by Choi et al. showed that it was not possible to predict which of the two morphologic varieties would be found at surgery in 50 patients ill enough to warrant surgical exploration.[30] Some of these signs such as phosphalipase A_2 activity, endotoxin, complement, ultrasound, C-reactive protein, and granulocyte elastase activity are relatively recent and require more intensive study. Methemalbuminemia and fibrogen estimations, while still effective, have become unfashionable, while fluid sequestration, peritoneal lavage, and CT scan have emerged or returned.[18,30,38,59,77] Selective signs will be discussed in various sections of this chapter.

Hypocalcemia

Hypocalcemia, usually of marked severity, that is, calcium levels below 7 mg%, was considered to be evidence of gross fat necrosis with extensive saponification into calcium soaps. A serum calcium level below 4 mg% was regarded as uniformally fatal but was indeed rare. Even this highly fatal sign may be temporary, as evidenced by a patient with viral pancreatitis with myocardiopathy, peripheral neuritis, pancreatitis, and a serum calcium level of 2 mg% who survived the attack albeit after a fulminating course. We now know that the hypocalcemia is largely a reflection of hypoalbuminemia and the result of a reduction in protein-bound calcium levels. It would be necessary to measure levels of ionizable calcium, a test rarely available in most institutions, in patients with hypocalcemia disproportionate to the level of the serum albumin level or in whom evidence of tetany may be elicited.[4]

Methemalbuminemia

When first described, the presence of methemalbumin in the serum was regarded as a potential diagnostic sign of pancreatitis, as indeed it was.[64] However, various groups showed that methemalbuminemia could be found in any condition associated with intraabdominal hemorrhage, for example, ectopic pregnancy, ruptured aorta, intrahepatic hemorrhage, and even gut strangulation,[5,11,40,42,51,78] in which hyperamylasemia may occur. It thus became obvious that methemalbuminemia signifies hemorrhagic pancreatitis once the diagnosis of pancreatitis has been established and therefore has the same prognostic consequence of hemorrhagic or necrotic pancreatitis, that is, between 30% and 50% mortality when detected.

Phospholipase A_2

Despite the known importance of phospholipase A_2 in the pathophysiology of the initiation and progression of acute pancreatitis, measurements of phospholipase A_2 levels in the serum have not been found to be superior to measurements of levels of other enzymes as a diagnostic or prognostic measure, or to differentiate pancreatitis from other intraabdominal causes of hyperamylasemia (P. Banks and S. Bank unpublished data 1990). More recently, Buchler et al. have found a correlation between phospholipase A_2 activity (rather than concentration) and necrotic pancreatitis, the number of Ranson's signs, and pulmonary complications.[25] These studies deserve to be investigated further.

Fluid Sequestration

Although it was one of the early prognostic signs of Ranson, the fluid required in the first 24 to 48 hours was deemed important as a grave prognostic sign on its own. More recently, Sauven et al. have reevaluated the quantity of sequestrated fluid during the first 48 hours in 218 patients and found 86% mortality in 44 patients who sequestrated more than 2 L. However, the total mortality of 23% in their series suggests that they were dealing with a high incidence of fulminating attacks in all groups.[77]

Acute-Phase Reactants and Antiprotease Activity

In an unpublished study in 1975, Bank and Novis studied α_1-antitrypsin, α_1-chymotrypsin, and inter-α-antitrypsin values in the serum of patients with acute pancreatitis and suggested that patients who failed to show a rise in these acute-phase reactants during the attack (due to either an excess in trypsin binding or a genetic deficiency) tended to have more severe and even fatal attacks. The α_2-macroglobulin and C-reactive protein levels were also studied and found to be decreased and increased, respectively, in acute pancreatitis. Recently there has been renewed interest in correlating acute-phase reactants and products of cell degranulation to prognosis in acute pancreatitis; α_1-antitrypsin levels greater than 40 g/L and C-reactive protein levels greater than 120 mg/L have been claimed to be associated with a high incidence of fatal attacks and may in conjunction with Ranson's and Bank's signs prove prognostically extremely accurate. Granulocyte elastase and a new peptide-pancreatitis associated peptide (PAP) are currently being evaluated.

Although these individual signs of severity are still useful in predicting prognosis, they have been almost totally surpassed in prognostic value by multiple biochemical or clinical criteria.

Multiple Criteria

Early Objective Signs (Ranson's Signs) (Table 3-2)

The concept of using a single physical or biochemical sign to detect severity was superseded by Ranson's computerized evaluation of a large number of biochemical signs to assess which grouping would enhance the prognostic capability.[71] These 11 early objective signs, assessed in the first 48 hours, are now well

TABLE 3-2. RANSON'S EARLY OBJECTIVE SIGNS

		Alcohol and Other	Gallstone
	Age	>55 years	>70 years
	WBC	>16,000/mm^3	>18,000/mm^3
0-h	Blood sugar	>200 mg/100 ml	>220 mg/100 ml
	LDH	>350 U/L	>250 U/L
	AST	>250 U/L	>250 U/L
	HCT	↓10%	↓10%
	BUN	↑5 mg/100 ml	↑2 mg/100 ml
	Ca^{2+}	<8 mg/100 ml	<8 mg/100 ml
48-h	Pao_2	<60 mm HG	
	Base deficit	>4 mEq/L	>5 mEq/L
	Fluid sequestration	>6000 mL	>4000 mL

↓ decrease ↑ increase

known and the most used of the newer signs, despite some difficulty in recalling all the signs and the relative frequency of poor or delayed documentation of all the signs in the patient chart with regard to the exact time relationships, blood collection, fluid replacement, and other factors. Ranson's original contention was based on utilizing the severity score to stratify individual patients into prognostic groups to assess the value of peritoneal dialysis in those patients with severe disease. This spawned a whole new era in evaluating therapeutic measures based upon prognostic signs of an attack.[16,70,73,74] It has become apparent that assessment of the 11 early prognostic signs correctly predicts severity in some 60% to 80% of patients compared with visual clinical assessment or utilizing single physical or biochemical parameters that predict severity in some 30% to 40%. However, it should be emphasized that certain single signs such as shock, severe ileus, or evidence of hemorrhagic pancreatitis individually provide evidence of severe or fulminating disease. Ranson's prognostic signs provided the opportunity for various groups to explore, add, delete, and vary the signs under the pretext of (1) simplifying the signs to improve recall, (2) increasing the specificity and sensitivity of the signs, (3) modifying them to account for the pancreatic population and availability of tests in specific geographic areas, and (4) determining differences in signs for various etiologic groups; it also allowed groups to (1) investigate the reliability of the signs with regard not only to mortality but also to subsequent complications, (2) compare the signs to more conventional clinical criteria, and (3) assess the value of newer signs such as ultrasonography or radiology, singly or in combination, that have been said to be prognostically important. To this end, Ranson himself has modified his original early prognostic signs into two other groups, that is, for patients with gallstone pancreatitis (Table 3-2) and for those with impending abscess formation.

Clinical and Biochemical Follow-up on Ranson's Early Objective Signs (Fig. 3-1)

The most widely quoted modified signs are those of Imrie, which are used extensively in England. These vary from Ranson's signs largely by the inclusion of serum albumin levels as an important prognostic factor.[16] This theme of hypoalbuminemia has also been emphasized by other investigators including Jacobs, Blamey, Corfield, Harness, and Goulbourne.[16,33,44,45,49] Figure 3-1 provides a bird's-eye view of the early prognostic factors among various authors and provides a summation of what appear to be the common denominators among the signs. Thus, excluding those authors who have reverted to a single sign, that is, Sauven et al., who use fluid sequestration only,[77] and Larvin and McMahon's Acute physiologic score,[53] or those with tests rarely considered (such as C-reactive protein and α_1-antiproteinase, etc.) the prevalence of the signs are as follows: BUN levels in 11 studies, calcium levels in 10, LDH levels in 9, WBC counts in 8, blood sugar levels in 8, Pa_{O_2} in 7, albumin levels in 6, hematocrit in 5, AST levels in 4, fluid sequestration in 4, base excess in 2, creatinine levels in 2, amylase levels in 1, prothrombin time, bilirubin levels in 1, temperature in 1, and chest x-ray films in 1. The best fit among the groups thus seems to confirm the recent proposal by Cesar et al. from Lisbon, who arrived at a group of four signs by

	Ranson 1974	Jacobs 1977	Imre 1978	Harness 1981	Bank 1983	Blamey 1984	Corfield 1985	Damman 1987	Buchler 1987	Larvin 1987	Cesar 1987	Goulbourne 1987
AGE	1 2 55 75		+	+		+		+				
WBC	+ +	+	+	+	+	+	+					
GLUCOSE	+ +		+	+	+	+	+	+				
LDH	+ +		+	+		+	+	+	+		+	
SGOT	+ +		+	+			+					
HCT	+ +	+		+	+							
PO2	+		+	+	+	+	+				+	
BUN	+ +	+	+	+	+	+	+	+			+	+
CA^{++}	+ +	+	+	+	+	+	+	+			+	
BASE EXCESS	+ +			+								
FLUID SEQUEST	+ +			+								
ALBUMIN		+	+	+		+	+					+
CREATININE		+						+				
AMYLASE												+
α_1 ANTITRYPSIN									+			
α_2 MACROGLO.									+			
C.R. PROTEIN									+			
ENDOTOXIN								+				
CHEST X RAY												+
C.T.								+	+			
APS/PT/BIL.		++							+			
OTHER				Low B.P.				Ileus				

1) Original sign
2) For gall stones

Figure 3-1. Modifications of Ranson's signs.

Ranson. (1) refers to Ranson's original early prognostic signs. (2) is modified for gallstone pancreatitis.
Harness et al. Modified from McMahon, Ranson, Jacobs, and Goekas. Consider three Levels. Level 1 = Ranson's signs + temperature >101°F. Level 2 = BP <90 mm Hg. Level 3 = hemorrhagic signs or peritoneal lavage.
Damman et al. Modified Ranson's signs taken in conjunction with raised endotoxin level (>10 U/mL), ileus, and grade E or four CT signs. They claim a 90% correct prediction of severe disease.
Buchler et al. In predicting necrotizing pancreatitis examined five parameters—LDH, C-reactive protein, α_1-antitrypsin, α_2-macroglobulin, and CT scanning—and found all useful but LDH and C-reactive protein alone was 100% predictive.
Larvin and McMahon. Three objective illness-scoring systems—acute physiologic score (APS), simplified APS (SAPS), and the MRC sepsis score—were used; APS was superior, especially as an advance warning of complications.
Cesar et al. By discriminant analysis found LDH, Po_2, calcium, and BUN to give same predictive values as Ranson's, Blamey's or Bank's signs (PPV 44%; NPV 96%; therefore better in defining a mild attack.)
Goulbourne et al. Found amylase gradient (ratio of first amylase level to 24-hour amylase level < 2.0) among 57 variables to be important together with proteins, urea, and chest x-ray abnormality (two or more = 53% mortality).
Sauven et al. Found fluid sequestration of 2 L/day for greater than 48 hours to be a grave sign in 218 patients (86% mortality).
Agarwal and Pitchumoni* Simplified the clinical criteria (Bank) to include only cardiac, pulmonary, renal, and metabolic (Ca^{2+}, albumin). Related complications rather than mortality in a largely alcoholic group of patients (and thus, expectedly, found a low overall mortality).
McMahon et al.* Peritoneal lavage with 1 L of saline; severity is dependent on depth of color (red-chocolate opalescent).
Carter* Delineated signs that suggest a gallstone etiology that also included sex, AST, alkaline phosphatase, and high amylase levels. However, Goulbourne et al. found only sex, age, and ALT to correlate with a biliary etiology.

* The last three refer to clinical variations—not in figure.

discriminant analysis namely, Pa_{O_2}, BUN, LDH, and calcium levels.[29] However, clearly each group of pancreatologists have become proficient at applying their own set of criteria, and if the groups can use their own criteria to predict severity, there is no reason these criteria should not be used.[15,36] Nevertheless, there are some disquieting aspects of the use of the biochemical criteria. Although there can be little doubt that they have improved prognostic ability, the prognostic relationship between the criteria and mortality and morbidity still leaves much to be desired. Thus, the correct prognosis even with five or six of Ranson's criteria is in the region of 60% to 80%, and conversely even patients with fewer than three criteria occasionally progress to severe complications (such as abscess or hemorrhage) and may die. Clearly, therefore, there is a need for even more effective criteria, and this has led to a resurgence of the evaluation of clinical parameters and even exploration of a combination of clinical, biochemical, and more recently radiologic factors to enhance the prognostic capacity. The first of these arose from our own examination of extraabdominal organ involvement as a sign of impending complications and death and a comparison between these and Ranson's early prognostic criteria.

Clinical Criteria (Bank) (Table 3-3)

In 1983, Bank and his colleagues examined a group of criteria based on clinical evaluation of the patient (including the occasional readily available chemical test) in acute pancreatitis.[8,10,13] Because of the nature of the population in their hospital, the majority of acute attacks were unrelated to alcohol. The clinical criteria were compared with Ranson's early prognostic signs with regard to prognosis of mortality and intraabdominal complications. The clinical criteria are shown in Table 3-3 and as can be seen are dependent largely on the presence of evidence of extraabdominal organ involvement or complication.[19,26,28] Cardiac, pulmonary, and renal signs were the most common, but neurologic, hematologic, or metabolic disturbances were also frequent. These systemic effects are apparently related to some yet-unidentified circulating toxin elaborated by the chemical or inflammatory process. Popular incriminating factors to date are endotoxins,

TABLE 3-3. CLINICAL CRITERIA OF SEVERITY (Bank and Wise)

Cardiac	Shock, tachycardia >130, arrhythmia, ECG changes
Pulmonary	Dyspnea, rales, $Pa_{O_2} < 60$, ARDS (adult respiratory distress syndrome)
Renal	Urine output < 50 mL/h, rising BUN and/or creatinine level
Metabolic	Low or falling Ca^{2+}, pH, albumin
Hematologic	Falling HCT, (Diffuse intravascular coagulation), low platelets, split products
Neurologic	Irritability, confusion, localizing signs
	Hemorrhagic disease: On signs or peritoneal tap
	Tense distension: Severe ileus, fluid ++
Interpretation:	≧ 1 in any of the organ categories = severe disease; 60% mortality or more. (The greater the number of extra-abdominal organs involved the worse the prognosis)

circulating pancreatic enzymes or polypeptides, noxious prostaglandins, lysosomal proteins, and possibly even oxygen free radicals. The signs are often associated with hemorrhagic pancreatitis, free fluid in the abdomen, and ileus, but the clinical criteria were better indications of mortality or morbidity than the local manifestations of disease. Figure 3-2 shows the relative frequency of extraabdominal organ involvement in the first 48 hours of the acute attack, the contribution of that organ involvement to the mortality in the patients who died, and the overall mortality. It can be seen that pulmonary involvement is the most frequent extraabdominal risk factor (20%) followed by renal, cardiac, and then metabolic, hematologic, and neurologic, the latter being about equal at (3%). When these criteria were compared with Ranson's signs, it was found that there was an excellent agreement between five or more Ranson's signs and one criterion of Bank's signs (i.e., any evidence of extraabdominal involvement), that is, a mortality of 50% to 60%. In addition, the mortality from an intraabdominal complication, that is, abscess, bleeding, or cyst, was almost entirely dependent on whether the patient had poor risk factors rather than the complication itself. It should be noted that the mortality in our largely nonalcoholic group of patients (1978–83) was 13.5% and is comparable to most series from Britain or Germany[20] (i.e., ± 11%) and indeed with Ranson's nonalcoholic or fulminating postoperative group (20%) compared with the 5% to 7% mortality noted in series gathered from populations with largely alcoholic patients. The data from these latter series unintentionally or intentionally include a number of patients with established chronic pancreatitis with acute attacks, most of whom are in little danger of developing any signs or risk factors, and these patients can skew the data in many ways. Variations in a

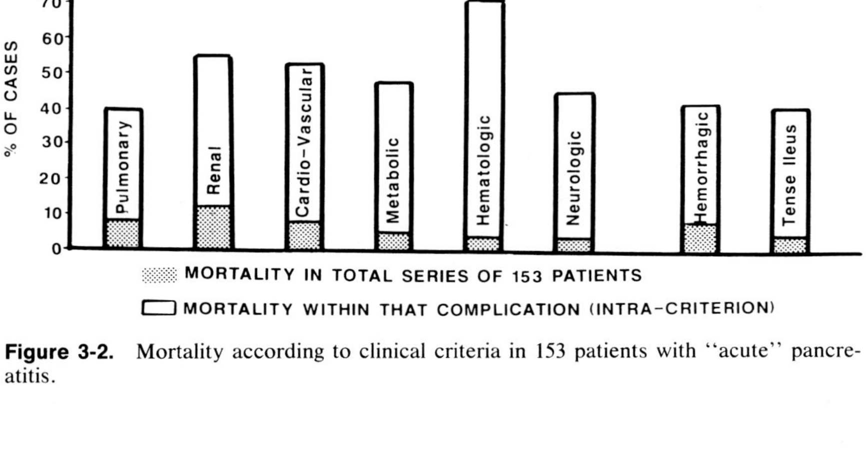

Figure 3-2. Mortality according to clinical criteria in 153 patients with "acute" pancreatitis.

return to clinical criteria have been proposed by Agarwal and Pitchumoni, and the acute physiologic score has been assessed by McMahon and his group.[3,53] Agarwal and Pitchumoni's series, which reduces the number of clinical criteria still further, had only two deaths and predicted intraabdominal complications rather than mortality. These modifications would have to be reevaluated in larger numbers and compared with Ranson's or Bank's signs to determine whether they apply to all etiologic groups and make a significant difference in prognosis compared with the earlier criteria.

Combinations of Clinical Criteria and Biochemical Tests

These have also been reassessed, and one group even found that a closer look at the fluctuations of serum amylase levels, that is, the rapidity of the reduction of amylase levels, had useful predictive value in association with some clinical signs and pleural disease.[44] This is of interest, as most pancreatologists have not regarded the intensity of the abdominal pain or the level of serum amylase to be of any prognostic importance, and in fact there have been a number of studies suggesting an inverse relationship between the serum amylase level and the severity of disease in acute pancreatitis, both clinically and when compared with CT scanning signs.

Assessment of Severity Based on Invasive Techniques

The presence of Grey Turner's, Cullen's, or hematologic signs (methemalbuminemia, hemoglobinuria) of hemorrhagic disease does not reflect the true incidence of hemorrhagic pancreatitis. This can be inferred from the peritoneal aspiration studies of Pickford and McMahon et al.[58,62,63,68] Their studies correlate the severity of the attack with the color and characteristics of aspirated fluid from the peritoneal cavity on admission. Even this may be an underestimate of hemorrhagic and/or necrotizing pancreatitis as one can only presume that the major site of bleeding or necrotic exudate is retroperitoneal rather than intraperitoneal.[32]

These authors in a largely nonalcoholic population of patients, have proposed and shown that peritoneal aspiration delineates the severe cases within 6 to 12 hours (as opposed to 0–48 hours in the early prognostic or clinical criteria) and therefore allows the choice of immediate peritoneal dialysis through the same catheter as that used for diagnosis or other rescusitative techniques. This proposal, although having much to commend it, has not gained much acceptance except in a few selected surgical centers in England presumably because of the following:

1. The occasional bowel perforation reported with intraabdominal catheterization (and we ourselves have had one; and one wonders how many more would occur in inexperienced hands).

2. The reluctance of physicians to be pressured into invasive procedures for benefits that are at best doubtful, thus having a high risk/benefit ratio.

3. The inability of some groups to show improved prognostic accuracy with an invasive procedure when compared with the more conventional noninvasive assessment, including early CT scanning and ultrasound.

4. The natural reluctance of most patients to have an invasive procedure done during mild attacks, thus skewing the overall results of the statistical reliability of the test. Clearly, if peritoneal aspiration reveals chocolate-colored fluid, a diagnosis of necrotizing or hemorrhagic pancreatitis is established.

Severity Based on Radiologic Findings

CT Scanning

CT assessment, the youngest entrant into the severity-prognostic field, and until now well recognized for its accuracy in diagnosing complications, has already generated diverse opinions of its value in predicting outcome. This once again demonstrates the importance of evaluating multiple similar studies, particularly in a disease with so many variables as acute pancreatitis. Recent studies have graded the CT scan findings in acute pancreatitis either from 0 to 4 or from 1 to 6 or from A to E. The lowest numbers and letters indicate normal or edema localized to the gland, and the highest numbers progressively more severe changes indicative of edematous or necrotic pancreatitis to extensive peripancreatic and more distal fluid and necrotic collections. The grading has been claimed by some groups to be of value in overall prognosis and predicting future abscess formation if CT is carried out early (e.g., Balthazar et al.)[6,52,72] Other groups in Germany (Buchler et al. and Damman et al.) have found a poor correlation between CT grading and clinical status of the patient and even progression to abscess formation.[24,36] Vernacchia et al. found that only 28% of patients with grade E CT findings eventually developed an abscess, and even the severity score correlated poorly with the complication rate.[84] London et al., in a review of 72 patients (31 with severe criteria according to Imre), found an abnormal scan in 70% but poor correlation between clinical severity and CT findings (sensitivity 23%, specificity 86%) and concluded that CT findings are not a useful prognostic examination.[54] Of course, this applies only to early diagnostic-prognostic CT, as it is clear that CT carried out at later stages of the disease, for complications, in which nonresolution of the attack is a problem, has perhaps been the greatest advance in diagnosis to date. Further, although CT morphologic change may lag well beyond the clinical recovery, we have suggested that on occasion, oral refeeding after a fulminating or severe attack is probably best delayed until CT resolution is evident if recurrence of the attack is to be avoided.[71] Contrast enhanced CT is essential in assessing necrosis in the gland.

Ultrasonography

This has not been critically assessed to date, one of the problems being difficulty in visualization of the pancreas in the presence of ileus, so common during bad attacks of pancreatitis.[34,60] Further evaluation of this simple and now readily available technique is required before it is regarded as nonhelpful because it is possible that early clear visualization of the gland may be an important indicator of a mild attack, and difficulty in visualization due either to ileus or to extensive necrosis may be a sign of severe disease.

Single Flat Plate

Although a single flat plate has not been critically assessed with regard to accuracy of prognostic indicators, the finding of marked ileus with multiple fluid levels is clearly a bad prognostic sign; but the relative infrequency of this sign as an early finding makes it insensitive.

ERCP

Until recently regarded as a virtually heretical study during the acute attack, endoscopic retrograde cholangiopancreatography (ERCP) has recently been reinvestigated by European endoscopists to ascertain whether one could diagnose areas of irreparable necrosis that may be amenable to surgical removal to improve prognosis, rather than to continue with the limited medical therapy available. Clearly, like all studies on surgical as against medical treatments, the number of cases evaluated would have to be large to overcome the statistical uncertainty of the relative value of the choice of the medical or surgical treatment if a decision had been made to use the other modality. The ERCP changes of necrotic pancreatitis are related to severe duct disruption, extravasation of dye into the parenchyma, and perforation into surrounding tissues or freely into the retroperitoneal cavity. Hemorrhage from the pancreatic duct is a particularly lethal sign designating penetration of a large vessel by the necrotic process. All these signs are very suggestive of severe pancreatitis from the view of both mortality and subsequent complications. Contrast enhanced CT may however be equally accurate and less invasive.

Skinny Needle Aspiration

The value of skinny needle aspiration for pus cells or bacteria in areas of suspected necrosis or masses also needs further assessment with regard to predicting severity. Most of the studies have been carried out against historical controls or have brought obvious cases of clinical abscess formation into the series. Thus, at this stage it is not possible to confirm whether these techniques have improved assessment of severity and the mortality of patients with pancreatitis over and above assessment of risk factors of suspected phlegmon or abscess taken in conjunction with CT scanning alone. However, the technique appears to be safe and may obviate the need for surgery if no bacteria or pus is aspirated. Severity and mortality need to be examined in a blinded controlled fashion in the light of more recent evidence that abscess formation if properly treated has a far better prognosis than previously documented, especially in those patients in whom the severe prognostic signs have either not occurred with the attack or have subsided by the time the abscess develops.

TABLE 3-4. MORTALITY IN ACUTE PANCREATITIS WITH MISCELLANEOUS CAUSES

	No.	Mortality	%
Postoperative	5	4	80
Hyperlipemia	6	2	33
Carcinoma	4	2	50
Drug-related 3; traumatic 2;			
Other miscellaneous -nonfatal	congenital anomalies 3; previous surgery 3; intestinal obstruction, viral, diabetic, duodenal ulcer, hypercalcemia, Crohn's disease, and sarcoidosis, 1 each.		

RELATIONSHIP OF ETIOLOGIC GROUPS TO SEVERITY (TABLE 3-4)

Despite numerous studies that relate etiologic groups to mortality in acute pancreatitis, it is likely that the prognosis is related to the severity of the attack as judged by biochemical or clinical criteria and only rarely to etiology. However, the evidence to date would suggest that certain groups of patients have a greater tendency to have severe attacks and thus by extrapolation a greater risk of dying. Thus, postoperative and hyperlipemic pancreatitis appear to have inordinately high mortalities compared with alcoholic, gallstone, drug-related, and idiopathic forms of the disease.[16,21,47,87] The data even on postoperative and hyperlipemic pancreatitis have to be viewed with caution because of the relatively small numbers in statistically relevant series of acute pancreatitis. From an etiologic standpoint then, the risk factors seem to be of little value. Therapeutically, however, risk factors may be helpful in delineating patients who are likely to have a gallstone etiology and in whom immediate stone removal may be expedient.

PROGNOSTIC SIGNS AND MORTALITY WORLDWIDE

The mortality of acute pancreatitis (based on the Marseilles classification) is in the region of 9% to 15% in various series. The vast majority of patients survive after a relatively uncomplicated course lasting 3 to 7 days, and 10% to 15% after a prolonged course of delayed resolution, abscess, or cyst formation, gastrointestinal hemorrhage, pancreatic fistula formation, and so forth. The variation in mortality based on single, multiple, or clinical prognostic signs varies widely from series to series, but it appears generally agreed that (1) based on a single sign (e.g., fluid sequestration, hypocalcemia, shock) without utilizing multiple biochemical or clinical criteria provides an indicator of potentially lethal disease in 15% to 50% of cases; (2) patients with five or more of Ranson's signs or one organ complication by Bank's criteria have a mortality of 50% to 60% with a severity index accuracy between 60% and 80%;[8,16] (3) frank hemorrhage or discolored abdominal fluid has the same type of prognosis as 2,[63] and (4) a combination of clinical, biochemical, and radiologic (i.e., CT scanning) criteria gives a 90% indication of fulminating necrotic disease and the mortality rate of some 60% (Damman et al.).[36] It thus seems clear that some 5% to 15% of patients will be regarded as having a relatively minor attack at the onset of the clinical course and nevertheless progress to either greater severity or, more commonly, abscess formation, cyst, or hemorrhage. However, it is clear that the high mortality rates for these complications nearly always occur in patients with severe attacks by Ranson's or Bank's signs. It has thus become clear that most abscesses or hemorrhages are now treatable and that the patient will survive if the signs of fulminating disease are not present. It is also imperative that newer investigations and newer modalities of therapy be equated against the severity scores before they are regarded as having changed the course of the disease. Clearly, ultrasonography, CT scanning, and skinny needle aspiration have made a dramatic difference in selecting patients for surgery and assessing the site and best treatment of cyst and abscess, but whether mortality has improved is yet uncertain. Angiography and embolization have clearly affected mortality from bleeding.

THE RELATIONSHIP OF COMPLICATIONS AND PROGNOSTIC SIGNS (TABLE 3-5)

The relationship between Ranson's objective signs, the clinical criteria, and the major complications of the acute attack are shown in Table 3-5. As expected, intraabdominal complications occurred in a high percentage of patients with more than three of Ranson's signs and one or more of Bank's signs. In alcoholic pancreatitis, the curtailed clinical criteria proposed by Agarwal and Pitchumoni were intimately associated with abscess and cyst formation rather than a predictor of mortality. Although the various indicators of severity can alert one to the potential of abscess or cyst formation, confirmation of abscess is occasionally difficult. Thus, Ranson has suggested a variation of his prognostic signs to include the likelihood of abscess; CT is of obvious benefit; Warshaw and Lee consider radioimmunoassay for ribonuclease to be a sensitive test for the development of abscess; and Block et al. recently described fever >38.5°C, base excess −4 mmol/L, hematocrit <35%, and Pa_{O_2} <60 mm Hg to have an 83% predictive value.[14,17,31,35,86] Gerzof, et al. have shown the value of skinny needle aspiration for pus cells and bacteria in pancreatic masses[41] but have not correlated its value

TABLE 3-5. CLINICAL COURSE IN RELATION TO RISK FACTORS

Early Objective Signs				Clinical Criteria			
		Course				Course	
Number Positive	Number of Cases	Simple	Complicated	Number Positive	Number of Cases	Simple	Complicated
0	16	14	2	0	58	47	11
1–2	24	20	4	≧1	7	1	6
3–5	20	14	6				
6–8	5	0	5				
Total	65	48	17		65	48	17

with the severity of the attack or whether it is necessary in patients with less severe attacks in whom the prognosis of abscess would appear to be good.[85]

VALUE OF ASSESSING RISK FACTORS

Therapeutic Value

"If a patient comes into the emergency room and has three or more of Ranson's signs or one or more Bank's signs, the patient must be admitted to the intensive care unit. If the physician in charge of the ICU says there are no beds in the unit, you then tell him or her that that is his or her problem and you are removing your responsibility for the patient." This advice to my fellows and interns reflects my personal feeling about the importance of critical care monitoring for patients with severe or impending severe signs. It is probably true to say that meticulous ICU monitoring and appropriate and timely intervention for extraabdominal organ complications or intraabdominal local complications remains the only effective therapy that has reduced the mortality of the acute attack from some 80% to 90% for fulminating attacks to 40% to 50% and thus the overall mortality for acute attacks of pancreatitis to 5% to 7% in all groups including alcohol and 8% to 10% for groups excluding alcohol in acute pancreatitis. Tables 3-6 and 3-7 show the difference in mortality in two 4-year time periods as assessment of severity and ICU therapy has been used more frequently. Although the numbers are small, it does seem to show a trend to decreased mortality in patients even with severe disease in the last 4-year period. As we have no way at present to predict which of the patients with severe signs within the risk criteria will live or die, this emphasizes the importance of an impeccable critical care approach. Thus, even patients who are desperately ill with eight Ranson's signs or a number of organ failure signs may be salvaged. Clearly, patients with multiple signs, apart from the usual intensive care regime, should also be subject to a Swan Ganz catheter and other sophisticated monitoring measures. Harness et al. have looked at various levels of severity in an attempt to regulate therapy (Table 3-8).[45] The German workers in Ulm have recently reported remarkably low mortality rates of some 8% to 22% in fulminating pancreatitis with careful evaluation of clinical

TABLE 3-6. ACUTE PANCREATITIS; MORTALITY IN TWO 4-YEAR PERIODS

	1978–1982			1983–1987			Total		
	No.	Mortality	%	No.	Mortality	%	No.	Mortality	%
Alcohol	8	2	25	17	0	0	25	2	8
Gallstones	26	2	8	35	1	3	61	3	5
Idiopathic	15	3	20	8	1	12	23	4	17
Miscellaneous	26	3	11	18	4	22	44	7	16
Total	75	10	13.5	78	6	8	153	16	10.5

TABLE 3-7. SEVERITY AND MORTALITY IN ACUTE PANCREATITIS USING RISK FACTORS

	1978–1982		1983–1987	
	Ranson (%)	Bank (%)	Ranson (%)	Bank (%)
Severe *	24	22	20	19
Mortality in "severe" group	50	56	38	40
Mortality in "mild" group	4	2	0	0
Overall mortality	13.5%		8%	

* Ranson's early objective signs: five or more.
Bank's clinical criteria: one or more.

prognostic signs, sepsis signs, necrosectomy, and prolonged retroperitoneal drainage. This enviable result will hopefully become universal.

Value in Being Forwarned of Local Complications

Although abscess and cyst rarely complicate a seemingly mild attack of pancreatitis, they may occur. However, the incidence of these complications with severe attacks varies among series from 30% to 60%. Clearly then, patients who continue to be ill or have recovered from an initial attack with multiple criteria need to be followed up and probably need at least a CT scan and skinny needle aspiration soon after the attack to elucidate whether they have any fluid collec-

TABLE 3-8. THERAPEUTIC VALUE OF SIGNS OF RISK FACTORS (HARNESS)

Level	Definition	Initial Treatment
I	2 risk factors	Nasogastric suction Fluid resuscitation Pain medication
II	3–4 risk factors or BP < 90 mm Hg	Intensive monitoring in unit Respiratory care Aggressive fluid resuscitation
III	5 risk factors, or methemalbumin in serum or peritoneal fluid, or peritoneal free fluid >10 mL, or peritoneal lavage fluid the color of dark beer, or "prune juice" peritoneal fluid, or peritoneal fluid total protein >5.0 g/mL CNS coma	Peritoneal dialysis Intensive monitoring in unit Respiratory care Aggressive fluid resuscitation Nutritional support
IV	Uncertain diagnosis Rapid deterioration in level II or III Etiologic factor amenable to operation Complications indicating operation	Operation

tions or abscess formation. The earliest indication of gastrointestinal hemorrhage requires endoscopy to ascertain where the bleeding is coming from. Special attention should of course be given to the short gastric veins in the fundus of the stomach, which may become varicose depending on the amount of compression of the splenic vein by the enlarged pancreas or abscess formation.

Value in Treatment of Various Etiologic Groups

While a number of the prognostic signs such as age and levels of LDH, alkaline phosphatase, AST, and of course bilirubin may be useful in suggesting a gallstone cause of the attack, the question is whether an assessment of severity can assist in management.[61,66] There has clearly been a tendency to earlier stone removal in acute pancreatitis among some surgeons and endoscopists. In 1984, at the second Marseilles Symposium on the classification of pancreatitis and again at the World Congress in Gastroenterology in San Paulo, Brazil in 1986, we suggested that patients with known gallstones or diagnosed as having gallstones during the attack should be treated according to the following scheme[8,66] (Table 3-9):

1. If the attack is assessed as mild, fewer than three of Ranson's signs or none of Bank's signs, common duct visualization and biliary surgery should be carried out at any time during the hospital stay, preferably within the first few days.

2. If the attack was mild on admission and while being observed or awaiting operating time the patient develops increasing Ranson's signs or any of Bank's signs, operation or endoscopic sphincterotomy and stone retrieval should be undertaken as a matter of urgency.

3. If there are more than five of Ranson's signs or one or more Bank's signs, the patient should be monitored and treated in the ICU, allowing cardiac, renal, pulmonary, and metabolic therapy to be undertaken to improve the patient's general condition and, if possible, allowing the attack to subside before biliary surgery is undertaken. If progressive deterioration occurs instead of improvement, an urgent cholecystotomy, or if the expertise is present, an urgent sphincterotomy, may be necessary. This approach has also been proposed by Verizen and Prorok in a group of 180 patients with acute biliary pancreatitis in Pennsylva-

TABLE 3-9. THERAPY BASED ON ASSESSMENT OF PROGNOSTIC SIGNS IN ACUTE BILIARY PANCREATITIS

Ranson's Prognostic Signs	Bank's Clinical Criteria	Therapy
<5	0	Elective surgery, endoscopic sphincterotomy
>5	1 or more	Careful monitoring until clinical improvement, then surgery or ERCP
$<5 \rightarrow 5$ or more	$0 \rightarrow 1$ or more	Urgent surgery or endoscopic sphincterotomy

nia, where they compared the complication rate and mortality following surgery in 79 patients with mild pancreatitis as against 29 with severe pancreatitis and concluded that surgery was indeed hazardous in those patients with severe disease.[83] Clearly, the place of endoscopic sphincterotomy in these latter patients with fulminating disease as opposed to watchful expectancy and operating after the attack has subsided requires extensive further experience.[50,75,82] Other authors suggest duct exploration or at least visualization in all patients with pancreatitis in whom a cause is not apparent.[2,65] The prognostic signs do not appear to play a role in any of the other etiologic groups of acute pancreatitis except perhaps the rare cases of pancreatitis due to periampullary diverticulum, in which stenting the common duct may allow improved biliary and pancreatic flow by deflecting the angle between the biliary and pancreatic systems.[80,81]

The Value of Risk Factors in Therapeutic Trials

Pancreatitis has long been considered an unpredictable disease rendering controlled and even uncontrolled trials of various diagnostic and therapeutic measures of limited value and difficult to interpret. Although this still holds true today in some respects, there can be little doubt that classification of patients with regard to the severity of the attack according to one or other of the biochemical or clinical risk factors has greatly facilitated stratification into mild or rarely fatal attacks and those that are severe and frequently become complicated with a mortality in the region of 50%. Thus, the outcome is in fact much more predictable since the advent of the prognostic signs, making therapeutic, medical, endoscopic, or surgical initiatives and controlled trials much more meaningful.

Previous trials that did not include any assessment of risk factors can virtually be discarded as meaningless.[22,37,39,46,76] These include various early trials related to nasogastric suction; antibiotics; oxygen therapy; steroids; drugs such as glucagon, somatostatin, and aprotinin; even the mortality of early surgery, abscess, and cyst; and more recently, uncontrolled trials of the value of early stone removal by surgery or endoscopy in gallstone-associated pancreatitis. More recent studies have included a comparison of subjects within the various prognostic groups, and although most of these studies tend to be recent and as yet undecided, it does seem clear that the mortality from abscess and bleeding is heavily weighted according to the severity of the attack and that antibiotics and hyperalimentation are probably beneficial for severe, prolonged attacks. It is now also clear that peritoneal lavage will decrease the early mortality, (i.e., within the first 10 days of severe attacks) although perhaps not materially affecting the overall mortality. Perhaps the most promising of all is what appears to be a true reduction in the overall mortality of acute pancreatitis since the advent of attention to the risk factors and appropriate intensive care therapy. The recognition of the clinical criteria, especially with regard to attention to alteration in cardiac, pulmonary, renal, metabolic, and hematologic changes and their correction, appears to have decreased the mortality of the severe attack from 50–56% to 40% or less in the present series spanning two 4-year time periods, the first from 1978 to 1982 and the second from 1983 to 1987, and the overall mortality from 13.5% to 8%. Furthermore, the mortality now seems to be largely confined to the elderly and patients with concomitant severe disease, that is, collagen disease, lymphoma, and cardiac disease, in the last 4-year period in our series. This seems to be in accord with other reported series, mainly from Damman and his group in Ulm. Clearly, the lower mortality is due to improved ICU and other modalities of treatment but it all seems to have come during the time of more meticulous consideration of prognostic factors for the attack.

For the future, it is clear that studies of medical or surgical measures in acute pancreatitis, either diagnostic or therapeutic, should not be passed for publication by editorial boards of journals if stratification into the criteria used for judging the severity of the attack is not specified.

Risk Factors and Postpancreatitis Functional Reserve

There are a few studies that relate the severity of the attack to eventual pancreatic exocrine and endocrine function. Marks et al. found that 10% of patients with gallstone pancreatitis who were reinvestigated either for subsequent symptoms or routinely months or years after an attack of acute gallstone pancreatitis had some abnormality of pancreatic exocrine function (in a formal secretin cholecystokinin pancreatic function test) and that these patients tended to have had severe attacks.[56] Bank et al. noted decreased insulin reserve to glucose, glucagon, and tolbutamide stimulation months after severe acute gallstone pancreatitis in patients with normoglycemia. This was interpreted as indicating either temporary or permanent morphologic damage.[12] Perhaps the best evidence of the relationship between severity and morphology was the finding of persistent histologic changes (including calcification) in rats in which hemorrhagic-necrotic pancreatitis had been produced as against complete recovery in experimental edematous pancreatitis. More recent excellent follow-up studies by Buchler et al., Paez et al. appear to substantiate the probability that morphologic and subclinical exocrine and even endocrine dysfunction may still be present months and perhaps even years after severe necrotizing pancreatitis but rare after edematous pancreatitis.[23,57,67] To make these studies more meaningful, it is best to leave alcohol-induced pancreatitis out of consideration in their series because of the difficulty in knowing whether alcoholic patients have subclinical endocrine-exocrine insufficiency even before their first attack; then it is not surprising that a number of these latter patients manifest diabetes and/or steatorrhea even after a first attack (e.g., as in our definition of precalcific pancreatitis). When only the biliary group in Buchler's series is considered, and despite a progressive improvement between the first and second investigation, morphologic (ERCP, ultrasound, or CT) changes occurred in 47% and exocrine or endocrine dysfunction in 30% and 22%, respectively, of these patients 13 to 14 months after the attack. However, clinically manifested diabetes or steatorrhea is exceedingly uncommon as a consequence of gallstone or nonalcoholic acute pancreatitis, and we have seen only two cases of steatorrhea and two of persistent diabetes (where it was not known before) in nonalcoholic acute pancreatitis after the first acute attack. It therefore does seem clear that persistent pancreatic abnormality by testing may be more common after severe pancreatitis or massive necrosis than previously suspected but that clinically overt insufficiency is practically confined to those patients who developed massive necrosis on a background of alcohol-induced pancreatitis.

SUMMARY

Signs of fulminating or severe pancreatitis have been recognized for many years and have indeed always been a guide to the intensity of monitoring and therapy of the attack. However, single signs that include shock, ileus, evidence of hemorrhagic disease, hypoalbuminemia, hypocalcemia, hypoxemia, and so forth, had a limited prognostic range because they occurred as an early manifestation in only fewer than 20% of patients. However, it should be remembered that it was appreciated then, as now, that the presence of one of these signs anticipated a high mortality and morbidity. Newer single signs such as the level of acute-phase reactants and granulocyte degradation products may be shown to be prognostically accurate.

Introduction of more accurate criteria, both Ranson's early prognostic signs and more refined clinical criteria and many modifications of these over the last decade have clearly enhanced assessment up to levels approaching 60% to 80% for a severe attack within 24 to 48 hours and possibly up to 90% with the combined use of age, a group of biochemical and clinical signs, and CT scanning. A few patients will obviously escape detection and run a fulminating course despite absence of the prognostic signs early on, and it seems likely that differentiation between edematous and necrotizing pancreatitis will always be difficult other than by surgery in many patients. Clearly, various groups have become comfortable with these or their own "risk signs" that predict prognosis, and provided that the predictive value of their own criteria is high, they should be used in their particular environment. There may in fact be differences in the frequency of predictability of the criteria in various etiologic groups and geographic areas.

Having established the prognostic value and predictability of the signs with regard to mortality and the potential of developing an intraabdominal complication, it is basic to return to the initial question: Has delineation of the signs of severity been an interesting intellectual exercise, or has it contributed to reduction in the mortality of the acute attack? This is a difficult question to answer as it involves careful consideration of mortality rates from many centers. The British average of some 11% compares with that of our hospital (8% to 13.5%), which includes two 4-year periods, from 1978 to 1982 and from 1983 to 1987, with virtually identical numbers in each period. There was a reduction of mortality from 13.5% to 8% over the later period, when consideration of risk factors became commonly accepted and recognized by the physicians and surgeons on the staff. As no new dramatic specific therapeutic measures have been introduced and peritoneal lavage is only very seldomly performed at this hospital, this improved mortality may be due to a rapid recognition of "risk factors" and immediate and intensive therapy aimed at curtailing the extra abdominal and intraabdominal complications. The German group has reported remarkably low mortality rates with rapid and prolonged drainage or necrosection based on Ranson's and Bank's signs. It remains to be seen conclusively whether the utilization of prognostic signs as a guide to the urgency of intervention in gallstone pancreatitis or percutaneous skinny needle aspiration for the diagnosis of pancreatic infection will further decrease the mortality of acute severe pancreatitis. At present, these techniques are virtually confined to certain centers of enhanced enthusiasm for the techniques. Lastly, no study pertaining to acute pancreatitis today can be regarded as statistically valid without reference to one or other of the prognostic categories to stratify the "risk" potential of the attack.

REFERENCES

1. Aaron J, Bank S, Kumari S, Rosenblum G, Ackert G. Clinical vs CT findings as an indication for refeeding after acute pancreatitis. Gastroenterology 80:847(A), 1985.
2. Acosta JM, Rossi R, Oscar MRG, et al. Early surgery for acute gallstone pancreatitis: Evaluation of a systematic approach. Surgery 83:367–370, 1978.
3. Agarwal N, Pitchumoni CS. Simplified prognostic criteria in acute pancreatitis. Pancreas 1:69–73, 1987.
4. Allam BF, Imrie CW. Serum ionized calium in acute pancreatitis. Br J Surg 64:665–668, 1977.
5. Anderson MC, Toronto IR, Needleman SB, Gramatica L. Assessment of methemalbumin as a diagnostic test for acute pancreatitis. Arch Surg 98:776–780, 1969.
6. Balthazar EJ, Ranson JHC, Naidich DD, et al. Acute pancreatitis: Prognostic value of CT. Radiology 156:767–772, 1985.
7. Bank S. Acute and chronic pancreatitis. In: Dent TL, ed. Pancreatic Disease. New York, Grune & Stratton, 1981, pp. 167–188.
8. Bank S. Risk factors in acute pancreatitis—Towards a classification based on clinical criteria. In: Gyr K, Singer M, Sarles H, eds. Pancreatitis: Concepts and Classification. Amsterdam, Excerpta Medica, Elsevier, pp 389–394.
9. Bank S. Gallstone pancreatitis: Pathogenesis, concepts and clinical aspects in advances in hepato-biliary-pancreatic surgery. In: Post Grad Course Syllabus. Eighth World Congress of Gastroenterology, San Paulo, Brazil, 1986, pp 12–15.
10. Bank S, Wise L. Risk factors in acute pancreatitis. Am J Gastroenterol 77:680, 1981.
11. Bank S, Barbezat GO, Marks IN, Silber W. Methemalbuminemia in acute abdominal emergencies. Br Med J 2:86–88, 1968.
12. Bank S, Marks IN, Vinik AI. Clinical and hormonal aspects of pancreatic diabetes. Am J Gastroenterol. 64:13–22, 1975.
13. Bank S, Wise L, Gersten M. Risk factors in acute pancreatitis. Am J Gastroenterol. 78:637–640, 1983.
14. Banks PA. Sepsis indicators in acute pancreatitis. Pancreas 2:497–498, 1987.
15. Berry AR, Taylor TV, Davies GC. Diagnostic tests and prognostic indicators in acute pancreatitis. J R Coll Surg Edinb 27:345–352, 1982.
16. Blamey SL, Imrie CW, O'Neill J, Gilmour WH, Carter DC. Prognostic factors in acute pancreatitis. Gut 25:1340–1346, 1984.
17. Block S, Buchler M, Bittner R, Beger HG. Sepsis indicators in acute pancreatitis. Pancreas 2:499–505, 1987.
18. Block S, Maier W, Beger HG, et al. Identification of pancreas necrosis in severe acute pancreatitis—Imaging procedures vs clinical staging. Gut 27(9):1035–1042, 1986.
19. Bradley EL. Complications of pancreatitis: Medical and surgical management. Philadelphia, WB Saunders, 1982, pp 51–72, 154–203.
20. Bradley EL. Overview—Mortality in complications of pancreatitis: Medical and surgical management. Philadelphia, WB Saunders, 1982, pp 11–13.
21. Buch A, Buch J, Carlsen A, Schmidt A. Hyperlipidemia and pancreatitis. World J Surg 4:307–314, 1980.

22. Buchler M, Block S, Krautzberger W, Bittner R, Beger HE. Necrotizing pancreatitis: Peritoneal lavage or local lavage of the lesser sac? Dig Dis Sci 29:944(A), 1984.
23. Buchler M, Hauke A, Malfertheiner P. Follow-up after acute pancreatitis, morphology and function. In: Berger HG, Buchler M, eds., Acute pancreatitis. New York, Springer-Verlag, 1987, pp 367–374.
24. Buchler M, Malfertheiner P, Beger HG. Correlation of imaging procedures biochemical parameters in clinical stage in acute pancreatitis. In: Malfertheiner P, Ditschuneit H, eds. Diagnostic Procedures and Pancreatic Diseases. Berlin, Springer-Verlag, 1986.
25. Buchler M, Malfertheiner P, Schadlich H, Nevalainen T, Beger HG. The role of phospholipase A2 in human acute pancreatitis, speculation or truth. Dig Dis Sci 32:1160(A-3), 1987.
26. Buchler M, Malfertheiner P, Unl W, Beger HG. A new staging system in patients with acute pancreatitis. Gastroenterology 81:1331(A), 1986.
27. Bunao RM, Meyer KK. Pancreatitis with encephalomalacia and ascites. Am J Gastroenterol 55:145–151, 1971.
28. Carey LC. Extra abdominal manifestations of acute pancreatitis. Surgery 86:337–342, 1979.
29. Cesar M, Marques A, Deus J, et al. Prognostic criteria in acute pancreatitis—A critical evaluation Gut 28:368(A), 1987.
30. Choi TK, Ng WS, Wong J. Surgery during acute pancreatitis: Observations on 50 patients. Am J Surg 153:369–373, 1987.
31. Collins REC, Frost SJ, Spittlehouse KE. The P3 iso-enzyme of serum amylase in the management of patients with acute pancreatitis. Br J Surg 69:373–375, 1982.
32. Cooper MJ, Williamson RCN, Pollock AV. The role of peritoneal lavage in the prediction and treatment of severe acute pancreatitis. Ann R Coll Surg Engl 64:422–427, 1982.
33. Corfield AP, Williamson RCN, McMahon MJ et al. Prediction of severity in acute pancreatitis: Prospective comparison of three prognostic indices. Lancet 24:403–407, 1985.
34. Cotton PB, Lees WR, Vallon AG. Grayscale ultrasonography and endoscopic pancreatography in pancreatic diagnosis. Radiology 134:453–459, 1980.
35. Crass RA, Meyer AA, Brooke JR, et al. Pancreatic abscess: Impact of computerized tomography on early diagnosis and surgery. Am J Surg 150:127–131, 1985.
36. Damman HG, Dreyer TA, Gebhard J, Grabbe E. Prognostic indicators in acute pancreatitis. Clinical experience and limitation. In: Beger HG, Buchler M, eds. Acute pancreatitis. Berlin, Springer-Verlag, 1987, pp 181–197.
37. Diaco JF, Miller LD, Copeland EM. The role of early diagnostic laparatomy in acute pancreatitis. Surg Gynecol Obstet 129:263–269, 1969.
38. Foulis AK, Murray WR, Galloway D, et al. Endotoxemia and complement activation in acute pancreatitis in man. Gut 23:656–661, 1982.
39. Geokas MC, Olsen H, Barbour B, et al. Peritoneal lavage in the treatment of acute hemorrhagic pancreatitis. Gastroenterology 58:950(A), 1970.
40. Geokas MC, Rinderknecht H., Walberg CB, Weissman R. Methemalbumin in the diagnosis of acute hemorrhagic pancreatitis. Ann Intern Med 81:483–486, 1974.
41. Gerzof SG, Banks PA, Spechler SG, et al. Role of guided percutaneous aspiration in the early diagnosis of pancreatic sepsis. Dig Dis Sci 30:950(A), 1984.
42. Goodhead B. Significance of methemalbuminemia in acute abdominal emergencies. Arch Surg 101:376–378, 1970.
43. Gordon D, Calne R. Renal failure in acute pancreatitis. Br Med J 3:801–803, 1972.
44. Goulbourne IA, Dixon JM, Duffy S, Davies GC. Risk of death from acute pancreatitis Gut 28:370(A), 1987.
45. Harness JK, Hoverstein GH, Knoc JA. Acute pancreatitis: Surgical therapy. In: Dent TL. Pancreatic Disease. New York, Grune & Stratton, 1981, pp 189–204.
46. Howes R, Zuidema GD, Cameron JL. Evaluation of prophylactic antibiotics in acute pancreatitis. J Surg Res 18:197–200, 1975.
47. Imrie CW, McKay AJ, Benjamin IS, Blumgart LH. Secondary acute pancreatitis: Aetiology, prevention, diagnosis and mangement. Br J Surg 65:399–402, 1978.

48. Jacob HS, Goldstein IM, Shapiro I, et al. Sudden blindness in acute pancreatitis: Possible role of complement-induced retinal leukoembolization. Arch Intern Med 141:134–136, 1981.
49. Jacobs ML, Daggett WM, Civetta JM, et al. Acute pancreatitis: Analysis of factors influencing survival. Ann Surg 185:43–51, 1977.
50. Kelly TR, Swaney PE. Gallstone pancreatitis. The second time around. Surgery 92:571–575, 1982.
51. Kelly TR, Klein RL, Porquez JM, Homer GM. Methemalbumin in acute pancreatitis: An experimental and clinical appraisal. Ann Surg 175:15–18, 1972.
52. Kivisaari L, Somer K, Standetskjöld-Norderstam CG, et al. Early detectors of acute fulminant pancreatitis by contrast-enhanced computed tomography. Scand J Gastroenterol 18:39–41, 1983.
53. Larvin M, McMahon MJ. Serial objective measurements of severity in acute pancreatitis Gut 28:369(A), 1987.
54. London NJM, Neoptolemos JP, Bailey I, James D. Serial CT scanning in acute pancreatitis. Gut 28:368(A), 1987.
55. Louw JH, Marks IN, Bank S. The management of severe acute pancreatitis. Postgrad Med J 43:31–44, 1961.
56. Marks IN, Bank S, Louw JH. The diagnosis and management of pancreatitis. In: Glass JBT, ed. Progress in Gastroenterology. New York, Grune & Stratton, 1982, vol II, pp 412–472.
57. Martin F, Pederzoli P, Marzoli GP. Short and long-term results after necrotizing pancreatitis. In: Berger HG, Buchler M, eds., Acute pancreatitis. New York, Springer-Verlag, 1987, pp 375–376.
58. Mayer AD, McMahon MJ. The diagnostic and prognostic value of peritoneal lavage in patients with acute pancreatitis. Surg Gynecol Obstet 160:507–512, 1985.
59. Mayer AD, McMahon MJ, Bowen M, Cooper EH. C-reactive protein: An aid to assessment and monitoring of acute pancreatitis. J Clin Pathol 37:207–211, 1984.
60. McKay AJ, O'Neill J, Imrie CW, Duncan JG. Is an early ultrasound scan of value in acute pancreatitis? Br J Surg 69:369–372, 1982.
61. McMahon MJ, Pickford IR. Biochemical prediction of gallstones early in an attack of acute pancreatitis. Lancet 2:541–543, 1979.
62. McMahon MJ, Pickford IR, Playforth MJ. Early prediction of severity of acute pancreatitis using peritoneal lavate. Acta Chir Scand 146:71–175, 1980.
63. McMahon MJ, Playforth MJ, Pickford IR. A comparative study of methods for the prediction of severity of attacks of acute pancreatitis. Br J Surg 67:22–25, 1980.
64. Northam BE, Rowe DS, Winstone NE. Methaemalbumin in the differential diagnosis of acute haemorrhagic and oedematous pancreatitis. Lancet 1:348, 1963.
65. Osborne DH, Imrie CW, Carter DC. Timing of biliary surgery in gallstone associated acute pancreatitis. Gut 21:924(A), 1980.
66. Osborne DH, Imrie CW, Carter DC. Biliary surgery in the same admission for gallstone-associated acute pancreatitis. Br J Surg 68:758–761, 1981.
67. Paez O, Uscanga L, Nogyeron G, Galvan E, Robles-Diaz G. Functional impairment after severe acute pancreatitis. Dig Dis Sci 32:1181(A-24), 1987.
68. Pickford IR, Blackett RL, McMahon MJ. Early assessment of severity of acute pancreatitis using peritoneal lavage. Br Med J 2:1377–1379, 1977.
69. Ranson JHC. Timing of biliary surgery in acute pancreatitis. Ann Surg 189:654–663, 1979.
70. Ranson JHC, Pasternack BS. Statistical methods for quantifying the severity of clinical acute pancreatitis. J Surg Res 22:79–91, 1977.
71. Ranson JHC, Rifkind KM, Roses DF, et al. Objective early identification of severe acute pancreatitis. Am J Gastroenterol 61:443–451, 1974.
72. Ranson JHC, Balthazar EJ, Cacavale R, Cooper M. Computed tomography and the prediction of pancreatic abscess in acute pancreatitis. Ann Surg 201:656–664, 1985.
73. Ranson JHC, Rifkind KM, Roses DF. Prognostic signs and the role of operative management in acute pancreatitis. Surg Gynecol Obstet 138:69–81, 1974.

74. Ranson JHC, Rifkind KM, Turner JW. Prognostic signs and non-operative peritoneal lavage in acute pancreatitis. Surg Gynecol Obstet 143:209–219, 1976.
75. Safrany L, Cotton PB. A preliminary report: Urgent duodenoscopic sphincterotomy for acute gallstone pancreatitis. Surgery 89:424–428, 1981.
76. Satiani B, Stone HH. Predictability of present outcome and future recurrence in acute pancreatitis. Arch Surg 114:711–716, 1979.
77. Sauven P, Playforth MJ, Evans M, Pollock AV. Fluid sequestration: An early indicator of mortality in acute pancreatitis. Br J Surg 73:799–800, 1986.
78. Schow PD, Englert E. Methemalbumin and pancreatitis: A warning. Ann Intern Med 82:281–282, 1975.
79. Sharf B, Bental E. Pancreatic encephalopathy. J Neurol Neurosurg Psychiatry 34:357–361, 1971.
80. Stark B, Bank S, Greenberg R. Duodenal diverticula and pancreaticobiliary disease: To stent or not to stent. Gastrointest Endosc 154(A), 1986.
81. Thomas E, Reddy KR. Cholangitis and pancreatitis due to juxtapapillary duodenal diverticulum. Endoscopic sphincterotomy is the other alternative in selected cases. Am J Gastroenterol 77:303–304, 1982.
82. Van Der Spuy S. Endoscopic sphincterotomy in the management of gallstone pancreatitis. Endoscopy 13:25–26, 1981.
83. Verazin GT, Prorok JJ. Prognostic signs in acute biliary pancreatitis. Am J Gastroenterol 82:970(A), 1987.
84. Vernacchia FS, Jeffrey RB, Federle MP, et al. Pancreatic abscess. Predictive value of early abdominal CT. Radiology 162:435–438, 1987.
85. Warshaw AL, Jin G. Improved survival in 45 patients with pancreatic abscess. Ann Surg 202:407–417, 1985.
86. Warshaw AL, Lee KH. Serum ribonuclease elevations and pancreatic necrosis in acute pancreatitis. Surgery 86:227–234, 1979.
87. White TT, Morgan A, Hopton D. Postoperative pancreatitis. A study of seventy cases. Am J Surg 120:132–137, 1970.

CHAPTER

4

DIAGNOSIS OF THE ACUTE ABDOMEN ASSOCIATED WITH HYPERAMYLASEMIA

Simmy Bank and Gerard P. Burns

CONTROVERSY

The presence of a raised serum amylase level is for many physicians a sine qua non for the diagnosis of acute pancreatitis. However, the serum amylase level is nonspecific and is elevated in many other conditions. Amylase clearance tests were introduced to allow compensation for renal function but have not clarified the problem. Assays for isoamylases have enabled separation into pancreatic and nonpancreatic amylase and have been of some value in differentiating pancreatic disease. These and other unresolved issues are discussed in this chapter.

The cause of an elevated amylase level in patients with abdominal pain can be difficult to determine. The problem, of course, is usually the differentiation of pancreatitis from other diseases. In acute abdominal emergencies this may be crucial. This chapter reviews the biochemical tests that attempt to differentiate these two groups. It is clear that the tests may be unhelpful in difficult cases, in which laprotomy may be required.

The diagnosis of pancreatitis is conventionally made on a combination of a clinical history, raised serum amylase levels, and a flat plate of the abdomen to exclude nonpancreatic causes of abdominal pain. Despite the availability of estimations of other enzymes such as lipase, trypsin, esterase, ribonuclease, phospholipase A_2, and isoamylase fractionation by both chemical and radioimmunoassay techniques, measurement of amylase remains by far the most common diagnostic blood test performed. To this end Steinberg et al.[29] has investigated the specificity and predictive value of amylase, isoamylase, lipase, and trypsin levels in acute pancreatitis and found little difference between the tests, thus validating the value of amylase levels as the time-honored diagnostic test. The problem, of course, is that hyperamylasemia is common to pancreatitis and a large variety of other acute abdominal emergencies and unrelated diseases with an abdominal pain component.[2–4,7,15,16,20,30,34] The purpose of this chapter is to discuss the common clinical problems arising from the detection of hyperamylasemia.

HYPERAMYLASEMIA IN ACUTE ABDOMINAL EMERGENCIES

Clearly, the most diagnostically frequent and important question concerning hyperamylasemia results from the frequency of hyperamylasemia in acute abdominal conditions other than pancreatitis (see Table 4-1).

1. *Incidence of hyperamylasemia:* The incidence of finding a high amylase level in these conditions varies from high (60%–100%) in perforated peptic ul-

TABLE 4-1. CAUSES OF HYPERAMYLASEMIA

Acute Abdominal Emergencies
Perforated peptic ulcer without radiologic free air
Acute cholecystitis with hyperamylasemia
Intestinal obstruction with incipient strangulation
Intestinal infarction
Ruptured aortic aneurysm or dissection
Ruptured ectopic pregnancy
Acute salpingitis
Torsion of ovarian cyst or carcinoma
Abdominal trauma with hematoma formation
Perforated diverticulitis
Postgastrectomy afferent loop obstruction
Crohn's disease
Carcinoma of the ovary
Physiologic
Pregnancy
? Genetic S hyperamylasemia
Protein-Bound Hyperamylasemia
Inborn macroamylasemia attached to albumin or globulin, macroamylase
IgA-bound: celiac disease, lymphoma, IPSID
IgG-bound: chronic infections, liver disease
Immune-complex-bound: AIDS, collagen disease, Sjögren's syndrome
Decreased Excretion of Amylase
Acute and chronic renal failure
Tumor-Associated Amylase
Cancer of the ovary
Cancer of the lung
Lymphoma
Hematologic malignancy
Other tumors
Miscellaneous
Salivary gland disease, e.g., mumps, tumors
Diabetic ketosis
Postictal
Post-ERCP

TABLE 4-2. DIAGNOSTIC GROUPS AND NO. OF PATIENTS WITH HYPERAMYLASEMIA, HYPERAMYLASURIA, OR BOTH

Diagnosis	Serum Samples	Elevated Serum Amylase	Urine Samples	Elevated Urine Amylase	Hyperamylasemia and/or Hyperamylasuria
Acute biliary disease	24	5 (21%)	18	9 (50%)	10 (42%)
Intestinal obstruction	20	5 (25%)	17	2 (12%)	8 (40%)
Acute appendicitis	20	3 (15%)	15	5 (33%)	8 (40%)
Acute diverticulitis	10	2 (20%)	7	3 (43%)	4 (40%)
Perforated peptic ulcer	6	3 (50%)	5	3 (60%)	5 (83%)
Acute pancreatitis	5	5 (100%)	3	3 (100%)	5 (100%)
Acute gastroenteritis	4	1 (25%)	2	0 (0%)	1 (25%)
Ruptured aortic aneurysm	3	3 (100%)	3	1 (32%)	3 (100%)
Tuboovarian disease	3	2 (66%)	3	1 (33%)	3 (100%)
Miscellaneous*	5	3 (60%)	4	2 (50%)	3 (60%)
Total	100	32 (32%)	77	29 (38%)	50 (50%)

* One patient each with pneumonia, saddle embolus, gastric carcinoma with obstruction, acute lymphadenopathy, and renal failure with associated cardiac failure.

cer[13,26,22] and intestinal strangulation and infarction (9) to relative rarity in appendicitis and diverticulitis.[21,23]

2. *Magnitude of the elevation:* The amylase level may vary from minor elevations to 20 to 30 times the upper limit of normal. The innumerable variations in amylase methods contribute to these variations on occasion. The higher levels are often associated with specific causes of disease such as acute cholecystitis, perforated peptic ulcer, intestinal infarction, or ruptured aneurysm;[24] and the lower levels with appendicitis, Crohn's disease, and infective gastroenteritis.[32,33]

3. *Interval between the onset of disease and measurement of amylase levels:* Amylase levels decrease with increasing duration of the disease in pancreatitis and cholecystitis and are highest after a more prolonged interval in intestinal obstruction, perforation, and infarction.

4. *Variation from study to study:* Incidence of hyperamylasemia in acute abdominal disease varies between 10% and 50%, with most studies reporting a 15% to 30% range. The high incidence of hyperamylasemia in these conditions is often irrelevant as many of the clinical conditions become clinically obvious. The important questions are how often hyperamylasemia presents a real diagnostic dilemma between pancreatic and nonpancreatic emergencies, and whether we have any clinical or biochemical methods to distinguish between a surgically correctable cause and one in which surgery may be unnecessary, for example, pancreatitis or Crohn's disease, or totally contraindicated, for example, infective gastroenteritis; a misdiagnosis could be lethal.

In a personal series the incidence of hyperamylasemia in nonpancreatic true abdominal emergencies was of the order of 30% (Table 4-2).[23] However, the diagnosis of perforated ulcer, appendicitis, cholecystitis, or ruptured aneurysm was fairly obvious after history, physical examination, abdominal flat plate, and routine blood analysis in some 90%. Thus, a true diagnostic dilemma occurred in about 10%, still a relatively high incidence of possible diagnostic error. Few studies have investigated the true diagnostic difficulty, but a laparotomy rate of 3% to 20% to make the diagnosis has been reported.

5. *Mechanism of hyperamylasemia:* In some of these nonpancreatic abdominal emergencies, the mechanism for the raised amylase level is obvious, but in others, it is enigmatic. In perforated ulcer, bowel perforation, and intestinal strangulation, intraluminal enzymes escape into the large absorbing surface of the peritoneal cavity. In acute cholecystitis, the gross predominance of the P-isoamylase suggests that subclinical pancreatitis is the predominating pathogenesis.[11,31] In inflammatory conditions such as Crohn's disease and gastroenteritis, increased vascularity of the bowel promotes amylase absorption. However, the mechanism in ruptured aortic aneurysm, diabetic ketoacidosis, and intestinal obstruction without strangulation is not immediately apparent.

APPROACH TO DIFFERENTIATING PANCREATIC FROM NONPANCREATIC HYPERAMYLASEMIA IN ABDOMINAL EMERGENCIES

The various tests that have been used in an attempt to differentiate these two conditions are as follows:

- Level of amylase
- Use of other enzymes
- Amylase/creatinine ratio
- Urine amylase level
- Isoenzymes of amylase
  - Absolute values
  - Ratio of P to S
  - Level of individual enzymes
- Amylase level in exudates, e.g., ascites, pleural fluid
- Amylase thermolability (no longer in use)

Level of Amylase

Historically, the earliest conventional and most used test to differentiate these two conditions has been the amylase level. The first level considered diagnostic was 1000 U, or 9 to 10 times the upper level of normal for the Somogyi method. In other emergencies (Table 1) the level can be even higher, whereas in acute fulminating pancreatitis, the level may occasionally be lower. However, it remains a useful cutoff level for the diagnosis of acute pancreatitis.

The next level considered diagnostic was an amylase level three times the upper limit. In a recent study, Lim et al. found that only 2% of 24 nonpancreatic hyperamylasemic states exceeded three times the upper reference limit (URL) for their laboratory in patients with intraabdominal disease (21). However (this is a good lesson in careful reviewing), when one looks at the individual data on their scattergraphs, it is clear that nonemergency cases are lumped with potentially fatal disease, and in fact, perforated ulcer had an incidence of 1 in 8 (12%) with small bowel disease and presumably infarction of 1 of 2 (50%) had level greater than three times the upper limit of normal and abdominal injury 3 of 17 (18%). In addition, 5 of 32 patients with grade I or obvious pancreatitis but none with grade II had levels below three times the upper limit of normal. In our own series, these conditions including ruptured aneurysm would give the greatest concern in diagnosis.

Other Enzymes

The literature is replete with comparisons between levels of amylase, lipase, trypsin, and, more recently, esterase, ribonuclease, and phospholipase (S. Bank and P. Banks, unpublished data). Although these are extremely useful measures when the hyperamylasemia is due to nonemergent disease or macroamylasemia or "S" amylasemia, they are of little differentiting value in surgically significant conditions causing hyperamylasemia. Even in pancreatitis, Steinberg has shown the same sensitivity, specificity, and predictive value for amylase, lipase, trypsin, and isoamylases, so that even consideration of these predicted values would not be useful.

Amylase/Creatinine Ratio

When first described by Levitt et al.[19] and extended by Warshaw and Fuller,[35] this test was considered specific for acute pancreatitis. As the ratio has the urine amylase level as the numerator and the creatinine level is not a very large number, it is obvious that the ratio would not be of greater value than the urine amylase level, which unfortunately is elevated in nonpancreatic hyperamylasemia as much as in acute pancreatitis. Conversely, renal involvement in fulminating pancreatitis decreases the amylase excretion, thus lowering the ratio (when the ratio was first described, this happened in the first two patients with pancreatitis for which one of the authors [S. B.] determined the ratio; thus it was dropped from our diagnostic armamentarium); it is also unreliable in diabetic ketoacidosis and in conditions that produce S-hyperamylasemia.[8,18] The ratio is of course useful in macroamylasemia, but here again, a comparison between serum and urine amylase levels should make the diagnosis obvious. For reasons that are not yet apparent (possibly glucagon, prostaglandins, etc.), acute pancreatitis results in increased glomerular filtration and excretion of amylase.

Urine Amylase Level

The urine amylase level when greater than 1000 U/L per hour is clearly useful, but other causes of nonpancreatic hyperamylasemia may also produce these levels. It may have the advantage of remaining elevated longer than serum levels.

Serum and Urine Isoamylase Estimations

Absolute Values

Studies carried out in our department on serum P-amylase levels in acute abdominal emergencies were in agreement with Steinberg et al. in that isoamylase levels had the same predictive value as total amylase levels in acute pancreatitis. Lin et al. found that P-amylase levels were virtually the same as total amylase levels in the differentiation of acute pancreatitis from other diseases with acute abdomen. Spot urine amylase levels of greater than 750 U/L for total amylase and 410 U/L for P-amylase were suggestive of acute pancreatitis in our studies.[6,25]

Ratio of P- to S-amylase

In 27 patients with acute pancreatitis, we found that the P-amylase accounted for at least 75% of the total amylase in all cases, not infrequently being 100% of the total amylase. This ratio of P to S exceeded 75% in 56% of patients with nonpancreatic hyperamylasemia with acute abdomen and was less than 75% in 44% (Table 4-3). This latter 44% could be confidently designated nonpancreatic surgical emergencies and treated accordingly. However, the value over 75% was

TABLE 4-3. ISOAMYLASE VALUES IN PATIENTS WITH HYPERAMYLASEMIA AND/OR HYPERAMYLASURIA

Diagnosis	Patients with Hyperamylasemia and/or Hyperamylasuria	P-Isoamylase < 0.75
Acute biliary disease	10	1 (10%)
Intestinal obstruction	8	3 (38%)
Acute appendicitis	8	6 (75%)
Acute diverticulitis	4	3 (75%)
Perforated peptic ulcer	5	2 (40%)
Acute pancreatitis	5	0 (0%)
Acute gastroenteritis	1	1 (100%)
Ruptured abdominal aortic aneurysm	3	1 (33%)
Tuboovarian disease	3	2 (66%)
Miscellaneous	3	3 (100%)
Total	50	22 (44%)

obviously nondiagnostic and compatible with pancreatitis or a nonpancreatic cause.

Amylase in Effusions and Exudates

The finding of high amylase values in ascitic or pleural effusions is, of course, very helpful in the diagnosis of pancreatitis. However, this is a reflection of serum amylase levels and is elevated in other conditions including macroamylasemia, and "S" amylasemia, particularly ovarian disease.[28]

Summary

Although consideration of the amylase level alone will diagnose and distinguish the vast majority of cases, the addition, if available, of tests for other enzymes, isoamylases, and the P/S ratio will further help in differential diagnosis between pancreatitis and nonpancreatic disease in the individual patient. However, the diagnosis may still be uncertain based on history, biochemical tests, and even fluid aspiration. What approach should one adopt if there is any question about the differential diagnosis? An emergency CT scan will certainly be helpful, although about 20% of patients with acute pancreatitis have a normal CT scan. However, a normal scan is highly unlikely in the patient with fulminating disease in danger of imminent death. If any doubt still exists, laparotomy should be undertaken. Previous studies regarding the possible deleterious effects of laparotomy on mortality are probably invalid, as the patients who died were not stratified into risk factors as assessed by Ranson's early objective signs or Bank's clinical criteria. It is likely that the patients who died after surgery would probably have died with medical treatment.

HYPERAMYLASEMIA IN PATIENTS WITH ABDOMINAL PAIN AND RENAL DISEASE

Because of inability to filter or reabsorb amylase, hyperamylasemia due to acute or chronic renal disease presents one of the most difficult diagnostic problems in patients with acute abdominal conditions.[5,27] All the biochemical tests mentioned may be fallacious, and one usually has to resort to ancillary tests such as sonography, CT scanning (which may be contraindicated because of dye problems), and even MRI to exclude acute pancreatitis. Peritoneal aspiration or laparotomy may become diagnostically expedient. Hyperamylasemia in renal disease rarely exceeds three times the upper limit of normal, and levels of this magnitude were observed in only 3 of 35 patients by Royse et al.[27] However, we have certainly seen patients with levels higher than 1000 U/L. A high serum and low urine amylase level is specific for renal disease in the absence of macroamylasemia. The amylase/creatinine ratio is meaningless. An S-amylase level greater than the P-amylase level in the urine occurred in 18 of 20 patients with renal failure investigated by us. This occurs only in renal disease and severe chronic pancreatitis, as in normal controls and hyperamylasemia with other causes, P-amylase levels always exceed those of S-amylase in the urine.[1,2] Despite these tests, the combination of hyperamylasemia with renal failure and abdominal pain can thus be an insuperable diagnostic problem.

HYPERAMYLASEMIA IN PATIENTS WITH NONEMERGENT ABDOMINAL PAIN

In these patients, the abdominal disease may be subacute or chronic, thus permitting a more leisurely investigation of the elevated amylase level.

Nonemergent Abdominal Disease With or Without Renal Disease

Hyperamylasemia may be found in patients with chronic peptic ulcer, Crohn's disease, and intestinal adhesions and presents a problem in interpretation. Standard clinical investigational procedures usually lead to clarification of the dilemma.

Tumor-associated Amylase

Four neoplastic conditions that are frequently associated with abdominal pain may be associated with very high amylase levels, and confusion with pancreatitis is not uncommon. These are pancreatic carcinoma, carcinoma of the ovary (particularly with ascites), lymphoma, and hematologic malignancy. Carcinoma of the ovary and lymphoma, in particular, may be associated with amylase values in the thousands, and in the high thousands in effusions. The most relevant test in all these conditions is isoamylase determination, the predominance of S-amylase being the diagnostic feature. On chromatography, abnormal and anion-migrating bands of amylase that consist of either tumor-associated amylase or deaminated S-amylase in serum and especially in effusions are pathognomonic of tumor-associated amylase.[17] Of the other tests, urine amylase levels and creatinine amylase ratio are unhelpful as S-amylase is excreted in the urine. Clearly, elevations of levels of the enzymes lipase, trypsin, esterase, and so forth, would mitigate against amylase emanating from nonpancreatic sources. However, we have found high trypsin values in some carcinomas, and levels of the other enzymes have not really been tested in sufficient patients. Occasionally the predominant amylase is of the P type in hematologic malignancies and, of course, in pancreatic carcinoma. The finding of significant S-amylase in an asymptomatic patient should alert one to the possibility of a hidden malignancy.[1]

Pancreatitis-producing Medications in Patients with Abdominal Pain

6MP or azathioprine (Imuran) in patients with Crohn's disease, steroids in patients with collagen diseases, diuretics in patients with renal disease or cirrhosis, sulfasalazine (Azulfadine) in inflammatory bowel disease, and tetracycline in gastroenteritis are but some of the drugs that could cause pancreatitis in patients with abdominal diseases that produce pain and in which hyperamylasemia may occur from the disease itself. If the predominant amylase is S-type, pancreatitis can be excluded. In many cases the diagnosis will depend on clinical progress of the disease, and even then the diagnosis of pancreatitis may have to be speculative.

Abdominal Pain in Pregnancy

The differentiation of physiologic hyperamylasemia of pregnancy from pregnancy with abdominal pain is almost entirely dependent on isoenzyme fractionation in S-hyperamylasemia. This is particularly important with regard to the high frequency of gallstones in pregnancy and the rare patient with pregnancy-associated pancreatitis.[14]

Protein- and Immunocomplex-bound Hyperamylasemia—Macroamylasemia

Protein-bound macroamylasemia occurs in about 2% of the population in whom no disease is found and often results in an erroneous diagnosis of pancreatitis in patients with nonpancreatic abdominal pain.[12] This year alone one of the authors (S. B.) has seen two patients who have had endoscopic retrograde cholangiopancreatography (ERCP) for macroamylasemia but who were suffering from irritable bowel syndrome. This is even more surprising when the relative ease of diagnosis is considered, namely, normal urine amylase levels and amylase/creatinine ratio in the presence of hyperamylasemia. To confirm the diagnosis, gel filtration, chromatography, and thermolability techniques are required.[10]

Circulating amylase may also become attached to isolated serum proteins; for example, to IgA in high-IgA states such as celiac disease, immunoproliferative small intestinal disease, and abdominal lymphoma; to IgG in chronic inflammatory states and cirrhosis; and to immune complexes in AIDS and collagen diseases. Again, pancreatitis is frequently the first diagnosis in these conditions when abdominal pain and hyperamylasemia are the presenting features. The diagnosis is made on an awareness of these states, low urine amylase levels, and the presence of macroamylase on serum chromatography and gel filtration.

CONCLUSIONS

Hyperamylasemia in patients with abdominal pain is common to many diseases, and it may require great skill and ingenuity to determine the cause. In many diseases, particularly those in which the main amylase produced is of the S type or a physiologic or pathologic protein-bound macroamylase, the decision is nonurgent and time is available to determine the cause of the hyperamylasemia. This usually requires urine amylase determinations, chromatography, and gel filtration techniques to establish the nature of the amylase.

In those conditions in which time is of the essence to distinguish pancreatitis from a surgically correctable intraabdominal emergency, the level of hyperamylasemia, other enzyme estimations, isoenzyme levels, and the ratio of P- to S-amylase result in a high rate of diagnostic accuracy. However, it is axiomatic that if any doubt about the diagnosis exists, an emergency contrast CT examination may be diagnostic, and if not, laparotomy should be carried out without delay.

REFERENCES

1. Amman RW, Berk E, Fridhandler L, et al. Hyperamylasemia with carcinoma of the lung. Ann Intern Med 78:521–525, 1973.
2. Bank S. Acute and chronic pancreatitis. In: Dent TL, ed. Pancreatic Disease. New York, Grune & Stratton, 1981, pp 167–188.
3. Bank S. Alcoholic and non-alcoholic chronic pancreatitis—Differences in natural history? Pancreas 2:365–367, 1987.
4. Bank S. Chronic pancreatitis: Clinical features and medical management. Am J Gastroenterol 81:153–167, 1986.
5. Bank S, Pandya H, Anfang C, Lendvai S, Urivetsky M: The relationship between P (pancreatic) and S (salivary) amylase in controls, chronic pancreatitis and renal failure. Gastroenterology 82:1013(A), 1982.
6. Bank S, Pandya H, Lendvai S. Single random urine specimen in the diagnosis of pancreatic disease using isoamylases. Gastroenterology 78:136(A), 1980.

7. Belfiore F, Napoli E. Interpretation of hyperamylasemia in diabetic coma. Clin Chem 19:387–389, 1973.
8. Belfiore F, Vecchio LL, Napoli E. Serum enzymes in diabetes mellitus. Clin Chem 19:447–452, 1973.
9. Burnett W, Ness TD. Serum amylase and acute abdominal disease. Br Med J 2:770, 1955.
10. Ellis CJ, Meier PB, Levitt MD. Temperature dependence of macroamylase binding. Pancreas 2:48–52, 1987.
11. Fung WP, Murray RN, Massarei JRL, et al. P3 amylase isoenzyme with cholelithiasis. Am J Gastroenterol 76:52–55, 1981.
12. Helfat A, Berk JE, Fridhandler L. Prevalence of macroamylasemia, further study. Am J Gastroenterol 62:54–58, 1974.
13. Imrie CW, Whyte AS, Frew EMS. A pattern of serum amylase concentration in the initial 24 hours after perforation of duodenal ulcers. JR Coll Surg Edinb 19:370–373, 1974.
14. Jouppila P, Mokka R, Larmi TK. Acute pancreatitis in pregnancy. Surg Gynecol Obstet 138:879–882, 1966.
15. Kelly ML. Elevated serum amylase level associated with ruptured ectopic pregnancy. JAMA 164–406, 1957.
16. Knight AH, Williams DN, Ellis G, Goldberg DM. Significance of hyperamylasemia and abdominal pain in diabetic ketoacidosis. Br J Surg 3:128–131, 1973.
17. Kosches DS, Sosnowik D, Ledvai S, Bank S. Unusual anodic migrating isoamylase differentiates malignant from non-malignant ascites. J Clin Gastroenterol 11:43–46, 1989.
18. Levitt MD, Johnson SG. Is the Cam/Ccr ratio of value for the diagnosis of pancreatitis? Gastroenterology 75:118–119, 1978.
19. Levitt MD, Rapoport M, Cooperband SR. The renal clearance of amylase in renal insufficiency, acute pancreatitis, and macroamylasemia. Ann Intern Med 71:919–925, 1969.
20. Lewison EF. The clinical value of the serum amylase test. Surg Gynecol Obstet 72:202, 1941.
21. Lin XZ, Wang SS, Tsai YT, et al. Serum amylase, isoamylase, and lipase in the acute abdomen. J Clin Gastroenterol 11:47–52, 1989.
22. Mahaffey JH, Brockman L, Jordan GL, Howard JH. A study of the serum amylase concentration in patients with acute presentation of gastrointestinal ulcers. Surg Genecol Obstet 101:129–132, 1955.
23. Pace BW, Bank S, Wise L, Burson LC, Borrero E. Amylase isoenzymes in the acute abdomen: An adjunct in those patients with elevated total amylase. Am J Gastroenterol 80:898–901, 1985.
24. Paloyan D, Simonowitz D. Diagnostic considerations in acute alcoholic and gallstone pancreatitis. Am J Surg 132:329–331, 1976.
25. Pandya H, Bank S, Lendvai S, Kranz V. Isoamylase ratios in urine—its value in acute pancreatic disease. Annual convention and course in post-graduate gastroenterology of the American College of Gastroenterology, October 1980. Am J Gastroenterol 74:88, 1980.
26. Rogers FA. Elevated serum amylase: A review and an analysis of findings in 1000 cases of perforated peptic ulcer. Ann Surg 153:228–260, 1961.
27. Royse VL, Jensen DM, Corwin HL: Pancreatic enzymes in chronic renal failure. Arch Intern Med 147:537–539, 1987.
28. Skude G, Mardh PA, Westrom L. Amylase of the genital tract, I: Isoamylases of genital tract tissue homogenates and peritoneal fluid. Am J Obstet Gynecol 126:652–656, 1976.
29. Steinberg WM, Goldstein SS, Davis ND, Shamma'a J, Anderson K. Diagnostic assays in acute pancreatitis—A study of sensitivity and specificity. Ann Intern Med 102:576–580, 1985.
30. Sudo K, Kanno T. Properties of the amylase produced in carcinoma of the lung. Clin Chem Acta 73:L1–12, 1976.

31. Swensson EE, King ME, Malekpour A. A serum amylase isoenzyme alterations in acute abdominal conditions. Ann Emerg Med 14:421–423, 1985.
32. Swensson EE, Maull KI. Clinical significance of elevated serum and urine amylase levels in patients with appendicitis. Am J Surg 142:667, 1981.
33. Thomson HJ. Clinical significance of moderate elevation of serum amylase. J R Coll Surg Edinb 29:303–306, 1984.
34. Warshaw AL, Imbembo AL, Civetta JM, Diaggett WM. Surgical intervention in acute necrotizing pancreatitis. Am J Surg 127:484–491, 1974.
35. Warshaw AL, Fuller AF. Specificity of increased renal clearance of amylase in the diagnosis of acute pancreatitis. N Engl J Med 292:325–329, 1975.

CHAPTER

5

THE ROLE OF RADIOLOGY IN THE DIAGNOSIS AND FOLLOW-UP OF ACUTE PANCREATITIS

Jack Farman and Richard M. Schaffer

EDITORIAL COMMENT

The authors have intentionally started their chapter with some of the more forgotten aspects of radiology in acute pancreatitis, namely those in common use before the availability of ultrasound and CT scanning. It should not be forgotten that flat plate, gastrointestinal series, barium enema, and intravenous pyelogram may all be important ancillary investigations in problematic acute pancreatitis, investigations that are relatively rarely performed today. At the other end of the spectrum, although ERCP is rarely used in acute pancreatitis in the United States (as evidenced by its omission from discussion in this chapter), it should be stated that certain centers in Europe consider it a relatively safe and important investigation in delineating areas of severe necrosis or duct disruption, which may require therapy. The authors state that ultrasound may be normal in 20% and CT in 30% of patients with an acute attack. These are really disappointing numbers and should perhaps be correlated with (1) whether the pancreatitis is acute or chronic according to the Marseilles classification and (2) the relationship of the attack to severity as judged by either Ranson's or Bank's criteria. One would then hope that ultrasound with or without CT may be diagnostic in close to 100% of severe, acute cases, particularly in those patients with abdominal pain and hyperamylasemia in whom the differential diagnosis is not immediately apparent on clinical examination. One would hope that ultrasound and CT carried out immediately might avoid the necessity for laparotomy to make an unquestionable diagnosis. Finally, the authors stress the value of ultrasound and CT in differentiating blood from fluid collections and both of these from pseudocysts. Fluid collections tend to reabsorb spontaneously while cysts have somewhere in the region of a fifty-fifty chance of requiring surgical intervention.

CONTROVERSY

There have been such rapid advances in the role of the radiologist in the diagnosis of an attack of acute pancreatitis and in monitoring its course that a review is timely. Such newer techniques as contrast-enhanced CT and percutaneous drainage of abscesses have revolutionized diagnosis and treatment. However, the relative values of ultrasound versus CT scanning remain somewhat controversial particularly in relation to cost, mobility of the patient, screening versus definitive anatomic diagnosis, and repeated follow-up studies. Is there a place for the more conventional studies, that is, abdominal flat plate, barium, or water soluble contrast studies, intravenous pyelography, or angiography?

The approaches to confirming the diagnosis of acute pancreatitis are as varied as the modalities presently available for investigating the pancreas itself. Plain x-ray, sonography, computerized axial tomography (CT), and barium studies of both the upper and lower gastrointestinal tract as well as endoscopic retrograde cholangiopancreatography (ERCP) can provide significant information for the investigator. Magnetic resonance does offer some helpful information, though, as yet, it remains limited and insufficient for diagnostic purposes.

PLAIN FILM FINDINGS

Valuable information regarding the presence of pancreatitis may be obtained from routine chest and abdominal radiographs. Information so gleaned tends to be ignored or neglected as investigators concentrate on more sophisticated and elaborate investigations.

Helpful plain film findings include pancreatic calcification, gallstones, focal areas of small bowel dilatation, ascites, and the presence of upper abdominal masses. Pancreatic calcification is optimally demonstrated by obliquing the patient 15 degrees in either direction from either the supine or the prone position. Small foci of calcification in the head and body are best visualized off the lumbar spine and not obscured by bone density.

Additional information includes the presence of fat lucencies that develop as a result of necrosis of fat tissue in the peritoneal cavity and retroperitoneum. The development of stippled lucencies grouped together outside the confines of the normal colon or small bowel indicates the development of a pancreatic abscess.

The "airless" abdomen is a common finding in severe pancreatitis. Small bowel loops, usually filled with small amounts of air, are not visualized as air is displaced and dilated intestinal loops fill with fluid. The differential diagnosis of these findings includes high small bowel obstruction and infarction.

Dilatation of the colon may occur in focal form or more dramatically as a "cutoff" in the column of distended large bowel at the splenic flexure.[6] This finding is the result of accumulation of pancreatic exudate in the left upper quadrant leading to edema and spasm surrounding the colon and at that site (Fig. 5-1).[16] The radiographic appearance mimics colonic obstruction by an annular carcinoma.

A significant finding is the presence of a soft tissue mass that impresses the stomach and displaces it from the colon because of pancreatic phlegmon; this can be confirmed by sonography or CT scanning.[14,15] Frequently the colon is narrowed and shows a scalloped appearance when outlined by air.

Information obtained from the chest radiograph includes pleural effusion, more common on the left side than on the right. Though usually moderate in

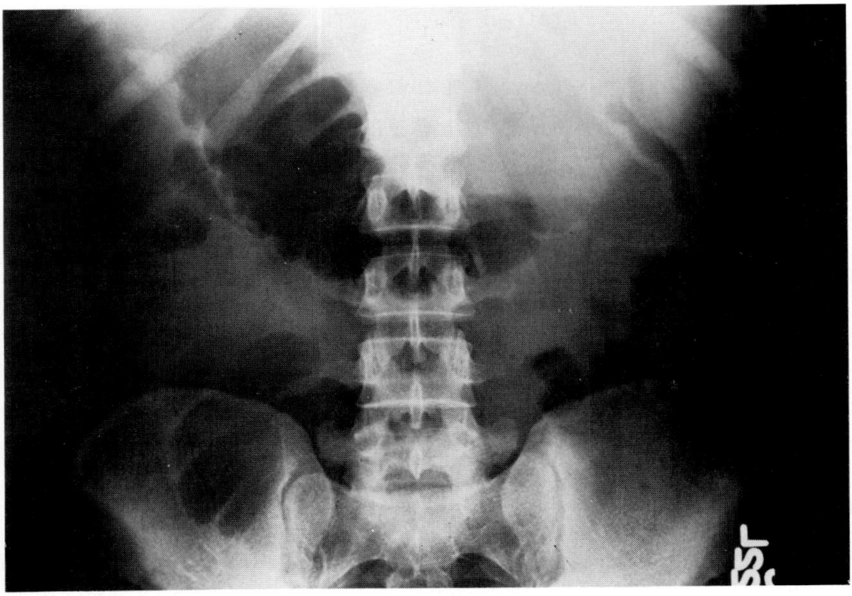

A

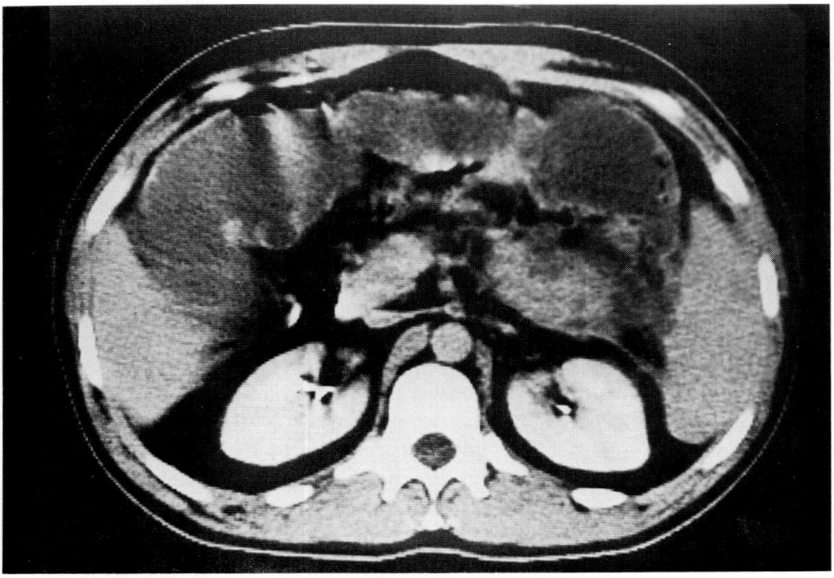

B

Figure 5-1. (A) Plain film of the abdomen. "Cutoff" of the air column in the transverse colon in the region of the splenic flexure secondary to acute pancreatitis. (B) CT scan. Markedly dilated colon extending to the splenic flexure. The adjacent tail of the pancreas is swollen and edematous. Thickening of Gerota's fascia is seen on the left side.

degree, these effusions may be extensive and obscure much of the hemithorax. In addition, the cardiac outline may increase in size and shape as a result of the development of a pericardial effusion from contiguous pancreatitis. With improvement and resolution, the effusions resorb, and the lungs, as well as the cardiac contour, return to normal.

Infradiaphragmatic fluid may track into the chest, usually through the esophageal or aortic hiatus. The former route is commoner. A posteriorly situated patent foramen of Bochdalek is another portal of entry of exudate into the chest. Rarest of all, the diaphragm undergoes necrosis, leading to communication between the pleural space and peritoneal cavity with fluid tracking freely between the two regions.

Pseudocysts that develop in the chest appear as masses or collections that may compress and displace the esophagus and cause dysphagia.[22] The exudate has been known to track through the loose connective tissue of the mediastinum as far proximally as the cervical region and present as a swelling in the supraclavicular fossa.[22] Large exudative collections may be responsible for dysphagia when there is a sizable accumulation in the esophagogastric region. The barium swallow in these patients reveals narrowing of the distal esophagus as well as a mass effect on the fundus and edema of gastric mucosa in the adjacent area. These findings can be confirmed on CT scanning as well.

THE UPPER GI EXAMINATION

The upper gastrointestinal (UGI) series has presently assumed second place to the CT scan; however, the latter examination does not provide complete information regarding the nature of anatomic changes, masses, subtle findings of small or large bowel obstruction, or the development of ischemic change. Barium studies provide better documentation of detailed effects on the stomach, duodenum, and small bowel and the inflammatory nature of the changes produced (Figs. 5-2 to 5-5).

A single-contrast barium study is the preferred examination for these patients. The presence of excess fasting secretions and food residue together with mucosal edema of the stomach, duodenum, and proximal small bowel prevent satisfactory coating by the denser barium suspensions required in the double-contrast examination. In addition, patients are frequently on intravenous supportive therapy and are too ill to maneuver and rotate easily to ensure an optimal examination.

While water-soluble contrast media required in CT scanning does outline and demonstrate masses well, the investigator should be aware of the limitations of these studies in providing details of ulceration, spasm, and edema.

Duodenal deformities are numerous and varied, ranging from edema and deformity of the duodenal bulb to widening of the duodenal sweep with dilatation and sluggish peristalsis. Duodenal bulb deformities may be misinterpreted as peptic ulceration, especially when pancreatitis is associated with UGI bleeding. Pancreatic exudates may collect along the medial aspect of the duodenal sweep, extend into the retroperitoneum, and form masses that can compress the duode-

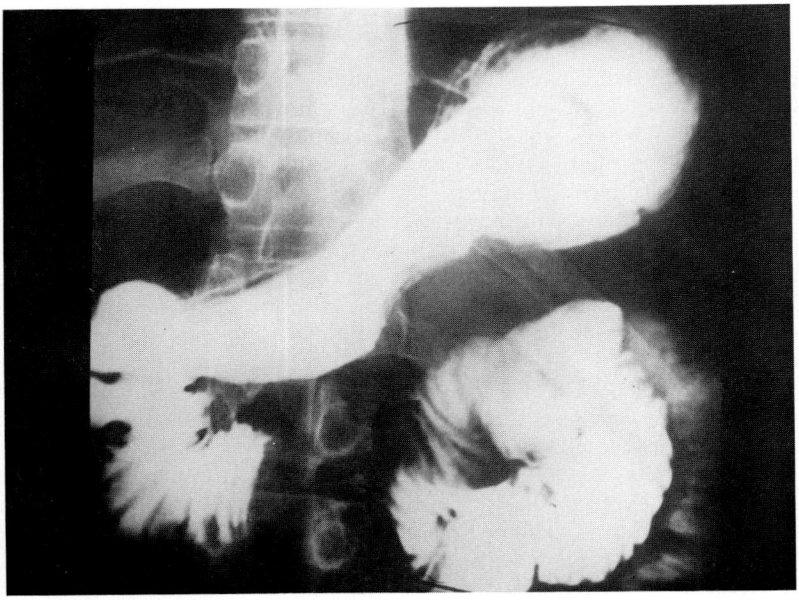

A

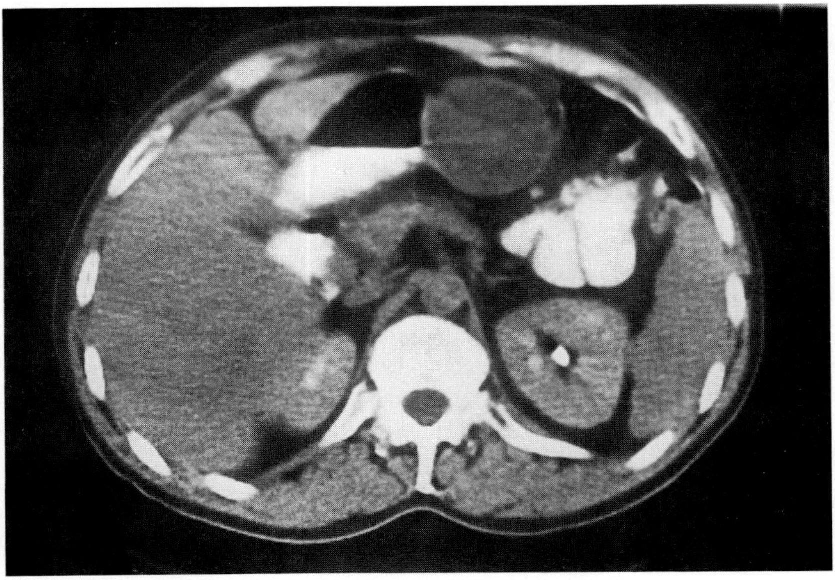

B

Figure 5-2. (A) Upper GI series. The crescentic mass effect on the greater curve of the stomach is due to pressure from a pancreatic pseudocyst. (B) CT scan. Circumscribed and well-defined pancreatic pseudocyst adjacent to the stomach and separate from the atrophic pancreas. (Courtesy of E. Balthazar, M.D., New York University Medical Center.)

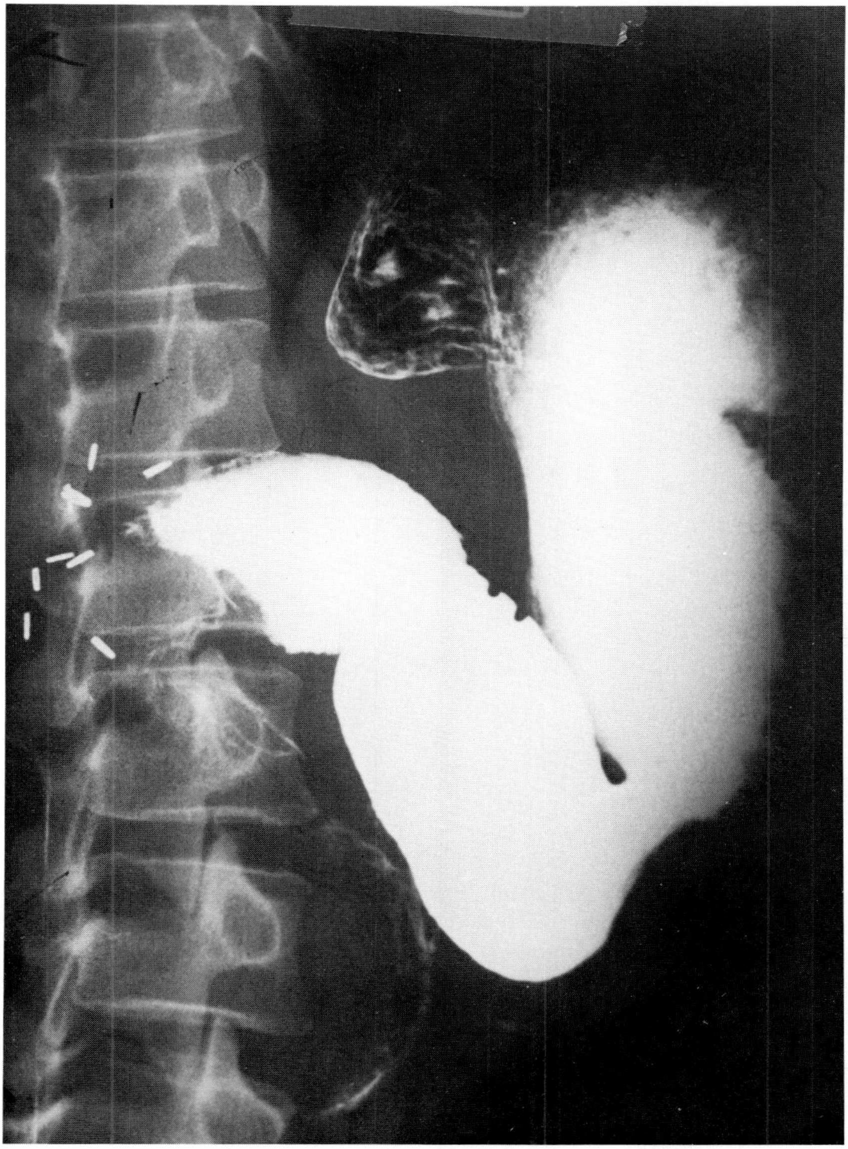

Figure 5-3. Upper GI series. A large mass involving the descending duodenum, compressing and obstructing both the stomach and the duodenum.

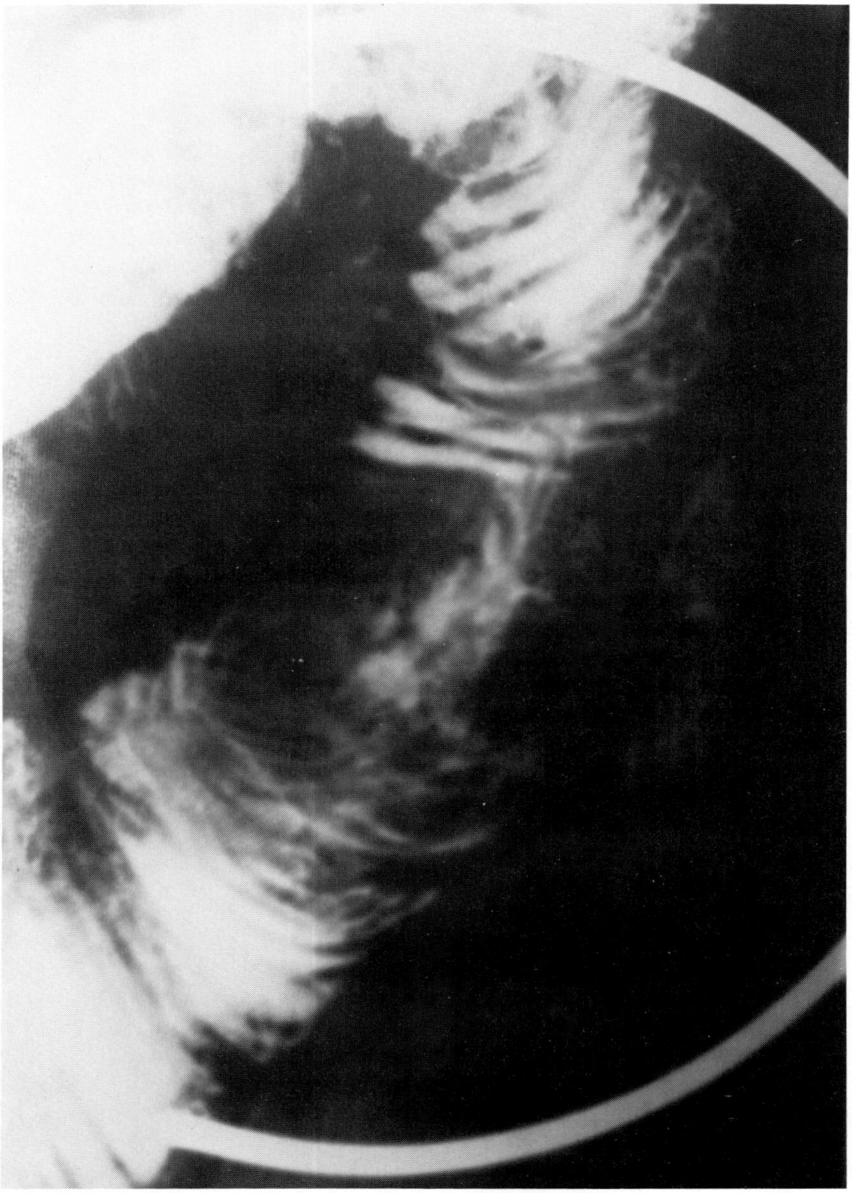

Figure 5-4. Barium study. Localized view of a jejunal stricture just beyond the duodenojejunal junction. Note the well-defined margins and "shoulders" with intact mucosa. The appearances, the result of pancreatitis confirmed at laparotomy, resolved with conservative treatment.

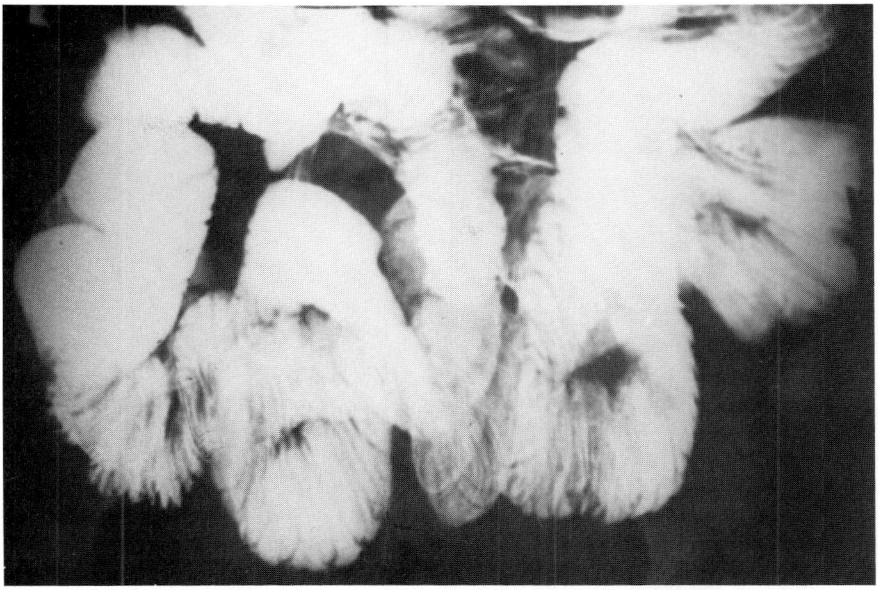

Figure 5-5. Small bowel follow-through. Dilated, edematous small bowel loops displaced superiorly by a large pelvic pseudocyst.

num from the posterior and lateral aspects of the second and third parts especially. Significant UGI obstruction may be shown on barium series (Fig. 5-3).

The small bowel may show involvement of jejunal or ileal loops as pancreatic exudate extends from the retroperitoneum and accumulates in the small bowel mesentery.[16] When a localized accumulation of exudate encircles a segment of the small bowel, it can produce dramatic narrowing, especially when associated with peritonitis, omental adhesions, and spasm (Fig. 5-4).

Careful fluoroscopic evaluation of the strictures usually confirms an intact mucosa and a distensible lumen indicating the inflammatory nature of the process (Fig. 5-4). Exudates may accumulate distally in the right iliac fossa and form masses large enough to be palpable. Compression and displacement of the terminal ileum, cecum, and ascending colon can be confirmed by barium studies.[6]

Spontaneous evacuation of a pseudocyst into the stomach,[21] duodenum, or small bowel is not uncommon and easily identified on barium study. Sudden diminution of an abdominal swelling together with an improvement in symptoms is often associated with the passage of a blood-tinged, diarrheic stool. Occasionally a pseudocyst may evacuate simultaneously into two adjacent viscera, such as duodenum and colon.[19]

Rare complications of acute pancreatitis include emphysematous gastritis as well as gastric abscess formation. The development of a pseudocyst anterior to the stomach, which may be large enough to displace it posteriorly, is uncommon

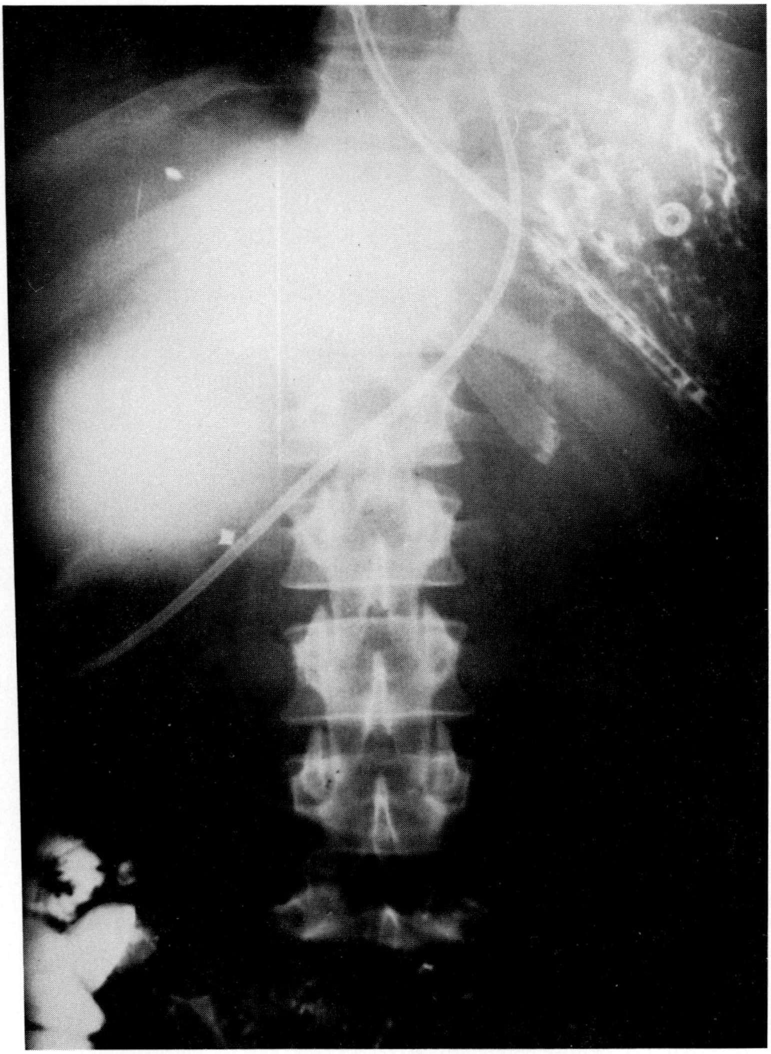

Figure 5-6. (A) Anteroposterior and (B) lateral radiographs of a barium-outlined stomach. Water-soluble contrast medium has been injected into an enormous anteriorly placed pseudocyst. On the lateral view this displaces the stomach posteriorly. Drainage was achieved percutaneously. (Courtesy of Dr. R. Surapaneni, Brooklyn VA Hospital, New York.) (*Figure continues.*)

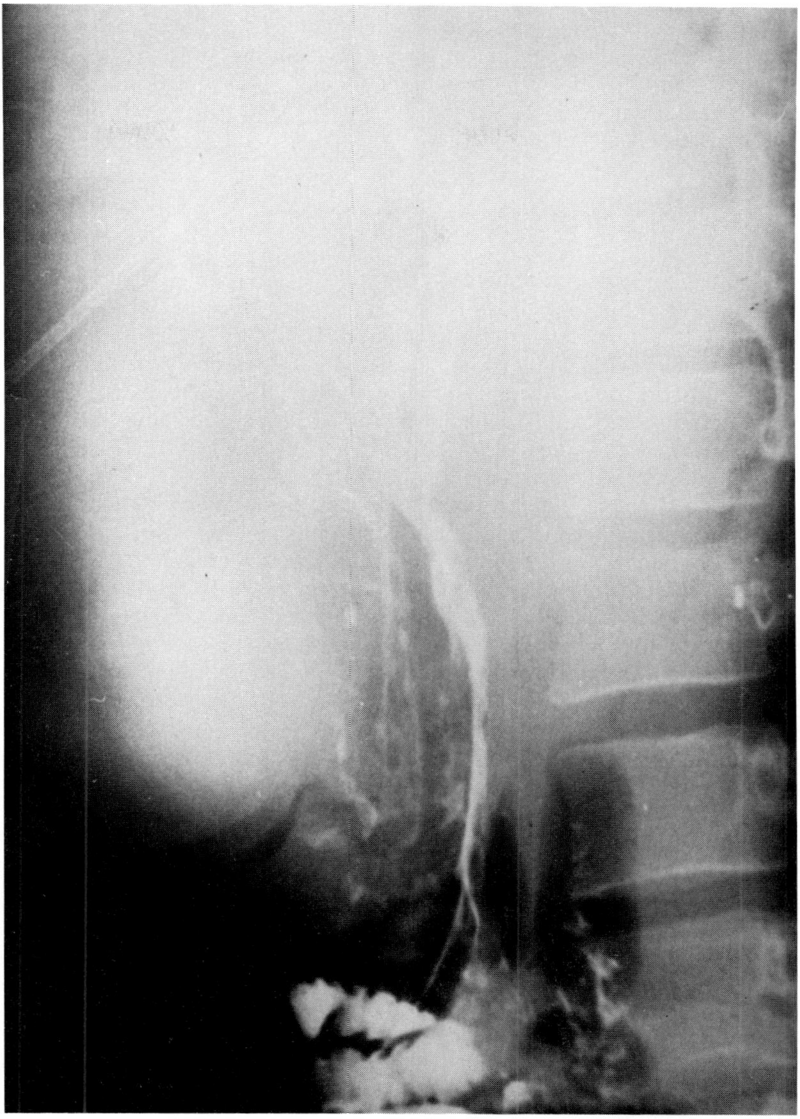

B

Figure 5-6. *(continued)*

and rarely recognized as a cause for displacement. If exudate escapes from the retroperitoneum and lesser sac by eroding through peritoneal coverings, a pseudocyst can form in the peritoneal cavity and, if large enough, produce the posterior displacement of the stomach described above (Fig. 5-6). In these patients a CT scan is all-revealing.

COLONIC CHANGES IN PANCREATITIS

Extension of pancreatic exudate into the transverse colon produces edematous changes as the colon is bathed in the irritating exudate released as a result of phlegmonous inflammation. Large collections in a developing pseudocyst may abut on the colon, especially along its superior aspect where it produces a crescentic mass impression and edema of the colonic wall. Erosive changes produced through pressure and necrosis of the bowel wall by a pseudocyst can result in spontaneous evacuation of the pseudocyst into the colon. This carries with it significant mortality and morbidity as well as the dangers of severe hemorrhage.

Accumulations in the paracolic gutters result in spasm and edema of the adjacent colon. The splenic flexure is especially likely to be involved, the medial aspect more so than the lateral wall.[6,16] Localized circumferential narrowing and edema may resemble tumor involvement. These areas need to be carefully evaluated at fluoroscopy for evidence of change and distensibility. Frequently surgeons exploring the abdomen in this phase of the disease may be uncertain whether they are dealing with a benign process or malignancy. Significant accumulation of exudate in the retroperitoneum may displace the ureter in the loin and collect in the pelvis. The sigmoid is involved too by accumulation of exudate via the mesocolon as well as by adjacent mass. Rectal displacement by pelvic extension of a pseudocyst (Fig. 5-7) has been recorded.[7]

Mesenteric vascular occlusion, either arterial or venous; arterial encasement; and pressure effects on the splenic and mesenteric veins are common. Splenic vein thrombosis, which may be confirmed by ultrasonography (US), is a complication leading to the development of varices and collateral venous flow. Portal and mesenteric venous thrombosis may occur as well. Acute vascular occlusions may induce significant ischemic changes including bowel necrosis, perforation, and peritonitis.[6]

SPLENIC INVOLVEMENT IN ACUTE PANCREATITIS

Pseudocysts that develop in the body and tail of the pancreas can extend through the splenic hilum and enlarge within the spleen (Fig. 5-8).[24] Abscess formation and secondary hemorrhage are common. Not all intrasplenic pseudocysts, however, demonstrate a recognizable connection with the pancreas.

Exudates may enter the splenic hilum along the course of the splenic vessels and lymphatics and a pseudocyst form and develop in this manner. The lateral aspect of the spleen is a common site for pancreatic exudate to accumulate too (Fig. 5-14C).

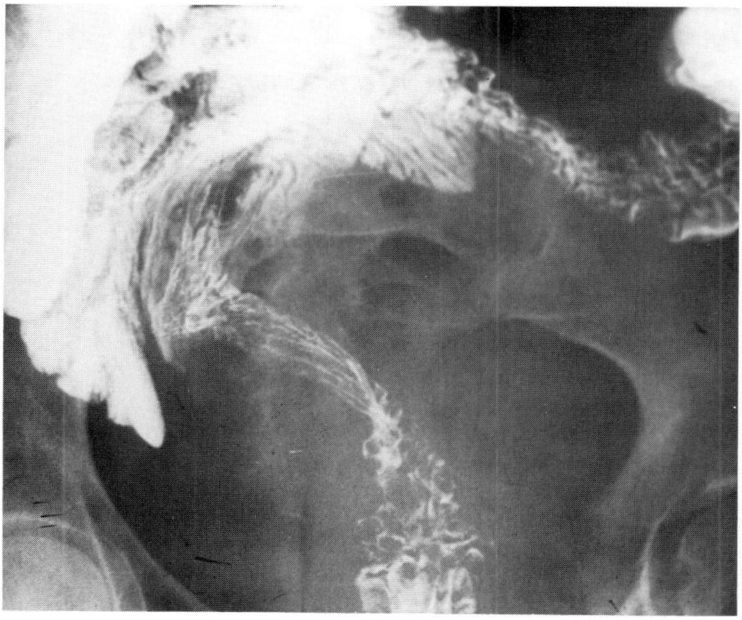

A

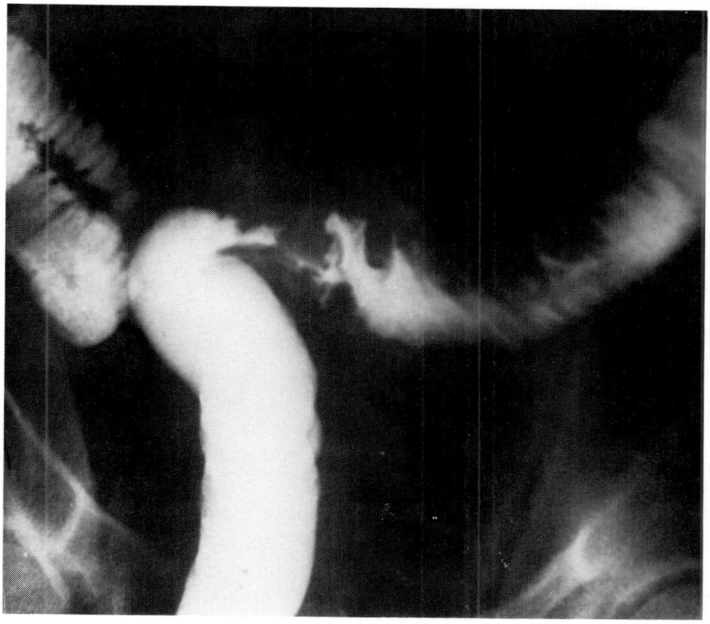

B

Figure 5-7. (A) Barium enema. Large pseudocyst in the pelvis compressing and "splinting" the rectum and elevating the sigmoid out of the pelvis. (B) Barium enema. Edema and pressure changes on the sigmoid colon are evident. The rectum is displaced to the right. (From Farman et al.[7] with permission.)

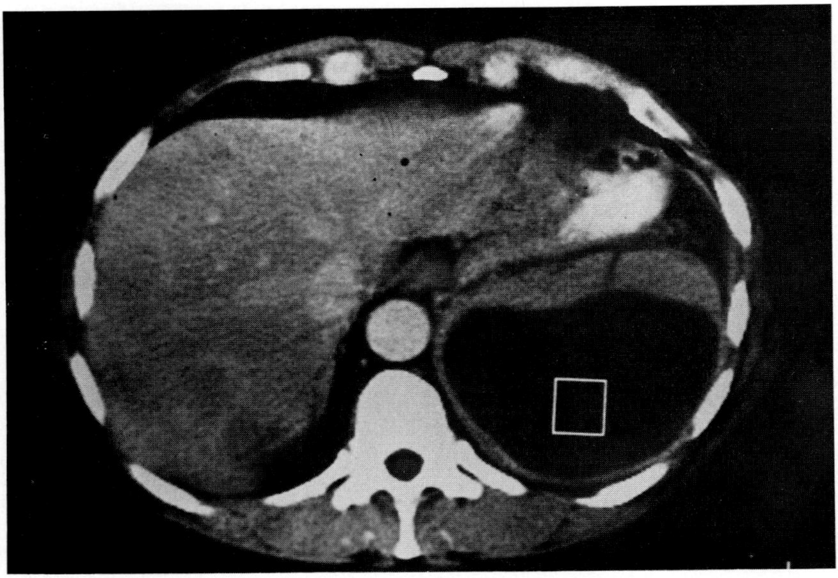

Figure 5-8. CT scan of the liver and spleen. A large intrasplenic pseudocyst is seen compressing splenic tissue.

The development of a splenic artery pseudoaneurysm leading to severe, life-threatening hemorrhage is a common complication requiring immediate diagnostic confirmation by angiography and ligation of the involved artery.[18]

The interventional radiologist plays an important role in the percutaneous drainage of collections, pseudocysts, and abscesses including those that involve the spleen.[3,10,11,17,23]

ERCP AND CHOLANGIOGRAPHY

The investigation of acute pancreatitis by ERCP is usually unrevealing in the early attacks. It requires several episodes of pancreatitis to produce ductal changes of stricture, deformity, and dilatation. Just how frequent and how severe the attacks have to be for changes to occur is unknown.

Injections of iodinated contrast medium into the pancreatic duct is not without risk; it can induce pancreatitis that may be severe and on occasion fatal.[4]

A pseudocyst may be shown by ERCP to communicate with adjacent viscera including the stomach, duodenum, and liver (Fig. 5-9).[5,19,21] An obstructing gallstone or pancreatic calculus may be identified as the cause of pancreatitis. A cutoff in the pancreatic duct by a carcinoma may, in a small percentage of cases, lead to pancreatitis as the presenting symptom. Difficulty may arise in differenti-

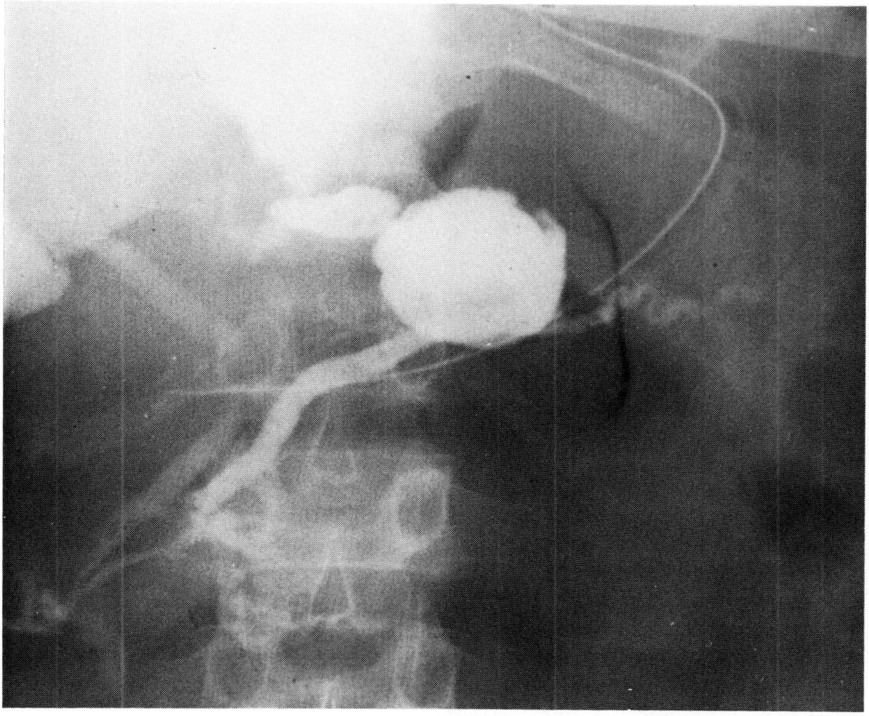

Figure 5-9. ERCP. The pancreatic duct has been filled, and contrast medium has entered a pseudocyst that connects with a more proximal collection extending superiorly into the mediastinum.

ating carcinomatous obstruction from that due to inflammatory disease, as the radiologic appearances can be identical (see chapter 10).

ERCP is most useful in identifying the site of ductal rupture in patients with pancreatic ascites and provides valuable information for surgical intervention (Fig. 5-10). Occasionally, during an acute attack or in the presence of jaundice, ERCP or transhepatic cholangiography (THC) may be necessary for evaluating the biliary tree (Fig. 5-11).

GENITOURINARY COMPLICATIONS

The body and tail of the pancreas are in anatomic approximation with the kidney hilum and upper pole of the kidney on the left side. On the right side, the head of the pancreas lies within the C loop of the duodenum and is an anterior relation of the medial aspect of the kidney, as well as its hilum and pelvis. It is possible,

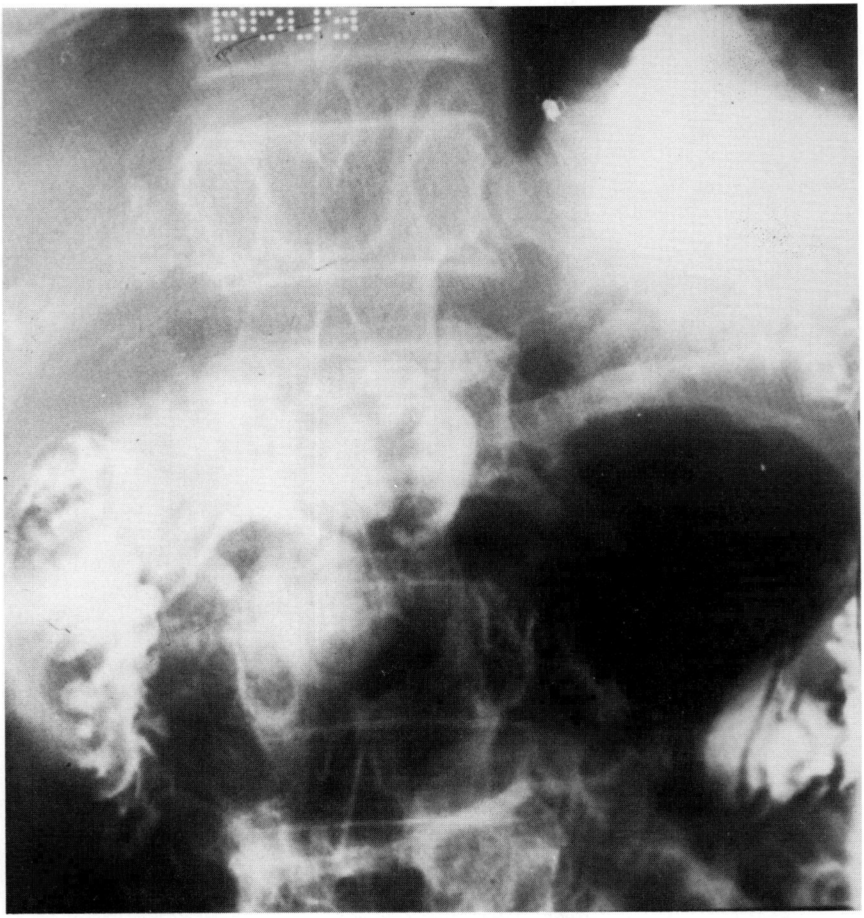

Figure 5-10. ERCP in pancreatic ascites. Contrast medium has been injected to outline a short segment of the pancreatic duct within the head. The duodenum, stomach, and proximal small bowel have been outlined. There has been free spill of contrast medium into the peritoneal cavity.

therefore, that pancreatic exudate and pseudocysts may compress and flatten either kidney, but they are more likely to do so on the left side.

Spasm of the vessels in the renal hilum may result in differential excretion (Fig. 5-16). A large exudate or collection in the perirenal tissues can tilt the axis of the kidneys as well as produce effects by compression. These changes are best identified by intravenous pyelography IVP, CT scanning, and US. Pseudocysts involving the renal parenchyma are rare, produce filling defects, renal enlargement, and excretory changes that need to be differentiated from tumor as well as

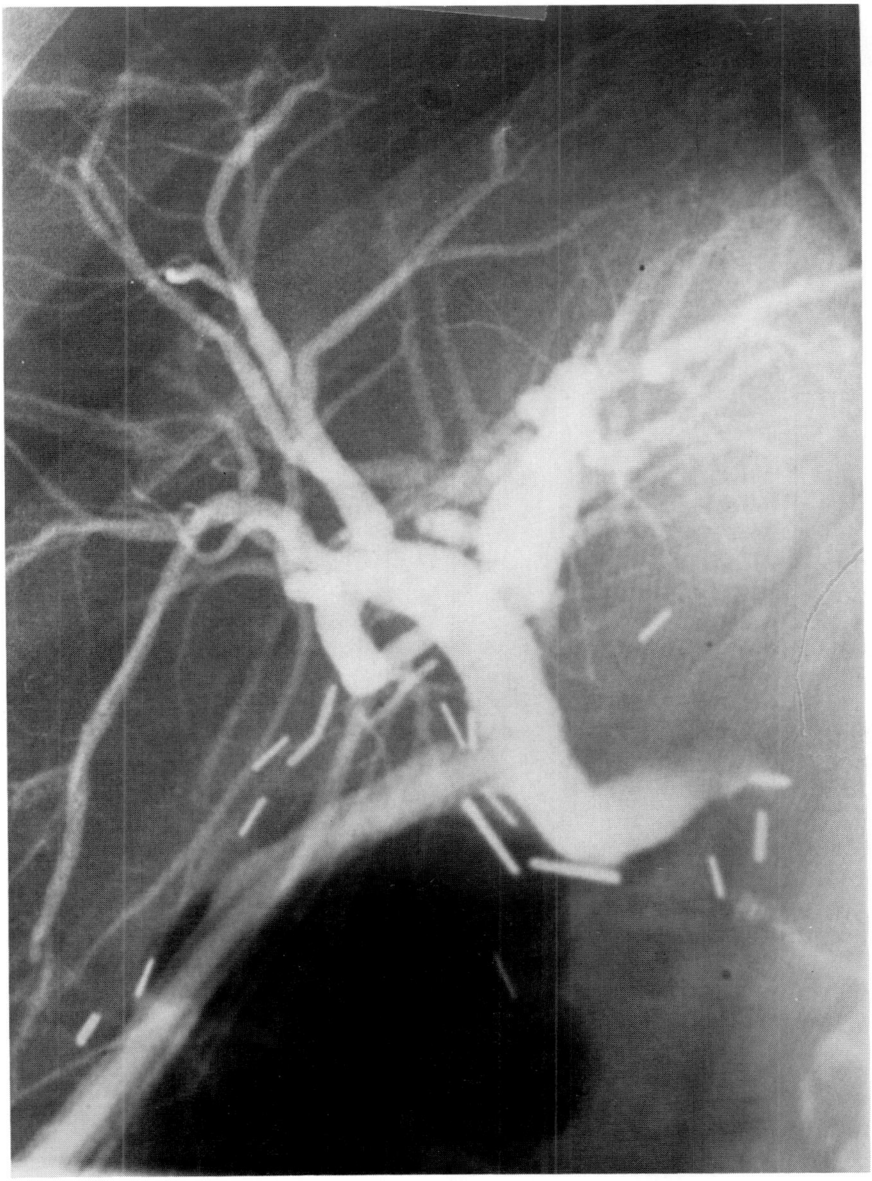

Figure 5-11. Postoperative T-tube cholangiogram. Acute pancreatitis that has produced total obstruction of the common bile duct by a large pancreatic phlegmon.

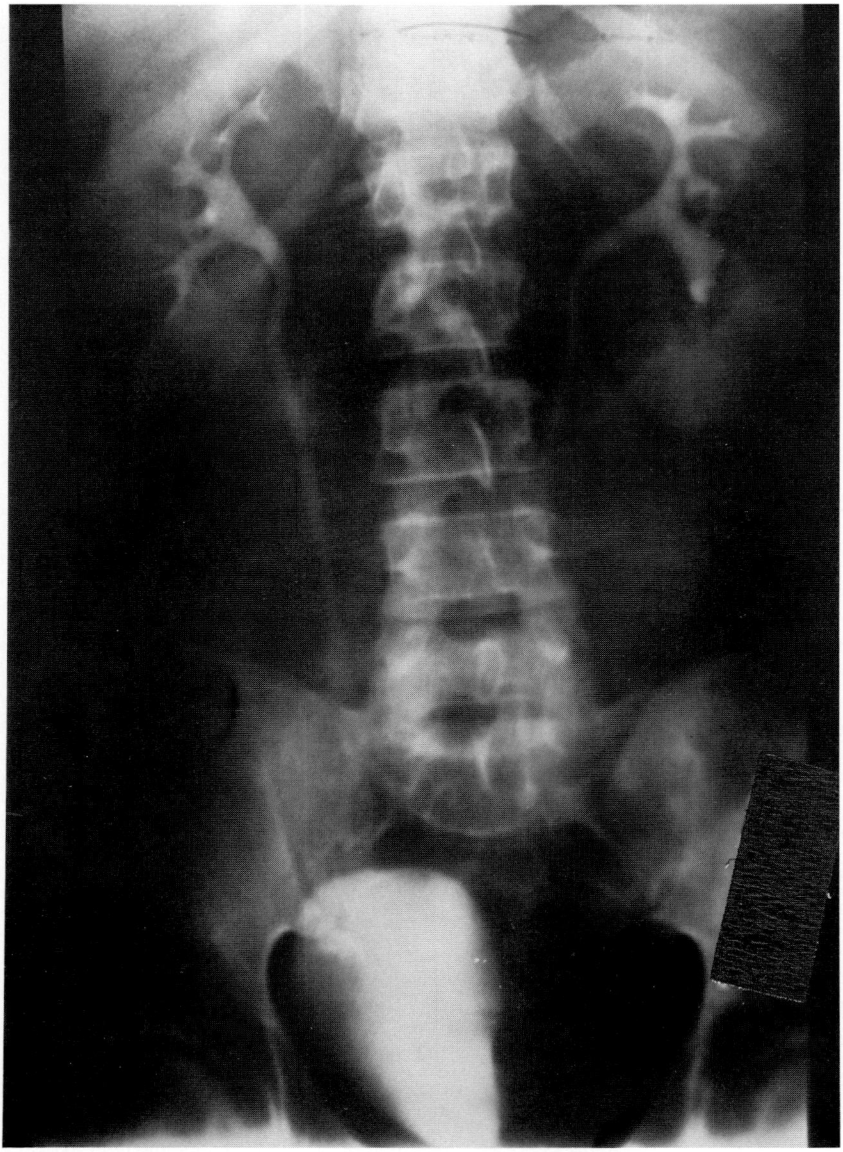

Figure 5-12. IVP. A large left-sided pseudocyst is present displacing the left ureter medially and the bladder to the right side. (From Farman et al.[7] with permission.)

abscess (Fig. 5-17). Displacement and obstruction of the ureter has been recorded as well.[7] Rarely, the pseudocyst may descend into the pelvis and produce mass effect and displacement of the bladder (Fig. 5-12).

BONES AND JOINTS

Both bone and joint changes may occur in acute pancreatitis. The metaphyseal area is most often involved. Fat necrosis occurs in the marrow, probably assisted by vascular occlusion. Lytic changes with periosteal reaction are more easily identified in children and may mimic the appearances encountered in metastatic disease. With healing, the bone changes improve or resolve but may result in a bony infarct developing. The bones around the hip joints, knees, and ankles are most often involved. Less frequently the smaller bones of the hands and feet are subject to these changes.

ULTRASONOGRAPHY AND CT OF ACUTE PANCREATITIS

Currently available US equipment affords superb resolution and allows a simple and accurate study of the pancreas. It has been estimated that the pancreas may be satisfactorily imaged in 90% of patients. Patient preparation includes fasting prior to the exam; this decreases the amount of bowel gas present that otherwise would limit the diagnostic accuracy. The CT is not affected by bowel gas, which, in fact, serves as an excellent natural contrast agent for delineating loops of bowel. Oral contrast material is necessary prior to CT to opacify adjacent bowel loops, thereby avoiding confusion with a peripancreatic mass. Intravascular contrast material is suggested for CT primarily for the delineation of peripancreatic vessels. Neither oral nor intravascular contrast material is necessary for US.

Pancreatic US includes imaging the gallbladder, biliary tree, liver, spleen, and kidneys; it is also recommended to survey the peripancreatic spaces, the paracolic gutters, and the lower abdomen. One can also examine the costophrenic angles for pleural effusion and the pelvis for ascites and for fluid collections.

Ultrasonography is generally regarded as a noninvasive and cost-effective method of evaluating patients with clinically suspected acute pancreatitis. It is an extremely accurate imaging modality for the confirmation of the clinical diagnosis, for the detection of complications of pancreatitis, and for the evaluation of patient's response to therapy. In the instances in which US is thought to be equivocal or is believed to have underestimated the extent of disease, the addition of CT is essential. The combination of US and CT allows a confident diagnosis in most patients.

Sonographically, the pancreas is a homogenous structure, but in older patients it may be heterogenous because of fatty infiltration. The CT appearance of the normal pancreas also reflects its composition, with a smoothly contoured homogeneous gland in younger patients and a lobulated heterogeneous gland with lobules of fat in elderly patients.

The spectrum of sonographic findings in pancreatitis runs from a normal-appearing gland in 20% of cases of mild acute (interstitial) pancreatitis to massive pancreatic enlargement and edema.[3] Pancreatic enlargement is usually global, but not infrequently only a portion of the gland is enlarged. The pancreas is usually of decreased echogenicity owing to interstitial edema. The CT findings parallel the sonographic findings in that it has been estimated that 30% of patients with acute pancreatitis will have a normal-appearing CT scan. However, US has a lesser incidence of false-negative scans because of its ability to detect subtle textural changes of edema in early or mild pancreatitis in a gland of essentially normal size before similar changes are noted on CT scans.[14] Thus, a normal-appearing pancreas on either US or CT does not exclude the diagnosis of acute pancreatitis in a patient with suggestive symptoms and supportive laboratory data. In more severe cases of pancreatitis, CT may show haziness of peripancreatic fat and thickening of peripancreatic fascial layers due to the inflammatory process extending beyond the pancreatic capsule.[15] The fat planes surrounding the mesenteric vessels are preserved in pancreatitis and serve as a useful sign in the differentiation from pancreatic carcinoma. Ultrasonography is incapable of demonstrating these changes in the peripancreatic fat.[1,14]

In the most severe types of pancreatitis, the ultrasonographic appearance is modified in several ways. In hemorrhagic pancreatitis, the pancreas may be more echogenic than usual because of the presence of blood in the interstitium of the pancreas. Peripancreatic fluid may also be more echogenic secondary to clot formation. This complication may be better demonstrated on CT, where blood has a characteristic higher attenuation than simple fluid. Phlegmonous pancreatitis is imaged on US as an irregular ill-defined echo-poor solid mass corresponding to the massive diffuse indurated pancreatic tissue migrating along fascial planes. Computed tomography images the full extent of the phlegmon more accurately than US. Ultrasound and/or CT may be used to follow the course of phlegmonous pancreatitis, determining which cases resolve spontaneously and which evolve into pseudocyst or abscess.[14,15]

Balthazar et al. correlated the initial CT appearance of pancreatitis with the risk of complications and patient prognosis and categorized the findings on CT into five groups.[2] In group A the CT appearance was normal. In group B there was focal or diffuse pancreatic enlargement. In group C there was evidence of peripancreatic inflammatory changes. Group D was associated with a single peripancreatic fluid collection, and in group E there were multiple fluid collections. The higher the grade, the greater the risk of abscess formation, the longer the hospital stay, and the greater the morbidity and mortality.

Sometimes ancillary findings on US or CT allow one to speculate on the underlying cause of acute pancreatitis. The presence of cholelithiasis raises the possibility of gallstone pancreatitis, although this is not a reliable association since many patients with pancreatitis have gallstones incidentally. The presence of choledocholithiasis, however, is much stronger evidence for gallstone pancreatitis. With meticulous technique, most stones in the common bile duct may be imaged sonographically. Choledocholithiasis along with focal enlargement of the pancreatic head in a patient without a history of alcoholism is virtually pathognomonic of gallstone pancreatitis. This may be differentiated from pancreatic carcinoma by the history, by serial examination, and frequently by US or CT-guided fine needle aspiration biopsy.[23]

Peripancreatic fluid collections refer to accumulations of fluid seen soon after the clinical presentation of acute pancreatitis. They are generally seen in patients with prolonged illness and carry an increased incidence of complications.[20] Pseudocyst refers to a more chronic peripancreatic fluid collection, generally seen several weeks after the acute episode, which does not resorb during therapy and establishes its permanence by forming a dense connective tissue capsule. Thus the difference between an acute peripancreatic fluid collection and a pseudocyst is important. The former has no fibrotic capsule, distends a preexisting anatomic department, and is a transient condition generally occurring early during the course of acute pancreatitis. A pseudocyst has a thick fibrous wall, is rounder, displaces or involves adjacent organs, and is more often associated with recurrent or chronic pancreatitis. Peripancreatic fluid collections may be located in any compartment in the body that has potential communication with the anterior pararenal space. Most collections, however, are located near the pancreatic bed, most often in the lesser sac and in the left anterior pararenal space. The fluid may also accumulate in the right anterior pararenal space, the posterior pararenal space, and the perinephric space. Posterior pararenal collections may involve the psoas muscle, may occasionally extend along the pelvic retroperitoneum, and may rarely travel inferiorly to the proximal thigh or as far inferiorly as the popliteal fossa, where they may mimic a Baker's cyst clinically. As mentioned previously, fluid collections may also migrate as far superiorly as the superior mediastinum, presenting clinically as a mediastinal mass, and they also involve intraabdominal viscera such as the liver and spleen.[10,22,24] As a general rule, any fluid collection in a patient with a history of alcoholism should have peripancreatic fluid collection or pseudocyst in the differential diagnosis, and if such a collection is aspirated its fluid content should be routinely assayed for amylase concentration.

The demonstration of one fluid pocket does not rule out the presence of others. In this respect, CT can most accurately provide a "road map" of the affected regions, since it is superior to US in demonstrating the size and extent of the fluid collections. However, US may easily detect fluid collections if they are within the pancreas or in a peripancreatic space not obscured by bowel. Either imaging modality may be used to monitor the resolution of peripancreatic fluid collections or their progression into pseudocysts. On US pseudocysts are round or elliptical masses with thick, sometimes irregular, walls (Fig. 5-13). They may be completely echo-free, reflecting their fluid content, or may be complex, containing some internal echoes, representing debris. They may be unilocular or multilocular. On CT, pseudocysts usually have the same density as water but may have increased density if hemorrhagic or superinfected. Gas bubbles or an air-fluid level in a pseudocyst may represent superinfection but may also indicate communication of the cyst with bowel. In such cases, the differentiation from pancreatic abscess is difficult. Pseudocysts that occasionally involve adjacent viscera may be demonstrated by US and CT (Fig. 5-14). With either US or CT, the thickness of the wall of the pseudocyst may be measured and varies directly with the age of the cyst. The demonstration of a thick wall usually implies a mature

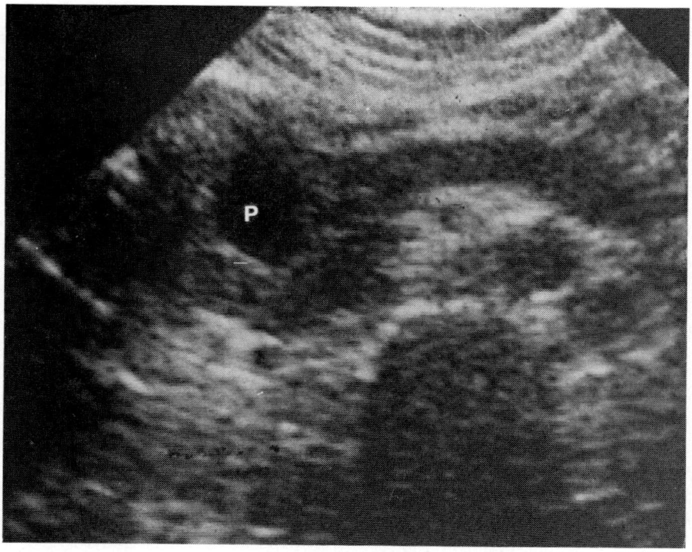

Figure 5-13. Pancreatic pseudocyst, transverse sonogram. There is an irregularly walled pseudocyst (P) located at the anterior aspect of the head of the pancreas.

cyst and a likely successful surgical outcome after anastomosis with bowel. Occasionally, an aneurysm of the splenic artery or gastroduodenal artery may simulate a pseudocyst on US and CT.[17]

In those patients who are not responsive to treatment, US or CT may demonstrate a complication of acute pancreatitis to account for their prolonged or intractable course. Pancreatic abscess is a complicaton in up to 10% of cases of severe necrotizing pancreatitis.[9–11] Although occasionally the diagnosis of pancreatic abscess may be made on plain radiography, this is too often a retrospective diagnosis. Abscess may be diagnosed by US but with limited specificity and sensitivity. To demonstrate abscess formation, CT is the most efficaceous study; the appearance is that of a fluid collection with an irregular wall and with surrounding "dirty" fat. The distinction between abscess and pseudocyst is difficult without aspiration, but the presence of gas in the collection implies infection. This is not absolute since fewer than half of abscesses contain visible pockets of gas, and since gas may be seen even in a sterile pseudocyst because of communication with bowel. In this respect, multiple scattered bubbles of gas within a fluid collection are more suggestive of abscess than is a single air-fluid level. Pockets of gas diffusely involving the pancreatic parenchyma are to be seen in cases of emphysematous pancreatitis. Pancreatic ascites may too be recognized on US or CT.[1,11,18] Splenic vein thrombosis is more often associated with pancreatic carcinoma, but bland thrombus in the splenic vein may rarely be seen with acute pancreatitis and may be demonstrated on US.[25]

If splenic vein thrombosis is not obvious on real time ultrasound, its absence should be confirmed with Doppler ultrasound, preferably using duplex instru-

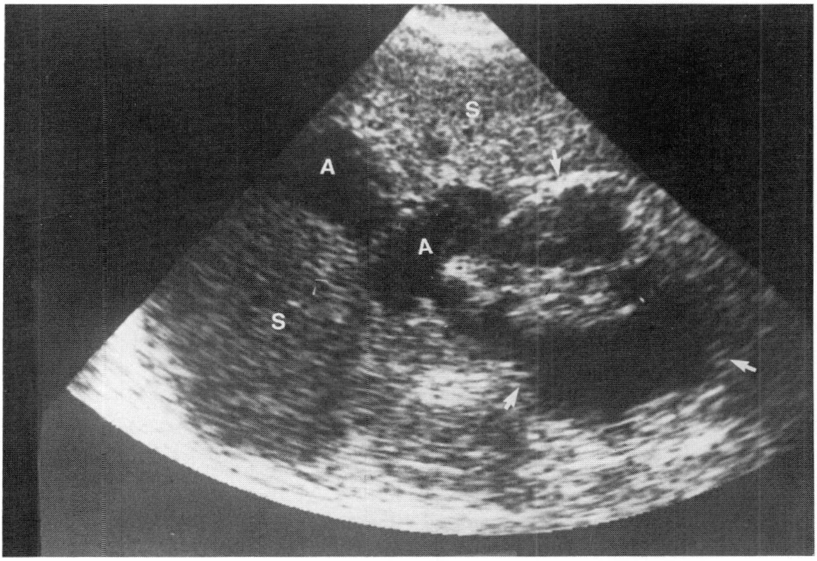

A

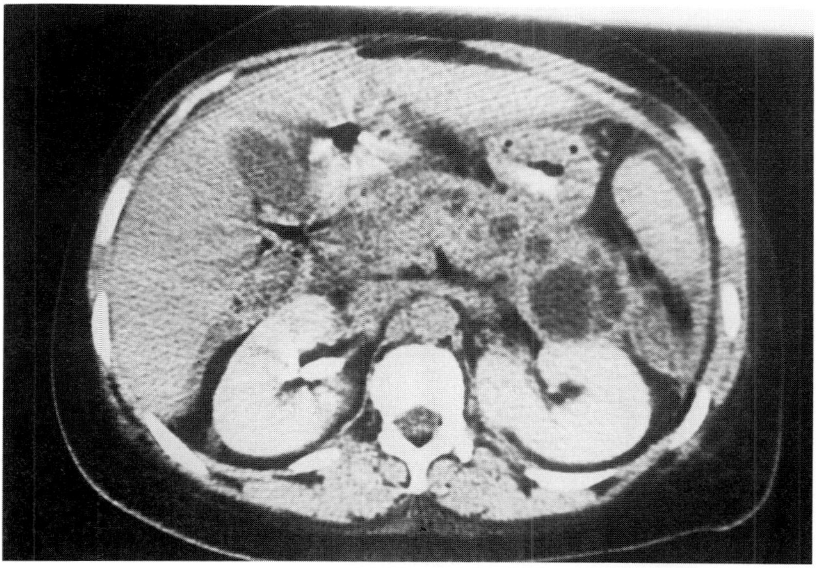

B

Figure 5-14 (A) Acute pancreatitis. The pancreas (arrowheads) is enormously swollen, containing several abscesses. One large abscess (A) extends into the spleen (S). (B) Transverse scan of the upper abdomen including the spleen, pancreatic body, and tail. Several pancreatic pseudocysts are present. An intrasplenic collection is present (C). At operation the large pseudocyst in both the tail of the pancreas and the spleen proved to be infected. (*Figure continues.*)

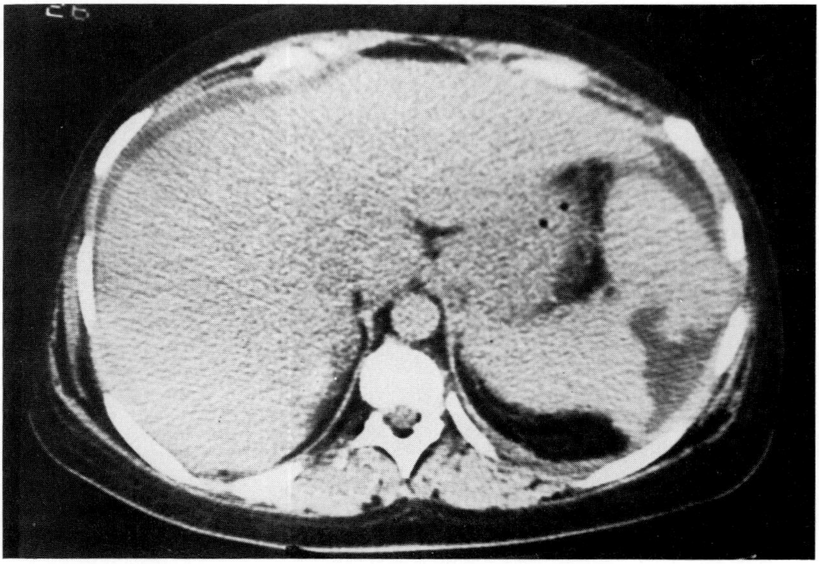

C

Figure 5-14 (*continued*). (C) An irregular triangular filling defect is seen on the posterolateral aspect of the spleen due to the intrasplenic pseudocyst.

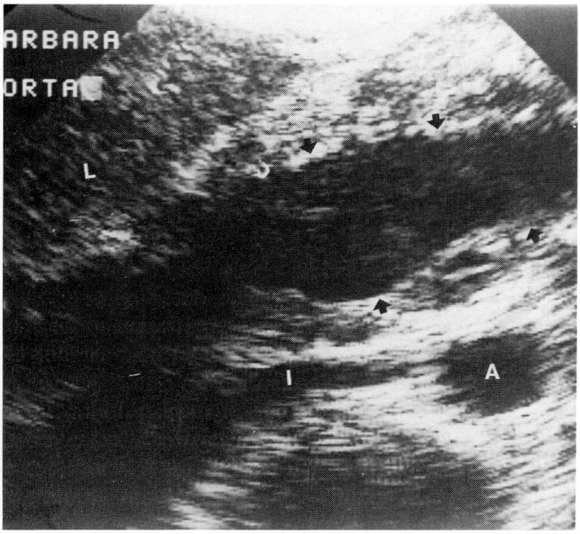

Figure 5-15. Splenic vein thrombosis, transverse sonogram. The lumen of the splenic vein is markedly enlarged because of thrombus (arrow). L = liver, A = aorta, I = inferior vena cava. (Courtesy of Linda Saunders, M.D., Columbia-Presbyterian Medical Center, New York.)

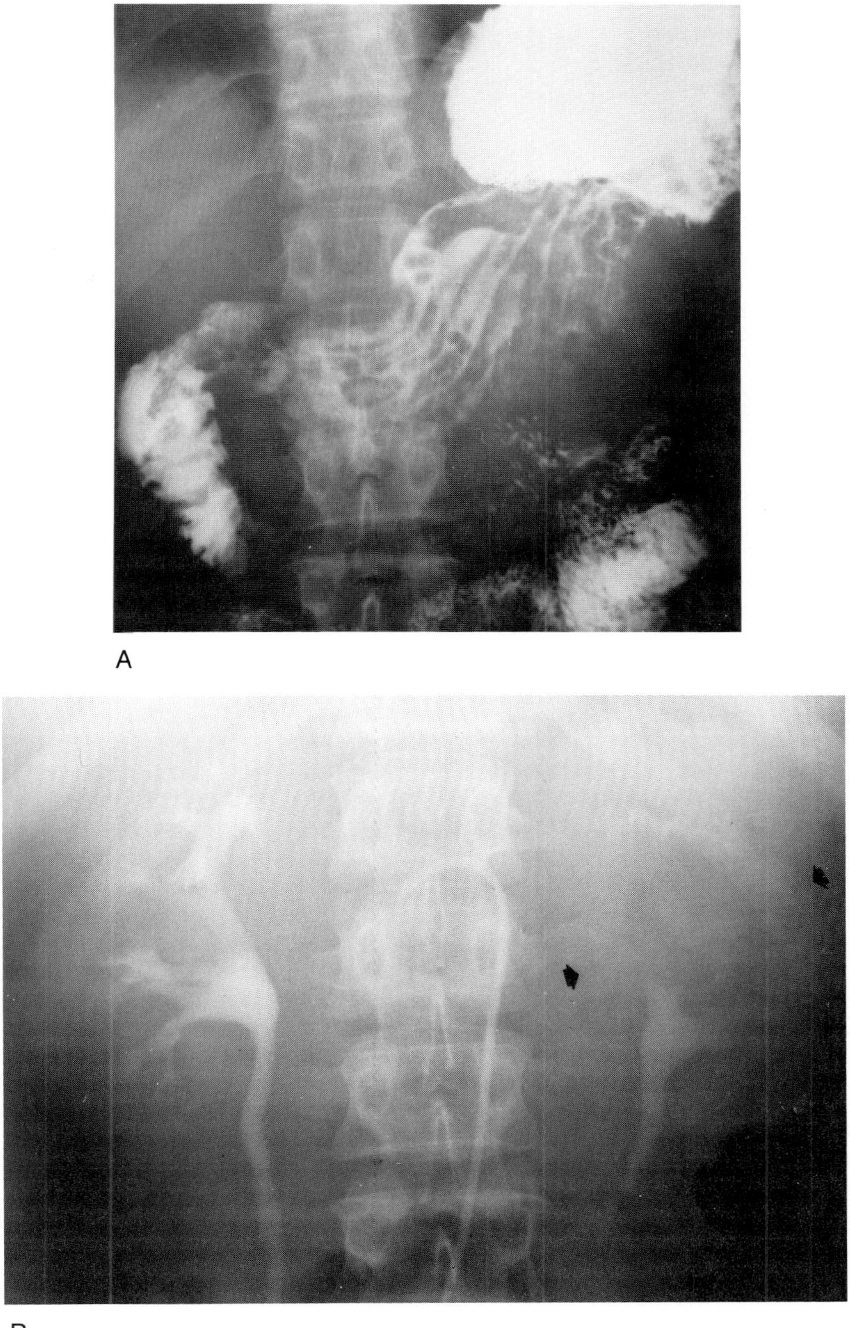

A

B

Figure 5-16. (A) A large pseudocyst is present, compressing the stomach from its posterior aspect and preventing adequate filling. The mass extends laterally to displace small bowel loops away from the greater curve. (B) IVP. Differential excretion due to compression of the left kidney, the medial and lateral margins of which are indicated by arrows.

ments which combine sonographic imaging with Doppler spectral analysis. If color flow imaging is available, it allows quick and accurate representation of flow.

Recently, magnetic resonance angiography (MRA) has emerged as a noninvasive high-resolution modality with which to image vessels throughout the body and can often obviate the need for contrast angiography in many patients. This holds much promise for imaging deep abdominal vessels including the splenic vein.

If jaundice is present, US is the most accurate modality for distinguishing between obstructive jaundice and hepatic parenchymal disease. Sonographically, the strictured duct of acute pancreatitis has a long, smooth, tapered appearance as opposed to the abrupt irregular configuration seen in pancreatic carcinoma.

In summary, either US or CT may be used for screening patients with suspected acute pancreatitis if confirmation of the clinical diagnosis is necessary (Figs. 5-15 to 5-17). If, however, one suspects complicated pancreatitis from the onset, CT should be the initial study employed. Either US or CT may be used to follow patients with complicated pancreatitis, but in general US is the preferred modality because it is less expensive, is less invasive, and meets with greater patient acceptance. For uncomplicated acute pancreatitis with full clinical resolution, no follow-up diagnostic study is necessary in most cases. These two imaging modalities are not mutually exclusive, and in many instances both examinations may be more helpful in reaching a confident diagnosis than either study alone.

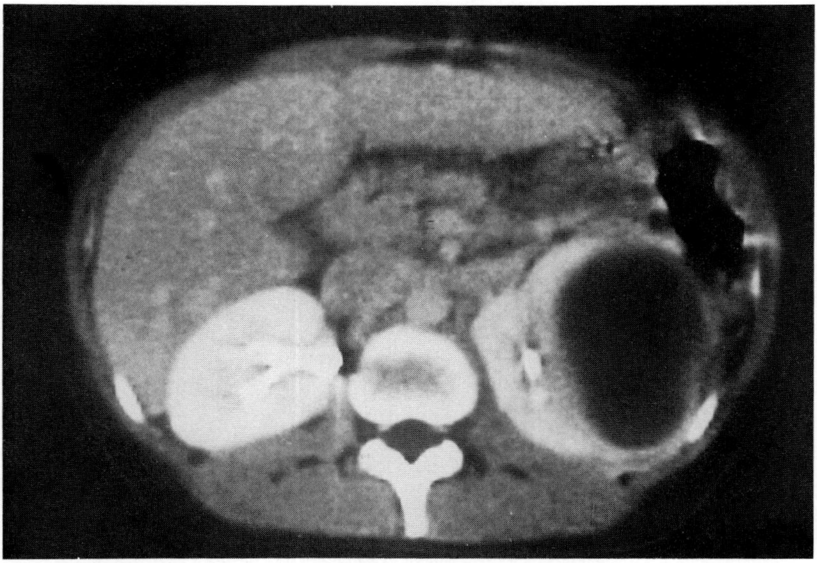

Figure 5-17. Large left-sided intrarenal pseudocyst in a 30-year old patient with severe pancreatitis. Two smaller exudative collections were also present in the diffusely enlarged inflamed pancreas on higher CT sections.

REFERENCES

1. Arger PH, Mulhern CB, Bonavita JA. An analysis of pancreatic ultrasonography in suspected pancreatic disease. J Clin Ultrasound 7:91–97, 1979.
2. Balthazar E, Ranson JHC, Naidich D, et al. Acute pancreatitis: Prognostic value of computed tomography. Radiology 156:767–772, 1985.
3. Barkin JS, Smith FR, Pereiras R, et al. Therapeutic percutaneous aspiration of pancreatic pseudocyst. Dig Dis Sci 26(7):585, 1981.
4. Bilbao MK, Dotter CT, Lee TG, et al. Complications of ERCP. Gastroenterology 70–314, 1976.
5. Dean S, Kendall MJ, Slaney G, et al. Pancreatic pseudocyst with gastric and colonic connections treated conservatively. Br J Surg 67:429–430, 1980.
6. Farman J. Colonic complications of pancreatitis. In: Marshak RH, Radiology of the Colon. Philadelphia, WB Saunders, 1980, pp 672–687.
7. Farman J. Unusual pelvic complications of a pancreatic pseudocyst. Gastrointest Radiol 3:43–45, 1978.
8. Freeny PC. Radiology of the Pancreas: Two decades of progress in imaging and intervention. AJR 150:975, 1988.
9. Gerzof SG, Banks PA, Robins AH. Early diagnosis of pancreatic infection by computed tomography aspiration. Gastroenterology 193:1315–1320, 1987.
10. Gerzof SG, Banks PA, Spechler SJ. Role of guided percutaneous aspiration in the diagnosis of early pancreatic sepsis. Dig Dis Sci 29(10):950, 1984.
11. Gerzof SG, Johnson WC, Robins AH. Percutaneous drainage of infected pancreatic pseudocysts. AJR 147:1007–1009, 1986.
12. Jeffrey RB Jr., Laing FC, Wing VW. Extrapancreatic spread of acute pancreatitis: New observations with real-time ultrasound. Radiology 159:707, 1986.
13. Karlson KB, Martin EC, Fankuchen EI, et al. Percutaneous drainage of pancreatic pseudocysts and abscesses. Radiology 142:619, 1985.
14. Lee JKT, Stanley RJ, Melson GL, et al. Pancreatic imaging by ultrasound and computed tomography: A general review. Radiol Clin North Am 27:1, 1979.
15. Lee JKT, Sagel SS, Stanley RJ, eds. Computed Body Tomography with MRI Correlation. New York, Raven Press, 1989, pp 564–577.
16. Meyers MA. Dynamic Radiology of the Abdomen, 3rd ed. Springer-Verlag, 1988, pp 344–355.
17. Miller CE, Cooperberg PL, Cohen M, et al. Pitfalls in the ultrasonic diagnosis of the pancreatic pseudocyst. J Clin Assoc Radiol 29:239–242, 1978.
18. Sankaran S, Walt AJ. The natural and unnatural history of pancreatic pseudocysts. Br J Surg 62:37, 1975.
19. Shatney CH, Sosin C. Spontaneous perforation of a pancreatic pseudocyst into the colon and duodenum. AJR 126:433–438, 1973.
20. Siegelman SS, Copeland BE, Saba GP, et al. Computed tomography of fluid collections associated with pancreatitis. AJR 134:1121–1132, 1980.
21. Sugawa C, Walt AJ, Sankaran S, et al. Pancreatic pseudocysts communicating with the stomach. Arch Surg 12:1050–1053, 1977.
22. Sybers MD, Shelp WD, Morrisey JF. Pseudocyst of the pancreas with fistulous extension into the neck. N Engl J Med 278(19):1058, 1968.
23. vanSonnenberg E, Wittich R, Casola C, et al. Complicated pancreatic inflammatory disease: Diagnostic and therapeutic role of interventional radiology. Radiology 155:355–340, 1985.
24. Warshaw AL, Chesney T, Evens GW, et al. Intrasplenic dissection by pancreatic pseudocysts. N Engl J Med 287:72–76, 1972.
25. Zalcman M, Van Gansbeke D, Matos C, et al. Sonographic demonstration of portal venous system thromboses secondary to inflammatory diseases of the pancreas. Gastrointest Radiol 12:114, 1987.

CHAPTER

6

THERAPEUTIC OPTIONS IN ACUTE PANCREATITIS

Benjamin W. Pace and Leslie Wise

EDITORIAL COMMENT

In the nonoperative treatment of acute pancreatitis, not one of the current modalities of treatment has been shown to influence the course of the disease or the incidence of complications. However, the controlled studies that have been published must be interpreted cautiously. The wide clinical spectrum of severity in acute pancreatitis with a preponderance of milder cases mandates that either large numbers of patients are studied in controlled trials or that there is adequate stratification for severity of disease. It should be stressed that in the individual patient the various therapeutic options may be used with considerable symptomatic benefit. For example, nasogastric suction will relieve severe nausea and vomiting, and cimetidine will decrease the risk of bleeding from stress ulceration. For patients at high risk of complications, we believe that antibiotics should be given and peritoneal lavage considered because of the symptomatic improvement that results, particularly in respiratory function.

There is no evidence to support routine early operative drainage in acute pancreatitis, although some recent reports have emphasized the importance of early diagnosis and debridement of pancreatic necrosis. In the absence of infection, necrosis may not be an urgent indication for operation. Conservative debridement of pancreatic necrosis is preferable to formal pancreatic resections, and recent studies suggest that the excised material often consists of nonpancreatic necrotic fat.

CONTROVERSY

Various therapeutic options are available for the management of acute pancreatitis. Most have been controversial at one time or another, and some have been the subjects of controlled clinical trials. The options have usually had a sound theoretical basis often not substantiated in the clinical application. For example, nasogastric suction was recommended to remove acid and thus decrease pancreatic stimulation, trypsin inhibitors to decrease enzyme activity and necrosis, antibiotics given early to prevent infection and abscess.

Controversy in the therapy of acute pancreatitis revolves around several key issues. Once identified as suffering from acute pancreatitis, all patients require resuscitation to a lesser or greater degree. In this regard, discussion surrounds the use of crystalloid versus colloid solutions as well as the role of total parenteral nutrition. Attempts to "place the gland at rest" usually follow, including attempts at decreasing hormonal stimulation of the pancreas via the gastrointestinal tract. Though this represents a logical theoretical approach, considerable debate surrounds this yet-unproven approach to treatment. Antibiotic therapy in acute pancreatitis is similarly common, yet controversial.

Further controversy surrounds the use of supportive therapy in the setting of acute necrotizing pancreatitis. Other proposed therapies include "triple-ostomy," drainage alone, resectional therapy, and peritoneal dialysis. The treatment of complications, especially hemorrhage, has slowly evolved, yet not without debate. Finally, one of the more recent controversial topics in acute pancreatitis is the application of vagotomy, with or without an associated drainage procedure, versus behavior modification in the prevention of recurrence of acute pancreatitis in the alcoholic patient. Each of these controversial areas is discussed in depth below.

The term *acute pancreatitis* describes a broad group of pathophysiologic derangements of the pancreatic gland. Acute pancreatitis manifests itself in a broad spectrum of severity, varying from the very mild to the life-threatening condition of acute necrotizing pancreatitis.[24,57,89] It is this diversity that makes the study of acute pancreatitis so difficult. The majority of patients with acute pancreatitis resolve their attack rapidly with conservative supportive management, and only 5% to 10% of patients require further diagnostic and therapeutic intervention.[96] Research appropriately focuses on this smaller group with a more severe form of disease. Because of the wide spectrum of severity and etiology of acute pancreatitis, the interpretation and application of presented data is at times difficult. Considerable weight is given to this "mixed-bag" contention by the not infrequent lack of reproducibility among different surgical investigators applying a given treatment to their individual study groups.

CONTROVERSIES IN CLASSIFICATION AS RELATES TO THERAPEUTIC TRIALS

Debate exists as to the applicability of the numerous classification schemes that exist in regard to acute pancreatitis. Their varied application, in the selection of patients for study and the interpretation of results, limits the conclusions that can be drawn from the research available (Chapter 2). In brief, the Marseilles classification divides acute pancreatitis into *acute* and *acute relapsing* based on the sequence of events.[96] Of greater utility, a classification based on etiology divides acute pancreatitis into that induced by overindulgence in alcohol, biliary tract disease, hyperlipidemia, precedent surgery, and a host of infrequent factors such as pancreas divisum, hypercalcemia, duodenal diverticulosis, parasitic infection, drug therapy, and so forth. This system has as its greatest benefit the identification of those etiologic factors that have individually associated proven treatments (cholecystectomy for biliary tract disease—Chapter 7—elimination of offending medication, etc.). Etiologic classification allows stratification of patients with a given pathophysiologic mechanism for research as well as therapy (alcoholic vs. nonalcoholic, etc.) (Chapters 2 and 12), as well as heightening the awareness of the clinician in certain cases by identifying patients at the highest risk (i.e., post-operative pancreatitis). Classifications based on the severity of the disease and associated risk factors (Chapter 3) also serve to heighten the awareness of the physician as to those patients at greatest risk. Clearly, clinical judgment alone has performed poorly in this regard. Corfield et al.,[14] reporting on 436 attacks in 418 patients, showed that clinical assessment identified only 34% of patients with complicated or fatal outcomes.[14] Risk factor analysis as popularized by Ranson and associates[72] and modified by Bank et al.[3] was a marked improvement in isolating those patients at high risk. However, the majority of studies on therapy in acute pancreatitis that disaggregate patients on severity alone often clump together patients with noncomparable pathophysiologic derangements, although all are seriously ill. This, as noted later, may render the results so obtained poorly reproducible.

Hollender and associates, from Strasbourg, France, recommend therapy based on the degree of pathologic change within the gland and surrounding tissue.[35] *First degree* refers to diffuse edema of the pancreas, which, when treated medically, almost universally resolves. *Second degree* identifies limited pancreatic necrosis, often poorly responsive to medical treatment, which can be attacked surgically with some success. *Third degree* represents diffuse pancreatic necrosis involving not only the pancreas but often peripancreatic tissue. This form is highly lethal. The problem with this system is that even the first step, the identification of acute pancreatitis in a patient presenting with upper abdominal pain, tenderness, guarding, and hyperamylasemia, may be difficult as we have demonstrated in our recent study (Chapter 4).[67]

CONTROVERSIES IN DIAGNOSIS

Radiology, peritoneal lavage, and laparotomy are all currently advocated controversial methods of diagnosing acute pancreatitis. The evidence supporting each modality is outlined below.

Radiologic Diagnosis

The role of radiology in the diagnosis of acute pancreatitis is discussed in depth in Chapter 5. Debate exists as to the use of ultrasonography versus computerized tomography (CT) as the principal radiologic modality. Suffice it to say here that though sonography may be used to confirm the clinical diagnosis, detect complications (e.g., pseudocyst), and identify associated biliary tract pathology, only CT has the potential to differentiate acute edematous pancreatitis from hemorrhagic pancreatitis as well as from acute necrotizing pancreatitis with or without extension into the peripancreatic spaces.[49] This, of course, is interpreter-dependent. In fact, in a prospective study of 51 patients, Nordestgaard and associates[65] were able to divide their findings into four grades: grade A, no abnormality; grade B, enlargement and inflammation of the pancreas; grade C, extension into one peripancreatic space; and grade D, extension into two or more peripancreatic spaces. Indeed, all patients with complications or a fatal outcome were characterized as grade C or D. Surprisingly, in this series, those patients dying of their disease were all in the group of Ranson signs 0 to 2. There were no deaths in the Ranson 3 to 5 or 6 or more categories.

Peritoneal Lavage

Peritoneal lavage in this setting is performed in a manner similar to that of its use in trauma. Though a number of treatment benefits have also been put forth (see discussion on peritoneal dialysis), the possible role of diagnostic peritoneal lavage is (1) to assess severity and prognosis (Chapter 3), (2) to distinguish acute pancreatitis from those entities in the differential diagnosis that present clinically in a similar manner (Chapter 4), and (3) to detect hemorrhagic fluid within the free peritoneal cavity. Bradley and associates reported on the role of microscopy of peritoneal lavage fluid.[9] They detected one case of biliary peritonitis and one case of mesenteric infarction originally diagnosed as acute pancreatitis (2%) among 96 other cases of acute pancreatitis when microscopic examination of the lavage fluid was used routinely. Additionally, Kauste and associates from Helsinki, Finland, reported that of 25 patients determined at autopsy or laparotomy to have hemorrhagic pancreatitis, only three (12%) were diagnosed as such, early, on routine therapeutic peritoneal lavage.[40] Despite these low yields, it is a simple matter to stain and scan microscopically any fluid obtained during prognostic or therapeutic peritoneal lavage, and we encourage its analysis under these circumstances. We have found no advocate of peritoneal lavage solely for diagnosis. The complication rate as well as the false-positive rate for diagnostic peritoneal lavage reported in the literature approaches that of the above-noted yields,[23] markedly limiting its usefulness in the setting of acute pancreatitis.

Laparotomy for Diagnosis

Controversy surrounds the use of diagnostic laparotomy in the setting of acute pancreatitis, not only vis-à-vis other diagnostic modalities but also regarding the potential deleterious effects of this procedure in an already-debilitated patient.[32]

For years the classic teaching warned of the added stress of an exploratory laparotomy in an already compromised patient with acute pancreatitis.[90] Pollack, however, in his review of 100 patients, found no difference in mortality comparing conservative therapy versus early laparotomy, despite the fact that the more severely ill patients had been subjected to surgery in this retrospective nonrandomized study.[69] Trapnell and Anderson retrospectively reviewed their large series involving 324 patients.[90] In this study, the indication for operation was most often the confirmation of the clinical diagnosis. They found a mortality of 24%, 24%, and 21% for conservative therapy, exploratory laparotomy alone, and exploratory laparotomy with an associated biliary procedure, respectively. It should be pointed out that in over 95% of cases the patients had either biliary or idiopathic causes assigned to their acute pancreatitis, alcoholism accounting for only 1% of their patients. Warshaw and Richter outlined their indications for diagnostic laparotomy as (1) clinical deterioration despite adequate conservative management, (2) increasing evidence of frank peritonitis, and (3) a laboratory picture inconsistent with classic acute pancreatitis.[96] We concur with these indications, and we feel that if laparotomy is performed for these indications then "if the patient has pancreatitis, little is lost; when some other diagnosis is revealed, much can be gained."[89] An error in diagnosis (e.g., missing a perforated viscus or necrotic bowel) may lead to a rapidly fatal outcome if left undetected.

CONTROVERSIES IN RESUSCITATION

From 5% to 10% of patients with acute pancreatitis suffer from a severe form with a high incidence of morbidity and mortality. Major fluid shifts are characteristic, early respiratory insufficiency occurs frequently, and multiple system failure may ensue. It is important to note that shock has been associated with a 50% to 90% mortality in this setting.[5,24] Once identified as high-risk according to any of the several assessment modalities available (Chapter 3), the patient should be placed in an intensive care unit where continuous monitoring is available. Resuscitation is begun and the patient is serially evaluated for the adequacy of volume restoration using Swan-Ganz monitoring. The type of fluid used for resuscitation as well as the use of total parenteral nutrition is a matter of debate.

Colloid Versus Crystalloid

Controversy exists as to the role of colloid agents in the resuscitation of patients with acute pancreatitis. Kellum et al. reviewed four cases of acute respiratory insufficiency secondary to acute pancreatitis in which albumin and diuretic therapy were employed.[43] Two patients (50%) survived, causing them to conclude, without apparent convincing evidence, that "pulmonary interstitial edema is mobilized by the use of albumin concentrates and diuretics." Ranson and associates, encouraged by this report, used albumin and diuretic therapy in a nonrandomized manner in 13 patients with respiratory insufficiency complicating acute pancreatitis.[75] In 4 of these 13 patients, the respiratory insufficiency rapidly resolved. To our knowledge, only two randomized studies of this subject in acute pancreatitis are available. Martin et al., using 25 dogs with experimentally produced and operatively confirmed necrotizing pancreatitis, found no difference between Ringer's lactate, 25% albumin, or hetastarch when each was transfused in adequate volume to maintain normal blood pressure, cardiac output, pulmonary capillary wedge pressure, and urinary output.[53] In a different approach, Sanfey et al., isolating the canine pancreas, found a marked diminution in pancreatic edema with the use of albumin versus Ringer's lactate when used in similar volumes along with blood in experimentally produced acute pancreatitis.[77] Our view is that respiratory insufficiency in acute pancreatitis does not differ significantly from that seen in sepsis, trauma, or the adult respiratory distress syndrome in which early increased capillary permeability or leak exists. Numerous studies performed over the past several years have shown an equal distribution of albumin, with its concomitant colloid oncotic pressure, to *all* extracellular compartments in these settings, making its use in resuscitation only more expensive rather than more effective compared with crystalloid solutions.[4,34,71,77]

Fresh-frozen plasma has also been advocated as an important part of the resuscitation regimen. Cuschieri, Wood, and associates reviewed 239 patients with acute pancreatitis with an overall mortality of 3.7%.[15] Of interest, in 96 attacks in 69 patients diagnosed as having *severe* pancreatitis by the criteria of Ranson and/or Imrie (Chapter 3), an admirable 4.2% mortality was recorded with the routine use of fresh-frozen plasma. The authors concluded that naturally occurring powerful proteinase inhibitors, present in the plasma, were responsible for this low mortality. This report is promising, suffering only from the lack of a control group.

Nutritional Support

The indication and timing of the use of nutritional support in acute pancreatitis is controversial. Since most cases of uncomplicated acute pancreatitis resolve within about a week with only supportive therapy, the *premature* institution of nutritional support by any means is probably unnecessary and may be potentially dangerous. Ranson and Spencer felt that the early reinstitution of oral feeding to patients prior to the complete resolution of pancreatic inflammation, especially in those high-risk patients with three or more risk factors, was associated with reactivation of the inflammatory process.[74] This, they felt, predisposed these patients to the formation of a pancreatic abscess.

Total parenteral nutrition (TPN) at any stage may be associated with complications, including pneumothorax secondary to line placement and line sepsis. Sax et al. reported a 10.5% catheter sepsis rate in patients with acute pancreatitis receiving TPN compared with a 1.5% rate for those on routine intravenous crystalloid therapy.[80] Goodgame and Fisher retrospectively analyzed their complications using TPN in the setting of acute pancreatitis, revealing a 17% catheter sepsis rate within the first 2 weeks.[31] Surgical research into the effects of starvation and metabolism has taught us that up to 2 weeks of starvation is adequately tolerated when peripheral glucose infusion therapy is used to minimize protein catabolism.[81] The noted high rate of spontaneous resolution of acute pancreatitis within 2 weeks, the line sepsis rate, and the diagnostic dilemma presented to the clinician in differentiating catheter-related infection from that of an infected pancreatic mass in cases of sepsis limit the use of TPN in early pancreatitis.

Controversy exists over the safety and efficacy of TPN (including lipids) in those patients with severe or complicated pancreatitis and a protracted process who require some form of nutritional supplementation. First, the concept of "resting" the pancreas (discussed in detail below) is logical but as yet of unproven benefit. Patients with pancreatic fistulas seem to represent the ideal model in which to study the controversial effects of nutritional support on pancreatic secretion. Klein and associates studied one patient with a pure pancreatic fistula.[45] The patient was first given dextrose solution in increasing concentrations followed by isolated amino acid solutions, 10% and 20% fat emulsions, and finally, TPN infusions. Concentrated glucose infusion (10%–20%) resulted in a significant reduction in the fistula output and amylase concentration. Amino acid therapy had no effect, while intravenous fat emulsion increased both parameters. These effects of glucose and amino acid infusions in pancreatic fistulas were confirmed by Bivins and associates.[7] Neither Bivins nor Grundfest et al. found any change with the administration of intravenous fat emulsion.[33] Silberman et al. gave lipid-based nutritional support to 11 patients suffering from acute pancreatitis with no clinical exacerbations.[82] Nitrogen balance was positive in the three patients in this series so tested. We support the use of TPN in severe and complicated acute pancreatitis in which a hospital course of greater than 2 weeks is likely. Unfortunately, the only prospective randomized trial stopped short of fully meaningful results by drawing conclusions at 8 days.[80]

THE "GLAND AT REST" CONTROVERSY

Nasogastric Suction

Most patients with acute pancreatitis require nasogastric suction for symptomatic relief. Therefore, all studies comparing nasogastric suction with a control group, must, of necessity, be restricted to patients with mild pancreatitis. In all these studies, nasogastric suction failed to reduce the duration or severity of abdominal pain, the interval until bowel function returned, the need for narcotic administration, the length of hospital stay, the need for intravenous therapy, or the lipase or amylase levels. These results are summarized in Table 6-1.

H_2 Antagonists

The studies available are summarized in Table 6-2. Cimetidine was of no benefit compared with routine intravenous therapy (Loiudice et al.,[52] Broe et al.,[10] Meshkinpour et al.[60]) or compared with nasogastric suction (Loiudice et al.,[52] Goff et al.,[30] Regan et al.[76]). The only benefit encountered was a reduction in the hospital length of stay (6.8 ± 2.7 vs. 8.5 ± 4.8 days) in the study by Goff. This benefit was not reproduced by Broe et al.[10] or Meshkinpour et al.[60] Again no

TABLE 6-1. RANDOMIZED PROSPECTIVE STUDIES ON THE EFFICACY OF NASOGASTRIC SUCTION IN ACUTE PANCREATITIS

Investigator	Year	No. of Patients	Conclusion	Comments
Levant[51]	1974	29	No benefit	
Naeije[63]	1978	58	No benefit	
Field[21]	1979	37	No benefit	
Fuller[25]	1981	21	No benefit	Nasogastric suction patients had a significantly longer duration of nausea and vomiting
Lange[47]	1983	50	No benefit	Compared with free intake of clear liquids
Loiudice[52]	1984	45	No benefit	Also compared nasogastric suction with cimetidine with no benefit
Sarr[78]	1986	60	No benefit	Other medications not used routinely
Total		300		

advantage was noted as related to abdominal pain and tenderness, ileus, fever, or amylase levels.

Glucagon

Similarly, the advocates of glucagon therapy have failed to obtain evidence of efficacy in controlled trials (Table 6-3). Kronborg et al. investigated 22 patients, all with severe nonbiliary pancreatitis, in a randomized double-blind trial of glucagon therapy.[46] There was no statistical difference in the rate of severe complications or mortality. Durr and associates from Germany, studying 59 patients in a

TABLE 6-2. RANDOMIZED PROSPECTIVE STUDIES OF CIMETIDINE THERAPY IN ACUTE PANCREATITIS

Investigator	Year	No. of Patients	Conclusion	Comments
Meshkinpour[60]	1979	27	No benefit	Also no harm noted for cimetidine
Regan[76]	1981	20	No benefit	Compared with nasogastric suction or combined therapy
Broe[10]	1982	116	No benefit	52.5% had nasogastric suction in place for vomiting
Goff[30]	1982	95	Only shorter length of stay noted	Compared with nasogastric suction, no other benefit found
Loiudice[52]	1984	45	No benefit	Also no benefit compared with nasogastric suction
Total		303		

TABLE 6-3. GLUCAGON THERAPY IN ACUTE PANCREATITIS

Investigator	Year	No. of Patients	Conclusion	Comments
Med. Res. Council[59]	1977	257	No benefit	Compared with aprotinin or aprotinin and glucagon
Durr[18]	1978	59	No benefit	
Gilsanz[27]	1978	62	No benefit*	Compared with anticholinergics
Kronborg[46]	1980	22	No benefit	All patients with severe pancreatitis (overall 37% mortality)
Debas[16]	1980	66	No benefit	
Total		466		

* More rapid abatement of abdominal pain in exchange for severe headache.

similar fashion, also concluded that there was no difference in the subjective evaluation of pain, the amount of analgesia and/or antispasmodic therapy required, the amylase level, the hospital length of stay, or the mortality.[18] This was further confirmed by Debas et al. also in a prospective randomized double-blind fashion; in 66 patients no difference was noted in the need for analgesia, the presence of abdominal signs, the persistence of ileus, or the length of stay in the hospital.[16] In a large multicenter British study, 257 patients were randomly assigned to glucagon, aprotinin, or combined therapy groups.[59] No control group was used. An overall 1% mortality rate was recorded. In the doses used, neither drug was found to diminish the associated mortality. Finally, a study from the University of Madrid comparing glucagon with anticholinergic therapy found no difference in the mortality or frequency of complications among 62 patients.[27] They did, however, find that the glucagon group had a more rapid abatement of abdominal pain, but this at the cost of quite severe headaches. In view of these studies, we do not feel glucagon therapy is indicated in the treatment of acute pancreatitis.

OTHER CONTROVERSIAL DRUG THERAPIES

Controversial drug therapies include the proteolytic enzyme aprotinin (Trasylol) and antibiotics. The available evidence is summarized below.

Aprotinin

Multiple prospective investigations have been undertaken on the value of antiproteolytic therapy in acute pancreatitis. These studies are summarized in Table 6-4. Aprotinin is an antiproteolytic agent that inhibits the activity of trypsin and the lysis of fibrin by human plasmin. Despite promising early experimental work, no clinical benefit has been shown for this therapy as noted. The only study

TABLE 6-4. RANDOMIZED PROSPECTIVE STUDIES OF APROTININ THERAPY IN ACUTE PANCREATITIS

Investigator	Year	No. of Patients	Conclusion	Comments
Trapnell[92]	1967	261	No benefit	Low-dose
Baden[2]	1969	49	No benefit	Early therapy intra- or post-operatively
Parkash[68]	1972	240	No benefit	
Trapnell[91]	1974	105	Decreased mortality	A 21% mortality for mild cases in the control group is unacceptably high, placing study in doubt
Med. Res. Council[59]	1977	257	No benefit	Also no benefit when combined with glucagon
Imrie[38]	1978	161	No benefit	
Total		1073		

showing some advantage (Trapnell et al., 1974[91]) appears flawed. The control group had 63% mild cases, yet 21% of these mild cases died. As concluded by Imrie and associates,[38] there is "no case for the continued use of Trayslol in the stated dosage in the future management of pancreatitis."

Antibiotics

Evidence of infection of necrotic pancreatic tissue with time is available. Yet the use of antibiotics in this setting is unproved and controversial. (Antibiotic use in pancreatic abscess is discussed in Chapter 9.) Howes et al. from Johns Hopkins studied the use of prophylactic ampicillin on acute pancreatitis, randomizing 104 patients prospectively into ampicillin versus no antibiotic therapy.[36] No significant difference was noted regarding fever, amylase, or rate of infection. Similarly, Finch and associates from Vanderbilt University studied ampicillin therapy in acute pancreatitis in a prospective randomized double-blind study.[22] Fifty-eight patients were evaluated, all receiving nasogastric suction and atropine. In the study group, ampicillin 500 mg intravenously every 6 hours was also given (1 g of cephalosporin intravenously every 6 hours in the penicillin-allergic patients). No significant difference in the length of stay or number of days the patient remained febrile was noted. More importantly, the complication and recurrence rates were similar. Yet in the more severe forms of pancreatitis, bacteria have been recovered from resected pancreatic tissue early on, suggesting a possible role for antibiotic therapy (not prophylaxis) in these patients.[95] Beger et al., in a recent prospective clinical study, cultured a broad spectrum of bacteria from 39% of operative specimens of pancreatic necrosis.[6] The organisms cultured included aerobic and anaerobic gram-negative organisms, aerobic gram-positive organisms, and *Mycobacterium tuberculosis* and *Candida*. Many of these organisms are obviously not sensitive to ampicillin. Little, therefore, can be concluded about the efficacy of antibiotic therapy from studies limited to ampicillin in mild forms of disease.

TABLE 6-5. ANTIBIOTICS AND OTHER DRUGS PROPOSED FOR THE THERAPY OF ACUTE PANCREATITIS

Medication	Year	No. of Patients	Prospective Double-Blind	Conclusions	Comments
Antibiotics					
Howes[36]	1975	104	Yes	No benefit	
Finch[22]	1976	58	Yes	No benefit	All patients given nasogastric suction, atropine, and antibiotics
Calcitonin					
Goebell[29]	1979	94	Yes	Less abdominal pain	Multicenter
Martinez[54]	1984	31	Yes	No benefit	All severe pancreatitis (Ranson signs ≥ 3)
Indomethacin					
Ebbehoj[19]	1985	30	Yes	Fewer opiate injections	Too small a study to evaluate effect on prognosis
Insulin					
Svenson[87]	1975	29	Yes	Less abdominal pain	80% pain-free within 4 hours of the onset of pain with insulin vs. 28.5% pain-free without insulin
Prostaglandins					
Standfield[84]	1983	66 mice	Animal	Markedly increased survival	32% mortality with PGE_2 compared with 100% mortality in the placebo group
Atropine					
Cameron[13]	1979	56	Yes	No benefit	
Phospholipase A_2					
Tykka[93]	1985	64	Yes	More rapid recovery	Group not well matched for age or etiology

Beger's group further reported on 114 patients with acute necrotizing pancreatitis without abscess. All patients included had failed conservative management, subsequently undergoing laparotomy and removal of necrotic pancreatic tissue. All tissue specimens were cultured. Time in hospital prior to surgery, extent of necrosis, and mortality were positively correlated with the presence of bacterial contamination. The contamination rate rose from 24% to 71% for those patients operated on during the first and second weeks of hospitalization, respectively. The extent of pancreatic and extrapancreatic necrosis was greater in the bacteriologically positive group, and this group had a 37% mortality compared with 9% for the bacteriologically negative group. Of all patients, 37% received antibiotic therapy once the clinical diagnosis of infection was entertained during the phase of conservative management.

In interpreting these results, Beger implicates the presence of bacterial contamination in the further extension of pancreatic necrosis with a resultant increase in mortality. We question the validity of this assumption. It is possible that the more extensive pancreatic and extrapancreatic necrosis facilitated the seeding of bacteria. Indeed, the severity of the disease process may be the factor influencing mortality rather than the bacterial status. In conclusion, though we feel the studies presented fail to show clear benefit for the use of antibiotics in acute pancreatitis, these studies are quite limited, and we continue to use antibiotics when clinical evidence of pancreatic infection exists.

Miscellaneous

Other drug therapies used in patients with acute pancreatitis are summarized in Table 6-5. One animal study (Standfield[84]) is included as it shows great promise for the use of prostaglandins. Mice with experimentally induced acute pancreatitis has a 100% mortality in the placebo group compared with a 32% mortality for those mice given prostaglandin E_2 (PGE_2). This remains to be reproduced in humans. The other trials are generally disappointing, including recent trials with the latest entrant octrestide (Sandostatin).

SUMMARY OF THE CONTROVERSIES OF RESUSCITATION, PLACING THE GLAND AT REST, AND OTHER DRUG THERAPIES

Crystalloid infusion appears as effective as colloid infusion in the volume resuscitation required in acute pancreatitis and is less expensive. Nasogastric suction is instituted only for nausea and/or vomiting. Hyperalimentation, in general, should be avoided for up to 2 weeks, at which point the anticipation of a protracted hospital course justifies its implementation. Early assessment of risk is undertaken, and those patients with a more severe form of the disease are treated as discussed below. All patients should be examined initially by sonography to confirm the diagnosis and evaluate the patient for possible associated biliary pathologic lesions. Careful serial assessment of those patients deemed originally to be at little risk is undertaken. This to identify promptly those cases advancing to a more severe form requiring alternative therapy or those in whom alternative diagnoses need to be entertained.

CONTROVERSIES IN THE THERAPY OF ACUTE NECROTIZING PANCREATITIS

The benefits of various aggressive interventional therapies versus supportive therapy for severe forms of acute pancreatitis have been debated in the literature for decades.

Supportive Versus Surgical Therapy

Moynihan in 1925 advocated operation upon the pancreas and gallbladder with drainage of each in all cases of acute pancreatitis.[62] The prohibitively high associated mortality led later investigators to recommend conservative management for uncomplicated mild pancreatitis with relative success. However, nonoperative supportive therapy when applied to acute necrotizing pancreatitis with infection carries an associated mortality approaching 100%. Gliedman and associates reviewed 48 patients so treated; all 48 patients died.[28] This dismal result was reproduced by Jordan and Spjut 2 years later in 30 patients treated supportively.[39] In a recent report Aldridge et al., reviewing the literature, found the mortality to approach 80% for conservative therapy.[1] In contrast to this 80% to 100% nonoperative mortality, Gliedman, Jordan, and Aldridge found their operative mortality to be 33% to 51%. Yet operative therapy is not the only alternative available. Peritoneal dialysis, most often via catheters placed during diagnostic laparotomy, rivals resection as the modality of choice. The evidence supporting each of these is discussed in detail below.

Triple-Ostomy Therapy

In 1970, Lawson et al. proposed *triple-ostomy* as the ideal operation for acute necrotizing pancreatitis.[48] In a pathophysiologic approach to treatment, gastrostomy, cholecystostomy, and jejunostomy were employed to reduce stimulation of pancreatic secretion, treat possible primary or secondary biliary pathologic lesions, and serve as a feeding route, respectively. In addition, drainage of the lesser sac was employed to remove collecting toxins and debris. In their study, 15 severely ill patients were treated with triple-ostomy therapy, 3 (20%) having a systolic blood pressure below 80 mm Hg on admission and 11 (74%) having a systolic blood pressure below 90 mm Hg prior to operation despite aggressive management in the hospital. A mortality of 26% was noted for the whole group despite an earlier study noting an 87% mortality rate for similar patients in shock. Waterman et al. treated 10 patients confirmed at operation as having acute hemorrhagic pancreatitis with triple-ostomy and sump drainage of the pancreas and the lesser sac with a remarkable 10% mortality.[97] Several years later, Warshaw and Richter reported on triple-ostomy therapy, instituting this in approximately 5% of their patients.[96] Eleven patients judged clinically to be "dying" after 24 to 48 hours of supportive therapy had triple-ostomies and drainage performed. The predicted mortality for the group was 90%, based on previous experience, yet 81% rapidly improved with an ultimate mortality of only 36%. Ranson et al. expressed their concern that triple-ostomy therapy may lead to bacterial contamination of a susceptible necrotic pancreatic bed.[72] It has been well shown that in up to 30% of cases the gallbladder harbors bacteria under routine conditions,[17,41,42] further supporting Ranson's contention. McCarty and Dickerman reported on complications of triple-ostomy therapy in 40 patients (not every patient received the full triple decompression as outlined by Lawson).[57] An overall 55% mortality was noted, being 60% in those with acute hemorrhagic pancreatitis. Of 36 Stamm gastrostomies, 8 (22%) were inadequate, requiring supplemental nasogastric suction, and 3 patients (8.3%) developed peristomal abscesses requiring incision and drainage. Of 37 patients who had undergone cholecystostomy, 14 had a concomitant radiographic evaluation of the biliary tree via the drainage tube, this being normal in 57%. When 30 jejunostomy feeding tubes were placed, 9 (30%) were clamped and never used and 1 fell out immediately after surgery. In 33%, jejunostomy feedings were not tolerated because of vomiting. In two patients, the jejunostomy became the site of small bowel obstruction, and, most seriously, in one patient, it became the origin of myonecrosis of the abdominal wall leading eventually to death. In addition to these complications, 14 (35%) of the 40 triple-tube patients required reoperation for ongoing sepsis. We feel that one needs to compare critically the results of triple-ostomy and drainage (Table 6-6) to that obtained with drainage alone, drainage with peritoneal dialysis, and resectional therapy (see Tables 6-7 to 6-9).

Drainage Alone

One aspect of the controversy over triple-ostomy therapy has been whether the benefits of this procedure are derived from the extensive pancreatic drainage it provides with little benefit derived from the triple decompression procedure. Three retrospective studies on the use of drainage alone are reviewed here (see

TABLE 6-6. TRIPLE-OSTOMY THERAPY WITH DRAINAGE FOR SEVERE ACUTE PANCREATITIS

Investigator	Year	No. of Patients	Mortality (%)	Comments
Waterman[97]	1968	10	10	
Lawson[48]	1970	15	26	
Warshaw[96]	1974	11	36.4	
McCarty[57]	1982	40	55	60% in acute hemorrhagic pancreatitis
Total		76	41	

TABLE 6-7. RESULTS OF DRAINAGE WITH OR WITHOUT BILIARY DECOMPRESSION IN ACUTE NECROTIZING PANCREATITIS

Investigator	Year	No. of Patients	Mortality	Comments
Jordan[39]	1972	21	57%	
			50% drainage alone	
			50% drainage and cholecystectomy	
			50% drainage, cholecystectomy, and common bile duct exploration	
			100% drainage, gastrostomy, and feeding jejunostomy	
Gebhardt[26]	1981	63	59%	39% for resection
			72% drainage alone	All hemorrhagic necrotizing pancreatitis
			56% drainage and biliary decompression	
			45% drainage, irrigation, and biliary decompression	
Kivilaakso[44]	1981	42	69%	37% for resection
Total		126	62%	

TABLE 6-8. RESULTS OF RESECTIONAL THERAPY FOR ACUTE NECROTIZING OR HEMORRHAGIC PANCREATITIS

Investigator	Year	No. of Patients	Mortality (%)	Comments
Norton[66]	1974	4	25	All acute hemorrhagic pancreatitis with near total pancreatectomy
Edelman[20]	1974	187	39	10% mortality for sequestrectomy *early* once drainage failed
				Days in Hosp. prior to OR — Mortality (%)
				<3 — 47
				3–8 — 23
				>8 — 51
Kivilaakso[44]	1981	30	37	Nonoperative therapy, 96% mortality; operative drainage alone, 69% mortality
Hollender[35]	1981	49	37	67% mortality for proximal pancreaticoduodenectomy
Gebhardt[26]	1981	72	39	59% for drainage with or without biliary decompression
Aldridge[1]	1985	15	33	
Total		357	38	

TABLE 6-9. PERITONEAL DIALYSIS

Investigator	Year	No. of Patients	Mortality (%)
Ranson[75]	1974	103	83
Stone[85]	1980	70	15
Kauste[40]	1983	28	36
Mayer[56]	1985	91	27
Total		292	45

Table 6-7). The addition of biliary decompression when needed seemed to have little effect on outcome. The mortality rate in these studies is in the range of 60%. This rate appears prohibitively high compared with that for resectional therapy (see discussion below).

Resectional Therapy

Proponents of resectional therapy argue that the lowest mortality may be achieved not by drainage and/or decompression but rather by débridement or resection of necrotic pancreatic tissue. Proponents of resectional therapy for acute necrotizing pancreatitis do not, for the most part, disagree about total versus partial pancreatic resection. Their indications are based on the degree and extent of pancreatic necrosis found at laparotomy. Leger et al. noted that the surface changes often misrepresented the degree of central pancreatic necrosis present.[50] Nordbac et al. analyzed the histology slides of 54 patients who had undergone resection for acute disease.[64] Though all tissue debrided or resected was clinically identified as necrotic pancreatic tissue, they found that histologic evidence of parenchymal necrosis was present in from 0% to 100% of each resected specimen. Quite clearly, clinical visual examination of the mobilized pancreas by itself is inadequate. Based on these results, Nordbac et al. have suggested limiting resectional therapy to only the most extreme cases to avoid resection of normal tissue; other workers[2,35,44] have emphasized the importance of incising the pancreatic capsule to determine the true extent of the disease.

Once the pathologic lesion has been clearly delineated at laparotomy, the choice of resectional therapy includes débridement as in sequestrectomy for limited pancreatic necrosis or partial or subtotal pancreatectomy for extensive necrosis of the majority of the gland not including the head. For this type of pancreatic resection the reported overall mortality approximates 38% (see Table 6-8).

Peritoneal Dialysis

Advocates of peritoneal dialysis point to the markedly improved respiratory status of patients receiving this therapy as primary treatment in contrast to other therapeutic modalities (Table 6-9). Wall reported on peritoneal dialysis in acute pancreatitis in 1965.[94] Enzyme-rich toxic material elaborated by the pancreas undergoing parenchymal destruction would theoretically be eliminated via lavage prior to its absorption into the systemic circulation. Ranson and Spencer from New York University retrospectively categorized 103 patients with severe pancreatitis (three or more Ranson signs) into conservative therapy alone, percutaneous lavage, lavage via operatively placed catheters, and diagnostic operation without lavage.[73] Seventy percent of their patients were alcoholics, and all received ampicillin and nasogastric suction. There were no early deaths during the first 10 days in the lavage groups, while 45% of those in the nonlavage groups died during this period, most often from cardiovascular and respiratory failure. Unfortunately, late death secondary to sepsis and multisystem failure ensued in many in the lavage groups, and the overall mortality was comparable between the lavaged and nonlavaged groups, being 83% versus 84% respectively. Nonoperative patients had a 19% abscess rate, while those explored had a 68% incidence of abscess irrespective of whether or not they were lavaged. In conclusion, these data support the positive effects of peritoneal lavage in preventing early death while failing in the prevention of late pancreatic sepsis. Mayer et al., in a 1985 multicenter trial involving 24 hospitals, prospectively randomized 91 patients into peritoneal lavage within 38 hours of admission or supportive treatment.[56] The lavage group received 2 L of peritoneal lavage per hour for 3 days. All patients received nasogastric suction, intravenous fluid, plasma, and oxygen as needed. Here again, there was no difference in mortality between the control group and the lavage group, being 28% in each. The complication rates were also similar between the two groups. In light of these results, Mayer et al. have concluded that "the lavage did not appear to modify the survival rate, the incidence of pancreatic collections (pseudocyst or abscesses), or the plasma amylase concentration." They point to another unpublished study by several of the co-authors suggesting that enzymes are delivered to the systemic circulation via the lymphatics and veins draining the gland rather than by absorption from the peritoneal cavity. This contention is certainly consistent with their results in the present study.

In contrast, Kauste et al. studied 28 patients in whom lavage was the *primary* treatment in proven cases of acute necrotizing or hemorrhagic pancreatitis.[40] In addition to lavage, these patients received hyperalimentation in a surgical intensive care unit. The overall mortality was 36%. Lavage alone appeared effective in 20 of the 28 patients (71%) with an associated mortality of only 30%. Eight patients deteriorated despite primary lavage therapy, requiring a 60% to 90% pancreatic resection in each case with an overall 50% mortality. The authors also note that "a striking feature was observed in all patients. When the peritoneal lavage functioned properly, no respiratory failures were encountered," despite the fact that these patients all had severe pancreatitis by the criteria of Ranson. Stone and Fabian from Emory University School of Medicine randomized 70 patients with severe pancreatitis into initial supportive therapy or peritoneal dialysis therapy.[85] Of 34 patients initially treated by dialysis, only five (15%) died. In contrast, 23 (64%) of 36 patients treated by initial conservative therapy deteriorated to the point where, in 17 of these patients, peritoneal lavage was instituted as a "lifesaving measure." Of these 17 patients, 36% survived. These results as well as those of Kauste et al., in contrast to those of Mayer et al., support peritoneal dialysis as an effective primary therapy or adjunctive measure for patients with severe and/or necrotizing pancreatitis compared with supportive therapy. For those patients deteriorating despite this therapy, additional measures are required.

SUMMARY OF THE CONTROVERSIES OF THERAPY IN ACUTE NECROTIZING PANCREATITIS

While supportive therapy is an important part of the treatment of any patient with acute pancreatitis, it appears to be inadequate for those with severe and/or necrotizing pancreatitis. A mortality rate in this setting approaching 80% to 100% has been noted for conservative therapy. With the exception of Ranson, a 15% to 36% mortality rate (Table 6-9) for patients with severe acute pancreatitis treated by peritoneal dialysis has been achieved. This is a satisfactory result and, in each series, represented a marked advantage over conservative therapy. Certainly in the British experience, where severity assessment is most often via a peritoneal tap, the immediate institution of peritoneal dialysis using the same catheter, in those assessed as high risk, is relatively simple. The American experience of clinical and laboratory severity assessment, as championed by Ranson, makes peritoneal dialysis an additional and invasive component of therapy. However, the studies discussed above, several of which show a significant improvement in the survival of patients with lavage therapy, should not be ignored. We believe that initial lavage therapy should be considered in all high-risk patients to help decrease the risk of the development of respiratory insufficiency. In those who then go on to show signs of deterioration, early operative intervention should be entertained with resectional therapy based on the location and extent of disease. This, hopefully, would avoid the late mortality demonstrated by Ranson. Routine application of triple-ostomy therapy or drainage alone appears to be unsatisfactory.

THERAPY FOR COMPLICATIONS

Pancreatic Pseudocyst and Abscess

Controversies surrounding these are discussed in detail in Chapters 11 and 12.

Acute Ascites and Hydrothorax

The indications and timing of conservative versus interventional therapy for ascites and hydrothorax secondary to acute pancreatitis is controversial. Peritoneal and retroperitoneal collections as well as their extensions into the chest, mediastinum, neck, scrotum, and so forth, are most often innocuous unless secondary to the rupture of a pancreatic pseudocyst. This rupture releases the previously contained fluid rich in enzymes and toxic material (see Chapter 12). In the experience of Cameron et al., 80% of ascitic collections were secondary to such a rupture, 10% were classified as idiopathic, and 10% had no identified cause.[11,12] In approximately 50% of cases, the ascites clears permanently within 2 weeks of the institution of paracentesis, nasogastric suction, hyperalimentation, acetazolamide (Diamox), and atropine therapy. Approximately 20% of the patients so treated, however, had fatal complications such as gastrointestinal bleeding, hyperalimentation catheter sepsis, and unexplained sudden death. Based on these results, Cameron et al. advise a 3-week trial of the outlined therapy. For nonresponders they advise surgical correction with the actual therapy guided by the results of preoperative endoscopic retrograde cholangiopancreatography (ERCP). Weaver et al.[98] also suggest therapeutic paracentesis, reporting results similar to those of Cameron et al.

Hydrothorax in this setting is simply an extension of the collected fluid into the chest; as with ascites, treatment is aimed at the pancreatic source. For hydrothorax, therapy similar to that outlined above for ascites will result in a 60% success rate.[12] In those in whom therapy fails, ERCP and surgery upon the pancreas are undertaken as noted above.

Intestinal Obstruction

Bradley and Clements noted 9 cases of duodenal obstruction among 878 cases of acute pancreatitis (1.0%).[8] In each case, the duodenal mucosa was proved intact by endoscopy performed to rule out tumor as the cause of the pancreatitis. Four of these patients (44%) had sudden onset of duodenal obstruction during the acute phase, all resolving spontaneously within 3 weeks. The other five patients (56%) had an insidious onset of duodenal obstruction felt to be secondary to chronic fibrosis. No obstruction in this group resolved spontaneously within 4 weeks despite restriction of oral intake and hyperalimentation, a bypass procedure being required in each case. Hunt and Mildenhall reviewed the pathologic findings on 13 cases of proven obstruction of the transverse colon; all were due to ischemia.[37] Of 13, 12 were at or just proximal to the splenic flexure, the area most commonly involved in ischemic colitis of any cause. Certainly ileus and transient or permanent obstruction may occur, varying in the degree of ischemia and its resolution. Here, as in ischemic colitis, expectant therapy is employed, with operative treatment undertaken as indicated.

Intestinal Fistula

Should intestinal fistulas secondary to acute pancreatitis be treated expectantly or surgically? Intestinal fistulization, most commonly from a pancreatic abscess, occurs, though infrequently. Decompression of the abscess cavity is often incomplete. Mason et al., reporting on seven cases of proven intestinal fistulization, found that in three cases, the abscess cavity required further surgical drainage and débridement.[55] In addition, internal fistulization was associated with gastrointestinal hemorrhage, occurring in one of the seven patients of Mason et al. (see the discussion on hemorrhage below and the discussion on pancreatic abscess and pseudocyst in Chapters 11 and 12).

Hemorrhage

The mode of therapy and the role of angiography are controversial. Hemorrhage occurs most often after drainage of an infected pancreatic pseudocyst. However, the occasional erosion of a major peripancreatic artery, probably by enzymatic pseudoaneurysm formation, has also been reported.[83] Well-controlled studies on the use of angiography, embolization, and/or surgery in this setting are lacking. Stabile et al. found that preoperative angiography routinely identified the offending vessel.[83] Warshaw and Richter noted the site of bleeding to be the splenic, gastroduodenal, or inferior pancreaticoduodenal arteries in 45%, 17%, and 11% of cases, respectively.[96] They noted that isolated reports of nonoperative control of bleeding via transcatheter embolization are available, but in general, definitive surgical therapy is still advised. Postoperative hemorrhage carried the worst prognosis, with a 60% mortality compared with 34% mortality for spontaneous bleeding. Also, bleeding in the region of the head of the pancreas, with its abundant collateral blood supply, carried a 43% mortality compared with a 16% mortality for bleeding from the body and tail of the gland with its limited blood supply and greater possibility for resectional therapy.

CONTROVERSIES IN THE PREVENTION OF RECURRENCE

The timing of interventional therapy in gallstone pancreatitis and pancreatic divisum are the subject of Chapters 7 and 8. But what of the alcoholic patient with acute relapsing pancreatitis? Debate exists about the role of vagotomy, with or without an associated drainage procedure, versus behavior modification in the prevention of recurrences in acute alcoholic pancreatitis. Efforts in these and other alcoholic patients to reduce or eliminate alcohol ingestion have failed miserably. Thompson et al.[88] report a 51% recurrence rate among 61 patients; this high rate was also reported by Satiani and Stone.[79] Three clinical studies on surgical therapy to prevent recurrences are available from our review of the literature. McCleery et al. reported on vagotomy without an associated drainage procedure in the management of recurrent acute pancreatitis.[58] In each case, recurrent attacks had been recorded over a 2- to 10-year period. During a 13-month median follow-up period, improvement was noted in all patients. Of 11 patients, 10 had resumed work, the last patient suffering from tuberculosis. A concomitant 2- to 70-lb weight gain was noted (mean 22.8 lb).

In separate studies, Stone et al.[86] and Pradhan et al.[70] performed vagotomy and antrectomy with Billroth II reconstruction in an attempt to prevent recurrence of disease. The hypothesized benefit of this procedure is the elimination of acid and alcohol contact with the duodenal mucosa that might hormonally stimulate pancreatic secretion. Both studies were limited to patients with alcohol-induced pancreatitis. Pradhan et al. studied 14 patients so treated with a median 4-year follow-up.[70] Five patients (35.7%) were classified as having a good result with no recurrence or complication. Six patients (42.8%) were classified as having a fairly good result without recurrence, but other complications of alcohol abuse including cirrhosis, pancreatic insufficiency, and malnutrition became manifest. Lastly, three patients (21.4%) had a fair result, with two cases of a mild transient relapse and one case of severe hemorrhagic pancreatitis. Stone et al., in a well-controlled prospective randomized study, segregated 66 patients into an operative therapy group receiving a truncal vagotomy and Billroth II gastrectomy or a control group given intensive encouragement to abstain from alcohol.[86] Of the patients included for study, 80% had had relapses of acute pancreatitis in an average of 14 months. At 24-month follow-up, a marked difference was noted in the recurrence rates of the two groups ($p < .001$). The recurrence rate remained unchanged in the control-encouragement group (73%). In marked contrast, only 2 of 31 patients (6%) developed recurrence within 24 months in the group treated surgically. Two patients in this group were lost to follow-up, but, even including these as recurrences, marked improvement was achieved.

Although these results seem promising, at the present time vagotomy with or without an associated drainage procedure should only be carried out in an experimental setting.

REFERENCES

1. Aldridge MC, Orenstein N, Glazer G, Dudley HA. Pancreatic resection for severe acute pancreatitis. Br J Surg 72:796–800, 1985.
2. Baden H, Jordal K, Lund F. Prophylactic and curative action of Trasylol in pancreatitis. A double-blind trial. Scand J Gastroenterol 4:291–295, 1969.
3. Bank S, Wise L, Gersten M. Risk factors in acute pancreatitis. Am J Gastroenterol 78(10):637–640, 1983.
4. Baudendistel L, Dahms TE, Kaminski DL. The effect of albumin on extravascular water in animals and patients with low pressure pulmonary edema. J Surg Res 33(4):285–293, 1982.
5. Becker V. Acute pancreatitis: Pathological anatomy and pathogenesis. World J Surg 5(3):303–313, 1981.
6. Beger HG, Bittner R, Block S, Buchler M. Bacterial contamination of pancreatic necrosis. A prospective clinical study. Gastroenterology 91(2):433–438, 1986.
7. Bivins BA, Bell RM, Rapp RP, Toedebusch WH. Pancreatic exocrine response to parenteral nutrition. JPEN 8:34–36, 1984.
8. Bradley EL III, Clements JL. Idiopathic duodenal obstruction. An unappreciated complication of pancreatitis. Ann Surg 193:636–648, 1981.
9. Bradley JA, Bradley P, and McMahon MJ. Diagnostic peritoneal lavage in acute pancreatitis—The role of microscopy of the lavage fluid. Br J Surg 68:245–246, 1981.
10. Broe PJ, Zinner MJ, Cameron JL. A clinical trial of cimetidine in acute pancreatitis. Surg Gynecol Obstet 154:13–16, 1982.
11. Cameron JL, Anderson RP, Zuidema GD. Pancreatitic ascites. Surg Gynecol Obstet. 125:328–332, 1967.
12. Cameron JL, Brawley RK, Bender HW, Zuidema GD. The treatment of pancreatic ascites. Ann Surg 170:668–676, 1969.

13. Cameron JL, Mehigan D, Zuidema GD. Evaluation of atropine in acute pancreatitis. Surg Gynecol Obstet 148:206–208, 1979.
14. Corfield AP, Cooper MJ, Williamson RC, et al. Prediction of severiity in acute pancreatitis: A comparison of the prognostic indices. Lancet 2(8452):403–407, 1985.
15. Cuschieri A, Wood RA, Cumming JR, Meehan SE, Mackie CR. Treatment of acute pancreatitis with fresh frozen plasma. Br J Surg 70(12):710–712, 1983.
16. Debas HT, Hacock AJ, Soon-Shiong P, Smythe HA, Cassim NM. Glucagon therapy in acute pancreatitis: Prospective randomized double-blind study. Can J Surg 23(6):578–580, 1980.
17. Delikaris PG, Michail PO, Klonis GD, et al. Biliary bacteriology based on intraoperative bile culture. Am J Gastroenterol 68:51–55, 1977.
18. Durr HK, Maroske D, Zelder O, Bode JC. Glucagon therapy in acute pancreatitis. A report of a double-blind trial. Gut 19:175–179, 1978.
19. Ebbehoj N, Friis J, Svendsen LB, Bulow S, Madsen P. Indomethacin treatment of acute pancreatitis. Scand J Gastroenterol 20(7):798–800, 1985.
20. Edelman G, Boutelier PH. Le traitement des pancreatitis aigues, necrosantes par l'ablation chirugicale précoce des portions necrosées. Chirurgie 100:155–167, 1974.
21. Field BF, Hepner GW, Shabot MM, et al. Nasogastric suction in alcoholic pancreatitis. Dig Dis Sci 24:339–344, 1979.
22. Finch WT, Sawyers JL, Schenker J. A prospective study to determine the efficacy of antibiotics in acute pancreatitis. Ann Surg 183:667–671, 1976.
23. Fischer RP, Beverlin BC, Engrav LH, et al. Diagnostic peritoneal lavage, fourteen years and 2586 patients later. Am J Surg 136:701–704, 1978.
24. Foster PD, Ziffren SE. Severe acute pancreatitis. Arch Surg 85:252–259, 1962.
25. Fuller RK, Loveland JP, Frankel MH. An evaluation of the efficacy of nasogastric suction treatment in alcoholic pancreatitis. Am J Gastroenterol 75:349–353, 1981.
26. Gebhard C, Gall FP. Importance of peritoneal irrigation after surgical treatment of hemorrhagic necrotizing pancreatitis. World J Surg 5:379–385, 1981.
27. Gilsanz V, Oteyza CP, Rebollar JL. Glucagon vs. anticholinergics in the treatment of acute pancreatitis. A double-blind controlled trial. Arch Intern Med 138:535–538, 1978.
28. Gliedman ML, Bolooki H, Rosen RG. Acute pancreatitis. Curr Prob Surg 7:1–52, 1970.
29. Goebel H, Ammann R, Herfarth C, Horn J. A double-blind trial of synthetic salmon calcitonin in the treatment of acute pancreatitis. Scand J Gastroenterol 14:881–9, 1979.
30. Goff JS, Feinberg LE, Brugge WR. A randomized trial comparing cimetidine to nasogastric suction in acute pancreatitis. Dig Dis Sci 27:1085–1088, 1982.
31. Goodgame TT, Fisher JF. Parenteral nutrition in the treatment of acute pancreatitis: Effects on complications and mortality. Ann Surg 186:651–658, 1977.
32. Grana W, Wise L. Role of emergency laparotomy in acute pancreatitis. Ann Surg 43:128–134, 1976.
33. Grundfest S, Steiger E, Selinkoff P, Fletcher J. The effect of intravenous fat emulsions in patients with pancreatic fistula. JPEN 4:27–31, 1980.
34. Grundmann R, Heistermann S. Postoperative albumin infusion therapy based on colloid osmotic pressure. A prospectively randomized trial. Arch Surg 120(8):911–915, 1985.
35. Hollender LF, Meyer C, Marrie A, Costa JdaS, Castellana JG. Role of surgery in the management of acute pancreatitis. World J Surg 5:361–368, 1981.
36. Howes R, Zuidema GD, Cameron J. Evaluation of prophylactic antibiotics in acute pancreatitis. J Surg Res 18(2):197–200, 1975.
37. Hunt DR, Mildenhall P. Etiology of strictures of the colon associated with pancreatitis. Am J Dig Dis 20:941–946, 1975.
38. Imrie CW, Benjamin IS, Ferguson JC, et al. A single-centre double blind trial of Trasylol therapy in primary acute pancreatitis. Br J Surg 65:337–341, 1978.
39. Jordan GL, Spjut HJ. Hemorrhagic pancreatitis. Arch Surg 104:489–493, 1972.
40. Kauste A, Hocherstedt K, Ahonen J, Tervaskari H. Peritoneal lavage as a primary treatment in acute fulminant pancreatitis. Surg Gynecol Obstet 156:458–463, 1983.

41. Keighley MRB. Microorganisms in bile. A preventable cause of sepsis after biliary surgery. Ann R Coll Surg Eng. 59:328–334, 1977.
42. Keighley MRB, McLeish AR, Bishop HM, et al. Identification of the presence and type of biliary microflora by immediate gram stains. Surgery 81:469–72, 1977.
43. Kellum JM Jr, DeMeester TR, Elkins RC. Respiratory insufficiency secondary to acute pancreatitis. Ann Surg 175:657–662, 1972.
44. Kivilaakso E, Fraki O, Nakki P, Lempinen M. Resection of the pancreas for acute fulminant pancreatitis. Surg Gynecol Obstet 152(4):493–498, 1981.
45. Klein E, Shnebaum S, Ben-Ari G, Dreiling DA. Effects of total parenteral nutrition on exocrine pancreatic secretion. Am J Gastroenterol 78:31–33, 1983.
46. Kronborg O, Bülow S, Joergensen PM, Svendsen LB. A randomized double-blind trial of glucagon in the treatment of first attack of severe acute pancreatitis without associated biliary disease. Am J Gastroenterol 73:423–425, 1980.
47. Lange P, Pederson T. Initial treatment of acute pancreatitis. Surg Gynecol Obstet 157:332–334, 1983.
48. Lawson DW, Daggit WM, Civetta JM, et al. Surgical treatment of acute necrotizing pancreatitis. Ann Surg 172:605–617, 1970.
49. Lawson TL. Acute pancreatitis and its complications. Computerized tomography and sonography. Radiol Clin North Am Sept 21(3):495–513, 1983.
50. Leger L, Chiche B, Louvel A. Pancreatic necrosis and acute pancreatitis. World J Surg 5:315–317, 1981.
51. Levant JA, Secrist DM, Resin H, et al. Nasogastric suction in the treatment of alcoholic pancreatitis. A controlled study. JAMA 229:51–52, 1974.
52. Loiudice TA, Lang J, Mehta H, Banta L. Treatment of acute alcoholic pancreatitis. The role of cimetidine and nasogastric suction. Am J Gastroenterol 79(7):553–558, 1984.
53. Martin DT, Kopolvic R, Grower WR, et al. Crystalloid vs. colloid resuscitation in experimental hemorrhagic pancreatitis. Surg Gynecol and Obstet 159:445–9, 1984.
54. Martinez E, Inaverrete F. A controlled trial of synthetic salmon calcitonin in the treatment of severe acute pancreatitis. World J Surg 8(3):354–359, 1984.
55. Mason DW, Forgash A, Balch HH. Internal fistula complicating pancreatic abscess. Surg Gynecol Obstet 140:39–43, 1975.
56. Mayer AD, McMahon MJ, Corfield AP, et al. Controlled clinical trial of peritoneal lavage for the treatment of severe acute pancreatitis. N. Engl J Med 312:399–404, 1985.
57. McCarty MC, Dickerman RM. Surgical management of severe acute pancreatitis. Arch Surg 117:476–480, 1982.
58. McCleery RS, Kesterson JE, Schaffarzick WR. A clinical study of the effect of vagotomy on recurrent acute pancreatitis. Surgery 30:131–145, 1951.
59. Medical Research Council. Death from acute pancreatitis. Medical Research Council multicentre trial of glucagon and aprotinin. Lancet Sept 24:632–635, 1977.
60. Meshkinpour H, Mollinari MD, Gardner L, et al. Cimetidine in the treatment of acute alcoholic pancreatitis. Gastroenterology 77:687–690, 1979.
61. Miller JM. Trasylol in acute pancreatitis. Br J Surg 65:887–888, 1978.
62. Moynihan B. Acute pancreatitis. Ann Surg 81:132–142, 1925.
63. Naeije R, Salingret E, Clumeck N, de Troyer A, Davis G. Is nasogastric suction necessary in acute pancreatitis? Br Med J 2:659–660, 1978.
64. Nordbac I, Pess T, Auvinen O, Autio V. Determination of necrosis in necrotizing pancreatitis. Br J Surg 72:225–227, 1985.
65. Nordestgaard AG, Wilson SE, Williams RA. Early computerized tomography as a predictor of outcome in acute pancreatitis. Am J Surg 152:127–132, 1986.
66. Norton L, Eisman B. Near total pancreatectomy for hemorrhagic pancreatitis. Am J Surg 127:191–195, 1974.
67. Pace BW, Bank S, Wise L, Burson LC, Borrero E. Amylase isoenzymes in the acute abdomen: An adjunct in those patients with elevated total amylase. Am J Gastroenterol 80(11):898–901, 1985.
68. Parkash O. A statistical and clinical evaluation of the efficacy of the enzyme inhibitor Trasylol in the treatment of acute forms of pancreatitis. Digestion 7:200–226, 1972.

69. Pollock AV. Acute pancreatitis—analysis of 100 patients. Br Med J 1:6–14, 1959.
70. Pradhan DJ, Leveque HL, Juanteguy JM, Seligman AM. The role of vagotomy, antrectomy and BII gastroenterostomy in the treatment of alcoholic pancreatitis. Am J Surg 124:21–27, 1972.
71. Rackow EC, Falk JL, Fein IA, Siegal JS. Fluid resuscitation in circulatory shock: A comparison of the cardiorespiratory effects of albumin, hetastarch and saline solutions in patients with hypovolemic and septic shock. Crit Care Med 11(11):839–850, 1983.
72. Ranson JHC, Riffkind KM, Roses DF, et al. Prognostic signs and the role of operative management in acute pancreatitis. Surg Gynecol Obstet 139:69–81, 1974.
73. Ranson JHC, Spencer FC. The role of peritoneal lavage in acute pancreatitis. Ann Surg 187:565–575, 1978.
74. Ranson JHC, Spencer FC. Prevention, diagnosis and treatment of pancreatic abscess. Surgery 82(1):99–106, 1977.
75. Ranson JHC, Turner JW, Roses DF, Rifkind KM, Spencer FC. Respiratory complications in acute pancreatitis. Ann Surg 179:557–566, 1974.
76. Regan PT, Malagelada JR, Go VL, Wolf AM, DiMagno EP. A prospective study of the antisecretory and therapeutic effects of cimetidine and glucagon in human acute pancreatitis. Mayo Clin Proc 56:499–503, 1981.
77. Sanfey H, Broe PJ, Cameron JL. Experimental ischemic pancreatitis: Treatment with albumin. Am J Surg 150(3):297–330, 1985.
78. Sarr MG, Sanfey H, Cameron JL. Prospective randomized trial of nasogastric suction in patients with acute pancreatitis. Surgery 100(3):500–504, 1986.
79. Satiani B, Stone HH. Predictability of present outcome and future recurrence in acute pancreatitis. Arch Surg 114:711–716, 1979.
80. Sax HC, Warner BW, Talamani MA, et al. Early total parenteral nutrition in acute pancreatitis: Lack of beneficial effects. Am J Surg 1:117–124, 1987.
81. Sheldon GF, Way LW. Surgical metabolism and nutrition. In: Way LW, ed. *Current Surgical Diagnosis and Treatment.* Los Angeles, Lange Medical Publications, 1985, p 149.
82. Silberman H, Dixon NP, Eisenberg D. The safety and efficacy of a lipid-based system of parenteral nutrition in acute pancreatitis. Am J Gastroenterol 77:494–497, 1982.
83. Stabile BE, Wilson SE, Debas HT. Reduced mortality from bleeding pseudocysts and pseudoaneurysms caused by pancreatitis. Arch Surg 118:45–51, 1983.
84. Standfield NJ. Prostaglandins and acute pancreatitis—Experimental and clinical studies. Br J Surg 70(10):573–576, 1983.
85. Stone HH, Fabian TC. Peritoneal dialysis in the treatment of acute alcoholic pancreatitis. Surg Gynecol Obstet 150:878–882, 1980.
86. Stone HH, Mullins RJ, Scovill WA. Vagotomy plus Billroth II gastrectomy for the prevention of recurrent alcohol-induced pancreatitis. Ann Surg 201(6):684–689, 1985.
87. Svenson JO. Role of intravenously infused insulin in the treatment of acute pancreatitis. A double-blind study. Scand J Gastroenterol 10:487–490, 1975.
88. Thompson JA, Durich JR, et al. Relapsing pancreatitis in alcoholic and nonalcoholic patients. Surgery 42:841–845, 1957.
89. Trapnell JE. The natural history and prognosis of acute pancreatitis. Ann Coll Surg Engl 38:265–287, 1966.
90. Trapnell JE, Anderson MC. Role of early laparotomy in acute pancreatitis. Ann Surg 165(1):49–55, 1967.
91. Trapnell JE, Rigby CC, Talbot CH. A controlled trial of Trasylol in the treatment of acute pancreatitis. Br J Surg 61:177–182, 1974.
92. Trapnell JE, Talbot CH, Copper WM. Trasylol in acute pancreatitis. Am J Dig Dis 12:409–412, 1967.
93. Tykka HT, Vaittinen EJ, Mahlberg KL, et al. A randomized double-blind study using $CaNa_{2EDTA}$, a phospholipase A2 inhibitor, in the management of human pancreatitis. Scand J Gastroenterol 20(1):5–12, 1985.
94. Wall AJ. Peritoneal dialysis in the treatment of severe acute pancreatitis. Med J Aust 2:281–283, 1965.

95. Warshaw AL, Imbembo AL, Civetta JM, et al. Surgical intervention in acute necrotizing pancreatitis. Am J Surg 127:484–491, 1974.
96. Warshaw AL, Richter JM. A practical guide to pancreatitis. Curr Probl Surg 21(12):1–79, 1984.
97. Waterman NG, Walsky R, Kasdan ML, et al. The treatment of acute hemorrhagic pancreatitis by sump drainage. Surg Gynecol Obstet 126:963–971, 1968.
98. Weaver DW, Walt AJ, Sugawa C, Bouwman DL. A continuing appraisal of pancreatic ascites. Surg Gynecol Obstet 154:845–848, 1982.

CHAPTER

7

THE TIMING OF INTERVENTIONAL THERAPY IN GALLSTONE PANCREATITIS

John H. C. Ranson

EDITORIAL COMMENT (Chapters 7 and 8)

The timing of surgical removal of gallstones in patients with "acute obstructive pancreatitis" is currently in a state of flux. Although it is now universally agreed that stone removal should be carried out during the initial hospitalization and not delayed for 2 to 3 months, it is the timing, either *early* or *intermediate*, and method of treatment that are currently controversial. Dr. Classen and his colleagues, who are extremely adept at therapeutic endoscopy, advocate immediate or early ERCP to determine whether a stone is present in the common bile duct, and extraction if present, and are not perturbed by injection of contrast material into the pancreatic duct. Others advocate early surgical removal (i.e., within 72 hours of admission) of impacted stones. Dr. Ranson points out that when the patient's clinical course or laboratory studies lead to uncertainty about the diagnosis, and when life-threatening extrapancreatic disease (such as perforated peptic ulcer or gangrenous cholecystitis) cannot be reasonably excluded, emergency celiotomy is required. Otherwise he recommends avoiding early intervention because of the increased morbidity and mortality, allowing the pancreatitis to subside and performing exploration late during the same hospital admission (intermediate approach).

Most studies of early intervention have either no controls or historical controls only and do not stratify the severity of the pancreatitis according to early prognostic signs or clinical criteria, or any of the other risk factors (see chapter 3). Thus, mortality rates of 0% to 1% in the early endoscopic or surgical intervention series suggest that the patients have very mild pancreatitis at the onset and mortality rates of 16% to 40% for the intermediate therapy probably indicate more severely ill patients. Patients with high amylase levels but no risk factors or CT changes can be operated on at any time and if symptoms should get worse, be treated emergently. It seems clear that successful removal of stones either endoscopically or surgically may still be followed by a continuing severe pancreatitis. However, the bottom line is that a large multicenter control trial is needed addressing endoscopic or surgical therapy, the timing of such therapy, and, most importantly, the mortality related to the severity of the initial attack. The only such trial from Liverpool tends to support a lower mortality with early endoscopic intervention, although it is not statistically significant.

CONTROVERSY

Recent studies have suggested that urgent removal of common duct stones may prevent a deterioration or ameliorate an attack of acute pancreatitis. Stone removal may be surgical or endoscopic and may have a very low mortality. Most studies have been either uncontrolled or have used historical controls and have not compared the severity of the individual attacks. One study used severity scores and seems to favor early stone removal. On the other hand, some pancreatologists and surgeons favor an approach of allowing the pancreatitis to improve and then investigating for stones and removing them during the same hospital admission. Endoscopic therapists have achieved excellent results in the management of acute calculous cholangitis, but their role in gallstone pancreatitis is less clear.

The association of gallstones with acute pancreatitis has been recognized at least since the end of the 19th century[41] and was firmly established by the work of Opie.[35] He suggested first that pancreatic inflammation was initiated by obstruction of the pancreatic duct by a gallstone. Later he proposed that reflux of bile into the pancreatic duct following obstruction of a common biliary and pancreatic channel was responsible for pancreatitis.[36] The more recent studies of Acosta and Ledesma[1] and Kelly[23] have demonstrated that gallstones can be identified in the stool of 85% to 94% of patients with gallstone-associated pancreatitis. Furthermore, the occurrence of gallstone pancreatitis has been reported to be associated with the presence of a large cystic duct, the presence of small, light gallstones, and the frequent presence of a common biliary and pancreatic channel.[23,31,51] While it seems probable that pancreatitis is initiated by passage of a gallstone through the ampulla of Vater, it is not clear whether the injury is related to obstruction of the pancreatic duct[1,41,53] or to the consequences of obstruction of a common biliary and pancreatic channel.[8,14,20,36,39,40] Acosta has suggested that the severity of pancreatic inflammation may be related to the duration of ampullary obstruction.[2] However, the incidence of persistent choledocholithiasis in a collected series of 1005 patients undergoing biliary surgery after subsidence of pancreatitis ranged from 8% to 48% (average 21%).[19] This, combined with the finding of stones in the stool, suggests that in most patients, ampullary obstruction is transient.

Whatever the mechanisms by which cholelithiasis initiates pancreatic inflammation, gallstones are present in approximately 60% of nonalcoholic patients with acute pancreatitis. Interventional measures may be considered in these patients for four general purposes: (1) diagnosis, (2) to ameliorate pancreatic inflammation or prevent its sequelae, (3) to treat complications of pancreatitis, and (4) to prevent recurrent pancreatitis. In clinical settings, it is often impossible to separate these objectives. However, this classification is convenient for purposes of discussion. Intervention to treat complications of acute pancreatitis is necessary most commonly for management of pancratic abscess or pseudocysts and is beyond the scope of the present discussion.

DIAGNOSIS

From a practical clinical viewpoint, a diagnosis of acute pancreatitis can be arrived at with reasonable certainty in most patients on the basis of routine clinical, radiographic, and biochemical features. In those with known or suspected cholelithiasis, the differentiation of acute pancreatitis from acute biliary disease with hyperamylasemia is usually of little consequence since both conditions generally respond well to standard noninterventional treatment. In some patients, however, it is impossible to differentiate acute pancreatitis from other acute life-threatening conditions such as obstructive cholangitis, mesenteric infarction, or gangrenous cholecystitis. These patients may require diagnostic celiotomy. In this regard, it should be stressed that strong positive evidence of pancreatitis, such as findings on computed tomography (CT), does not exclude concomitent life-threatening extrapancreatic disease in an occasional patient.

In patients with known or suspected cholelithiasis and possible pancreatitis, it may be important to exclude obstructive cholangitis or gangrenous cholecystitis. In most cases, a rapid response to standard therapy makes life-threatening biliary disease a remote possibility. However, if the patient is severely ill or does not respond rapidly to noninvasive treatment, accurate anatomic information about the status of the biliary tree may be essential. Available methods for this purpose include ultrasonography, oral cholecystography, intravenous cholangiography, ^{99m}Tc HIDA scans, endoscopic cholangiography, and percutaneous transhepatic cholangiography. Ultrasonography is valuable in patients with acute pancreatitis for demonstration of possible cholelithiasis. In addition, the ultrasonographic demonstration of distension of the gallbladder and thickening of its wall may suggest acute cholecystitis. Unfortunately, these findings are frequently seen in acute pancreatitis without true intrinsic acute cholecystitis. Ultrasonic techniques do not provide reliable information about possible choledocholithiasis. Successful visualization of the gallbladder by oral cholecystography requires absorption, excretion, and concentration of the contrast material in the gallbladder, and this is rarely possible in acutely ill patients. Intravenous cholangiography has been successful in visualizing a portion of the biliary tree in 65% of patients with acute pancreatitis in whom this study was undertaken during the first 7 days of treatment.[21] However, delineation of the common duct is often incomplete, and it is often the most severely ill patients in whom visualization is poorest. Biliary scanning techniques are usually valuable in determining the patency of the cystic duct. However, in patients with acute pancreatitis, the gallbladder may fail to visualize without intrinsic cholecystitis[13] or even cholelithiasis.

Endoscopic retrograde cholangiography provides excellent visualization of the biliary anatomy but may be complicated by exacerbation of pancreatitis or even the introduction of contaminated contrast material into devitalized pancreatic tissue. Percutaneous transhepatic cholangiography using current techniques provides excellent visualization of the biliary tree. It does not depend on hepatic function or require instrumentation of the ampulla of Vater. The reported success of this technique in visualizing the nonobstructed biliary tree is 70% and rises to 99% in the presence of biliary dilation.[15,50] Complications such as bleeding, bile leakage, or cholangitis may occur in 3% of patients, and it is clear that this technique should not be used unless adequate information cannot be achieved by safer noninvasive methods and the benefits of the information sought justify the potential morbidity. I have, however, found this technique to be a valuable measure in a small, highly selected group of patients. Table 7-1 shows the clinical and laboratory data in a group of 14 patients who had cholelithiasis in whom percutaneous transhepatic cholangiography was undertaken. Nine patients eventually were demonstrated to have acute pancreatitis with gallstones, and five had acute biliary disease without evidence of pancreatitis. The similarity of the two groups is emphasized by the data shown. Figure 7-1 shows the cholangiographic findings in a patient who was thought clinically to require diagnostic celiotomy for possible life-threatening biliary disease. Following this study, the patient was successfully managed by early nonoperative means for severe acute gallstone pancreatitis. Conversely, in patients with cystic or common duct obstruction, this study allows appropriate management of potentially life-threatening biliary pathologic lesions. It must, however, be emphasized that this study is appropriate only in a very small, severely ill group of patients.

When chemical, biochemical, and radiographic features or the patient's course lead to significant uncertainty concerning the diagnosis, celiotomy is required to exclude or treat life-threatening extrapancreatic disease. When uncomplicated acute pancreatitis is found at early diagnostic celiotomy, I believe that the surgical procedure should be limited to careful exploration of the abdominal cavity to exclude other pathologic lesions. Drains should not be placed in the area of the pancreas since they seem to increase the risk of late pancreatic sepsis. However, a soft intraperitoneal catheter may be left for peritoneal lavage in the postoperative period.[43]

In patients who are found to have acute pancreatitis and cholelithiasis at early diagnostic celiotomy, definitive correction of biliary pathologic lesions can usually be accomplished safely at that time if the acute pancreatitis is mild. Such

TABLE 7-1. MEAN VALUES AND RANGE OF CLINICAL AND LABORATORY DATA IN PATIENTS WITH ACUTE PANCREATITIS OR ACUTE BILIARY DISEASE AT HOSPITAL ADMISSION

	Acute Pancreatitis		Acute Biliary Disease	
	Mean	**Range**	**Mean**	**Range**
Age (years)	66	44–88	55	28–88
Temperature (°F)	99.3	97–102.2	100.5	99–104
White cell count mm^3	14,300	10,900–20,400	9900	8300–12,100
Serum amylase (SU%)	3242	69–6920	2084	800–3000
Serum bilirubin (mg %)	1.8	0.8–6.4	4.4	0.6–9.2
Serum alkaline phosphatase (IU %)	126	70–236	227	158–284
Aspartate aminotransferase (SFU %)	215	28–788	168	55–304
Serum lactic dehyrogenase (IU/L)	359	160–696	390	116–1012

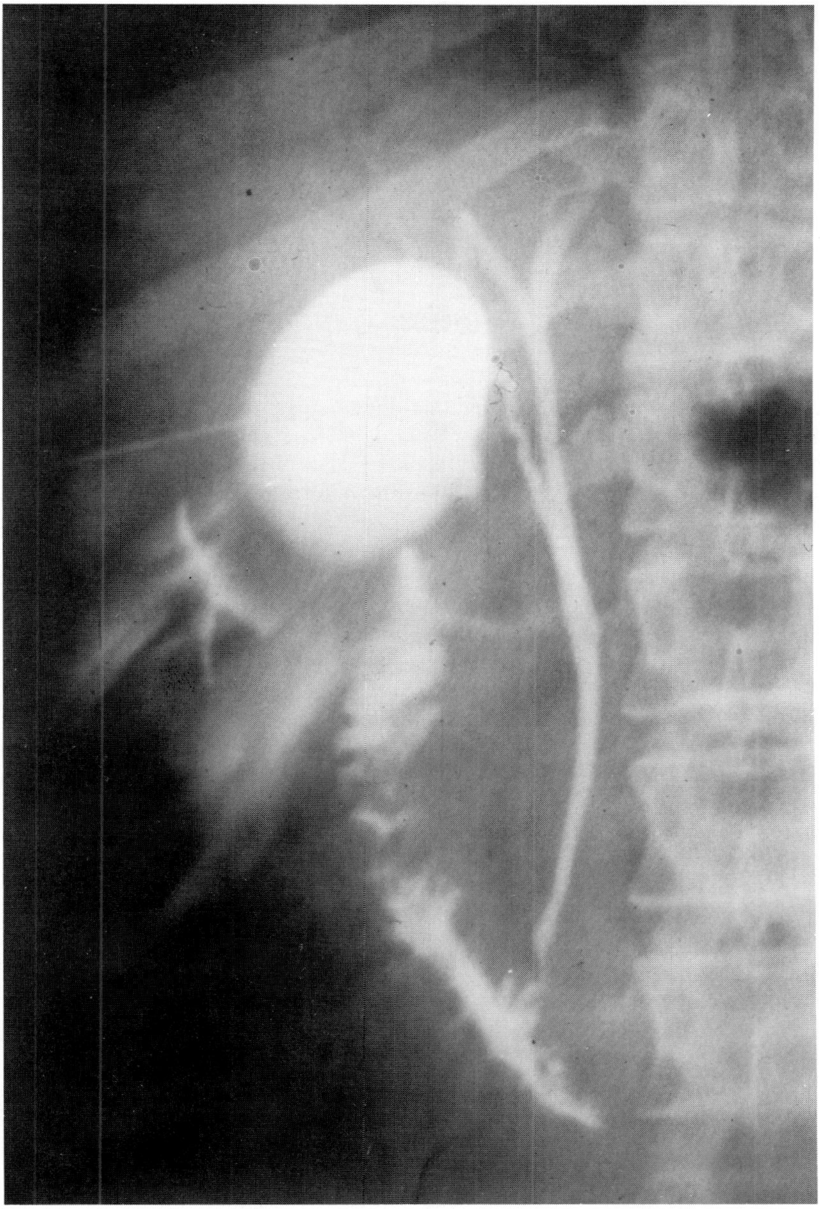

Figure 7-1. Percutaneous transhepatic Chiba needle cholangiogram in a patient with acute pancreatitis and gallstones revealing marked narrowing of the distal common bile duct with widening of the duodenal sweep.

surgery does not, in my experience, ameliorate the course of acute pancreatitis, but it does avoid the need for further treatment to prevent recurrent gallstone pancreatitis.[42] In patients who are found to have severe acute pancreatitis and gallstones at early celitomy, I prefer to limit biliary surgery to cholecystostomy and cholangiography. Definitive biliary surgery at this time has, in my experience, been hazardous in such patients and should be deferred.[42] There is no evidence that a cholecystostomy modifies the course of pancreatitis. However, high fevers and jaundice may occur in these patients, and radiographic access to the biliary tree simplifies their subsequent management.

AMELIORATION OF PANCREATIC INFLAMMATION

In patients with gallstone-associated pancreatitis, it is reasonable to hope that early biliary intervention might ameliorate the course of acute pancreatic inflammation. However, two major issues have clouded evaluation of this suggestion. The first is difficulty in determining the presence or absence of acute pancreatitis, and the second is the wide variability in the natural history of gallstone pancreatitis.

The unquestionable presence of acute pancreatitis can only be established by operation or autopsy, and, indeed, operative findings may be subject to differing interpretation. When peripancreatic fat necrosis or marked pancreatic edema or hemorrhage are found, most observers would agree that acute pancreatitis is present. Less marked pancreatic enlargement and some increased nodularity, especially in the head of the pancreas, are frequently encountered in patients with cholelithiasis. Clearly these findings may reflect some degree of pancreatic inflammation, but they rarely seem to be of any clinical consequence. It might be hoped that determinations of serum or urinary amylase or lipase levels might clarify the diagnosis of acute pancreatitis, and many authors consider that acute gallstone pancreatitis is present if the patient has abdominal pain, vomiting, elevated amylase levels, and demonstrated gallstones.[11,18,27,29,33,48,49,54] Unfortunately, 12.5% to 79% of such patients have no such evidence of pancreatitis at early operation or autopsy.[4,5,10,20,32,47] A review of 50 consecutive patients treated surgically for pathologically confirmed acute cholecystitis showed that initial serum amylase levels were elevated above 200 SU% in 16%, with a mean of 600 SU% and a range of 210 to 2320 SU%. Each of these patients underwent cholecystectomy within 5 days of amylase determination, but none had any significant pancreatic pathologic lesions at operation.

Some authors consider that pancreatitis is present if serum amylase levels exceed a value of 800 to 1200 IU/L,[24,25,32,37,38] while others have found that there is an inverse relationship between amylase level and pancreatic pathologic lesions.[4,29] Acosta et al.[2,3] and Kelly and Swaney[24–26] add the presence of jaundice to their criteria for diagnosing acute pancreatitis. Mean admission serum bilirubin levels in my patients with gallstone pancreatitis were only 2.6 mg % ($\pm$2.6 SD). Table 7-1 summarizes clinical and biochemical data in nine patients with acute pancreatitis with gallstones and five patients who had acute biliary disease without any gross evidence of pancreatitis at operation. These data are taken from a group of patients selected for percutaneous transhepatic cholangiography because the severity of their course made the differentiation of acute pancreatitis from acute biliary disease essential.[9] These are, thus, a highly selected group. They do, however, demonstrate that the differentiation of acute pancreatitis associated with gallstones from cholangitis or cholecystitis associated with elevated amylase levels can be extraordinarily difficult. In this particular group, the only patient with a normal serum amylase level had very severe pancreatitis at eventual surgery for infected pancreatic necrosis.

The second factor leading to confusion concerning the appropriate management of patients with acute gallstone-associated pancreatitis is wide variability in natural history. Among patients with true pancreatic inflammation, approximately 80% will recover uneventfully with most proposed therapeutic regimes. But 20% of patients have severe pancreatitis, and it is in this group that appropriate management may be a critical determinant of the clinical course and outcome. In 1974, we reported the 11 early objective prognostic signs listed in Table 7-2.[44] Each of these signs bears a statistical relationship to morbidity and mortality of acute pancreatitis. The relationship between the number of these signs that were present in individual patients and the risk of death or complications requiring more than 1 week of management in an intensive care unit is shown in Fig. 7-2.[42] In my group of patients selected on the basis of operative evidence of pancreatitis in 74% of cases and on the basis of strong clinical evidence of pancreatitis such as severe hypocalcemia, left upper quadrant tenderness, or a palpable epigastric mass in 26%, 71% had fewer than three positive prognostic signs. In this group only one patient (2%) died. In the 29% of patients who had three or more positive signs, 17% died and a further 30% developed complications requiring at least 1 week of intensive care.[42] In my studies, some patients with mild pancreatitis who survived but did not come to operation may have been overlooked.

In another series in which the diagnosis of pancreatitis was made on the basis of elevated amylase levels,[12] three or more positive prognostic signs were present in only 3% of 153 patients. Overall mortality in this report was 2%, and, undoubt-

TABLE 7-2. PROGNOSTIC SIGNS USED TO ESTIMATE THE SEVERITY OF ACUTE PANCREATITIS

At Admission or Diagnosis
Age over 55 years
White blood cell count over 16,000/mm^3
Blood glucose level over 200 mg/100 mL
Serum lactic dehydrogenase level over 350 IU/L
Serum aspartate aminotransferase level over 250 SFU %*
During the Initial 48 Hours
Hematocrit fall greater than 10 percentage points
Blood urea nitrogen rise more than 5 mg/100 mL
Serum calcium level below 8 mg/100 mL
Arterial P_{O_2} below 60 mm Hg
Base deficit greater than 4 mEq/L
Estimated fluid sequestration more than 6000 mL

* SFU = Sigma Frankel units.

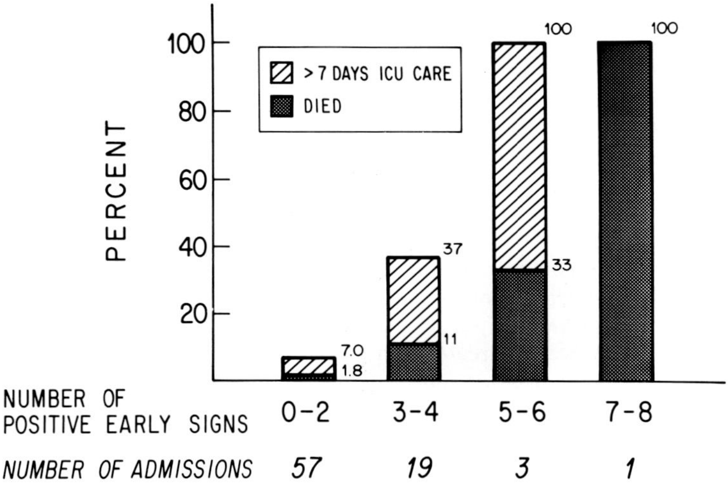

Figure 7-2. The morbidity of acute pancreatitis associated with cholelithiasis related to the number of positive prognostic signs.

edly, many patients without any significant pancreatic pathologic lesion were included.

By contrast, another study included only patients who had gallstones and elevated amylase levels together with "severe abdominal pain and systemic illness."[16] In this study, 56% of patients had three or more positive prognostic signs, and 50% of this group died. Only 1 of 11 patients with fewer than three positive signs died. He died of myocardial infarction 3 weeks after hospital discharge.[16]

In the past, most patients with acute gallstone pancreatitis were initially managed nonoperatively, and definitive biliary surgery to prevent pancreatitis was recommended after an interval of 2 to 4 months.[24] With improvement in the diagnosis of gallstones, it became clear that surgical correction of cholelithiasis could be undertaken safely during the same hospital admission once evidence of acute pancreatitis had subsided.[10,11,17,22,38] Further delay in biliary surgery only exposed the patient to a 25% to 50% risk of recurrent acute pancreatitis. Emergency operation was usually only recommended for diagnostic purposes or for patients who did not appear to be responding to nonoperative treatment.

In 1978, Acosta and associates published a review advocating early definitive biliary surgery within 48 hours of the onset of symptoms.[3] They examined a series of 86 patients who were managed initially by nonoperative methods between 1964 and 1972. Nineteen of these patients were operated upon between day 3 and day 14. Of this group 16% died and the mean hospital stay was 25 days. Forty-six subsequent patients were operated on within 48 hours of the onset of symptoms. Cholecystectomy, common duct exploration, and transduodenal sphincterotomy were undertaken as indicated. In this group, mortality fell to 2% and mean hospital stay was 13 days. In 72% of the more recent group of patients, a stone was found impacted at the ampulla of Vater. The authors interpreted these findings as indicating that persistent calculous obstruction of the ampulla of Vater was responsible for progression of pancreatic inflammation. Early surgical relief of such obstruction was urged. In a later study, Acosta et al. found stones impacted in the ampulla of Vater in 75% of patients undergoing operation during the initial 48 hours and in 45% of those operated on from day 2 to day 4 after the onset of symptoms.[2] Acosta's patients were treated in Argentina. However, in a group of 24 patients operated upon by Kelly in Ohio within the initial 72 hours of disease, an impacted ampullary stone was found in 63%.[24] An ampullary stone was found in only 5% of patients operated on between days 5 and 7. In evaluating the high incidence of early ampullary stone impaction in the reports of Kelly and Acosta et al., it is important to remember that elevated bilirubin levels are one of their criteria for the diagnosis of gallstone pancreatitis. In patients selected because of the presence of jaundice, a high incidence of bile duct obstruction may be clearly anticipated. In our experience with both operative and cholangiographic evaluation of the bile ducts, we have not observed a stone impacted in the ampulla of Vater in association with severe acute pancreatitis.[9] Patients with distal bile duct stones may be severely ill from cholangitis and have high serum amylase levels, but rarely do they have significant pancreatic inflammation. On the other hand, none of our patients with severe pancreatitis associated with gallstones have, up to this time, had operative or cholangiographic evidence of ampullary obstruction.

In the study of Acosta et al., 8 of 55 patients (14.5%) who underwent surgical relief of ampullary obstruction within 48 hours of the onset of symptoms had pancreatic "hemorrhage," "massive necrosis," "abscess," or a "pseudocyst."[2] By contrast 18 of 23 patients (78.3%) operated on more than 48 hours after the onset of symptoms had one of these findings. The authors believe that this demonstrates the importance of persistent ampullary obstruction in determining the severity of pancreatic pathologic lesions. Unfortunately, we are not told how many patients survived early nonoperative treatment uneventfully. In general, those who are operated upon after 48 hours come to surgery because of "failure of medical management." Patients operated upon because of secondary clinical deterioration do not reflect the overall spectrum of pancreatitis.

In Kelly's study of similarly selected patients, 24 patients were operated on within 72 hours.[24] Three (12%) of these patients died, and 25% developed complications. In the same study, 146 patients underwent operation after clinical evidence of pancreatic inflammation had subsided between days 5 and 8 after admission. In this group, there were no deaths and only 7% developed complications.

Stone et al., in 1981, reported a controlled clinical trial in which patients were randomly assigned either to early (<72 hour) cholecystectomy, transduodenal sphincteroplasty, and pancreatic septotomy or to early nonoperative management followed by elective surgery at 3 months.[49] The results of this study are summarized in Table 7-3. Jaundice was not a prerequisite for admission to this study, and ampullary obstruction was present in only 2 patients undergoing early surgery. Of the 36 patients who underwent early surgery, there was 1 death (2.8%), and 13.9% had major complications. None of the patients treated nonoperatively died, and their average hospital stay was 3 days shorter.

TABLE 7-3. EARLY (0–73 HOURS) VS. LATE (3–6 MONTHS) BILIARY SURGERY FOR GALLSTONE PANCREATITIS*

	No. of Patients	Hospital Days	Abscess (%)	Death (%)	Impacted Ampullary Stone (%)
Early operation	36				
Late operation	29				
Initial morbidity		10.7	0	0	
Secondary morbidity		12.1	6.9	6.9	
Total morbidity		13.5	5.6	2.8	5.6

* From Stone et al.[49]

These data convincingly demonstrate that in unselected patients with abdominal pain, hyperamylasemia, and gallstones, early operative intervention does not reduce the morbidity of the acute illness. Stone, however, combined the morbidity of elective surgery with that of the initial stay and concluded that early surgery was preferable. This interpretation is clouded by the fact that in this study, elective biliary surgery was associated with a mortality of 6.9%, a 6.9% incidence of subphrenic abscess, and one duodenal fistula. This is clearly an unacceptable morbidity for such surgery. Furthermore, a sample of patients selected by the presence of abdominal pain and elevated amylase levels would include a great majority of patients with either no pancreatitis or very mild disease. In these groups, early biliary surgery would be safe.

In 1979, I reviewed my experience with 80 episodes of gallstone-associated pancreatitis (Fig. 7-3).[42] It must be stressed that only patients with clear operative or clinical evidence of pancreatitis are included. In that review, early biliary surgery was associated with one death (9.1%) in patients with fewer than three positive prognostic signs but was associated with a high mortality in patients with severe disease on the basis of early objective criteria. Early nonoperative treatment was better tolerated in all groups. These results reflected a period when we had deliberately pursured a policy of early operative intervention in patients with severe, acute gallstone pancreatitis (Fig. 7-4). During that period, the overall mortality was 29%. Among 66 patients treated after that period, there was only 1 death (1.4%). This patient had undergone cholecystectomy and negative common bile duct exploration within a few hours of admission.

In a subsequent review, we examined the relationship of operation within the initial 48 hours of treatment to overall morbidity and mortality. The results of that review are shown in Fig. 7-5. The findings are very similar to those in Fig. 7-4. In our experience the overwhelming majority of patients with gallstone pancreatitis recover from their acute illness without biliary surgery. In severely ill patients, it is important to exclude obstructive cholangitis and gangrenous cholecystitis if nonoperative management is to be pursued. As discussed above, percutaneous cholangiography has been valuable in this regard.[9]

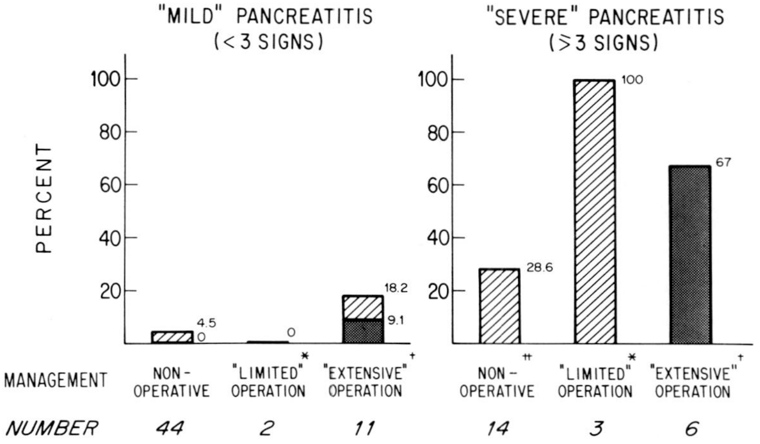

Figure 7-3. Overall morbidity and mortality related to the early management (days 0–7) in mild (0–2 positive signs) and severe (≥3 positive signs) acute pancreatitis. (*Cholecystostomy and/or peritoneal lavage; †cholecystectomy and/or common duct exploration or pancreatic resection; ‡included nonoperative peritoneal lavage in two.)

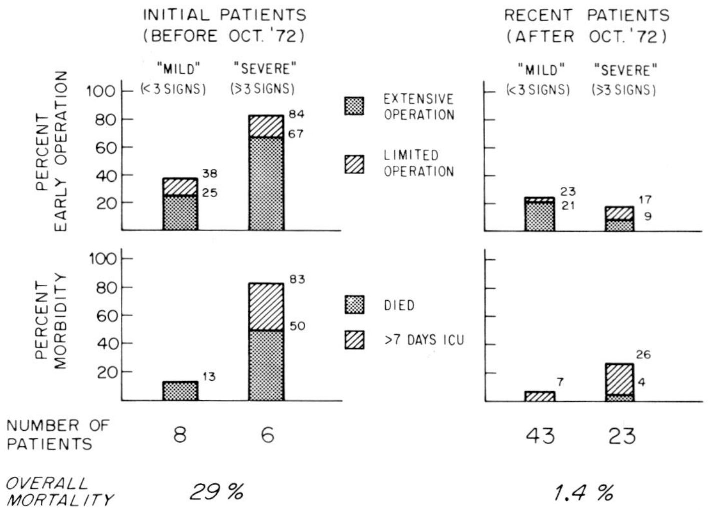

Figure 7-4. Early (days 0–7) operative management, morbidity, and mortality in 14 episodes of gallstone pancreatitis treated before October 1972 and in 66 more-recent episodes. "Extensive" and "limited" operations are listed in Fig. 7-3.

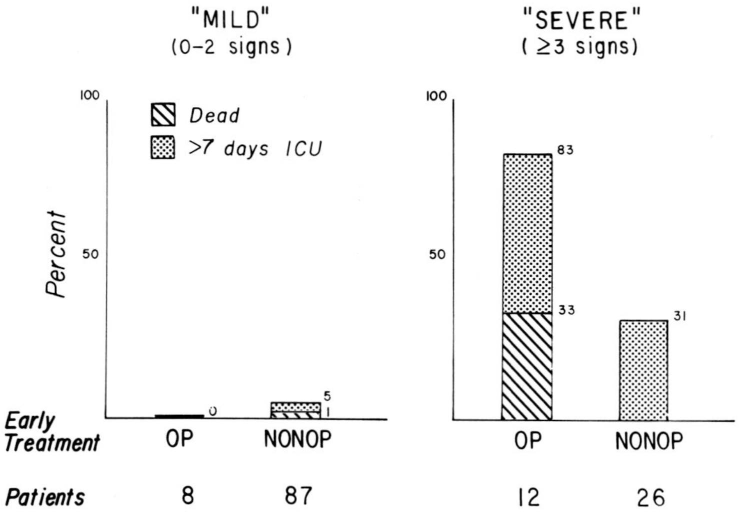

Figure 7-5. The relationship between initial 48-hour management, morbidity, and mortality in patients with "mild" (0–2 signs) and "severe" (3–11 signs) gallstone pancreatitis.

The reviews of Osborne et al.,[37] Welch and White,[54] Tondelli et al.,[52] Ong et al.,[34] and Kelly[24] all support an initial nonoperative approach followed by correction of biliary disease after signs of pancreatitis have subsided but during the same hospital admission in most cases. Mercer et al.[33] reported that 28 patients who were found to have mild pancreatitis at operation within 24 hours of hospital admission all survived and concluded that early operation was beneficial. A further report by Heij et al.[16] found that in patients with fewer than three positive prognostic signs, mortality was 14% after early surgery and 0% after delayed surgery. In patients with three or more positive prognostic signs, mortality was 50% in both treatment groups. He concludes that early surgery does not harm those with mild pancreatitis and may benefit those with severe disease. These conclusions do not appear to be supported by the data reported.

Gallstone Pancreatitis in Pregnancy

Cholelithiasis is the major etiologic association of acute pancreatitis that develops during pregnancy.[30,55] In patients who develop pancreatitis during pregnancy, gallstones can be diagnosed by ultrasound. Initial treatment should be nonoperative if possible. If pancreatitis has occurred in the first trimester, cholecystectomy and common duct exploration should be planned for the second trimester. If gallstone-associated pancreatitis develops during the second trimester, biliary surgery should be undertaken once evidence of pancreatitis has subsided.

In the third trimester, surgical correction of cholelithiasis should, if possible, be postponed until after delivery.[30]

Endoscopic Sphincterotomy

Endoscopic sphincterotomy or papillotomy has been increasingly used in the treatment of common bile duct stones, especially if the gallbladder has been previously removed. In patients who have recovered from an episode of pancreatitis associated with such stones, endoscopic papillotomy is one of the available methods for treating the underlying cholelithiasis for the purpose of preventing recurrent pancreatitis or other complications of choledocholithiasis.[53]

It has been suggested that endoscopic sphincterotomy carried out early during the acute episode of pancreatitis may ameliorate the course of pancreatitis. Evaluation of this suggestion is clouded by the same problems as the evaluation of early surgical procedures, namely difficulty in determining the presence or absence of pancreatic inflammation and wide variation in the natural history of acute pancreatitis.

In a review in 1978, it was reported that 58 patients had been treated for common duct stones and pancreatitis by endoscopic sphincterotomy without exacerbation of pancreatitis.[7] Safrany and Cotton[46] reported a series of 11 patients who had undergone urgent endoscopic sphincterotomy during acute pancreatitis. Two patients (18.2%) died, one of multiorgan failure and one of liver abscesses. Another patient had a 1.5-L bleed.

A report by Rosseland and Solhaug[45] compared early sphincterotomy during acute pancreatitis to delayed procedures carried out after the acute illness. Fourteen patients who underwent delayed sphincterotomy recovered without major complications, although one required repeat papillotomy and one required surgical intervention for removal of residual stones. Two other patients underwent subsequent surgical removal of their gallbladders. The 15 patients who underwent early sphincterotomy were all reported to have "prompt and marked improvement." Nonetheless, one (6.7%) died 5 days later of "heart failure" and one (6.7%) required repeated operative intervention for pancratic necrosis and sepsis. Three patients required cholecystectomy for acute cholecystitis.

The major concerns about endoscopic cholangiography and papillotomy are the risks of exacerbation of pancreatitis or of introducing contrast material with bacterial contamination into an area of devitalized pancreas. The magnitude of these risks is unknown. Following endoscopic retrograde cholangiopancreatography the overall incidence of pancreatitis is approximately 1% and of pancreatic sepsis, 0.3%.[6] The risk of pancreatitis appears to be substantially higher if endoscopic sphincterotomy is carried out.[28]

At present, endoscopic sphincterotomy and relief of calculous obstruction may be a reasonable approach to the management of obstructive cholangitis with or without elevated amylase levels, especially if the gallbladder is absent. There is, however, no evidence that this measure ameliorates the course of acute pancreatitis. Since in two reports of sphincterotomy during acute pancreatitis, the incidence of pancreatic sepsis was 7% and 9%, the procedure may be harmful in this setting.[45,46]

Conclusions

In patients with gallstones and acute pancreatitis, there is no convincing evidence that early surgical intervention or endoscopic sphincterotomy during the acute illness reduces morbidity and mortality. In those with severe pancreatitis, morbidity may be increased. Nonoperative early treatment should therefore be pursued if life-threatening extrapancreatic disease can be excluded. Surgical correction of cholelithiasis may safely be undertaken to prevent recurrent pancreatitis as soon as evidence of pancreatitis has subsided in most patients.

Prevention of Recurrent Pancreatitis

Although correction of associated biliary lithiasis does not appear to ameliorate the course of gallstone pancreatitis, recurrent acute pancreatitis can be anticipated in 25% to 63% of patients if cholelithiasis is not corrected.[11,20,22,27,38] If cholelithiasis is corrected, recurrent pancreatitis is seen in 0% to 9.3% of cases.[10,20,22,27,47]

In the past it was recommended that operative intervention to correct cholelithiasis be postponed for a period of 6 weeks to 3 months after an episode of pancreatitis. Such waiting, however, exposes the patient to a significant risk of recurrent acute pancreatitis.[37] Several reports have documented the fact that surgical correction of cholelithiasis to prevent recurrent pancreatitis can be safely accomplished in most patients as soon as clinical evidence of acute pancreatitis has subsided.[11,20,22] This is usually within the first several days of hospitalization. Since a longer delay has no benefit and some risk of further pancreatitis, I favor surgical correction of cholelithiasis at this time. One exception to this general approach is the patient who has been severely ill with acute pancreatitis and who has developed a large inflammatory pancreatic mass. This may be recognized by palpation or by CT. Adequate exploration of the common bile duct can be technically difficult in such patients. Accordingly, if they are clinically stable, I prefer to allow a period of several weeks or even months for resolution of the inflammation before undertaking biliary surgery. Such patients are, however, uncommon.

Surgical treatment of cholelithiasis in patients who have had pancreatitis follows conventional practice, but manipulation of the distal bile ducts and pancreas should be especially gentle. It has been suggested that the routine addition of transduodenal sphincterotomy and pancreatic septotomy may reduce the risk of recurrent biliary pancreatitis.[49] This procedure, however, involves additional risks to the patient, and there is no evidence whatever that it would improve the results of standard biliary surgery in these patients. In most patients with recurrent pancreatitis after biliary surgery, either there is a persistent or recurrent cholelithiasis or there is another cause of pancreatitis, such as alcohol abuse or hyperlipidemia. Thus, if cholecystectomy is undertaken in patients who have had pancreatitis but no gallstones are present, the incidence of recurrent pancreatitis is 38% to 75%.

CONCLUSIONS

Interventional measures may be required for diagnostic purposes within the first day or two of management of patients with suspected acute pancreatitis and gallstones. In selected patients, percutaneous transhepatic cholangiography may help to exclude cystic or common duct obstruction. However, if life-threatening extrapancreatic disease cannot be reasonably excluded by nonoperative means, diagnostic celiotomy is needed. There is, at present, no convincing evidence that early biliary intervention, either by surgical or endoscopic means, ameliorates the course of gallstone-associated pancreatitis. Recurrent acute pancreatitis can be expected, however, unless cholelithiasis is corrected in patients surviving acute gallstone pancreatitis. In these patients, correction of the underlying disease can usually be safely undertaken as soon as clinical and laboratory evidence of pancreatitis has subsided.

REFERENCES

1. Acosta JM, Ledesma CL. Gallstone migration as a cause of acute pancreatitis. N Engl J Med 290:484, 1974.
2. Acosta JM, Pelligrini CA, Skinner DB. Etiology and pathogenesis of acute biliary pancreatitis. Surgery 88:118–125, 1980.
3. Acosta JM, Rossi R, Galli OMR, et al. Early surgery for acute gallstone pancreatitis: Evaluation of a systematic approach. Surgery 83:367–370, 1978.
4. Adams JT, Libertino JA, Schwartz SI. Significance of an elevated serum amylase. Surgery 63:887, 1968.
5. Bernard HR, Criscione JR, Moyer CA. The pathologic significance of the serum amylase concentration. Arch Surg 79:311, 1959.
6. Bilbao MD, Dotter CT, Lee TG, Katon RM. Complications of endoscopic retrograde cholangiography (ERCP). Gastroenterology 70:314–320, 1976.
7. Classen M, Ossenberg FW, Wurbs D, Hagenmüller. Pancreatitis—An indication for endoscopic papillotomy? Endoscopy, 10:223, 1978.
8. Coffey RJ. The relationship of acute and chronic cholecystitis to acute pancreatitis. South Med J 47:448, 1954.
9. Coppa GF, LeFleur R, Ranson JHC. The role of Chiba-needle cholangiography in the diagnosis of possible acute pancreatitis with cholelithiasis. Ann Surg 193:393–398, 1981.
10. Dixon JA, Hillam JD. Surgical treatment of biliary tract disease associated with acute pancreatitis. Surg Gynecol Obstet 129:263–268, 1969.
11. Elfstrom J. The timing of cholecystectomy in patients with gallstone pancreatitis. Acta Chir Scand 144:487–490, 1978.
12. Frei JG, Frei VT, Thirlby RC, McClelland RM. Biliary pancreatitis: Clinical presentation and surgical management. Am J Surg 151:170–174, 1986.
13. Glazer G, Murphy F, Clayden GS, et al. Radionuclide biliary scanning in acute pancreatitis. Br J Surg 68:766–770, 1981.
14. Glenn F, Frey C. Re-evaluation of the treatment of pancreatitis associated with biliary disease. Ann Surg 160:723, 1964.

15. Harbin WP, Mueller PR, Ferrucci JT. Transhepatic cholangiography Complications and use patterns of the fine needle technique. Radiology 135:15–22, 1980.
16. Heij HA, Veen HF, Eggink WF, Obertop H. Timing of surgery for acute biliary pancreatitis. Am J Surg 149:371–374, 1985.
17. Hermann RE, Hertzer NR. Time of biliary surgery after acute pancreatitis due to biliary disease. Arch Surg 100:71–75, 1970.
18. Howard JM. Pancreatitis associated with gallstones. In: Howard JM, Jordan GL, eds. Surgical Diseases of the Pancreas. Philadelphia, JB Lippincott 1960.
19. Howard JM. Gallstone pancreatitis. In: Howard JM, Jordan GL Jr, Reber HA, eds. Surgical Diseases of the Pancreas. Philadelphia, Lea & Febiger, 1987.
20. Howard JM, Ehrlich EW. Gallstone pancreatitis: A clinical entity. Surgery 51:177, 1962.
21. Johnson HC, Minor BD, Thompson J, et al. Diagnostic value of intravenous cholangiography during acute cholecystitis and acute pancreatitis. N Engl J Med 260:158–161, 1959.
22. Kelly TR. Gallstone pancreatitis. Arch Surg 109:294–297, 1974.
23. Kelly TR. Gallstone pancreatitis: Pathophysiology. Surgery 80:488–492, 1976.
24. Kelly TR. Gallstone pancreatitis: The timing of surgery. Surgery 88:345–350, 1980.
25. Kelly TR. Gallstone pancreatitis. Ann Surg 200:479–485, 1984.
26. Kelly TR, Swaney PE. Gallstone pancreatitis: The second time around. Surgery 92:571–575, 1982.
27. Kim U, Sheth M. Optimal timing of surgical intervention in patients with acute pancreatitis associated with cholelithiasis. Surg Gynecol Obstet 150:499–501, 1980.
28. LeFerla G, Gordon S, Archibald M, Murray WR. Hyperamylasemia and acute pancreatitis following endoscopic retrograde cholangiopancreatography. Pancreas 1:160–163, 1986.
29. Linos DA, Adson MA. Gallstone pancreatitis. Int Surg 68:153–156, 1983.
30. McKay AJ, O'Neill J, Imrie CW. Pancreatitis, pregnancy and gallstones. Br J Obstet 87:47–50, 1980.
31. McMahon MJ, Playforth MJ. The relationship betwen gallstones and cystic duct anatomy in acute pancreatitis. Br J Surg 65:361, 1978.
32. Mackie CR, Wood RAB, Preece PE, Cuschieri A. Surgical pathology at early elective operation for suspected acute gallstone pancreatitis. Br J Surg 72:79–181, 1985.
33. Mercer LC, Saltzstein EC, Peacock JB, Dougherty SH. Early surgery for biliary pancreatitis. Am J Surg 148:749–753, 1984.
34. Ong GB, Adisehiah M, Leong CH. Acute pancreatitis associated with recurrent pyogenic cholangitis. Br J Surg 58:891–894, 1971.
35. Opie EL. The relation of cholelithiasis to disease of the pancreas and to fat necrosis. Johns Hopkins Hosp Bull 12:19, 1901.
36. Opie EL. The etiology of acute hemorrhagic pancreatitis. Johns Hopkins Hosp Bull 12:182, 1901.
37. Osborne DH, Imrie CW, Carter DC. Biliary surgery in the same admission for gallstone-associated acute pancreatitis. Br J Surg 68:758–761, 1981.
38. Paloyan D, Simonowitz D, Skinner DB. The timing of biliary tract operations in patients with pancreatitis associated with gallstones. Surg Gynecol Obstet 141:737–739, 1975.
39. Poncelet PR, Thompson AG. Role of infected bile in spasm of the sphincter of Oddi. Am J Surg 126:387, 1973.
40. Poncelet P, Thompson AG. Action of bile phospholipids on the pancreas. Am J Surg 123:196, 1972.
41. Prince M. Pancreatic apoplexy with a report of two cases. Boston Med Surg J 107:28, 1882.
42. Ranson JHC. The timing of biliary surgery in acute pancreatitis. Ann Surg 189:654–662, 1979.
43. Ranson JHC. Conservative surgical treatment of acute pancreatitis. World J Surg 5:351–359, 1981.

44. Ranson JHC, Rifkind KM, Roses DF, et al. Prognostic signs and the role of operative management in acute pancreatitis. Surg Gynecol Obstet 139:69–81, 1974.
45. Rosseland AR, Solhaug JH. Early or delayed endoscopic papillotomy (EPT) in gallstone pancreatitis. Ann Surg 199:165–167, 1984.
46. Safrany L, Cotton PB. A preliminary report: Urgent duodenoscopic sphincerotomy for acute gallstone pancreatitis. Surgery 89:424–428, 1981.
47. Sanchez-Ubeda R, Rousselot LM, Giannelli S. The significance of pancreatitis accompanying acute cholecystitis. Ann Surg 144:44, 1956.
48. Semel L, Schrieber D, Fromm D. Gallstone pancreatitis. Arch Surg 118:901–904, 1983.
49. Stone HH, Fabian TC, Dunlop WE. Gallstone pancreatitis. Ann Surg 194:305–312, 1981.
50. Tabrisky J, Lindstrom RL, Hanelin LG, et al. Chiba percutaneous transhepatic cholangiography. A valuable method for visualizing the non-dilated biliary tract. Am J Roentgenol 126:755–760, 1976.
51. Thurston OG. Pathogenesis of gallstone pancreatitis. Am J Surg 129:301, 1975.
52. Tondelli P, Stutz K, Harder F, et al. Acute gallstone pancreatitis: Best timing for biliary surgery. Br J Surg 69:709–710, 1982.
53. van der Spuy S. Endoscopic sphincterotomy in the management of gallstone pancreatitis. Endoscopy 13:25–26, 1981.
54. Welch JP, White CE. Acute pancreatitis of biliary origin: Is urgent operation necessary? Am J Surg 143:120–126, 1982.
55. Wilkinson EJ. Acute pancreatitis in pregnancy. Obstet Gynecol Survey 28:281–303, 1973.

CHAPTER

8

ERCP AND EPT IN ACUTE OBSTRUCTIVE (BILIARY) PANCREATITIS

Meinhard Classen, Klaus Knyrim, Friedrich Hagenmueller, and Horst Neuhaus

There is a general agreement that acute pancreatitis (AP) is characterized by autodigestion of the gland by its own products. The pathogenetic role of anatomic variations (common channel, different duct openings), direction of flow of secretions, pressures in different compartments, chemical composition, and microbiology of secretions are not quite understood. According to clinical observations, obstruction of the ampulla of Vater seems to be a decisive factor. The following arguments favor this assumption:

1. Gallstones are found in the feces of many patients with AP of unclear origin.[1,13]

2. Biliary microliths 2 mm in diameter (or less), hardly detectable by radiology, are found in the biliary and the pancreatic ducts of many patients with AP.[20,7]

3. Endoscopic retrograde cholangiopancreatography (ERCP) and surgery in the acute phase of AP demonstrate biliary and ampullary stones much more frequently when compared with delayed procedures.[28]

4. Endoscopic or surgical treatment of the cause of obstruction not only leads to rapid healing of AP, but also prevents recurrences.[2,23,28]

Obstruction of the ampulla of Vater can of course be caused by a number of different lesions (gallstones, parasites, tumors, etc.).

We propose the term *acute obstructive pancreatitis* (AOP), as it embraces the acute stage of the disease clinicopathologically and the pathogenetic mechanism. The various controversies on diagnosis and treatment of AOP caused by gallstones and parasites will be reviewed in this chapter.

DIAGNOSTIC WORKUP AND DIFFERENTIAL DIAGNOSIS

A carefully taken history and a thorough clinical examination are very important (Table 8-1). Some observations concerning laboratory tests need to be made. Routine laboratory studies are not suitable for differentiating AOP from acute alcoholic pancreatitis (AAP), since a study by Goodman et al. showed patients with alcoholic pancreatitis to have elevated concentrations of serum bilirubin, alkaline phosphatase, and aminotransferases.[12] Schoelmerich et al. showed that none of the different laboratory tests assessed had sufficient sensitivity and specificity in patients with acute pancreatitis to determine the biliary origin, which was defined by means of ERCP, surgery, and autopsy.[26] Refinement of enzyme assays for the diagnosis of AP have little impact upon the diagnostic criteria used by many clinicians.

Ultrasonography

This method offers a distinct aid in the diagnosis and evaluation of AP. It may show edema, pancreatic enlargement, pseudocysts, and fluid collections. It may demonstrate stones and dilatation of the biliary system. Gas, frequently present in pancreatitis, interferes with the ultrasonic beam. Sensitivity and specificity of ultrasonography to delineate biliary obstruction are 78% to 97% and 93% to 100%, respectively, as long as intraabdominal gas does not interfere with the examination. Ultrasonography often does not permit a clear distinction between alcoholic and obstructive pancreatitis.[26,29] However, the demonstration of stones in the gallbladder, without dilatation of the bile ducts, is not proof of AOP.

Computed Tomography

This method provides detailed information of pathologic alterations of the pancreas. The CT changes in the early phase of AP indicate the severity of the later course possibly better than Ranson's criteria,[22] but CT offers poor aid in the detection of an acute obstruction of the ampulla of Vater.[26]

ERCP

The greatest accuracy for detecting calculi in the biliary tree and the only means for establishing the diagnosis of AOP is provided by endoscopic observa-

TABLE 8-1. FEATURES SUGGESTING AOP

Age beyond 60 years
Female
No alcohol addiction
History of biliary colicky pain
Jaundice associated with fever
Detection with ultrasound of biliary calculi and/or dilated bile ducts

tion of the papilla of Vater, cannulation, and contrast instillation into the biliary and pancreatic ducts (ERCP). Whereas previous investigators were reluctant to utilize ERCP in the examination of AP as they were afraid to aggravate the course of the disease, we believe this argument has been proved to be no longer valid. Several studies from Europe and the Far East[6,9,16,17,21,25] have shown that ERCP studies can safely be performed in the presence of AP, if applied by experienced endoscopists and provided that endoscopic treatment (extraction of calculi, etc.) is instituted immediately after the diagnostic study. If therapy is not applied immediately after the instillation of radiographic dye, a greater risk of cholangitis and worsening of the acute pancreatitis may occur. Safrany et al. have shown convincingly that inadvertent administration of contrast material into the pancreatic duct does not have an adverse effect in patients undergoing endoscopic papillotomy (EPT) for gallstone-associated pancreatitis.[25]

We recommend an ERC study in all patients with symptoms indicating AOP as early as possible. Preferably, the pancreatic duct should not be visualized in order to minimize the risk of the procedure. However, if CT shows signs of necrotizing pancreatitis, visualization of the pancreatic duct may be required if surgery is contemplated.[11] This aspect should, however, be subjected to a well-planned trial. We agree with Rösch's statement that the only indication for ERCP in acute pancreatitis is the relief of obstruction (mostly stones) by EPT.[24]

In some cases AOP takes an unfavorable course, even after removal of the obstruction. Figure 8-1 shows findings of the ERCP examination of a patient with necrotizing AOP. This patient developed a huge pseudocyst within the head of the pancreas that required pancreatic surgery, even following the endoscopic extraction of two calculi from the ampulla and the common bile duct.

Aside from the radiologic findings, the endoscopic appearance of the papilla of Vater constitutes an important diagnostic clue to the presence of AOP. The papilla in the presence of acute obstructive pancreatitis is enlarged (balloon papilla, Fig. 8-2) with erythema of the mucosa and may show lacerations caused by incarcerated stones. Pus may be discharging from the orifice. A normal endoscopic appearance of the papilla together with the inability to visualize the bile ducts by means of endoscopic cannulation is uncommon in AOP cause by ductal stones.

Endoscopic Therapy

The option offered by ERCP and endoscopic papillotomy was discussed by us in 1978[5] and later by us and others in several retrospective studies including more than 400 patients.[6,7,9,16,17,21,25] Endoscopic papillotomy has proved to be a safe approach in the emergency setting (less than 48 hours after admission).[21] Rates of complications and mortality for emergent EPT do not exceed the values of EPT for other indications (3% and 0.8%).

In the first controlled trial, 121 patients with gallstone-induced pancreatitis were prospectively randomized and allocated to ERCP (plus EPT in proven obstruction) and to conventional treatment.[21] Predicted mild courses of the disease showed no difference in outcome. In contrast, patients with predicted severe

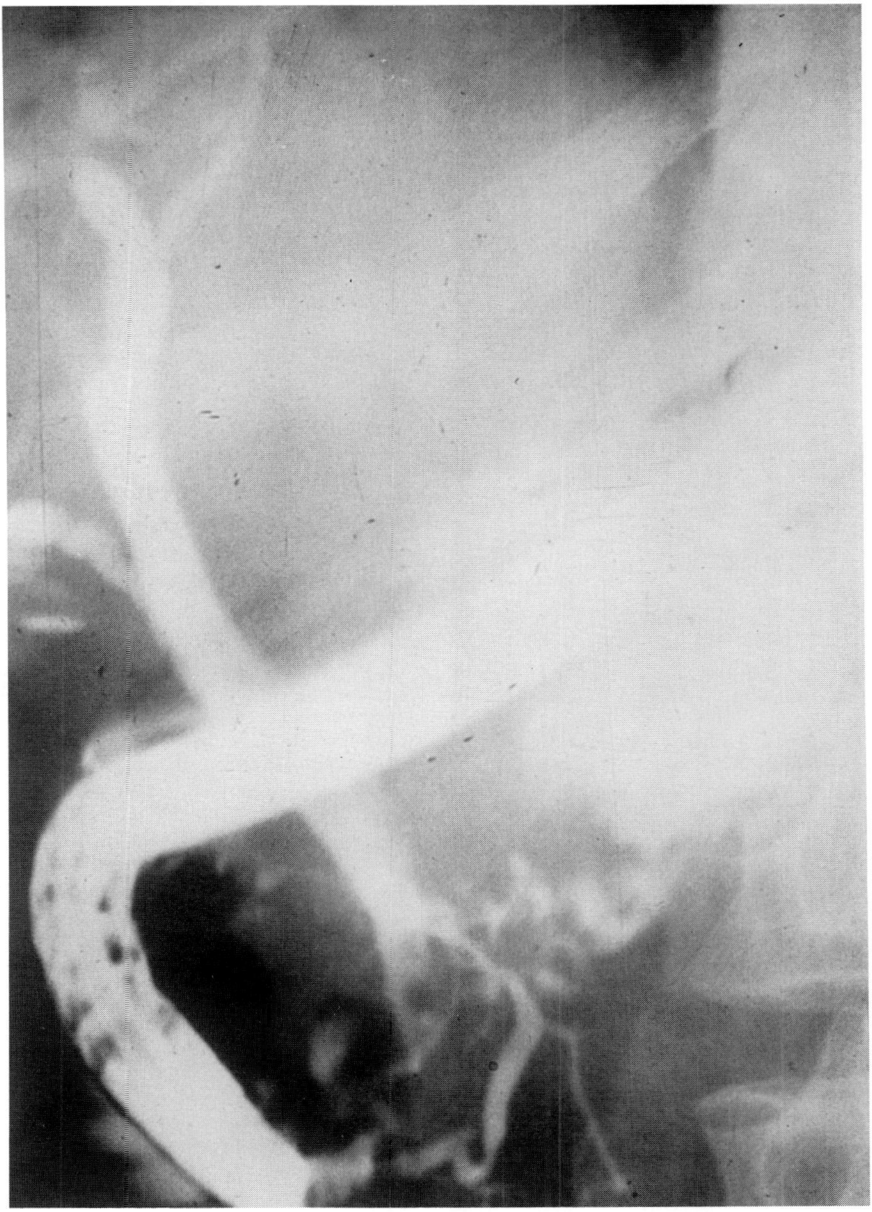

Figure 8-1. Acute biliary pancreatitis: two calculi in the distal common bile duct and a pseudocyst in the body of the pancreas. The pancreatic duct appears normal in the head of the pancreas. In the body of the pancreas the radiographic dye extravasates into a large pseudocyst.

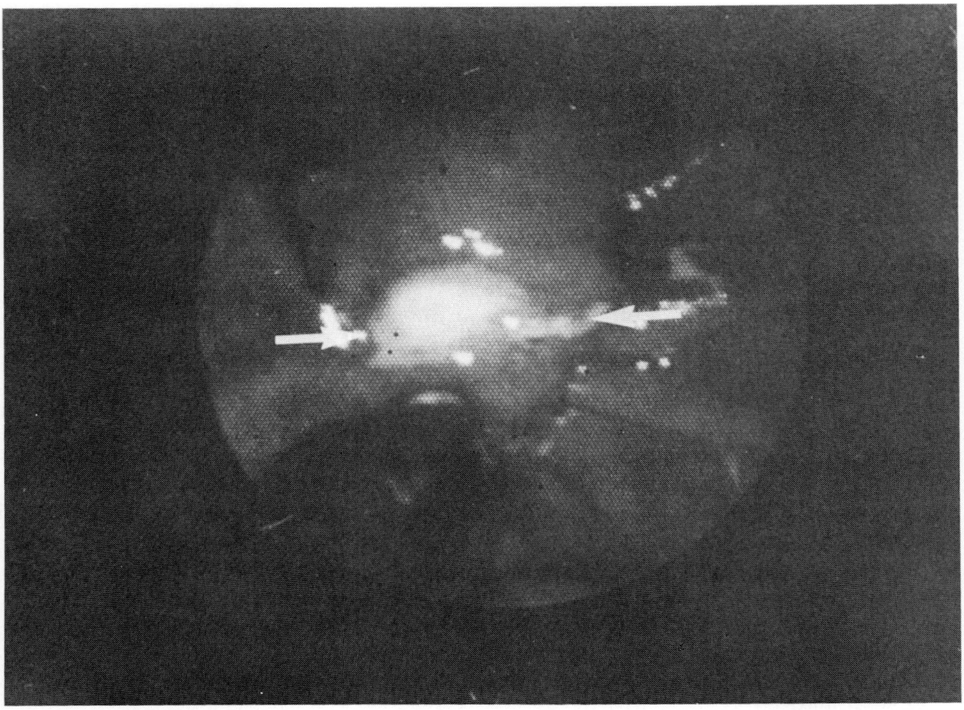

Figure 8-2. Endoscopic appearance of the papilla of Vater in acute biliary pancreatitis. The papilla is distended by an incarcerated stone. Erythema of the mucosa is present, and pus discharges from the orifice.

attacks benefited significantly from the endoscopic therapy. Complication rates (61%) and mortality (17.9%) in the conventionally treated group dropped to 24% and 1.7%, respectively, in the ERCP (EPT) groups (Table 8-2).

Our own results of endoscopic treatment of gallstone pancreatitis are included in a survey of Escourrou et al.,[9,8] which concerns 157 patients from five German and French centers. Duodenoscopy and ERC was done in 82% of the patients. The endoscopic appearance of the papilla (Table 8-3) was normal in only one third of the patients with biliary pancreatitis. In the majority of cases, inflammation of the papilla, visible stone impaction, "stiff orifice," or biliodoudenal fistula confirmed the clinical suspicion of biliary pathologic lesions as the cause of pancreatitis even without opacifying the duct systems. Small bile duct stones could not be proved radiologically in 23% of patients with AOP (Table 8-4). In the majority of these cases, microliths could be found in the bile after endoscopic papillotomy. This observation might justify papillotomy in patients with a clinical suspicion of AOP in combination with the endoscopic signs of "stone papilla"

TABLE 8-2. BILIARY PANCREATITIS: CONTROLLED TRIAL OF CONSERVATIVE TREATMENT VS. URGENT ERCP (EPT)*

	Conventional Management		Urgent ERCP (EPT)
Patients	62		59
Predicted mild outcome	34		34
Complications	12%		12%
Predicted severe outcome	28		25
Complications	61%	$p < .01$	24%
Mortality	8%		2%
Length of hospital stay (days)	17.0	$p < .05$	9.5

* From Neoptolemos et al.[21]

without radiologic proof. Our series contained only a small minority of patients in whom the indication for endoscopic papillotomy was based on endoscopic signs of "papillitis" without stones. Papillitis could occur due to an invisible "micro-stone" or following previous spontaneous stone passage. In Escourrou's multi-center survey, endoscopic papillotomy prompted healing of pancreatitis in 96% of cases (Table 8-5). In conclusion, patients with biliary pancreatitis benefit from endoscopic stone removal, and the manipulation does not promote complications.

Timing of Surgical Therapy for AOP caused by Ductal Stones

Until recently surgery was considered the only adequate therapy of gall-stone-associated pancreatitis. Today there exists general agreement that gall-stones in the common bile duct must be removed; however, the timing of surgery for AOP has been the subject of controversial discussions.[14,27] Three different time schedules have been suggested for treatment: emergency operation, defined as intervention performed within 48 hours of admission; *briefly delayed* operation, defined as performed later, but within the same hospital stay; and the *delayed approach* after complete remission of symptoms and carried out during a subsequent hospitalization.

TABLE 8-3. ENDOSCOPIC ASPECT OF THE PAPILLA IN BILIARY PANCREATITIS (n = 157)*

Normal	34%	
Inflammation	35%	
Impacted stone	14%	66%
"Stiff orifice"	10%	
Bilioduodenal fistula	7%	
Total	100%	

* From Escourrou et al.[9]

TABLE 8-4. ERCP IN BILIARY PANCREATITIS ($n = 157$)*

Stones	77%		
No stones	23%		
	Endoscopic finding	→	"Microlithiasis" 85%
		→	"Papillitis" 15%

* From Escourrou et al.[9]

Kelly stated that the emergency operation features a mortality rate of 12%,[13,14] whereas surgery after complete remission of pancreatitis is distinctly safer. This agrees with the findings of Frei et al.[10] showing postoperative complications occurring in 71% of the emergency groups compared with only 22% in the delayed surgery group. Also the rate of retained common duct stones in this study in the emergency group was as high as 14%.

Many other surgeons advocate delayed operative management for AOP because of the rather hazardous operative approach in the emergency setting. However, spontaneous recovery from AOP is not guaranteed, and necrotizing pancreatitis may occur. Additionally, 20% to 40% of patients may relapse after the first recovery.[13] Acosta et al. presented a study showing that early surgery resulted in a reduced operation mortality rate (2% vs. 16% for the delayed surgical approach).[6]

The current controversy regarding treatment of acute pancreatitis among surgeons was reinforced by two papers. In a study of 66 patients with pancreatitis due to gallstones, 11 patients were operated upon within 48 hours of admission, and 2 of them died. Further two patients on the waiting list for cholecystectomy also died from AP. There were no deaths in the group who received an operation for gallstones during the convalescent period (2–14 days after admission).[3] The authors state that the deaths of two patients from AP while waiting for an operation are an argument for immediate surgery in very ill patients. The safety of urgent operations for gallstones was shown by a study of 78 patients operated on during the early phase of AOP with no mortality.[23,3] An expert in the field of pancreatic surgery concludes that "the relative merits of urgent or somewhat later

TABLE 8-5. ERCP IN BILIARY PANCREATITIS ($n = 157$): CLINICAL COURSE*

First Days after EPT	
Healing	96%
Deterioration followed by delayed healing	2%
Death	1%
Follow-up after 1 Month	
Relapse of pancreatitis	6%
Recurrent common bile duct stone	4%
Cholecystitis	19% of patients with gallbladder
Elective cholecystectomy	33% of patients with gallbladder

* From Escourrou et al.[9]

intervention by the use of the knife or the endoscope will receive copious attention in the surgical literature over the course of the next few years.''[19]

AOP by Parasites

Ascaris lumbricoides is a common problem in many countries, and it is estimated that 25% of the entire world population is infested. Spontaneous appearance and disappearance in the bile duct can be diagnosed by ultrasound in many patients.[15] Sonography detected worms in the biliary tree in 24 of 28 (85.7%) and in the dilated pancreatic duct in 1 further patient. These findings were proved by ERCP.[15] Serial sonograms accurately demonstrated the spontaneous exit of worms in 18 of 28 patients and the persistence in 3 patients. The parasite may lodge in the biliopancreatic ductal system and cause AOP. Intestinal disease can be cured with anthelminthic drugs, but parasites inside the biliopancreatic system are resistant. They can be removed by EPT and basket extraction.[18] An interesting report from China describes the endoscopic removal of 15 live *Ascaris* worms from 14 patients with AP by means of a grasping forceps. In the patients the worm was visibly located in the ampulla of Vater and protruded into the duodenum. The patients recovered quickly after the endoscopic intervention. This paper supports our view of the pathogenetic mechanism of papillary obstruction in AOP.[4]

CONCLUSION

Opie's theory that ampullary obstruction (stones, parasites, etc.) can be the cause of AP is strongly supported by recent clinical observations. The term *acute obstructive pancreatitis* is proposed. It is not clear, however, why an intermittent or continuous obstruction of the ampulla leads to AP in some patients but not in others. Further careful studies concerning anatomic variations of the ampulla, direction of flow, chemistry, and microbiology of the secretions are urgently needed. Endoscopy will have to play an important role in these investigations.

Endoscopy with retrograde cannulation of the papilla of Vater (ERCP) allows one to establish the diagnosis of AOP. Recently published studies suggest that ERC studies can be safely done in case of AP if applied by an experienced endoscopist. An ERCP should be performed within 24 hours in patients with AP of unclear origin. Therapy should be instituted immediately, if required, by endoscopic means (EPT, stone extraction). Compared with other indications EPT has no greater risk in AOP. It is less invasive than surgery and is preferred by patients.

REFERENCES

1. Acosta JM, Ledesma CL. Gallstone migration as a cause of acute pancreatitis. N Engl J Med 290:484–487, 1974.
2. Acosta JM, Rossi R, Galli O, Pellegrini CA, Skinner DB. Early surgery for acute gallstone pancreatitis: Evaluation of a systemic approach Surgery 83:367–370, 1978.
3. Bell AM, O'Rourke MGE. Gallstone pancreatitis. Med J Aust 144:572–574, 1986.

4. Chen YS, Den BX, Huang BI, Xu LZ. Endoscopic diagnosis and management of ascaris—Induced acute pancreatitis. Endoscopy 18:127–128, 1986.
5. Classen M, Ossenberg FW, Wurbs D, Hagenmüller F. Pancreatitis—An indication for endoscopic papillotomy? Endoscopy 10:223, 1978.
6. Dupas JL, Delcenserie R, July JP. Early endoscopic sphincterotomy. An alternative to early surgery in gallstone pancreatitis. Dig Dis Sci 31(suppl):1199, 1986. Abstract.
7. Eimiller A, Neuhaus H, Schmidt F, et al. Ergebnisse der Notfallpapillotomie bei akuter Pankreatitis unterschiedlicher Genese. Gastroenterol 25:450, 1987.
8. Escourrou J. Treatment of gallstone pancreatitis. Abstract presented at the 8th World Congress of Gastroenterology, Sao Paulo, 1986.
9. Escourrou J, Liguory Cl, Boyer J, Hagenmüller F, Classen M. Emergency endoscopic sphinterotomy in acute biliary pancreatitis: Results of a multicenter study. Gastroenterology 92:1385 (abstract), 1986.
10. Frei SJ, Fsei VT, Thirlby RC, McClelland RN. Biliary pancreatitis: Clinical presentation and surgical management. Am J Surg 151:170–174, 1986.
11. Gebhardt CH, Riemann JF, Lux G: The importance of ERCP for the surgical tactic in hemorrhagic necrotizing pancreatitis. Endoscopy 15:55–58, 1983.
12. Goodman AJ, Neoptolemos JP, Carr-Locke DL, Finlay DBL, Fossard DP. Detection of gallstones after acute pancreatitis. Gut 26:125–132, 1985.
13. Kelly TR. Gallstone pancreatitis. Arch Surg 109:294–297, 1974.
14. Kelly TR. Gallstone pancreatitis—The timing of surgery. Surgery 88, 345–350, 1980.
15. Khuroo MS, Zargar SA, Mahajan R, Bhat RL, Javid G. Sonographic appearances in biliary ascariasis. Gastroenterology 93:267–269, 1987.
16. Leung JWL, Chung SCS, et al. The role of early ERCP and sphincterotomy in the management of acute biliary pancreatitis. Gastroenterology 92:1503, 1987.
17. Lux G, Riemann JF, Demling L: Biliäre Pankreatitis—Diagnostische und therapeutische Möglichkeiten durch ERCP und endoskopische Papillotomie. Gastroenterol 22:346–356, 1984.
18. Manialawi MS, Khattar NY, Helmy MM, Burcharth F. Endoscopic diagnosis and extraction of biliary *Ascaris*. Endoscopy 18:204, 1986.
19. McMahon MJ. Acute pancreatitis. Curr Opinion Gastroenterol 3:698–713, 1987.
20. Mouiel J, Bertrand JC, Mazarguil JP, Vedel JP, Coubier M. The role of millithiasis in the pathogenesis of acute pancreatitis. In: FL Hollender, ed. Controversies in Acute Pancreatitis. Berlin, Heidelberg Springer, 1982, pp 11–14.
21. Neoptolemos JD, Cass-Locke DC, London NJ, et al. Controlled trial of urgent endoscopic retrograde cholangiopancreatography and endoscopic sphincterotomy versus conservative treatment for acute pancreatitis due to gallstones. Lancet 2:979–983, 1988.
22. Nordestgaard AG, Wilson SE, Williams RA. Early computerized tomography as a predictor of outcome in acute pancreatitis. Am J Surg 152:127–130, 1986.
23. Prorok JJ, Frostle DR. Early definitive surgery for acute pancreatitis associated with choledocholithiasis. Am Surg 52:201–204, 1986.
24. Rösch W. ERCP in acute and chronic pancreatitis. In: Sivak MV Jr, ed. Gastroenterologic Endoscopy. Philadelphia, London, WB Saunders, 1987, pp 780–793.
25. Safrany L, Neuhaus B, Krause S, Portocarrero G, Schott B. Endoskopische Papillotomie bei akuter biliärer Pankreatitis. Dtsch Med Wochenschr 105:115–119, 1980.
26. Schelmerich J, Fross V, Johannesson BL, et al. Detection of biliary origin of acute pancreatitis. Comparison of laboratory tests, ultrasound, computed tomograpy, and ERCP. Dig Dis Sci 34:830–833, 1989.
27. Steer ML. Timing of surgery for gallstone pancreatitis. Gastroenterology 91:780–781, 1986. Selected summary.
28. Stone HH, Fabian TC, Dunlop WE. Gallstone pancreatitis: Biliary tract pathology in relation to time of operation. Ann Surg: 194:305–312, 1981.
29. Virjee J. Diagnostic radiology of pancreatobiliary tract. Curr Opinion Gastroenterol 3:655–663, 1987.

CHAPTER

9

THE RELATIONSHIP BETWEEN PANCREAS DIVISUM AND PANCREATITIS: MEDICAL ASPECTS

Charles J. Mitchell

EDITORIAL COMMENT (Chapters 9 and 10)

There are perhaps few areas as controversial in pancreatology today as the relationship of pancreas divisum to acute and chronic pancreatitis. This condition is the latest candidate proposed for an etiologic role in idiopathic pancreatitis, and it may be expected that the division between the proponents and those yet unconvinced will remain wide until more evidence from controlled trials of interventional procedures in pancreatitis associated with pancreas divisum are carried out. The main concern among the unconvinced is the relative frequency of pancreas divisum as an incidental anatomic abnormality at autopsy and ERCP (estimated at 4%–6%) as against the rarity of pancreatitis in these patients and that it may be no more than an incidental finding in patients with acute or chronic pancreatitis. This does not exclude the etiologic role in selected patients: there are very similar circumstances in medicine in which disease is only expressed in a small number of patients with an underlying abnormality. In this regard, it is difficult to explain otherwise the development of recurrent acute attacks in young patients in whom no other cause can be found and in whom pancreas divisum is present on ERCP. The editor (S. B.), has recently seen with Dr. David Dreiling such a patient, who has had recurrent attacks since the age of 16 with progressive decrease in secretin-stimulated pancreatic exocrine function over a 10-year period, suggesting progression to a chronic (? obstructive) type of pancreatitis. Despite this, the variable symptomatic response to endoscopic or surgical accessory sphincterotomy makes therapeutic decisions difficult with regard to the timing of therapy. If the symptoms are related to flow against a somewhat obstructed sphincter, the use of cholecystokinin-receptor antagonists or high doses of proteinase inhibitors may decrease secretion and should have some therapeutic benefit. If surgical therapy is contemplated, it should be reserved for younger patients with recurrent acute attacks in whom evidence of a dilated pancreatic duct can be visualized by CT scanning or secretin untrasound study and carried out by experienced surgeons.

Dr. Warshaw's careful studies of patients with pancreas divisum and abdominal symptoms suggest a chronic progressive or recurrent nonsevere pancreatitis. In selected patients demonstrating a positive secretin ultrasound study, the results of accessory papillotomy in his hands is beneficial in 75% to 80%. Perhaps more precise diagnostic methodology for elucidating papillary dysfunction and intermittent ductal obstruction may be developed. An unoperated group should serve as controls in future studies to permit a rational analysis of this problem.

CONTROVERSY

The embryologic abnormality of pancreas divisum is found in up to 6% of normal individuals at autopsy. Faced with this frequency, physicians find disease states attributed to this anatomic variation difficult to evaluate. It is thus not surprising that opposing views exist, varying from incriminating pancreas divisum as a cause of acute obstructive pancreatitis and even chronic pancreatitis to skepticism of the role of pancreas of the role of pancreas divisum in any disease state.

Pancreas divisum (PD) is increasingly encountered in clinical practice largely because endoscopic retrograde cholangiopancreatography (ERCP) has become widely available. The anomaly is caused by a failure of fusion of the dorsal and ventral pancreatic primordia in embryologic life so that the larger dorsal portion of the pancreas drains through the accessory ampulla separately from the smaller ventral portion, which drains through the main ampulla. Particular clinical interest has focused upon the possibility that PD causes or predisposes to the development of pancreatitis. Pancreas divisum is not a new discovery[39] and was documented in autopsy studies by Graaf in 1667. It was not until this century that systematic autopsy studies of the pancreatic duct system were carried out, which enabled the frequencies of the various anatomic arrangements to be more clearly defined. The use of ERCP has enabled large numbers of patients to be studied; early studies considered PD to be clinically irrelevant, but later authors have felt that the anomaly caused pancreatitis, leading some to embark upon surgical management of the condition. More recent studies have once again cast doubt upon the relationship between pancreatitis and PD, so that the pendulum has again swung back and confusion reigns once more about the most appropriate management of the condition.

The purposes of this chapter are to

1. Describe the anomaly and its anatomy
2. Assess the incidence of PD
3. Review the evidence for its relevance to the development of pancreatitis
4. Discuss the management of PD

EMBRYOLOGIC DEVELOPMENT

Meckel was the first to provide an embryologic interpretation of PD.[22] The pancreas develops from two distinct primordia—the dorsal and ventral anlagen—which arise from the duodenal diverticulum at an early stage of gestation (Fig. 9-1A). By the seventh week of intrauterine life the ventral anlage has rotated clockwise to be adjacent to the dorsal anlage (Fig. 9-1B) and the two have fused

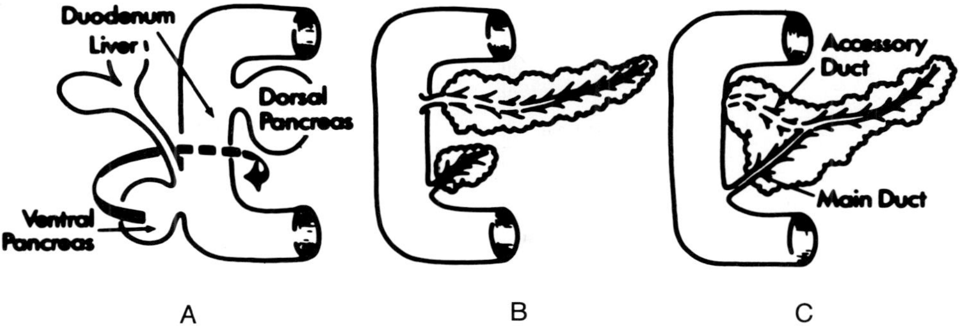

Figure 9-1. Embryologic development of the pancreas. (From Mitchell,[24] with permission.)

(Fig. 9-1C). Fusion of the two anlagen also means that in most instances the two duct systems also amalgamate. As a result, the main pancreatic duct is derived from both anlagen so that the dorsal pancreas contributes the main duct in the body and tail of the gland and the ventral pancreas provides the main duct in the head of the pancreas; the remaining part of the pancreatic duct in the dorsal anlage (shown by interrupted lines in Fig. 9-1C) provides the accessory duct. Thus, the normal anatomic arrangement is for the majority of the pancreatic duct system to drain through the ampulla of Vater together with the common bile duct, and the accessory duct drains through a small ampulla that is situated more proximally in the duodenal loop. Autopsy studies have demonstrated that this is the normal arrangement in 90% of specimens; an accessory duct is demonstrated in 85%, and communication between the two ducts is variable, occurring in 33% to 90% of specimens.

On some occasions the two duct systems on the ventral and dorsal anlagen fail to fuse, leaving the arrangement as shown in Fig. 9-1B, and this is the anomaly referred to as PD; examples are shown in Fig. 9-2. The result is that the larger dorsal part of the gland drains exclusively through the smaller accessory ampulla. Although PD is an unusual anomaly, it is certainly much commoner than an annular pancreas. More confusingly, the isolated ventral portion of the pancreas may only be vestigial (or even absent) or there may only be a minor connection, via secondary or tertiary duct branches, between the dorsal and ventral pancreas—*partial* PD. Illustrative examples are shown in Fig. 9-3.

INCIDENCE OF PD

The summarized results of a representative selection of the reported autopsy studies are shown in Table 9-1. It can be seen that the overall incidence is of the order of 7% (range 1%–11%).[2,3,10,23,31,40] These figures are similar to those reported for ERCP series (see Table 9-2) but do require some care in their interpretation. There is evidence that the incidence of PD shows geographic variation,

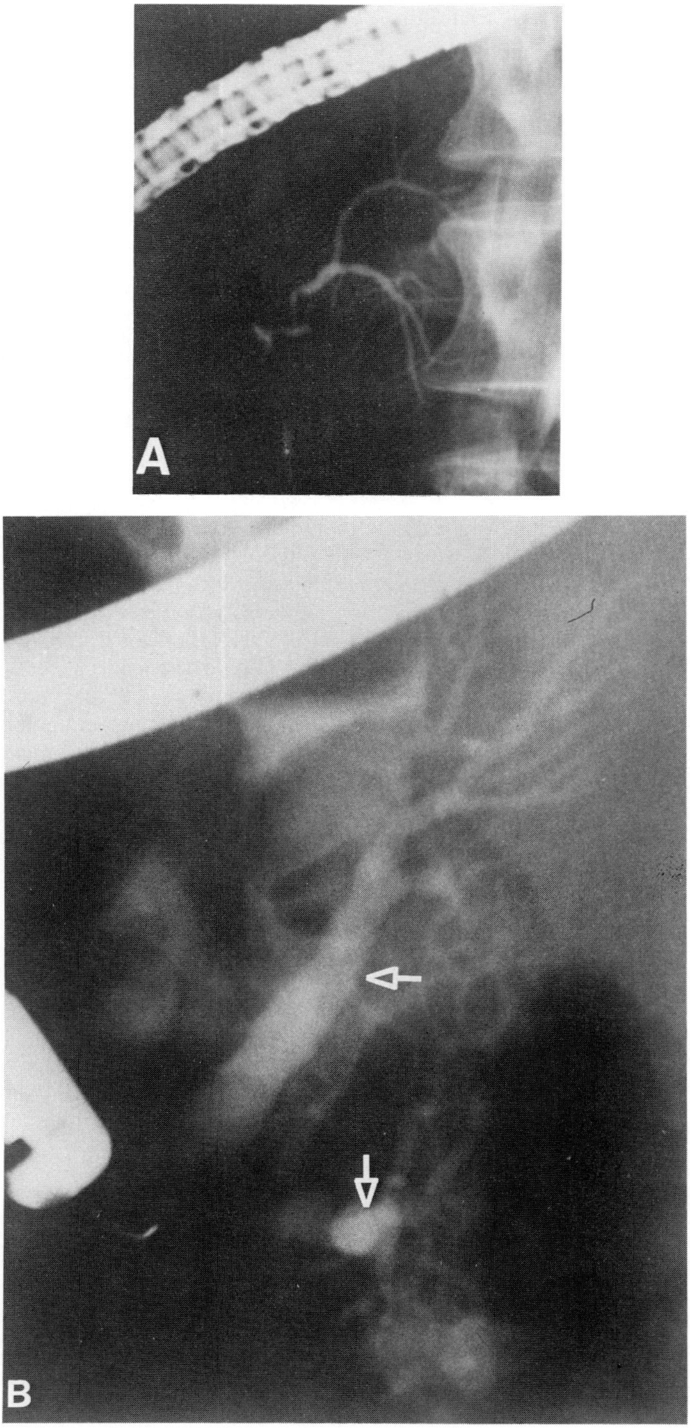
A
B

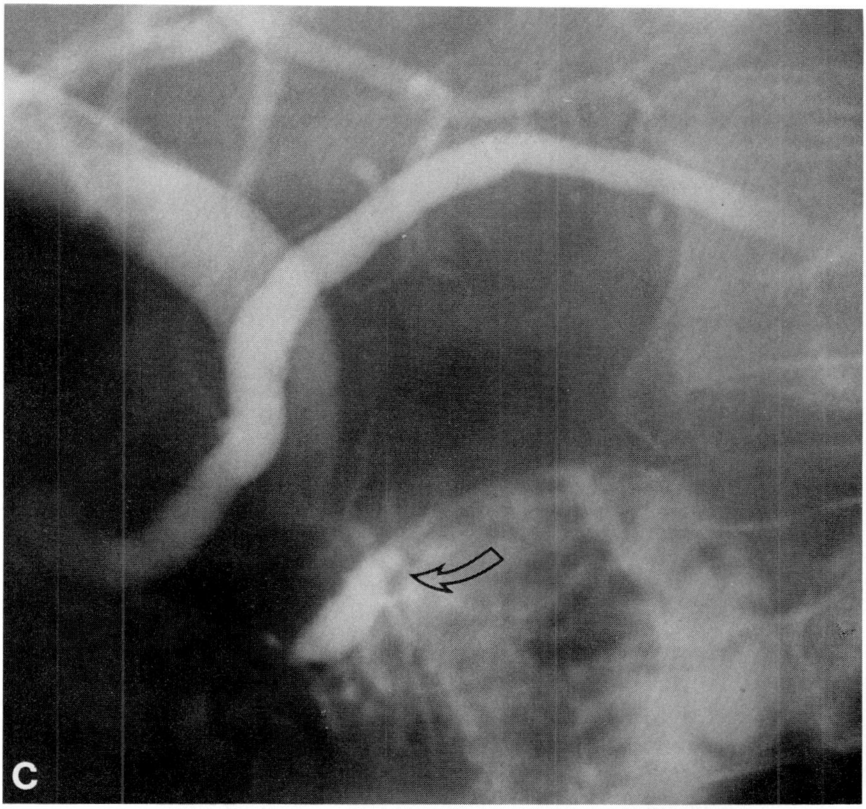

Figure 9-2. (A) A small ventral duct system. (B) An unusual extensive duplex ventral duct system (arrows) filled by cannulation of the main ampulla. (C) Demonstration of both ventral and dorsal duct systems after sequential cannulations of the main and the accessory ampulla. A small ventral duct system (arrow) is shown, as well as the separate dorsal duct. Contrast material is also present in the biliary tract. Note that side branch changes are present in both ducts in this patient with idiopathic chronic pancreatitis.

TABLE 9-1. INCIDENCE OF PD IN AUTOPSY SERIES

Author	Total Studied	Total PD, %
Baldwin[2]	76	5 (6.6)
Reinhoff and Pickrell[31]	100	11 (11.0)
Millbourn[23]	200	11 (5.5)
Berman et al.[3]	130	1 (0.8)
Dawson and Langman[10]	120	9 (7.5)
Stolte and Trommsdorff[40]	325	25 (7.7)

TABLE 9-2. INCIDENCE OF PD AT ERCP

Author	Total ERCP	Total PD, %
Thompson et al.[42]	850	11 (1.3)
Tulassy and Papp[43]	2377	33 (1.4)
Phillip et al.[29]	666	18 (2.7)
Gregg[12]	1100	33 (3.0)
Rosch et al.[33]	1850	63 (3.4)
Mitchell et al.[25]	449	21 (4.7)
Richter et al.[30]	519	26 (5.0)
Sahel et al.[36]	812	41 (5.0)
Cotton[8]	810	47 (5.8)
Ott and Rosch[28]	2389	140 (5.9)
Kruse[19]	700	41 (6.0)
Delhaye et al.[11]	3672	253 (6.9)

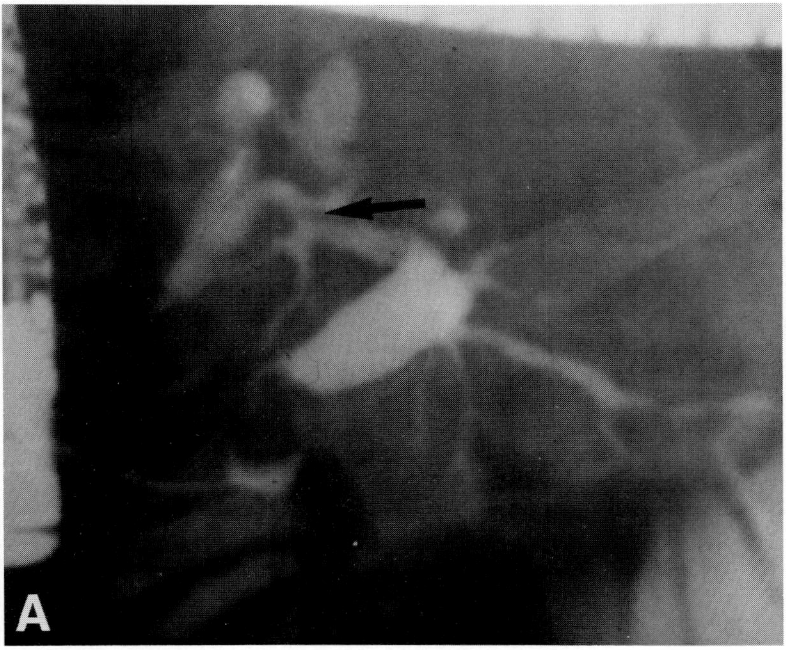

Figure 9-3. Partial fusion of the pancreatic duct system. (A) Cannulation of the main ampulla has filled a small, rather bulbous, duct system (the filling defect at the ampulla is a pancreatic stone). There is only a tertiary connection (arrow) with the dorsal duct, which is only partly filled, and is obviously abnormal. (B) A peculiar arrangement in a partially fused duct system. Cannulation of the main ampulla has filled the main duct. A larger distal accessory duct (arrow) arises as a side branch from a much narrower proximal portion, which crosses the main duct to drain the ventral pancreas. Florid changes of chronic pancreatitis are present throughout in this alcoholic patient. (*Figure continues.*)

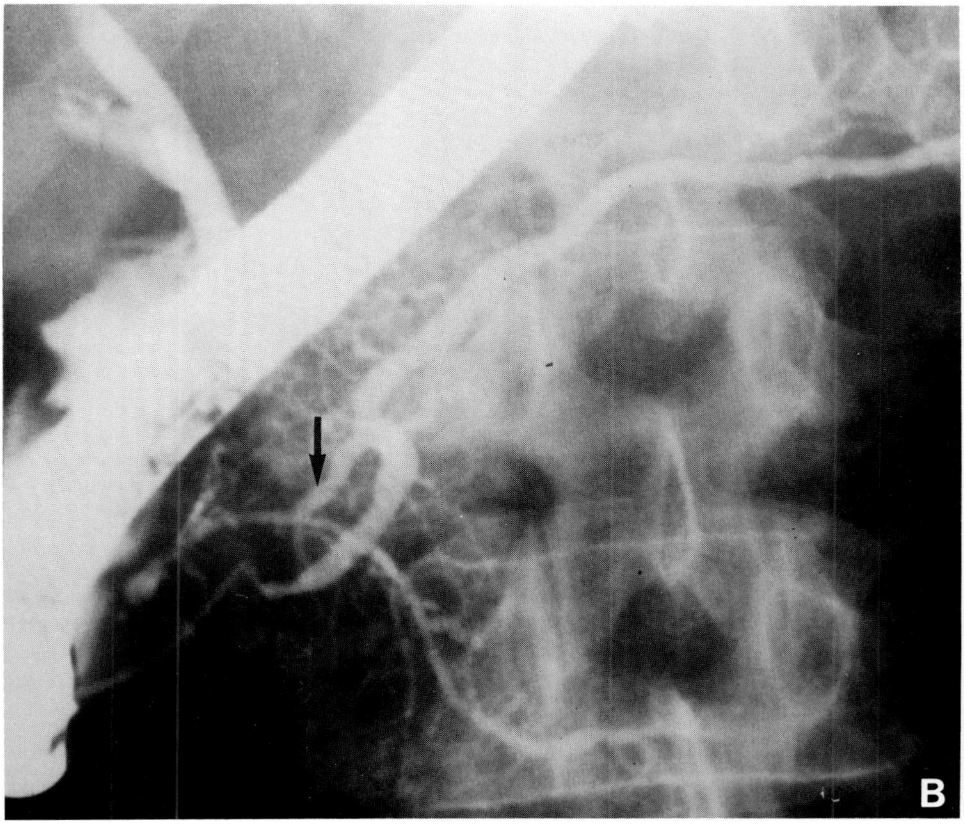

Figure 9-3. *(continued)*

particularly being less common in Hungary and Japan (where, interestingly, pancreatitis is uncommon). Delhaye et al. have found that incidence of PD detected by them has risen with increasing expertise at ERCP to a level of about 9%.[11]

PRACTICAL IMPLICATIONS

Regardless of whether one considers PD to be clinically significant, there are some important practical points for all who undertake ERCP. The separate ventral duct system filled by cannulation of the main ampulla is variable in size but always of small capacity, so that acinar filling, with the consequent risk of pancreatitis, is easily produced. Furthermore, careful radiologic screening during the injection of contrast material is required to demonstrate the anomaly consistently since the duct system may be tiny and not otherwise recognized. Failure to produce a pancreatogram (which may be due to an absent or vestigial ventral

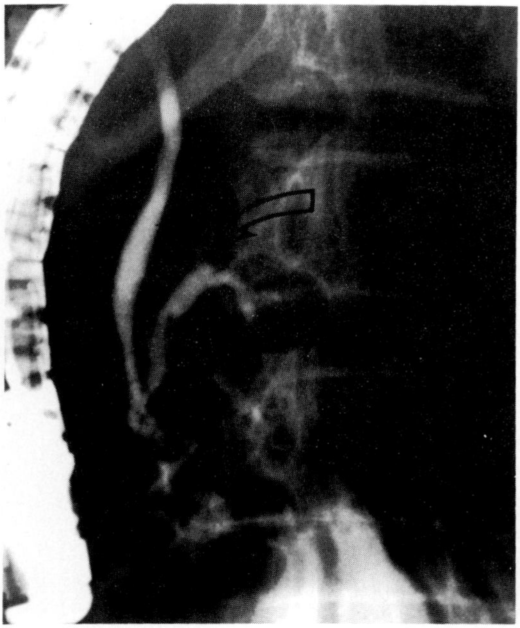

Figure 9-4. False PD. The pancreatic duct has been partially filled and terminates abruptly (arrow). The danger is to misinterpret this appearance as PD, when it is as likely to be due to cancer or pancreatitis. In fact further contrast injection showed terminal arborization rather than an obstructed main duct.

duct) or the demonstration of PD indicates the need to attempt accessory cannulation. This is difficult, but with experience, success rates of up to 80% are now being reported.[11,27] Usually a fine needle tipped catheter, such as the Cremer cannula, is required, and the accessory orifice can be rendered more visible after administration of intravenous secretin.

There are also other difficulties that may lead to diagnostic confusion. The most important is that a proximal duct occlusion by carcinoma,[24] or less commonly chronic pancreatitis,[46] can be misinterpreted as the anomaly–*false* PD (see Fig. 9-4), but in this situation there is usually an absence of terminal arborization of the ventral duct to give the clue. Also, PD may be incomplete (see Fig. 9-3) with only a secondary branch connection between the two main ducts, and this can look very like encasement due to a small tumor.[44] The presence of a double ventral duct system (see Fig. 9-2B) or carcinoma in the presence of PD may lead to bizarre appearances and further difficulties.

PANCREAS DIVISUM AND PANCREATITIS

The main interest in PD relates to whether or not it causes or predisposes to the development of pancreatitis. The eminently reasonable hypothesis is that in the presence of PD, major pancreatic drainage from the bulk of the gland is via the small accessory ampulla; this results in relative obstruction to secretory flow causing obstructive pancreatitis in the dorsal segment or "pancreatic pain." Current opinion as to the validity of this hypothesis remains sharply divided, and the purpose of this section is to review the available evidence from a rapidly proliferating literature.

Unfortunately, there are major problems in the interpretation of available data, as has previously been pointed out.[9,24] ERCP is performed in highly selected patient groups, and most reports reflect local interest and expertise. Furthermore, there is a distinct difficulty in providing realistic control groups, since normal subjects are understandably not studied; the use of patients with purely biliary disease as controls may not be valid and neither may be the use of those patients subsequently found to have no pancreatic disease, since the initial indication for ERCP must at least have suggested an underlying pancreatic lesion. Increasing numbers of ERCPs are performed for purely biliary indications (when pancreatography is frequently not attempted) and analysis of only those who did have a successful pancreatogram leads to bias that underestimates the incidence of PD in what is frequently used as a control group. Current tests for pancreatitis are insensitive, particularly in the diagnosis of early pancreatitis. Even when PD is demonstrated, accessory cannulation is frequently unsuccessful, particularly in earlier published series, and apparent cannulation failures contain some patients with an absent ventral pancreas. Further problems in the analysis of data include the possibility that PD may actually protect patients from the development of biliary pancreatitis or be an important cofactor with alcohol abuse in the production of pancreatitis. The problems of assessing whether there is really a relevant etiologic factor, notably alcohol, for pancreatitis in an individual patient is familiar to all who have worked in this field, and the reclassification of only small numbers of patients from idiopathic to alcoholic pancreatitis in a given series would markedly affect the conclusions.

Finally it is generally agreed that PD is clinically irrelevant in the great majority of cases (over 80%) and that it is only in the context of pancreatitis (or possibly undiagnosed abdominal pain) that the anomaly may be causative. One has to analyze some 25,000 pancreatograms to yield 1000 cases of PD, and since the anomaly will be clinically irrelevant in most, there will only remain about 200 patients with PD who also have pancreatitis, of whom at least half will have a recognized cause, leaving under 100 with idiopathic pancreatitis. The problems of statistical analysis after such "data dredging" have been pointed out by Langman[9] and are further confused by referral patterns to individual centers.

The large volume of published work supports the concept that PD causes pancreatitis, but few papers stand up to a detailed analysis. Cotton described 47 cases and found that 40% of these patients also had idiopathic pancreatitis compared with only 8% with normal duct anatomy;[8] conversely the incidence of PD in patients with idiopathic pancreatitis was impressively high at 25% compared with a control group with biliary tract disease, in whom the incidence was only 3.6%. A large study,[43] recently updated,[45] provided further support, because 46% of patients with PD had a previous history of acute pancreatitis compared with only 31% of patients with normal duct anatomy—a statistically significant difference; possible reservations about this work include the low incidence of PD in the series as a whole, the criteria used to diagnose pancreatitis, and the fact that the quoted relative risk has halved between the initial study and subsequent update. Another careful study showed a significantly higher incidence (13%) of PD in pancreatitis compared with those with nonpancreatic disease.[5]

Excepting these reports, the evidence for a causal association becomes less convincing. Gregg, who is often quoted, found that 39% of his patients with pancreatitis had PD,[12] but unfortunately he did not relate this figure to the total ERCP experience, and neither did Kruse,[19] who reported a 20% incidence of PD in chronic pancreatitis, similar to other reported incidences for normal duct anatomy.[25,45] Likewise, the Marseilles group in a study of 63 cases of PD found that 30% had acute or recurrent pancreatitis,[6] but again data for the incidence of pancreatitis with normal duct anatomy are not recorded.

Other widely quoted papers are open to considerable criticism. While Richter et al. showed a significantly higher incidence of PD in pancreatitis compared with controls (12% versus 3%),[30] 8 of the 15 with PD and pancreatitis also suffered from gallstones, cancer, or alcohol abuse; therefore, the incidence of PD in *idiopathic* pancreatitis in this series is only 6%, and conversely the 28% incidence of pancreatitis in PD was similar to that found in patients with normal duct anatomy (22%). A further paper from the same group appears to rely upon the same data.[47]

Another quoted study largely concerns the surgical management of PD and does not compare the incidence of PD and of normal duct systems in pancreatitis:[8] note that in only 4 of these 21 patients with PD was no other cause for their symptoms found. In two small studies most of the patients with PD and pancreatitis had another recognized cause for their disease.[4,17] Other studies likewise concerned few patients[1,16] or did not even claim to address the epidemiologic aspects.[21,42]

Therefore, the evidence in favor of the hypothesis is not as convincing as the number of reports implies. What, then, is the evidence for the converse view? The first large series reported 63 cases of PD, and only 8 patients had radiologic signs of pancreatitis, of whom 4 had disease in both anlagen;[33] other information is sparse, and the overall incidence of pancreatitis in the series is not quoted. A report from our own center again failed to show that PD caused pancreatitis—a view that we still hold after experience with over 100 cases—since the anomaly occurred equally in patients with and without pancreatitis;[25] furthermore, idiopathic pancreatitis was no more common in patients with PD (16%) than without (12%). A justified criticism of this study is that accessory cannulation was only rarely achieved, so that dorsal pancreatitis at ERCP was not excluded, but in over 80% of the patients with the anomaly an alternative, nonpancreatic, cause for their symptoms was found. A larger but infrequently quoted series of 140 cases of PD was reported in 1983;[28] only 38 of these cases had pancreatitis, which was idiopathic in 13 patients, that is, 9% of the total with PD. Pancreatitis was no more common in the presence of PD than with normal duct anatomy (27% vs. 25%). The largest study by Delhaye et al. comprises 304 patients with PD,[11] and it is important that the authors were able to achieve accessory cannulation with increasing frequency (overall in 62%). They found that PD was no more common in pancreatic disease than in other conditions. In the presence of chronic pancreatitis, the prevalence of PD was similar for alcoholic and idiopathic causes (7.2% vs. 4.6%), and in acute pancreatitis the anomaly was significantly commoner in alcoholic than in idiopathic pancreatitis (15% vs. 6.7%), but patients with biliary pancreatitis were less likely to have PD. The authors argue that in alcoholic pancreatitis an acute attack represents a single episode in the course of chronic disease so that all alcoholic pancreatitis should be considered together and when this is done the prevalence of PD is similar for alcoholic and nonalcoholic pancreatitis. Criticism of this large and careful study has been muted, although some have contested the validity of comparing all alcoholic pancreatitis to nonalcoholic pancreatitis, but this author would consider this to be a valid concept in the light of our current knowledge. The most recent study, comprising 41 patients, found that only 2 (4%) had pancreatitis, whereas 5% of patients with normal duct anatomy had idiopathic pancreatitis.[41] The conclusions to be drawn from such conflicting data appear to be as follows:

1. There is no doubt that in the majority of patients (over 80%), PD is clinically irrelevant.

2. Much of the evidence purporting to show that PD causes pancreatitis does not bear detailed analysis and other quoted papers do not even claim to do so.

3. There remain a few careful studies that support the author's conclusions either for or against the hypothesis; the total case numbers, rather than the reports, now favor the null hypothesis.

4. There remains an impression, and little more, that PD could be an additional risk factor in the development of alcoholic pancreatitis. Pancreatic hypersecretion occurs in early alcoholic pancreatitis and its effects might be exacerbated by the presence of PD.

5. The hypothesis that PD may cause "obstructive pancreatic pain"—whatever that may be—is not substantiated and probably these patients have another cause for their symptoms.

EVIDENCE FOR ACCESSORY AMPULLA OBSTRUCTION

The alternative approach to sustain the hypothesis that PD causes pancreatitis is to provide evidence that functional obstruction and/or pancreatic damage is present in the dorsal segment. A variety of evidence has been provided, ranging from clinical observation to more objective pressure measurements. Several authors have noted that pancreatic secretion spurts from the accessory ampulla under "high" (but not measured) pressure after secretory stimulation or accessory papillotomy. It has also been observed that there is sometimes a delay in the drainage of injected contrast material from the dorsal duct, but this does not correlate with the presence or absence of dorsal pancreatitis. One might also expect the dorsal duct to be dilated when PD is causing pancreatitis, which again is not a consistent finding.

If pancreatitis was confined to the dorsal anlage, this would support the hypothesis. While dorsal changes alone occur more frequently, there are an important but consistent minority of patients (about 30%) in whom ventral duct disease alone is seen;[5,9,24] and both ducts are abnormal in significant numbers of patients, particularly alcoholics. The accepted radiologic criteria for pancreatitis in the presence of normal duct anatomy may not be applicable to PD. Histologic studies are infrequent, but Rhode et al. found pancreatitis confined to the dorsal anlage in 9 of 13 resected specimens, whilst the dorsal changes were more severe in the remainder with disease in both anlagen.[32] The latter observation, also reported by others, is hardly surprising because the dorsal pancreas constitutes much of the gland, particularly its exocrine secretory component. Direct measurement of the size of the accessory ampulla using calibrated probes has been advocated by Warshaw et al., who proposed a lower limit of normal of 0.75 mm,[47] but others have been less enthusiastic, and endoscopic measurement is unsatisfactory.[9] A less invasive method uses ultrasonographic measurement of the dorsal duct diameter after secretin stimulation: one report found that postsecretin dilatation was an excellent predictor of stenosis,[48] but this has not been confirmed by Lowes et al., who also found (as have others) that secretin caused duct dilatation in significant numbers of normal controls.[20] Finally, Staritz et al. have performed endoscopic retrograde manometry of the accessory ampulla in controls and patients with PD and pancreatitis and showed that pressure was significantly higher in the latter group.[38] However, the diameter of the pressure-recording device (1.7 mm) meant that only nonstenotic ampullae could be studied, and the difference could be caused by pancreatitis rather than PD. The finding of associated choledochal sphincter stenosis reported in 37 of 90 patients[14] provides the rationale for dual sphincteroplasty.

ANCILLARY INVESTIGATIONS

To date no reliable investigation of PD less invasive than ERCP has been developed. There are sporadic reports that the pancreatic head appears enlarged at ultrasound or computed tomography (CT) in a minority of patients with PD.[25,37,50] Usually, however, the CT or ultrasound appearances are normal. There are no serum markers of PD. Pancreatic function tests are not helpful in diagnosis of the anomaly. Systematic studies of pure pancreatic juice collection for either quantitative or qualitative analysis are not available. When endoscopic dorsal pancreatography has failed and a decision to operate has been made, prograde operative pancreatography has been used to determine the nature of surgical intervention.

The diagnosis of acute or chronic pancreatitis in the presence of PD follows standard lines. Evidence of morphologic abnormality should be sought using ultrasound and/or CT scanning and pancreatic calcification may be present on a plain abdominal x-ray film. Exocrine function tests will detect insufficiency; steatorrhea may be present or diabetes detected. Serum amylase levels have frequently been reported to be elevated in patients with PD and acute (recurrent) pancreatitis, as one might expect. The insensitivity of the tests—particularly for early chronic pancreatitis—will at times lead to a persisting clinical impression that significant disease is present in spite of normal investigations. This is quite a diagnostic dilemma since whether or not one believes that the PD itself should be tackled directly, it is a great help to know whether or not pancreatitis is truly present. A technique that we have recently found useful is percutaneous pancreatic biopsy under ultrasound guidance to provide a histologic, rather than cytologic, sample. This technique is still in its infancy, but initial reports suggest that it is both safe and accurate.[15,26] We have biopsied the dorsal pancreas in only three patients with PD but found that the information provided was extremely helpful in their subsequent management.

SURGICAL TREATMENT OF PANCREAS DIVISUM

The declared association between PD and pancreatitis has prompted efforts to improve accessory ampulla drainage and thus hopefully alleviate the problem. Endoscopic accessory sphincterotomy was the first procedure attempted, but it is technically difficult. A recent review[9] of 43 cases followed for 3 years[35,36] showed symptomatic improvement in half of those with recurrent acute pancreatitis but in none of those with chronic pancreatitis. Restenosis occurred in up to 75% of patients, and the procedure carried a 25% complication rate. Most centers have now abandoned this approach, but preliminary results of stent insertion in the accessory ampulla are encouraging.

Early surgical approaches to the problem consisted of various forms of sphincteroplasty. Most commonly, both ampullae have been drained, often with additional cholecystectomy. In 9 reported series[1,4,7,12,13,16,17,21,30] a good symptomatic result was achieved in 35 of the 56 (63%) patients. The indication for operation was intractable symptoms (such as pain), but many of those operated upon did not have documented pancreatitis, and these were the patients who derived least benefit. Up to half of the patients treated also had a diseased gallbladder removed,[20] so that one wonders whether cholecystectomy was actually the beneficial procedure. Two deaths[13,17] and significant morbidity—50% in one series[21] have been reported. Accessory sphincteroplasty alone achieved good short-term results in 16 of 21 patients (76%).[7,30,34,35] A recent series with more prolonged follow-up[18] demonstrated impressive results in 14 patients with acute or recurrent pancreatitis, of whom all but 1 had no recurrent attacks, although again few patients who had pain but no pancreatitis benefited. A larger series comparing both approaches in 29 patients gave good results in 68% regardless of whether single or dual sphincteroplasty was used.[47] A recent update of this series with twice the numbers of accessory sphincteroplasties confirms the earlier results.[49]

The alternative surgical approach has been to use traditional techniques of drainage or resection. Such operations have only been performed when sphincteroplasty has failed or if chronic pancreatitis is established. As might be expected, the results are similar to those for patients without pancreas divisum.[4,12,16,34,35,42]

The author's comments as a physician upon surgical management of PD would be as follows. In the light of experience to date, it is a brave person who contemplates sphincteroplasty for PD in patients with abdominal pain and no evidence of pancreatitis, particularly when there would appear to be a significant morbidity and mortality. The high proportion of patients with PD who have gallbladder disease is interesting and perhaps makes surgical attack toward this aspect more appropriate. One should also remember the enthusiasm with which sphincterotomy of the main ampulla was performed as a treatment for chronic pancreatitis some 30 years ago, yet this would now be regarded as inappropriate. Finally the initial good results of sphincteroplasty for PD were achieved at only short follow-up periods, and evidence is now accumulating that the longer-term results are much more disappointing. Once chronic pancreatitis is established, it would seem that operations directed toward the accessory ampulla are irrelevant and that the disease should be treated along standard lines.

MANAGEMENT OF PD: A PERSONAL VIEW

Many patients will have already been investigated before the anomaly is found at ERCP, and it will be irrelevant in most because an adequate cause for their symptoms will have been found. There remain some patients requiring further evaluation who can be divided into two groups, namely, those with undiagnosed abdominal pain and those with pancreatitis (acute or chronic).

Abdominal Pain

It is worth emphasizing that there are many other causes of abdominal pain, because in this situation the decision to perform ERCP means that pancreatic disease has been actively considered. There are no pathognomonic features of pain arising from the pancreas, and personally I remain unsure of what constitutes "classical pancreatic pain" so frequently used as an operative indication without other support for the presence of pancreatitis.

One should therefore return to the basics after demonstrating PD in a patient with undiagnosed abdominal pain. Careful review of the history, clinical examination, and the adequacy of prior investigations are mandatory. The most important diagnoses to be excluded are:

1. *Peptic ulceration.* A significant minority of patients prove to have a previously undiagnosed peptic ulcer.

2. *Gallbladder disease.* This is found in ≤25% of patients, all of whom become asymptomatic following cholecystectomy. Note the high frequency with which this condition is found at operation for PD.[21]

3. *Irritable bowel syndrome.* This is a much more difficult condition in which to make a positive diagnosis but is nevertheless prevalent in developed countries. My experience is that 42% of these patients respond to an aggressive regime directed towards this diagnosis so a therapeutic trial is worthwhile.

4. *Depression.* Psychiatric assessment if no organic disease is found leads to a diagnosis of depression in 10% of patients. Perhaps these patients are depressed because of their abdominal pain, but they respond to appropriate treatment nevertheless. Previously unsuspected alcohol abuse has occasionally been detected by this referral.

5. *Miscellaneous conditions.* These have been detected in a few (<5%). Diagnoses of aortic aneurysm, porphyria, hypercalcemia, and hyperlipidemia indicate the requirement to fully investigate these patients.

One is left with very few patients with no positive diagnosis and persisting symptoms, and in such cases second opinions from both a physician and a surgeon are appropriate. This approach is particularly recommended to surgeons, since review of the literature on PD strongly suggests that it is not routine practice before operation. Additionally, the patient should be examined personally during an attack of pain if this has not been done previously particularly if a patient has been referred from elsewhere. History and examination at this time may differ from earlier accounts, and investigations performed while the patient is symptomatic (notably endoscopy, amylase levels, and liver function tests) may provide an answer. Two of our patients examined at this time were found to be severely constipated.

In the absence of previous clinical indications, it is only at this point that I seek more evidence for pancreatitis. Plain x-ray films (for calcification), routine biochemical tests, pancreatic ultrasound examination (while looking for gallbladder disease), and ERCP will already have been performed. We would now perform a CT scan, an exocrine pancreatic function test, and accessory cannulation if not previously successful. The two patients in whom no conclusion had been reached by this stage underwent percutaneous pancreatic biopsy; one had pancreatitis and the other did not.

In no patient of this group has operation been performed. Fewer than 10% have recurrent pain, which is easily controlled without narcotic analgesia; it is too early to say whether they will develop pancreatitis in the future but they have yet to do so and I feel that the results, morbidity and mortality do not justify sphincteroplasty in these patients.

Pancreatitis

In this group of patients my personal approach is to answer three questions:

1. *Is the pancreatitis acute (and recurrent) or chronic?* Pancreatic calcification, exocrine or endocrine insufficiency, or an abnormal pancreatogram will demonstrate the latter, but I suspect that in the future one will also require a normal pancreatic biopsy while the patient is in remission with documented hyperamylasemia during an acute attack to establish a diagnosis of acute recurrent pancreatitis.

2. *Is the pancreatitis really idiopathic?* The established causes of pancreatitis are well known and should be diligently sought, acknowledging the difficulties over alcohol intake and remembering the frequency of gallbladder disease.

3. *Is the disease confined to the dorsal pancreas?* This is a difficult problem to resolve if dorsal pancreatography is unsuccessful, unless of course the ventral pancreas is seen to be diseased (30% of our cases). Operative pancreatography may otherwise be required, as I do not believe that the other diagnostic approaches are validated so far.

If chronic pancreatitis is demonstrated, standard medical management is instituted, and no patient of mine to date has required surgical intervention; this merely reflects local experience of chronic pancreatitis as a whole (a minority are alcoholic), rather than any special treatment, since I find that few of my patients come to operation. If intractable symptoms should occur, the decision to resect or drain would be made along conventional lines. A demonstrable cause for pancreatitis is treated appropriately.

I would consider sphincteroplasty only in those patients with idiopathic acute recurrent pancreatitis and a normal ventral duct system. Personal experience of such patients is paltry (three cases) and the success of sphincteroplasty mixed, so that it would be out of place to comment more fully. However, perhaps what this experience does indicate is that careful assessment of patients with PD plus pain or pancreatitis leads to only a tiny minority who cannot be managed successfully by conservative means. We must be wary of offering an expensive and potentially dangerous operative "placebo" to our patients.

ACKNOWLEDGMENTS

I am grateful to my radiological colleagues in Scarborough and Leeds for their assistance in the provision of radiographs and to Mrs. A. C. Pryde for preparing the manuscript.

REFERENCES

1. Aumais G, Chatti N, Jobin G, Archambault A. Pancréas divisum: Étude rétrospective de 980 catheterismes rétrogrades de la papille. Union Med Can 115:382–386, 1986.
2. Baldwin WM. The pancreatic ducts in man, together with a study of the microscopial structure of the minor duodenal papilla. Anat Rec 5:197–228, 1911.
3. Berman LG, Prior JT, Ambramow SM, Ziegler DD. A study of the pancreatic duct systems in man by the use of vinyl acetate casts of post-mortem preparations. Surg Gynecol Obstet 110:391–403, 1960
4. Britt LG, Samuels AD, Johnson JW. Pancreas divisum: Is it a surgical disease? Ann Surg 197:654–661, 1983.
5. Buhler H, Seefeld U, Deyhle P, Largiader F, Ammann R. Klinische Bedeutung des Pancreas divisum. Schweiz Med Wochenschr 113:320, 1983.
6. Chevillotte G, Sahel J, Pietri H, Sarles H. Pancréatites aiguës à rechutes, associées au pancréas divisum. Gastroenterol Clin Biol 8:352–358, 1984.
7. Cooperman M, Ferrara JJ, Fromkes JJ, Carey LC. Surgical management of pancreas divisum. Am J Surg 143:107–112, 1982.
8. Cotton PB. Congenital anomaly of pancreas division as cause of obstructive pain and pancreatitis. Gut 21:105–114, 1980.
9. Cotton PB. Pancreas divisum: Curiosity or culprit? Gastroenterology 89:1431–1435, 1985.
10. Dawson W, Langman A. An anatomical radiological study on the pancreatic duct pattern in man. Anat Rec 139:59–68, 1961.

11. Delhaye M, Engelholm A, Cremer M. Pancreas divisum: Congenital anatomic variant or anomaly? Gastroenterology 89:951–958, 1985.
12. Gregg JA. Pancreas divisum: Its association with pancreatitis. Am J Surgery 134:539–543, 1977.
13. Gregg JA, Monaco AP, McDermott WV. Pancreas divisum: Results of surgical intervention. Am J Surg 145:488–492, 1983.
14. Gregg J, Solomon J, Clark G. Pancreas divisum and its association with choledochal sphincter stenosis. Am J Surg 147:367–371, 1984.
15. Hall-Craggs MA, Lees WR. Fine needle biopsy: Cytology, histology or both? Gut 28:233–236, 1987.
16. Heiss FW, Shea JA: Association of pancreatitis and variant ductal anatomy: Dominant drainage of the duct of Santorini. Am J Gastroenterol 70:158–162, 1978.
17. Jacocks MA, Remine SG, Carmichael DH. Difficulties in the diagnosis and treatment of pancreas divisum. Arch Surg 119:1088–1091, 1984.
18. Keith RG, Shapero TF, Saibil FG, Moore TG. Dorsal duct sphincterotomy is effective long-term treatment of acute pancreatitis associated with pancreas divisum. Surgery 106:660–667, 1989.
19. Kruse A. Pancreas divisum. Schweiz Rundschau Med 70:2064–2067, 1981.
20. Lowes JR, Lees WR, Cotton PB. Pancreatic duct dilatation after secretin stimulation in patients with pancreas divisum. Pancreas 4:371–374, 1989.
21. Madura JA, Fiore AC, O'Connor KW, Lehmann GA, McCammon RL. Pancreas divisum: Detection and management. Surg 51:353–357, 1985.
22. Meckel JF. Handbuch Der pathologischen Anatomie. Leipzig, CH Reclam, 1812.
23. Millbourn E. On excretory ducts of pancreas in man, with special reference to their relations to each other, to common bile duct and to duodenum. Acta Anat 9:1–34, 1950.
24. Mitchell CJ. Pancreas divisum and pancreatitis. In: Mitchell CJ, Kelleher J, eds. Pancreatic Disease in Clinical Practice. Pitman Books, London, 1981, pp. 404–414.
25. Mitchell CJ, Lintott DJ, Ruddell WSJ, Losowsky, MS, Axon ATR. Clinical relevance of an unfused pancreatic duct system. Gut 20:1066–1071, 1979.
26. Mitchell CJ, Wai D, Jackson AM, MacFie J. Ultrasound guided percutaneous pancreatic biopsy. Br J Surg 76:706–707, 1989.
27. O'Connor KW, Lehmann GA. An improved technique for accessory cannulation in pancreas divisum. Gastrointest Endosc 31:13–17, 1985.
28. Ott H, Rosch W. Pancreas divisum—Ursache einer Pankeatitis? Med Welt 15:466–468, 1983.
29. Phillip J, Koch H, Classen M. Variations and anomalies of the papilla of Vater, the pancreas and the biliary system. Endoscopy 6:70–77, 1974.
30. Richter JM, Shapiro RH, Mulley AG, Warshaw AL. Association of pancreas divisum and pancreatitis and its treatment by sphincteroplasty of the accessory ampulla. Gastroenterology 81:1104–1110, 1981.
31. Reinhoff W, Pickrell K. Pancreatitis. An anatomic study of the pancreatic and extrahepatic biliary systems. Arch Surg 51:205–219, 1945.
32. Rode J, Lowes JR, Dhillon AP, Cotton PB. Pancreas divisum pancreatitis. J Pathol 1986.
33. Rosch W, Koch H, Schaffner P, Demling L. The clinical significance of the pancreas divisum. Gastrointest Endosc 22:206–207, 1976.
34. Rusnak CH, Hosie RT, Kuechler PR, et al. Pancreatitis associated with pancreas divisum. Results of surgical intervention. Am J Surg 155:641–635, 1988.
35. Russell RCG, Wong NW, Cotton PB. Accessory sphincterotomy (endoscopic and surgical) in patients with pancreas divisum. Br J Surg 71:954–957, 1984.
36. Sahel J, Boustiere C, Sarles JC, Chevillotte G, Sarles H. Traitement du "pancréas divisum." Résultats préliminaires. Gastroenterol Clin Biol 7:293–298, 1983.
37. Soulen MC, Zerhouni EA, Fishman EK, et al. Enlargement of the pancreatic head in patients with pancreas divisum. Clin Imaging 13:51–57, 1989.
38. Staritz M, Hütteroth T, Rambow A, Meyer zum Buschenfelde K-H. Intraduktale

Druckmessung bei Pancreas divisum und normalen Pankreasgangsystem. Schweiz Rundschau Med 75:1392–1394, 1986.
39. Stern CS. An historical perspective on the discovery of the accessory duct of the pancreas, the ampulla of 'Vater' and pancreas divisum. Gut 27:203–212, 1986.
40. Stolte M, Trommsdorff, L. Pancreas divisum und chronische Pankreatitis.
41. Sugawa C, Walt AJ, Nunez DC, Masuyama H. Pancreas divisum: Is it a normal anatomic variant. Am J Surg 153:62–67, 1987.
42. Thompson MH, Williamson RCN, Salmon, PR. The clinical relevance of isolated ventral pancreas. Br J Surg 68:101–104, 1981.
43. Tulassy Z, Papp J. New clinical aspects of pancreas divisum. Gastrointest Endosc 26:143–146, 1980.
44. Tulassy Z, Papp J. Diagnostic aspects of incomplete pancreas divisum. Gastrointest Endosc 32:428, 1986. Letter.
45. Tulassy Z, Papp J. Pancreas divisum and pancreatitis. Gastroenterology 91:267, 1986. Letter.
46. Warshaw AL, Cambria RC. False pancreas divisum: acquired pancreatic duct obstruction simulating the congenital anomaly. Ann Surg 200:595–599, 1984.
47. Warshaw AL, Richter JM, Shapiro R. The cause and treatment of pancreatitis associated with pancreas divisum. Ann Surg 198:43–52, 1983.
48. Warshaw AL, Simeone J, Shapiro RH, et al. Objective evaluation of ampullary stenosis with ultrasonography and pancreatic stimulation. Am J Surg 149:65–72, 1985.
49. Warshaw AL, Schapiro RH. Pancreas divisum and Pancreatitis. Surg Annu 20:101–120, 1988.
50. Zeman RK, McVay LV, Silverman PM, et al. Pancreas-divisum: Thin-section CT. Radiology 169:395–398, 1988.

CHAPTER

10

THE RELATIONSHIP BETWEEN PANCREAS DIVISUM AND PANCREATITIS: SURGICAL ASPECTS

Andrew L. Warshaw

Pancreas divisum (PD) is a term originated to describe the anatomic variant wherein the duct systems of the dorsal and ventral segments fail to fuse during embryologic development (Fig. 10-1).[37,39] In consequence the exocrine secretions of the dorsal and ventral segments empty through separate orifices, the minor (accessory) and major papillae, respectively. Recent usage has added another variant in which fusion occurs, but the subsequent regression of the ventral duct segment leaves the dorsal duct and accessory papilla as the only outflow tract for the whole pancreas.[8,37,39] If these two entities are considered together as PD, their combined prevalence is about 9% in the western populations at autopsy[12] or endoscopic pancreatography.[8] It may be considerably less common in the Orient.[7]

Interest in PD—and controversy—has arisen with the suggestion that the anomaly may cause recurrent pancreatitis and "pancreatic pain." Some studies have shown a significant relationship between PD and symptoms,[6,13,17,24,27,31,37,39] while others have not.[8,21,25] The resolution of the differing conclusions may lie in a restatement of the issue: the problem is not PD, at least by itself, but accessory papilla stenosis in persons with PD.

Since most persons with PD are indisputedly healthy and never develop pancreatitis, the separate drainage systems of their dorsal and ventral pancreatic segments are clearly adequate. Following the hoary dictum "If it ain't broke, don't fix it," there is no treatment, medical or surgical, required in this great majority. It was suggested, however, that some *few* people with PD *also* had an inadequate opening of the accessory papilla.[6,13,18,24,37,39] It is not known whether that stenosis might be congenital or acquired. In either event, accessory papilla

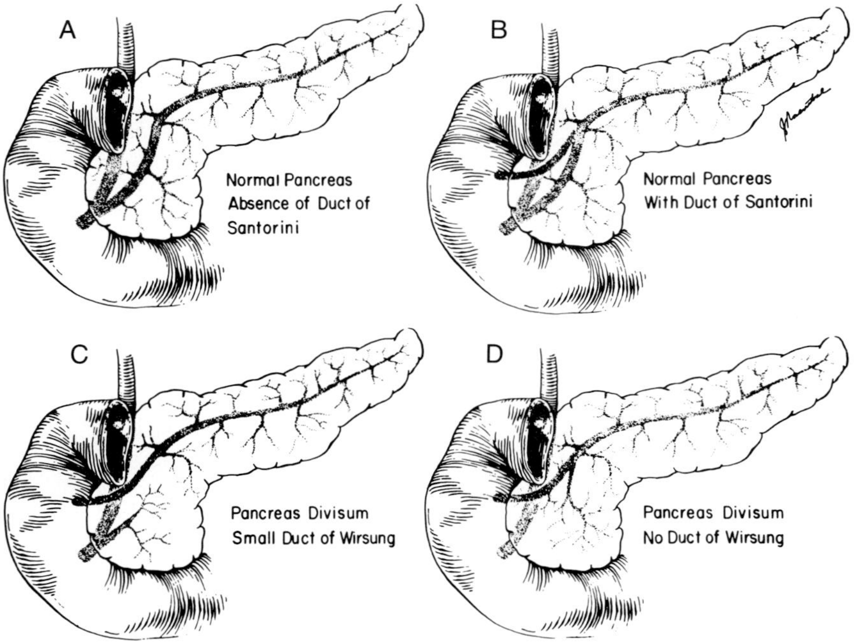

Figure 10-1. Variation in pancreatic duct anatomy. (A) Complete or nearly complete regression of the duct of Santorini (52% of the population). In an additional 9%, a small dorsal duct extends to the papilla but has no opening. (B) Fully communicating and equal ducts of Santorini and Wirsung (30%). In a variant of this, the communication may be small and functionally inadequate. (C) Complete nonunion of the dorsal and ventral ducts (5%). (D) Regression and absence of the ventral duct (4%). (C and D) In PD, most or all of the pancreatic secretions must exit via the dominant dorsal duct through the accessory papilla. (Statistics adapted from Grant.[12])

stenosis could assume importance only in the presence of PD or a dominant dorsal duct with an inadequate or absent ventral duct. When the dorsal and ventral segments communicate freely, as they normally do in 80% of people,[12] pancreatic secretions can exist via either the minor or the major papilla; and if the minor orifice is or becomes inadequate, the dorsal secretions simply drain via the ventral duct (or Wirsung) and major papilla (of Vater). However, when the anatomy obligates that the dorsal duct must discharge the bulk of pancreatic secretions through the accessory papilla, accessory papilla stenosis perforce leads to obstruction of the dominant dorsal pancreatic segment. This situation creates circumstances that give rise to a form of pancreatitis defined at the 1984 Marseilles Conference as obstructive pancreatitis.[28] Treatment of the condition is directed not at the PD but at improving the drainage at the accessory papilla.

The basic contention is, therefore, that it is not the prevalence of PD (a common phenomenon) that is important, but the prevalence of accessory papilla stenosis (an uncommon phenomenon) in persons who also have PD (a combination that is still more uncommon). If, hypothetically, one person in 10,000 had accessory papilla stenosis, no epidemiologic study yet done, including that of Delhaye et al., who performed pancreatography on almost 6000 patients in Brussels,[8] is powerful enough to show a significant relationship between PD and symptoms or disease. Thus, to deny the relationship on the basis of existing epidemiologic studies incurs the type II statistical error.

I have instead taken the empirical approach of studying symptomatic patients who are found to have PD. These constitute a very small, select minority of all those with the anomaly. The first burning question to be asked in each case is whether the symptoms are relevant to the PD. The second is what to do about it. In my opinion both questions center on the issue of accessory papilla stenosis: how to evaluate for it and how to eliminate it.

Nonetheless, before the acceptance of the thesis that a disease process may be associated with PD anatomy in some individuals, a word of caution is due because the consequent willingness to base a surgical act on that premise continues to entail considerable risk of failure. Reports of treatment of patients with PD have varied widely in their end results. Several of these reports contain only a few treated patients, little more than anecdotes, and are highly subject to idiosyncrasies of selection and statistical vagaries. If PD alone is the index for treatment, there is a great risk of irrelevancy, of the symptoms being due to a coincidental but unidentified cause. The largest published experience, which is my own, supports the association between PD, accessory papilla stenosis, and symptoms by the relatively good results from accessory papillotomy.[37,39] Even in our hands, however, the chance of persistence or recurrence of symptoms approaches 10% in the most favorable subgroup. If the basic premise is correct, those failures must indicate either that the selection of patients for operation was incorrect or that the operation itself failed to ensure unimpeded drainage through the dorsal duct orifice.

CLINICAL PRESENTATION

Most persons with PD anatomy (dominant dorsal duct with either an unfused or absent ventral duct) have no symptoms and never come to attention unless they are identified incidentally during study by pancreatography for some other condition. Potential confusion and mistaken assignment of importance of the PD may occur when the symptoms under scrutiny could be caused by pancreatitis. The anomaly in these people is coincidental, its only importance being the introduction of a misleading and confusing etiologic possibility.

Patients with symptoms that could be the consequence of PD and accessory papilla stenosis may have recurrent attacks of proven acute pancreatitis,[7,18,37] recurrent or persistent pain in the upper abdomen and back but without objective laboratory and roentgenographic correlates of pancreatitis.[6,24,37] or established chronic pancreatitis.[2,20,32] All these groups exist and must be considered. Symptoms may begin in childhood,[9,39,40] but the average age of onset has been about 33 years,[37,39] considerably lower than the age of patients with other forms of acute or chronic pancreatitis.[24] There is a strong predominance of the number of reported cases in women.[37,39] No familial associations have been recognized.[1]

The specific clinical signs and symptoms vary widely, but often I have observed a pattern of specific intermittent attacks, spaced weeks or months apart, gradually increasing in frequency and progressing toward constant daily pain. Hyperamylasemia is common early in the course during acute attacks but may become infrequent later and is generally absent in patients with chronic pain.[37] The virtual absence of clinically severe attacks or major complications of acute pancreatitis has been striking, but there was one notable instance of pancreatitis with severe generalized panniculitis (fat necrosis) cured by accessory papillotomy.[16]

Patients have been followed for periods exceeding 10 years. There is no convincing evidence in my own experience to indicate progression from acute to chronic pancreatitis (irreversible tissue changes). Others, however, have reported instances of PD in which biopsies or resection specimens show the dorsal segment to be fibrotic and damaged while the ventral segment is normal.[2,20] Thus the possibility remains that progressive cumulative damage to the pancreas may be a consequence of accessory papilla obstruction in some patients with PD.

The latter sequence raises the possibility that PD is the antecedent cause in some patients presenting with established chronic pancreatitis. While this possibility cannot be eliminated out of hand, it must be exceptional. Sahel et al. found no statistically significant association between chronic pancreatitis and PD in contrast to their observations on acute pancreatitis,[27] and lactoferrin levels in pancreatic secretions, said to be increased in chronic pancreatitis, were normal in patients with pancreatitis associated with PD.[10] In most patients with chronic pancreatitis, whether or not there is PD, both the ventral and the dorsal segments are involved.[7,37] To be convincing that accessory papilla stenosis is the pathogenetic factor, one would have to show a difference between dorsal and ventral duct morphology by pancreatography or a difference in the histologic appearance of the two segments.[2,20] Finally, we found accessory papillotomy ineffective when calcifications or pancreatography indicated chronic pancreatitis.[37] The pragmatic solution is to treat all patients with established chronic pancreatitis alike, whether the disease is caused by alcohol or PD or unknown factors. The surgical strategy should be determined primarily by the duct size and configuration,[34] not by the state of fusion of the dorsal and ventral systems. Presumably, but not necessarily, distal drainage by lateral pancreatojejunostomy (modified Puestow operation) will be as effective in patients with PD as in those with normally fused ducts,[36] but it is possible that some failures of the operation may occur because the ventral segment is not decompressed by dorsal duct drainage. In those cases resection of the pancreatic head by pancreatoduodenectomy may be necessary.

IDENTIFICATION OF CANDIDATES FOR SURGICAL TREATMENT

Whereas diagnosis of PD is relatively straightforward (and has been detailed in the previous chapter), it is much more difficult to gauge the functional size of the accessory papilla. Until recently even skilled endoscopists were unable to cannulate the accessory papilla regularly because of its location, angle, and size.[6,24] In my experience, that failure did not correlate either with the subsequent assessment of the size of the papillary orifice at operation or with the end results of accessory papillotomy. With the use of secretin (1 U/kg intravenously) to help identify the tiny papillary orifice and the new Cremer or similar fine-tipped catheters, dorsal duct pancreatograms can be obtained in 90% of persons with PD.[8] Because the technique involves impaction against the orifice or even puncture of the papilla, however, assessment of orifice size still cannot be made reliably. When deep cannulation is easy, it is probable that the accessory papilla is wide open, but that finding is rare unless the patient has already had a papillotomy.

The duct size and appearance are usually normal despite the small outflow tract. Only 1 of my 88 patients operated on for acute disease had even a slightly dilated duct, which shrank to normal after sphincteroplasty. Delayed emptying (more than 30 minutes) of contrast medium after pancreatography may be convincing evidence but occurs only rarely.

Other surgeons have been disturbed that the dorsal duct is not dilated as a general rule despite the concept of papillary stenosis. I assume that the stenosis is low-grade and may become important as a resistor only under high-flow conditions (such as after meals or after secretin administration—see below). My experience suggests that prominent duct changes suggestive of chronic pancreatitis (dilation of the main pancreatic duct, chain of lakes, secondary branch dilation, calcification, and stones) indicate the need for caution, for it is likely that accessory papillotomy will fail to relieve symptoms in such circumstances, no matter what their pathogenesis has been.[37]

Geenen et al. used endoscopic manometry to detect a hypertensive sphincter at the papilla of Vater with promising results.[11] Although Geenen applied it to the accessory papilla in a few instances,[7] the technique is of limited use here because of the diffculty inherent in cannulating the truly stenotic orifice and because the stenosis appears to be membranous rather than muscular (by our observation). It is not known for certain that there is a muscular sphincter component of the accessory papilla.

The size of the accessory papillary orifice can be measured directly at operation, but it is obviously more desirable to assess the functional adequacy of the papilla before deciding whether or not to operate. The morphine-prostigmine provocative test[19,22] has failed this challenge.[38] Our efforts have focused on noninvasive measurement of the change in pancreatic duct size under high-flow conditions induced by administration of secretin (Fig. 10-2).[38] The rationale for this test is that the abnormal resistance to flow through a too-small orifice causes prolonged congestive dilatation of the duct after strong secretory stimulation. Normally the effects of secretin, brief sphincter of Oddi contraction, and several minutes of stimulated pancreatic secretion[11] produce up to 3 minutes of mild pancreatic duct dilatation.[3] In contrast, the increase in duct diameter seen in patients with papillary stenosis is prolonged, lasting 15 to 30 minutes, and is often of greater magnitude (up to a 3-mm increase) and of greater longitudinal extent.[38] In patients with PD, of course, the action of the sphincter of Oddi is irrelevant,

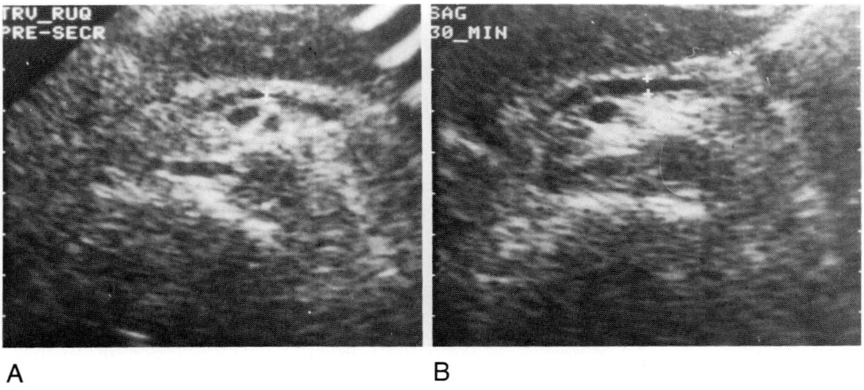

Figure 10-2. Secretin ultrasound provocative test. (A) A normal-sized pancreatic duct (presecretin). (B) A 3-mm increase in duct diameter sustained for 30 minutes after intravenous administration of secretin. The markers (+) indicate the pancreatic duct lumen.

and only the secretory stimulation and the accessory orifice size are likely to be determinants of the duct size response.

We give secretin, 1 U/kg intravenously, and measure the duct size before and at 1, 5, 15, and 30 minutes after injection. The increment in duct diameter is recorded at the head, body, and tail of the gland for purposes of scoring the grade of change: none, mild, moderate, or severe (Fig. 10-3). The dilatation induced by secretin is abolished after sphincteroplasty.[38] The observation supports the thesis

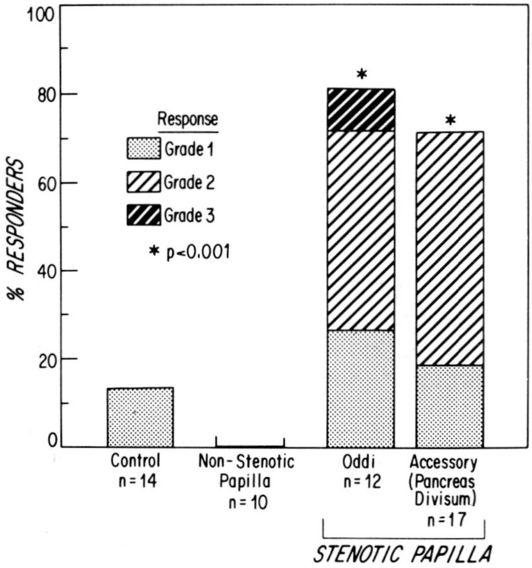

Figure 10-3. Pancreatic duct dilatation after secretin administration in patients serving as controls and in those with stenosis of the outflow tract at either the ventral or the dorsal duct (PD). Prolonged dilatation occurs mainly in those with stenosis. (From Warshaw et al.[38] with permission).

that relative obstruction of the papilla leads to prolonged duct dilatation after administration of secretin.

In my experience, now based on more than 250 tests, the secretin ultrasound test is about 70% sensitive in detecting surgically proved stenosis of the accessory papilla. Earlier we reported that nearly 90% of patients with a positive test (any grade) were relieved by accessory papillotomy, whereas only 20% to 25% of patients with a negative test had similar relief of symptoms.[38] Extension of that study indicates that at least 90% of patients with a positive test will benefit from accessory papillotomy.[39] The correlation tends to confirm that accessory papilla stenosis, indicated by a positive test, is responsible for the symptoms. From a pragmatic viewpoint we believe that this test, while not providing absolute guidelines, has been helpful in improving our decision making and selection of patients for surgical treatment.

NONSURGICAL TREATMENT

There are no controlled studies of patients with PD to assess the natural history of symptoms attributed to the anomaly. My own observations, perhaps biased by patterns of referral to a surgeon, suggest that pain often begins episodically, becomes more frequent, and may progress to constancy. We have not seen lasting regression or spontaneous resolution of symptoms. In some patients, documented attacks of pancreatitis may be interspersed among periods of pain without serum enzyme elevations or other objective signs. Despite persistence over many years, both life-threatening acute attacks and progression to true chronic pancreatitis appear to be rare: I have not seen either. Therefore, expectant treatment is probably fruitless but is unlikely to be hazardous. I have seen no evidence of successful drug treatment, either by oral pancreatic enzymes or by agents altering pancreatic or sphincter function. Enlargement of the opening of the accessory papilla has been attempted by a variety of endoscopic techniques, including balloon dilation, electrosurgical papillotomy, and stenting by endoprosthesis.[6,23,26,29] Experience with these has been disappointing on the whole. Too often the necessary catheters cannot be introduced through the tiny papillary opening. In fact, cannulation is most likely to be accomplished in just those patients who least need it, those with a papillary orifice that is already of adequate size. My analysis of collected anecdotes suggests that pancreatitis follows these manipulations fairly frequently, relief of symptoms is exceptional, and restenosis is the rule.[6,26] Although some endoscopists continue empirically to place endoprostheses into the dorsal duct, there is a paucity of evaluable published data.

SURGICAL TREATMENT

Surgical treatment of patients with PD is aimed either at reducing the volume of pancreatic secretions that must pass through the accessory papilla or at enlarging the papillary orifice. The former means distal pancreatectomy, with or without distal drainage into a Roux en Y loop of intestine, of which there are few reports and with which the experience has not been positive.[2,26] The latter usually means accessory papillotomy. Simultaneous sphincteroplasty of the major papilla has been advocated,[4,14,15,19] but the rationale for that approach is not apparent to me. My results for accessory papillotomy are the same with or without simultaneous sphincteroplasty of the major papilla.[37,39]

Accessory papillotomy is an often-difficult operation that must be performed meticulously. When feasible, it is desirable for technical ease and safety to perform the operation at a time when pancreatic inflammation is minimal. The technique has been described in detail elsewhere,[24,35,37,39] but certain aspects bear reemphasis (Fig. 10-4).

1. The accessory papilla lies in a constant location, 2 to 3 cm proximal and about 1 cm anterior to the major papilla on the medial duodenal wall. The configuration of the papilla is most commonly that of a small nipple 2 mm in diameter. It may be nearly flat rather than hemispheric. It is important to locate it quickly before traumatic edema and discoloration complicate the task. Intravenous administration of secretin, 1 U/kg, is helpful both to induce telltale flow and to make

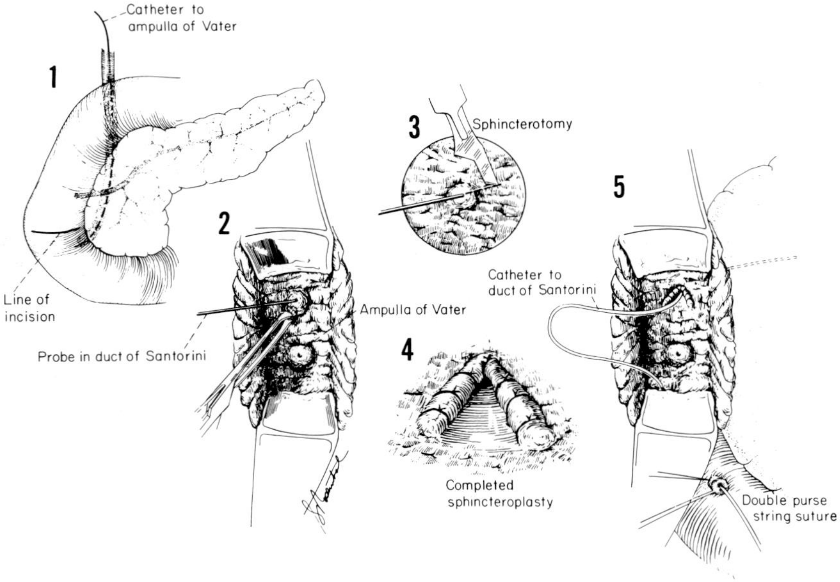

Figure 10-4. Technique for surgical sphincteroplasty of the accessory papilla. (1) The duodenum is opened transversely just above the major papilla (location may be facilitated by a catheter passed from above through the cystic duct if the gallbladder is being removed). (2) The accessory papilla is located a few centimeters proximal and anterior to the major papilla. A probe is placed into the dorsal duct lumen. (3) The anterior lip is opened with the probe in place to guide the incision. (4) The duodenal and pancreatic duct mucosae are approximated with fine absorbable sutures. (5) A 5 French catheter is left in the duct for postoperative drainage.

the papilla prominent. Palpation for the papilla may be more successful than a visual search. Exceedingly rarely (1 of 88 instances in my series) it may be necessary to resect the pancreatic tail for prograde catheterization of the dorsal duct in order to locate the accessory papilla.

2. Secretin-induced flow through the papilla provides some indication of the degree of stenosis: the efflux can range from nil to a jet. Visible estimates of flow before and after papillotomy may be strikingly different, attesting to functional stenosis.

3. An estimate of the size of the orifice can be made by calibrating with probes of different diameters. The opening of the normal duct of Wirsung is at least 1 to 1.5 mm, but the accessory papillary orifice ranges from 1 mm down to a barely visible pinpoint that does not admit any probe except by puncture. We call the orifice stenotic when a no. 1 lacrimal duct probe, which has a diameter of about 0.75 mm, does not pass easily into the duct.

4. The stenosis is short and membranous, occurring at the papilla, not higher up the duct. The papillotomy therefore need not be extensive. That is fortunate because the papillary segment of the duct, oriented at a right angle to the duodenal wall, is short and quickly dives into the pancreatic substance. This is in contrast to the oblique tunnel through which the ventral duct reaches its termination in the papilla of Vater. The papillotomy cannot easily be extended more than 1 cm, but that suffices.

RESULTS OF SURGICAL TREATMENT

The success rate for surgical treatment of PD has varied among institutions, ranging from dismal[5,14,26] to better than 70%.[18,37] The largest series previously reported (my own) was also among the most optimistic.[39] Discrepancies must be explained at least in part by differences in case selection. If all the patients with PD and abdominal pain, or even a partially selected group with proved pancreatitis, were to be treated with accessory papillotomy, the rate of successful relief would be predictably low in proportion to the prevalence of accessory papilla stenosis in the treated population. Conversely, if only patients with accessory papilla stenosis were chosen, surgical successes should be the rule, limited only by technical failures and restenosis.

I have performed accessory papillotomy on 88 patients with recurrent acute pancreatitis or pancreatic pain associated with PD: 66 women and 22 men, with an average age of 33 years. Any patient with calcification or duct pathomorphology suggesting chronic pancreatitis was eliminated from these considerations. Of the 88 patients, 65 were followed for a minimum of 2 years since the operation. I chose to wait at least this long to assess the outcome in order to avoid early nonspecific and placebo effects.

Overall, the condition of 45 of the 65 patients improved considerably. The patients were free of further attacks and nearly free of pain (not taking narcotics). In most instances, the relief was immediate and lasting, but some patients had one or two mild attacks during the first year after the operation, or sporadic pain that eventually subsided.

Of the 51 patients judged at operation to have a stenotic accessory papilla, 43 had a favorable course after papillotomy, whereas only 2 of 14 of those with a nonstenotic papilla had lasting benefit from the operation. These findings continue to fit with the thesis that accessory papillary stenosis is the key element in symptomatic PD.

The mode of presentation—discrete attacks versus chronic pain—seems to be of prognostic value. Patients whose course was characterized at the outset by isolated attacks, usually with hyperamylasemia, were more likely to be cured by accessory papillotomy than those who presented initially with continuous pain (80% vs. 50%).

Late failures do occur. Among the patients who had relapses, restenosis was documented in 6 patients of the 88, as far as we know. Restenosis in this 7% was heralded by return of pancreatic pain reminiscent of the original symptoms but usually of a steady nature rather than punctuations by discrete attacks. The restenosis was detected both by a reversion to a positive secretin ultrasound test and by inability to cannulate the accessory papillary orifices. In 5 patients, it was confirmed by pathologic findings at operation; 4 patients were treated by repeat papillotomy with two successes and two failures. The operation is difficult because the stricture is dense and fibrous, and there is little distance along the duct before it dives inaccessibly into the pancreatic substance. Obtaining a mucosa-to-mucosa approximation between fresh duodenal and pancreatic duct epithelium is a technically trying task. I leave a stent catheter through the reconstruction for several weeks in these instances.[33]

Attempts were made in one instance to dilate the structure with balloons and to stent it with an endoprothesis. These efforts were rewarded only with pancreatitis. The patient subsequently had a resection of the pancreatic head (Whipple operation) and later a total pancreatectomy before finally obtaining relief of pain. Fibrous stenosis of the pancreatic duct opening was noted in both resection specimens, along with dilated distal ducts and parenchymal atrophy.

Finally, one young woman had a series of endoscopic maneuvers including balloon dilatation and endoprostheses for recurrent symptoms attributed to restenosis. Her condition improved, but the follow-up period was short.

It is evident that when the original papillotomy fails, it is even harder to reestablish an adequate orifice. The first opportunity is the best and perhaps the only one. For recurrent stenosis, resection of the pancreatic head (Whipple-type pancreatoduodenectomy, preferably with preservation of the antrum and pylorus) may be the option most likely to succeed,[26] however radical it may seem. I have resorted to total pancreatectomy in two instances as a last resort—one of my own patients and one referred after failures of both papillotomy and distal drainage.

CONCLUSIONS

The proof of a genuine syndrome caused by PD and accessory papilla stenosis is empirical. In my experience, there are more persons with long-standing, persistent, and increasing symptoms who respond favorably to accessory papillotomy than chance or a placebo effect can reasonably explain. These same patients tend to have what is thought to be a pathologically increased resistance to excretion of pancreatic secretions through the accessory papilla (positive secretin ultrasound test), which is corrected by the accessory papillotomy (conversion to negative secretin ultrasound test). At operation, the orifice in the accessory papilla is tiny. Secretin-induced flow is only a trickle in these patients, but when the limiting membranous web is cut, pancreatic secretions gush forth. Symptoms present before the operation are perceived as absent as soon as the pain of operation has subsided enough to allow assessment. Symptoms recur if the papillary orifice restenoses.

Problems remain. Accurate selection of candidates for accessory papillomy is not yet possible because of the lack of a highly reliable test for accessory papilla stenosis. The secretin ultrasound test helps in this regard but still has a 10% to 20% false-positive and 30% to 35% false-negative rate. Patients with signs of irreversible chronic pancreatitis—and perhaps all alcoholics—should not be treated by papillotomy; they require a different kind of opeation, appropriate to their duct morphology. Accessory papillotomy demands meticulous technique to avoid failure and creation of even bigger problems with iatrogenic pancreatic duct obstruction. Restenosis may require pancreatoduodenectomy for palliation of symptoms.

The final caveat is this: PD as an anatomic form is common; PD as a cause of pancreatic symptoms is not common. Accessory papillotomy is no more of a panacea for abdominal pain than sphincteroplasty of the major papilla has been. Nonetheless, failures do not negate the successes. With appropriate care to patient selection and surgical technique, success can be the rule.

REFERENCES

1. Beggs I, Salmon PR. A case of hereditary pancreatitis and pancreas divisum. Eur J Radiol 4:71–73, 1984.
2. Blair AJ, Russell CG, Cotton PB. Resection for pancreatitis in patients with pancreas divisum. Ann Surg 200:590–594, 1984.
3. Bolondi K, Gaini S, Gullo L, Labo G: Secretin administration induces dilatation of main pancreatic duct. Dig Dis Sci 29:802–808, 1984.
4. Britt LG, Samuels AD, Johnson JW Jr. Pancreas divisum: Is it a surgical disease? Ann Surg 197:655–662, 1983.
5. Carey LC. International Workshop on Pancreas Divisum. Middlesex Hospital, London, England, 1984 (cited in reference 20).
6. Cotton PB. Congenital anomaly of pancreas divisum as cause of obstructive pain and pancreatitis. Gut 21:105–114, 1980.
7. Cotton PB. Pancreas divisum: Curiosity or culprit? Gastroenterology 89:1431–1435, 1985.
8. Delhaye M, Engelholm L, Cremer M. Pancreas divisum: Congenital anatomic variant or anomaly? Gastroenterology 89:951–958, 1985.
9. Forbes A, Leung JW, Cotton PB. Relapsing acute and chronic pancreatitis. Arch Dis Child 59:927–934, 1984.
10. Gaia E, Figarella C, Piantino P, Rocca G, Iuliano R, Calcamuggi G, Emanuelli G. Duodenal lactoferrin in patients with chronic pancreatitis and gastrointestinal diseases. Digestion 32:229–237, 1985.

11. Geenen JE, Hogan WJ, Dodds WJ, Stewart ET, Arndorfer RC. Intraluminal pressure recording from the human sphincter of Oddi. Gastroenterology 78:317–324, 1980.
12. Grant JCB. An Atlas of Anatomy, 4th ed. Baltimore, Williams & Wilkins, 1956, p. 140.
13. Gregg JA. Pancreas divisum: Its association with pancreatitis. Am J Surg 134:539–543, 1977.
14. Gregg JA, Monaco AP, McDermott WV: Pancreas divisum: Results of surgical intervention. Am J Surg 145:488–492, 1983.
15. Gregg J, Solomon J, Clark G: Pancreas divisum and its association with choledochal sphincter stenosis: Diagnosis by endoscopic retrograde cholangiopancreatography and endoscopic biliary manometry. Am J Surg 147:367–371, 1984.
16. Haber RM, Assaad DM. Panniculitis associated with a pancreas divisum. J Am Acad Dermatol 14:331–334, 1986.
17. Heiss FW, Shea JA. Association of pancreatitis and variant ductal anatomy: Dominant drainage of the duct of Santorini. Am J Gastroenterol 70:158–162, 1978.
18. Keith RG, Shapero TF, Saibel FG: Treatment of pancreatitis associated with pancreas divisum by dorsal duct sphincteroplasty alone. Can J Surg 25:622–626, 1982.
19. Madura JA. Pancreas divisum: Stenosis of the dorsally dominant pancreatic duct—A surgically correctable lesion. Am J Surg 151:742–745, 1986.
20. Marshall JB, Eckhauser ML. Pancreas divisum: A cause of chronic relapsing pancreatitis. Dig Dis Sci 30:582–587, 1985.
21. Mitchell CJ, Lintott DJ, Ruddell WSJ, et al. Clinical relevance of an unfused pancreatic duct system. Gut 20:1066–1077, 1979.
22. Nardi GL, Michelassi F, Zannini P. Transduodenal sphincteroplasty. 5–25 year follow-up of 89 patients. Ann Surg 198:453–461, 1983.
23. O'Connor KW, Lehman GA. An improved technique for accessory papilla cannulation in pancreas divisum. Gastrointest Endosc 31:13–17, 1985.
24. Richter JM, Schapiro RH, Mulley AG, Warshaw AL. Association of pancreas divisum and pancreatitis, and its treatment by sphincteroplasty of the accessory papilla. Gastroenterology 81:1104–1110, 1981.
25. Rosch W, Koch H, Schaffner O, Demling L. The clinical significance of the pancreas divisum. Gastrointest Endosc 22:206–207, 1976.
26. Russell RCG, Wong NW, Cotton PB. Accessory sphincterotomy (endoscopic and surgical) in patients with pancreas divisum. Br J Surg 71:954–957, 1984.
27. Sahel J, Cros RC, Bourry J, Sarles H. Clinico-pathological conditions associated with pancreas divisum. Digestion 23:1–8, 1982.
28. Sarles H. Revised classification of pancreatitis—Marseille 1984. Dig Dis Sci 30:573–574, 1985.
29. Soehendra N, Kempeneers I, Nam VC, Grimm H. Endoscopic dilatation and papillotomy of the accessory papilla and internal drainage in pancreas divisum. Endoscopy 18:129–132, 1986.
30. Traverso LW, Longmire WP Jr. Preservation of the pylorus in pancreaticoduodenectomy. A follow-up evaluation. Ann Surg 192:306–310, 1980.
31. Tulassay Z, Papp J. New clinical aspects of pancreas divisum. Gastrointest Endosc 26:143–146, 1980.
32. Turner LJ. Chronic pancreatitis and congenital strictures of the pancreatic duct. Am J Surg 145:582–584, 1983.
33. Warshaw AL. Postoperative catheter drainage of the pancreatic duct. Surg Gastroenterol 2:27–28, 1983.
34. Warshaw AL. Conservation of pancreatic tissue by combined gastric, biliary, and pancreatic duct drainage for pain from chronic pancreatitis. Am J Surg 149:563–569, 1985.
35. Warshaw AL. Accessory pancreatic duct sphincteroplasty. In: Litwin MS, ed. Atlas of Advanced Surgery. New York, Yorke Medical Books, 1986, pp 126–130.
36. Warshaw AL, Popp JW Jr, Schapiro RH. Long-term patency, pancreatic function, and pain relief after lateral pancreaticojejunostomy for chronic pancreatitis. Gastroenterology 79:289–293, 1980.

37. Warshaw AL, Richter JM, Schapiro RH. The cause and treatment of pancreatitis associated with pancreas divisum. Ann Surg 198:443, 1983.
38. Warshaw AL, Simeone J, Schapiro RH, Hedberg SE, Mueller PE, Ferrucci JT Jr. Objective evaluation of ampullary stenosis with ultrasonography and pancreatic stimulation. Am J Surg 149:65–72, 1985.
39. Warshaw AL, Simeone JF, Schapiro RH, Flavin-Warshaw B. Evaluation and treatment of the dominant dorsal duct syndrome (pancreas divisum redefined). Am J Surg 159:59–66, 1990.
40. Yedlin ST, Dubois RS, Philippart AI. Pancreas divisum: A cause of pancreatitis in childhood. J Pediatr Surg 19:793–794, 1984.

CHAPTER

11

APPROACH TO PATIENTS WITH PANCREATIC PSEUDOCYSTS AND ABSCESSES

Robert McGovern, Jamie S. Barkin, and Ira Agatstein

EDITORIAL COMMENT (Chapters 11 and 12)

Drs. McGovern, Barkin, and Agatstein begin their assessment of pancreatic abscess or cyst from the findings at CT and only secondarily from clinical and biochemical findings. This appears to the editors to be a very reasonable starting point at the present time. It is probably correct to say that under ideal conditions confirmation of abscess or cyst would be dependent in the end on the CT (and perhaps ultrasound) findings. Of course these techniques are not always available and accurate, and it is therefore just as well to be familiar with the clinical aspects of progression to abscess or cyst as suggested by Dr. Ranson or Dr. Beger. It now seems clear that the presence of Ranson's or Bank's severe signs either before or during the development of abscess is associated with a high mortality and that skinny needle aspiration for bacteria and leukocytes would assist in determining the need for immediate percutaneous or surgical drainage. The authors indicate that abscess formation is more common than previously thought in milder attacks, and these generally have a good outcome. It is therefore in infected necrosis (as opposed to abscess) that the mortality has to be reduced. These authors stress the importance of aspirating a number of areas to confirm infection. There are still two points that seem to need clarification even after the papers by the two authors:

1. What is the ultimate correct time to intervene in a cyst? It has become more obvious that it may not be necessary to wait 4 to 6 weeks for a wall to develop in patients with established chronic pancreatitis, but it is still uncertain whether a cyst communicating with a ductal system should be attended to earlier than one that does not. We have found that it is not usual for a complication such as rupture, infection, and bleeding to occur within 4 weeks. Perhaps this should be the cutoff time if significant evolution is not occurring, even if one has to resort to percutaneous aspiration or drainage or marsupialization rather than the more preferable internal drainage.

2. What is the optimal procedure for cyst or abscess? There seems to be a trend toward protection of turf, with radiologists pushing toward repeated aspirations or percutaneous drainage and reserving surgery only if these fail, and surgeons tending to recommend open drainage for abscess and internal drainage for all cysts. Gastroenterologists straddle the fence depending on their own expertise and that of the departments in their hospitals and are exploring endoscopic techniques such as transgastric and transduodenal drainage. It does seem that a number of multicentered trials free of political considerations would be relevant at this time.

Drs. Estakhri and Frey have demonstrated the importance of correct definition of pancreatic masses particularly with regard to distinction between infective necrosis (or infective phlegmon) and abscess. The former, having no real definable borders, tends to occur in patients with severe attacks, is nearly always fatal if not corrected early, and is best treated by extensive debridement with retroperitoneal drainage. Even with this, the mortality remains high. For noninfective necrosis the authors suggest aggressive nonsurgical treatment but not resection. However, even these patients do have a high mortality ranging from 59% to 93%. Herein lies the quandary, whether these latter patients are salvagable or whether a return to aggressive resection of all necrotic material (necrosectomy) now being reinvestigated by some European workers will be able to lessen the mortality. The authors stress the importance of bolus contrast medium on CT scanning to demonstrate areas of necrosis that have decreased enhancement and to guide percutaneous skinny needle aspiration of such areas to demonstrate whether the area is infected. On the other hand, abscess formation in those patients with less severe attacks has a good prognosis and can be treated by either percutaneous drainage or operation.

With regard to pancreatic cysts, the authors once again advocate watchful expectancy for 4 to 6 weeks and quote a figure of 40% spontaneous resolution, which is rather interesting when compared with the 20% to 28% reported by Dr. Barkin's group. Clearly we are in a gray area with regard to the actual definition of infective necrosis vis-à-vis severity of attacks, mortality, and relationship of early diagnosis (by skinny needle) to mortality. It would seem to the editors that again there is a need for multicenter trials to examine attack severity, timing of skinny needle aspiration and surgery, and mortality to at least get to grips with the true mortality data in the various groups.

CONTROVERSY

The diagnosis of infected pancreatic necrosis, abscess, or cyst has now been facilitated by skinny needle aspiration of a suspected lesion. It is generally agreed that the presence of infection mandates aspiration. However, there is some controversy whether percutaneous drainage suffices or surgical drainage is preferable. Cysts may be observed for several weeks. The reported incidence of spontaneous resolution varies widely, and again the question of aspiration or surgery remains somewhat unresolved.

The morbidity and mortality of patients with acute pancreatitis is caused by systemic complications such as cardiovascular, respiratory, and renal failure as well as the sequellae of pancreatic inflammation (pancreatic pseudocysts, abscesses, and necrosis). The focus of this chapter will be on these local inflammatory sequellae.

Our approach to patients with acute inflammatory pancreatic masses is then based upon the abdominal appearance on computed tomography (CT). This enables differentiation between solid and cystic masses but does not distinguish between infected and sterile lesions. Therefore CT should be combined with guided percutaneous needle aspiration. The latter allows the clinician to distinguish infected from noninfected lesions. The local lesions are classified into solid

TABLE 11-1. ABDOMINAL CT CHARACTERISTICS OF PANCREATIC MASSES

	Solid	Cystic
Inflammatory	Phlegmon (necrosis)	Pancreatic pseudocyst
	Early—Infected necrosis	
Infected	Late—Pancreatic abscess	Infected pseudocyst

or cystic lesions that are sterile or infected. Solid sterile inflammatory pancreatic masses are referred to as *pancreatic phlegmons* and have pancreatic necrosis as a major component. Solid infected lesions are referred to as *infected necroses* when they occur early in the course of acute pancreatitis and are labeled *pancreatic abscesses* when they become well localized, usually later in the patient's course. Cystic sterile lesions are *labeled pancreatic pseudocysts* and may include sterile blood collections in the acute phase of pancreatitis. Conversely, infected cystic lesions are labeled *infected pancreatic pseudocysts* (Table 11-1).

A pancreatic pseudocyst is a sterile fluid collection composed of necrotic debris, blood and pancreatic secretions surrounded by a nonepithelial wall. Pseudocysts are presumed to have a connection with a pancreatic duct at one point in their formation. This enables them to fill with pancreatic secretions; however, it is only demonstrable in one third to three quarters of the patients at the time of ERCP.[1,67,78] Impaired drainage through this pancreatic duct connection, along with the osmotic effect of the retained necrotic debris, contributes to the growth of the pseudocyst.[65] The pseudocyst may arise in any location within the pancreas and extend into the peripancreatic tissues. It may also dissect through the mesentery and be found virtually anywhere in the abdomen or chest. The majority of pseudocysts develop during the course of chronic pancreatitis, at times as a consequence of an attack of acute inflammation; however, in most cases they appear insidiously and cannot be clearly related to an acute attack. Fifty percent of pseudocysts are detected within the first 7 to 15 days following the acute episode of pancreatitis. However, their presence may not be detected for weeks if imaging studies are not performed, because they may be clinically silent.[2] The major causes of the underlying pancreatitis seen in patients with pseudocysts are the same as those in patients who do not develop pseudocysts.[2,72] Rarely, a pseudocyst can be seen in association with pancreatitis caused by an obstructing carcinoma of the pancreas.[49]

INCIDENCE

It is difficult to determine the true incidence of pancreatic pseudocysts because many previous studies were completed prior to the advent of the newer imaging techniques. In studies only using barium contrast medium, the incidence of detection of pseudocysts in patients with pancreatitis was between 1% and 10%.[59,86] However, when newer noninvasive imaging modalities such as ultrasonography (US) and CT are utilized, as many as 50% of patients who have experienced severe bouts of pancreatitis have been shown to have pseudocysts.[2] This increased incidence is secondary to improved detection of actual pseudocysts or possibly misinterpretation of the results of the newer techniques. The latter may occur as different lesions such as intra- and peripancreatic edema and fluid collection can simulate a pseudocyst by US.[46]

CLINICAL PRESENTATION

The symptoms of patients with an acute pseudocyst mimic those of acute pancreatitis. A pseudocyst should be suspected during the course of acute pancreatitis when the patient does not respond to conventional therapy, or when there is a persistently elevated serum amylase level despite clinical improvement. In addition to its presentation during the acute episode, a pseudocyst may present with recurrent symptoms subsequent to an episode of acute pancreatitis that had apparently resolved. Pseudocysts may arise in patients with chronic pancreatitis any time during the course of their disease. The pseudocyst may be asymptomatic or may mimic an acute exacerbation of chronic pancreatitis.

Although pseudocysts may occur at any age, they occur most commonly in the fourth and fifth decades of life.[60] This reflects the distribution of patients with acute pancreatitis. Abdominal pain is present in 80% to 90% of patients, and nausea, vomiting, and weight loss are also very common.[14,60]

On physical examination, a palpable abdominal mass is found in approximately 50% of patients.[14] This is probably an overestimation now that imaging shows us the presence of small pseudocysts. In addition, a large pseudocyst may not be palpable when it is located beneath the rib cage.

Unfortunately, the initial clinical manifestations of a pseudocyst may be a complication. These complications include retroperitoneal dissection, obstruction of intraabdominal hollow viscera, rupture into the peritoneal cavity or viscera, hemorrhage into the cyst or adjoining viscera, and infection.

NATURAL HISTORY

Since the advent and widespread utilization of the newer noninvasive imaging techniques of US and CT, our knowledge of the natural history of a pancreatic pseudocyst has been widely expanded. Prior to these developments, pseudocysts were suspected and possibly discovered in patients whose pancreatitis did not resolve as quickly as expected, whose elevated serum amylase levels persisted longer than usual, or in whom a palpable mass was found. Once their presence was confirmed by barium studies, the patient underwent surgical decompression. Therefore it was unknown previously whether a pseudocyst could resolve spontaneously.

Another difficulty in interpreting the literature regarding the natural history of pseudocysts prior to US and CT was that no distinction was made between intra- or extrapancreatic pseudocysts and palpable or nonpalpable pseudocysts.[53] Prior to the utilization of CT and US it was generally reported that spontaneous resolution of a pseudocyst occurred in 8% to 30% of patients.[14,19] However, one study reported that over 70% of pseudocysts spontaneously resolved in 3 weeks to 3 months, based on indirect evidence of barium studies or angiography.[12] This wide variation is a direct result of the inaccuracies of diagnostic studies. When resolution of pseudocysts was evaluated by US, approximately 20% were found to resolve spontaneously.[16] This resolution occurred in the first 6 weeks of detection in 90% of patients whose lesions subsequently resolved.[12]

A patient's history may help us to distinguish the presence of acute from chronic pseudocysts. This is clinically important, as the latter may be "mature" when they are discovered, and thus definitive treatment can be utilized during their initial evaluation. This avoids the risk of developing complications that occur more frequently with the continued presence of the pseudocyst. The history of an episode of acute pancreatitis within a period of 6 or more weeks preceding the diagnosis of the cyst favors the presence of an acute pseudocyst, whereas no history of recent events favors the presence of a chronic pseudocyst.[47,83] The appearance of the pseudocyst on CT helps us to determine which is less likely to resolve. Those with calcified walls do not usually resolve, and this is consistent with our concept that calcification of a pseudocyst represents a chronic process.[47] In addition, the presence of "thick walls" also seems to be associated with failure to resolve. The size of a pseudocyst that is likely to resolve spontaneously is undetermined. O'Malley et al. found that those less than 4 cm resolved spontaneously, agreeing with Aranha et al., who reported that the mean diameter of pseudocysts that resolved spontaneously was 4.2 ± 0.5 cm.[3,52] However, in the latter series it was found that approximately 15% of those greater than 6 cm resolved spontaneously; this compared to an overall spontaneous rate of resolution of 28%.[3]

DIAGNOSIS

The serologic diagnosis of a pseudocyst may be a reflection of the underlying pancreatic disease. If the patient has acute pancreatitis and develops a pseudocyst, the serum amylase level is usually elevated. However, only about half of patients with pseudocysts develop elevated serum amylase or lipase levels.[72] In contrast, as many as 80% of patients with pancreatic pseudocysts may have elevated levels of urinary amylase.[73] In addition to elevation of standard serum amylase levels, alterations of the amylase molecule that occur with stagnation of amylase-rich fluid in the pseudocyst may be detected in the serum of patients with pseudocysts and pancreatic ascites.[81,84] This may serve as a serologic marker that can direct our attention to the presence of a pseudocyst.

The procedures that are used for diagnosing pancreatic pseudocysts include US, CT, and endoscopic retrograde cholangiopancreatography (ERCP). Ultrasonography of the abdomen can detect approximately 85% of pseudocysts and can be easily used serially to determine the natural history of a pseudocyst.[64] It is generally felt that this is the initial procedure of choice for diagnosing pancreatic pseudocysts; however, it has a false-positive rate of 8.3% and a false-negative rate of 8.5%.[26] A major difficulty in using this technique in patients with acute pancreatitis is the inability to obtain a good-quality ultrasound picture because of overlying bowel gas or obesity. Endoscopic US has the potential to overcome this difficulty. This method is in a relatively early state of development.[31] Many intra- or peripancreatic lesions, including pancreatic abscess, hematoma, loculated ascites, pancreatic cystadenoma, cystadenocarcinoma, and aneurysms, may simulate a pancreatic pseudocyst by US.[46]

Abdominal CT gives a more detailed view of pancreatic pseudocysts, especially when they are in atypical areas such as the mediastinum, where US has limited usefulness. As with US, other pancreatic diseases including cystadenoma, cystadenocarcinoma, and/or necrotic carcinoma may mimic the CT appearance of a pseudocyst. When CT scanning was compared to US for detecting pseudocysts, it was found that CT detected pseudocyst formation twice as often as US.[37,39,66]

Endoscopic retrograde pancreatography (ERP) gives a detailed picture of the anatomy of the pancreatic ducts.[69] And ERCP is comparable to US for identifying pancreatic pseudocysts. The diagnostic accuracy is 85% for both techniques if definite and suspected pseudocysts are included in the calculations.[67] In a comparative study of US versus ERP, US failed to reveal the pseudocyst 25% of the time, compared with 11% by ERP.[69] An inherent problem with ERCP identification of pseudocysts is that contrast material only fills the pseudocyst in 33% to 80% of the cases.[10,43,51,57,67,78] The principal role of ERCP in patients with pseudocysts is in aiding the surgeon to plan an operative procedure and identify coexistent biliary disease. The major drawback in the use of ERCP in this setting is the potential of introducing infection, especially in pseudocysts that are larger than 3 cm.[43] At the time of laparotomy, O'Connor et al. found positive cultures in 62% of pseudocysts in patients who had undergone preoperative ERCP.[51] However, this risk may be minimized by performing ERCP 24 hours prior to surgery and possibly with the use of prophylactic antibiotics, as well as terminating filling of the pancreatic pseudocyst as soon as it is identified.[10] Recall that necrotic tumors may also be seen as extraductal cavities.[61]

DIFFERENTIAL DIAGNOSIS

Pancreatic diseases that may simulate a pseudocyst in both clinical and US features include inflammatory masses or peripancreatic fluid collections and a necrotic adenocarcinoma of the pancreas or "pseudopseudocysts".[39,61] In addition, both metastatic carcinoma to the pancreas and primary pancreatic carcinoma have been associated with the development of pancreatic pseudocysts, presumably from pancreatic ductal obstruction.[59] Many benign pancreatic lesions including cystadenomas, retention cysts, and hematomas as well as loculated ascites and aneurysms may also be mistaken for pseudocysts on US.[13] Distinguishing characteristics between pseudocysts and cystic neoplasms include cyst fluid amylase concentration, serum amylase levels, and the presence of communication with the pancreatic duct.[58,79]

The US features of an infected pancreatic pseudocyst cannot distinguish it from a sterile pseudocyst.[38] In addition, both may present clinical symptoms such as fever, leukocytosis, abdominal pain, and palpable mass, thereby preventing differentiation of these lesions. Therefore, in this situation percutaneous guided aspiration should be exercised in order to determine the presence of infection.[5]

COMPLICATIONS

During the time between discovery of the pseudocyst and planned definitive treatment, which is usually 6 weeks, a complication may occur. Overall, the complication rate varies between 30% and 40%.[12,60] These most frequently occur later in the course of the disease, with 90% occurring more than 3 weeks after the onset of the pseudocyst.[59] The complications of pseudocysts include dissection, obstruction, rupture, hemorrhage, and infection.

A pseudocyst may dissect upward into the pleural cavity, mediastinum, or neck, laterally into the spleen or kidney, and downward into the pelvis and thigh.[35,54,70] Dissection into the neck may cause a painful mass that mimics sialadenitis. A pseudocyst that extends into the pleural cavity frequently results in the development of a pleural effusion, rich in amylase and occasionally chylous in appearance. When a pseudocyst invades the mediastinum, it may simulate a mediastinal tumor and may cause esophageal obstruction and dysphagia. Lateral dissection into the spleen may cause splenic rupture or infarction. This complication may be mistaken for a splenic hematoma or neoplasm. Left kidney encroachment can mimic a renal tumor. If a pseudocyst dissects inferiorly, it may cause ureteral obstruction with resultant hydronephrosis and may also be confused with a pelvic neoplasm or even a hernia.

Pseudocysts can cause obstruction of intraabdominal viscera with predictable sequelae. These include common bile duct encroachment with resultant jaundice; antropyloric compression with gastric outlet obstruction; intramural extension or extrinsic compression of the duodenum that may present with abdominal pain and/or vomiting; and splenic and/or portal vein obstruction with portal hypertension, resulting in gastric and esophageal varices.[8,21,29,45,56,76,82] Finally, lymphatic obstruction can cause chylous ascites.[15] Obstruction of the CBD or intestine may require surgical decompression.[86]

The most common complication of a pseudocyst is spontaneous rupture, with equal occurrences into an adjacent abdominal organ or into the peritoneum. This occurs in fewer than 5% of patients with pseudocysts.[28] The rupture of a pseudocyst into a hollow organ, such as the stomach, duodenum, or colon, may result in temporary or permanent drainage. However, it is associated with an increased mortality ranging between 27% and 50%.[11,63] Severe hemorrhage can accompany rupture into any organ, while sepsis is encountered more frequently with colonic rupture.[63] A clue to the diagnosis of rupture into a viscus may be the sudden occurrence of diarrhea or vomiting accompanied by loss of a palpable pseudocyst. If the pseudocyst drains into the kidney, it may simulate a renal neoplasm. Acute ruptures of pseudocysts into the peritoneal cavity may be associated with a mortality rate as high as 70%.[48,63] This occurrence may simulate a perforated viscus, but radiographically, there may be no evidence of free air under the diaphragm. Conversely, when the leakage from the pseudocyst is slow with gradual accumulation of fluid, pancreatic ascites occur. Approximately 15% of pseudocysts have associated pancreatic ascites.[60]

Pseudocysts may erode into a major blood vessel, most commonly the splenic artery, and form pseudoaneurysms.[87] Catastrophic bleeding into the gastrointestinal tract may occur when the pseudoaneurysm erodes into the hollow viscera. Gastrointestinal bleeding may result also from blood tracking through the pancreatic duct and draining into the duodenum, so-called hemosuccus pancreaticus. The blood-filled pseudocyst may also rupture into the peritoneal cavity. Pseudoaneurysm formation should be suspected when a pseudocyst increases in size, with an associated decreasing hematocrit, especially if there is an accompanying bruit over the pseudocyst or a newly formed palpable mass.

Lastly, a pseudocyst may become infected either spontaneously or iatrogenically following ERCP or percutaneous aspiration.[85] The route of spontaneous infection is unknown but may be due to an apparent connection with the colon or other viscera. Other possible routes of infection include infected bile, hematogenous seeding, and spread along the lymphatics.[65]

TREATMENT

The timing and method of drainage of pancreatic pseudocysts is controversial. As more information on their natural history becomes available with the newer imaging techniques, it may be possible to decide exactly when drainage therapy should be initiated. Presently, if a pseudocyst complicates acute pancreatitis, therapy should be directed to the underlying pancreatitis. However, while treatment is not required, patients with asymptomatic, uncomplicated pancreatic pseudocysts should be observed for development of complications.[59]

If the patient is symptomatic, a period of bowel rest supplemented by peripheral or parenteral nutrition may allow resolution of pain. If a complication ensues during this therapy, specific treatment should be directed to this concurrent problem. The optimal time span between discovery and planned therapy of a pseudocyst would allow the maximal chance for spontaneous resolution and lowest chance of complications. This would also allow time for the pseudocyst wall to thicken and mature, so as to permit successful internal drainage if spontaneous resolution did not occur. This time interval is usually stated to be 6 weeks; however, Bradley et al. and Shatney and Lillchei have utilized a 4-week period with promising results.[12,62] Patients with chronic pseudocysts that are apparent on admission fare as well or even better with early intervention than patients with delayed operation.[20] Their low operative morbidity and mortality was confirmed by Crass and Way.[16]

If treatment is instituted, percutaneous therapeutic needle aspiration or prolonged catheter drainage may be curative.[38] We have shown that in 25% of the patients, needle aspiration alone may result in permanent resolution of pancreatic pseudocysts that were present for 6 weeks (Table 11-2).[6] Prolonged catheter drainage of pseudocysts that were present for 6 months to 1 year was successful in 100% of the patients, with a mean follow-up of 5 months.[61] VanSonnenberg achieved resolution of noninfected pseudocysts by needle or sheath drainage in 3

TABLE 11-2. SUMMARY OF PERCUTANEOUS DRAINAGE OF PANCREATIC PSEUDOCYSTS

	No.	Resolution
Aspiration or short-term catheter	22	6 (27%)
Catheter, long-term	63	49 (77%)

of 10 patients and by catheter drainage in 6 of 7 patients. The method that was used was determined by the presence or absence of communication of the pseudocyst with the pancreatic duct. Communication of the pseudocyst signifies that simple aspiration will not be curative and invariably the lesion will recur.[75] The same group recently reported 91% resolution of infected or sterile pseudocysts in 101 patients who had a mean drainage time of 20 days, which was slightly longer with communicating pseudocysts.[74]

Nonoperative external catheter drainage is usually performed by catheter placement directly into the cyst through an intraabdominal viscus. A modification of this technique is catheter placement via transgastric penetration, followed by prolonged drainage that allows formation of a communication between the stomach and the pancreatic collection. Nunez et al. reported eight pancreatic fluid collections that were successfully drained in six patients.[50] Kuligowska et al. also employed this approach without difficulty in six patients with a variety of pancreatic lesions.[41] A modification of this approach for drainage is percutaneous gastrocystostomy.[9,27] Its advantage is that it allows drainage of the pseudocyst internally, into the stomach. The percutaneous cystogastrostomy may be limited by the size of the internal drainage stent and the consistency of the cyst material and the needed location of the pseudocyst abutting against the stomach wall. Hancke and Henriksen reported the use of percutaneous cystogastrostomy in 18 patients whose cysts varied in diameter from 3 to 8 cm. Catheters were correctly positioned in 16 of the 18 patients. In these 16 patients, catheters were removed from 8 and remained in 8, and none of the cysts recurred during the mean observation period of 6 months.[27]

Drainage may also be accomplished by endoscopic approach if the pseudocyst compresses the stomach or duodenum, with the creation of an enterocystic fistula.[30,40] The largest series by Cremer and Deviere showed that endoscopic cystogastrostomy was successful in 13 patients and cystoduodenostomy in 5.[17] If these approaches are unsuccessful, elective surgical drainage will be necessary.

The diagnostic and therapeutic approach to the patient in whom a septic pancreatic process is suspected has been recently summarized by us.[4] It is important to determine the presence of pancreatic sepsis, because it has become the most common cause of death in the patient with acute pancreatitis.[55] One of the contributing factors is the inability to recognize its occurrence early in the course of acute pancreatitis. One might speculate that an infected pancreatic processes occurs only in severe pancreatitis. Thirty-eight of 65 patients in the series of Becker et al. and 6 of 21 in the series of Crass et al. had only mild pancreatitis when classified, using Ranson's criteria.[7,18] Overall, approximately half of the patients who develop septic pancreatic lesions have only mild pancreatitis. However, their mortality is related to the severity of the underlying pancreatitis.[18,33]

The clinical findings that are present in almost all patients with infected pancreatic lesions are spiking fevers, abdominal distension, and abdominal tenderness (73). Unfortunately, these are not specific for a pancreatic abscess and may be present in a patient with continuing necrotizing pancreatitis. Our findings agree with those of Warshaw et al. in that the individual features of the history and physical examination were unreliable for diagnosing pancreatic sepsis.[80] Bacteremia documented by positive blood cultures occurs 20% of the time. Although infrequent, its presence should suggest a pancreatic septic process.[7]

It has been suggested by Ranson et al. that there is a relationship of early CT findings to the development of late pancreatic sepsis.[55] They found that abscesses were most likely to occur in patients with more severe pancreatic abnormalities determined by CT, that is, inflammation confined to pancreatic and peripancreatic fat or fluid collection(s). However, Vernacchia et al. emphasize the poor predictive value of early CT for all patients with moderate or severe pancreatitis for development of pancreatic abscess.[77] While CT may not predict which patients progress to develop an abscess, it does serve as a guide for diagnostic procedures and, if applied early and combined with diagnostic needle aspiration, appears to be a factor in the improved survival of these patients.[18,36] Therefore, our initial diagnostic study is CT in a patient with abdominal pain and presumed pancreatic source of fever. We prefer CT examination to US because it not only allows us to distinguish a solid from a cystic pancreatic mass, but clearly delineates the degree of extension of the pancreatic inflammatory process into an adjacent organ, for example, colon. Unfortunately, it cannot determine whether a pancreatic mass is infected. Intrapancreatic air, a feature that was previously considered as the sine qua non for pancreatic abscess, may also be seen with pancreaticoenteric fistulas in individuals without abscess formation, as well as in patients with a patulous vaterian sphincter. In addition, it is not present in the majority of patients with abscesses.[34,36] Therefore, we use percutaneous needle aspiration guided by CT or US into the pancreatic mass(es) and/or fluid collection(s) to determine the presence of an infection[5,32] (Table 11-3). It is important to use guided needle aspiration of all cysts and in multiple areas of a septated cystic mass because one cannot

TABLE 11-3. SUSPICION OF "INFECTED" PANCREATIC LESION

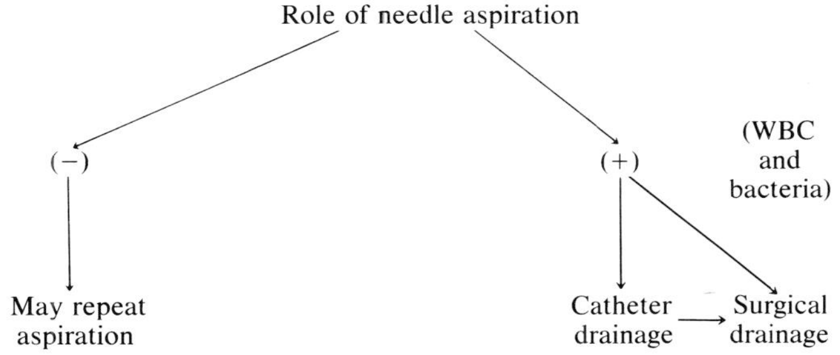

assume that infection is not present if only one of multiple cysts is aspirated. The aspirate must be gram-stained and cultured. The presence of organisms on a Gram stain with white blood cells is almost pathognomonic of a septic process, provided that the colon was not transgressed in the approach to the pancreas. Fluid white blood cell counts alone do not reliably separate a septic from a sterile inflammatory process. When organisms are visualized on Gram stain, catheter drainage of the mass is instituted. This has been employed for definitive therapy of infected cystic lesions and is successful in 70% to 90% of cases because they are usually localized. In addition, catheter drainage can be used as a temporizing measure in patients with solid pancreatic masses that have undergone subsequent liquification necrosis and are infected pancreatic abscesses.[24,25,68,71]

A solid inflammatory mass composed of indurated, edematous pancreas with infiltration of inflammatory cells involving adjacent retroperitoneal tissues is termed a *pancreatic phlegmon*. Tissue necrosis is not uncommon, making its differentiation from organizing pseudocyst or abscess sometimes difficult by CT. Tissue necrosis can be determined by using intravenous contrast material. Phlegmonous collections occur in up to 18% of all individuals experiencing bouts of acute pancreatitis. Their presence is associated with a greater likelihood of developing complications of pancreatitis.[42] A solid pancreatic lesion that yields no bacteria on Gram staining of an aspirate and a negative culture is managed best by supportive care including bowel rest, parenteral nutrition, and dietary advance depending on patient tolerance, whereas the finding of leukocytes with microbacterial organisms on needle aspiration of pancreatic tissue indicates pancreatic abscess formation. Management of such patients centers around surgical débridement of the pancreas with intraoperative pancreatic drain insertion. As one would surmise, mortality is high in such patients. Nonsurgical radiologically guided insertion of catheters with continued drainage has been reported to be a successful form of therapy for pancreatic abscesses.[74] However, most authorities feel that it should be used simply as a temporizing measure until the patient is more stable or should probably only be reserved for patients not deemed to be surgical candidates. It is this latter role that we favor.

In summary, if a clinician uses the above approach including CT with needle aspiration in the patient with acute pancreatitis and in whom a septic process may be present, these septic complications of pancreatitis could be recognized earlier, thereby decreasing their attendant morbidity and mortality.[22,23]

REFERENCES

1. Andersen BN, Hancke S, Neilsen SAD, et al. The diagnosis of pancreatic cyst by ERCP and ultrasonic scanning. Ann Surg 185:286, 1977.
2. Anderson MC. Management of pancreatic pseudocysts. Am J Surg 123:209, 1972.
3. Aranha GV, Prinz RA, Esgnerra AC, Greenlee HB. The nature and course of cystic pancreatic lesions diagnosed by ultrasound. Arch Surg 118:486–488, 1983.
4. Barkin JS, Kartsonis A. What approach do you suggest in the patient with fever and a tender abdominal mass (presumably pancreas) after an episode of acute abdominal pain associated with raised serum amylase? Am J Gastroenterol 83(1):13–14, 1988. Editorial.
5. Barkin JS, Hill M, Perreiras R, et al. Percutaneous guided aspiration for diagnosis of pancreatic abscess. Dig Dis Sci 27:1011–1014, 1982.

6. Barkin JS, Smith FR, Pereiras R, et al. Therapeutic percutaneous aspiration of pancreatic pseudocyst. Dig Dis Sci 26(7):585–586, 1981.
7. Becker JM, Pemberton JH, DiMagno EP, et al. Prognostic factors in pancreatic abscess. Surgery 96(3):455–461, 1984.
8. Bellon E, George C, Schreiber H, et al. Pancreatic pseudocysts of the duodenum. Am J Rad 133:827–831, 1979.
9. Bernardino ME, Amerson JR. Percutaneous gastrocystostomy: A new approach to pancreatic pseudocyst drainage. AJR 143:1096–1097, 1984.
10. Bilbao MK, Dotter CT, Lee TG, et al. Complications of ERCP. Gastroenterology 70:314–320, 1976.
11. Bradley EL, Clements JL. Transenteric rupture of pancreatic pseudocysts: Management of pseudocystenteric fistulas. Am Surg 42:827–837, 1976.
12. Bradley EL, Clements JL, Gonzales AC. The natural history of pancreatic pseudocysts: A unified concept of management. Am J Surg 137:135–141, 1979.
13. Caravati CM, Ashworth JS, Frederick P. Pancreatic pseudocysts: A medical evaluation. JAMA 197:572–576, 1966.
14. Cooperman A. Chronic pancreatitis. Surg Clin North Am 61(1):71, 1981.
15. Crandell W, Stueck G, McEvoy C. Chylous ascites due to a pancreatic pseudocyst. Surgery 14(1):83–111, 1953.
16. Crass RA, Way LW. Acute and chronic pancreatic pseudocysts are different. Am J Surg 142:660–663, 1981.
17. Cremer M, Deviere J. Endoscopic management of pancreatic cysts and pseudocysts. Gastrointest Endosc 32(5):367–368, 1986.
18. Crass RA, Meyer AA, Jeffrey RB, et al. Pancreatic abscess: Impact of computerized tomography on early diagnosis and surgery. Am J Surg, 150:127–131, 1985.
19. Czaja MJ, Fischer A, Marin GA. Spontaneous resolution of pancreatic masses (pseudocysts?) Arch Intern Med 135:558–562, 1975.
20. Ephgrave K, Hunt JL. Presentation of pancreatic pseudocysts: Implications for timing of surgical intervention. Am J Surg 151:749–753, 1986.
21. Farman J. Unusual pelvic complications of a pancreatic pseudocyst. Gastrointest Radiol 3:43–45, 1978.
22. Gerzof SG, Banks PA, Robins AH. Early diagnosis of pancreatic infection by computed tomography guided aspiration. Gastroenterology 193:1315–1320, 1987.
23. Gerzof SG, Banks PA, Spechler SJ. Role of guided percutaneous aspiration in the diagnosis of early pancreatic sepsis. Dig Dis Sci 29(10):950, 1984.
24. Gerzof SG, Johnson WC, Robins AH. Percutaneous drainage of infected pancreatic pseudocysts. Arch Surg 119:888–893, 1984.
25. Gerzof SG, Robins AH, Johnson WC, et al. Percutaneous catheter drainage of abdominal abscess: A five-year experience. N Engl J Med 305:653–657, 1981.
26. Gonzalez AC, Bradley EL, Clements JL. Pseudocyst formation in acute pancreatitis: Ultrasonographic evaluation of 99 cases. AJR 127:315–317, 1976.
27. Hancke S, Henriksen FW. Percutaneous pancreatic cystogastrostomy guided by ultrasound scanning and gastroscopy. Br J Surg 72:916–917, 1985.
28. Hanna WA. Rupture of pancreatic cysts: Report of a case and review of the literature. Br J Surg 47:495, 1960.
29. Hastings OM, Jain KM, Khadem M, et al. Intrasplenic pancreatic pseudocyst complicating severe acute pancreatitis. Am J Gastroenterol 69:182–186, 1978.
30. Hershfield NB. Drainage of a pancreatic pseudocyst at ERCP. Gastrointest Endosc 30(4):269–270, 1984.
31. Heyder N, Lutz H, Lux G, Demling L. Initial results of transgastric endoscopic ultrasonography in comparison with external ultrasound. Scand J Gastroenterol 19(suppl 94):85–90, 1984.
32. Hill MC, Dach JL, Barkin J, Isikoff MB, Morse B. The role of percutaneous aspiration in the diagnosis of pancreatic abscess. AJR 141:1035–1038, 1983.
33. Hurley JE, Vargish T. Early diagnosis and outcome of pancreatic abscesses in pancreatitis. Am Surg 53:29–33, 1987.
34. Itai Y, Ohtomo K, Kokubo T, et al. CT demonstration of gas in dilated pancreatic duct. J Comput Assist Tomogr 10(6):1052–1053, 1986.

35. Jaffe BM, Ferguson TB, Holte S, et al. Mediastinal pancreatic pseudocysts. Am J Surg 124:600–606, 1972.
36. Jeffrey RB, Grendell JH, Federle MP, et al. Improved survival with early CT diagnosis of pancreatic abscess. Gastrointest Radiol 12:26–30, 1987.
37. Kaplan JO, Isikoff MB, Barkin JS, et al. Necrotic carcinoma of the pancreas: The "pseudo-pseudocyst". J Comput Assist Tomogr 4(2):166–167, 1980.
38. Karlson KB, Martin EC, Fankuchen EI, et al. Percutaneous drainage of pancreatic pseudocysts and abscesses. Radiology 142:619–624, 1982.
39. Kolmannskog F, Kolbenstvedt A, Aakhus T. Computed tomography in inflammatory mass lesions following acute pancreatitis. J Comput Assist Tomogr 5(2):169–172, 1981.
40. Kozarek RA, Brayko CM, Harlan J, et al. Endoscopic drainage of pancreatic pseudocysts. Gastrointest Endosc 31(5):322–328, 1985.
41. Kuligowska E, Olsen WL. Pancreatic pseudocysts drained through a percutaneous transgastric approach. Radiology 154:79–82, 1985.
42. Lang EK, Springer RM, Lawrence WG. Abdominal abscess drainage under radiological guidance: Causes of failure. Radiology 159:329–336, 1986.
43. Laxson LC, Fromkes JJ, Cooperman M. Endoscopic retrograde cholangiopancreatography in the management of pancreatic pseudocysts. Am J Surg 150:683–686, 1985.
44. McCowin MJ, Federle MP. Computed tomography of pancreatic pseudocysts of the duodenum. AJR 145:1003–1007, 1985.
45. Mehta AI, McDowell DE. Pancreatic pseudocyst as a cause of jaundice. South Med J 71(12):1502–1506, 1978.
46. Miller CE, Cooperberg PL, Cohen MM. Pitfalls in the ultrasonographic diagnosis of the pancreatic pseudocyst. J Can Assoc Radiol 29:239–242, 1978.
47. Munn J, Altergott R, Prinz RA. Calcified pancreatic pseudocysts. Surgery 101(4):511–514, 1987.
48. Naftel W, Ravera J, Hevr HW. Pseudocyst of the pancreas stimulating a renal neoplasm. Urology 5(3):417–419, 1975.
49. Niccolini DG. Graham JH, Banks PA. Tumor induced acute pancreatitis. Gastroenterology 71:142–145, 1976.
50. Nunez D, Yrizarry JM, Russell E, et al. Transgastric drainage of pancreatic fluid collections. AJR 145:815–818, 1985.
51. O'Connor M, Kolars J, Ansel H, Silvis S, Vennes J. Preoperative endoscopic retrograde cholangiopancreatography in the surgical management of pancreatic pseudocysts. Am J Surg 151:18–24, 1986.
52. O'Malley VP, Cannon JP, Postier RG. Pancreatic pseudocysts: Cause, therapy, and results. Am J Surg 150:680–682, 1985.
53. Pollak EW, Michas CA, Wolfman EF. Pancreatic pseudocyst: Management in fifty-four patients. Am J Surg 135:199–201, 1978.
54. Prabhaker KN, Bennett DJ, Wright JS. Pseudocyst of the pancreas associated with hydrothorax: A case report and review of the literature. J Thorac Cardiovasc Surg 61(6): 885–890, 1971.
55. Ranson JHC, Balthazar E, Caccavale R, Cooper M. Computed tomography and the prediction of pancreatic abscess in acute pancreatitis. Ann Surg 201(5):656–665, 1986.
56. Reingold OJ, Walker JA, Barkin JS. Gastric outlet obstruction due to a pancreatic pseudocyst. Am J Gastroenterol 69:92, 1978.
57. Rohrmann CA, Silvis SE, Vennes JA. Evaluation of the endoscopic pancreatogram. Radiology 113:297–304, 1974.
58. Sachs JR, Deren JJ, Min S, Nusbaum M. Mucinous cystadenoma: Pitfalls of differential diagnosis. Am J Gastroenterol 84:811–816, 1989.
59. Sandy JT, Taylor RM, Christensen RM, et al. Pancreatic pseudocyst: Changing concepts in management. Am J Surg 141:574–576, 1981.
60. Sankaran S, Walt AJ. The natural and unnatural history of pancreatic pseudocysts. Br J Surg 62:37–44, 1975.
61. Shafer RB, Silvas SE. Pancreatic pseudo-pseudocysts. Am J Surg 127:320–325, 1974.
62. Shatney CH, Lillchei RC. The timing of surgical treatment of pancreatic pseudocysts. Surg Gynecol Obstet 152:809–812, 1981.

63. Shatney CH, Sosin H. Spontaneous perforation of a pancreatic pseudocyst into the colon and duodenum. Am J Surg 126:434–438, 1973.
64. Shetty AN. Pseudocysts of the pancreas: An overview. South Med J 73(9):1239–1242, 1980.
65. Siegleman SS. CT of fluid collections associated with pancreatitis. Am J Radiol 134:1121–1132, 1980.
66. Silverstein W, Isikorr MB, Hill MC, et al. Diagnostic imaging of acute pancreatitis: Prospective study using CT and sonography. Am J Radiol 137:497–502, 1981.
67. Silvis SE, Vennes JA, Rohrmann CA. Endoscopic pancreatography in the evaluation of patients with suspected pancreatic pseudocysts. Am J Gastroenterol 61:452–459, 1974.
68. Sostre CF, Flournoy JG, Bova JG, Goldstein HM, Schenker S. Pancreatic phlegmon: Clinical features and course. Dig Dis Sci 30:918–927, 1985.
69. Sugawa C, Walt AJ. Endoscopic retrograde pancreatography in the surgery of pancreatic pseudocysts. Surgery 86(4):639–647, 1979.
70. Sybers HD, Shelp WD, Morrissey JF. Pseudocyst of the pancreas with fistulous extension into the neck. N Engl J Med 278(19):1058–1059, 1968.
71. Torres WE, Evert MB. Percutaneous aspiration and drainage of pancreatic pseudocysts. AJR 147:1007–1009, 1981.
72. Tucker P, Webster PD. Traumatic pseudocysts of the pancreas: A report of ten cases Arch Intern Med 129:583–586, 1972.
73. Vajcner A, Nicoloff D. Pseudocysts of the pancreas: Value of urine and serum amylase levels. Surgery 66(5):842–845, 1969.
74. vanSonnenberg E, Wittich GR, Casola C, et al. Complicated pancreatic inflammatory disease: Diagnostic and therapeutic role of interventional radiology. Radiology 155:335–340, 1985.
75. vanSonnenberg E, Wittich GR, Casola G, et al. Percutaneous drainage of infected and non-infected pancreatic pseudocysts—Experience in 101 cases. Radiology 170:757–762, 1989.
76. Varriale P, Bonanno CA, Grace WJ. Portal hypertension secondary to pancreatic pseudocysts. Arch Intern Med 112:191, 1963.
77. Vernacchia FS, Jeffrey RB, Federle MP, et al. Pancreatic abscess: Predictive value of early abdominal CT-1. Radiology, 162(2):435–438, 1987.
78. Warshaw AL. Inflammatory masses following acute pancreatitis. Surg Clin North Am 54(3):621–636, 1974.
79. Warshaw AL, Rutledge PL. Cystic tumors mistaken for pancreatic pseudocysts. Ann Surg 205:393–398, 1987.
80. Warshaw AL, Jin G. Improved survival in 45 patients with pancreatic abscess. Ann Surg 202(4):408–417, 1986.
81. Warshaw AL, Lee KH. Aging changes of pancreatic isoamylases and the appearance of "old amylase" in the serum of patients with pancreatic pseudocyst. Gastroenterology 79:1246–1251, 1980.
82. Warshaw AL, Rattner DW. Facts and fallacies of common bile duct obstruction by pancreatic pseudocysts. Ann Surg 192:33, 1980.
83. Warshaw AL, Rattner DW. Timing of surgical drainage for pancreatic pseudocyst. Ann Surg 202(6):720–724, 1985.
84. Weaver DW, Bouwman DL, Walt AJ, et al. Aged Amylase. Arch Surg 117:707–711, 1982.
85. Wind GG, Rubin P, Waye J, et al. Pancreatic pseudocyst: Is endoscopic retrograde cholangiopancreatography contraindicated? Mount Sinai J Med 43(5):558–564, 1976.
86. Winship D. Moderator—Pancreatitis: Pancreatic pseudocysts and the complications. Gastroenterology 73:593–603, 1977.
87. Wolstenholme JT. Major gastrointestinal hemorrhage associated with pancreatic pseudocysts. Am J Surg 127:377–381, 1974.

CHAPTER

12

SURGICAL TREATMENT OF PANCREATIC NECROSIS, ABSCESSES, AND CYSTS

Mary E. Estakhri and Charles F. Frey

The sequelae of acute pancreatitis pose significant challenges to the surgeon in defining indications for operative intervention. Increased understanding of the pathogenesis and natural history of pancreatitis has allowed us to better define and describe some of these sequelae, which include pancreatic necrosis, infected pancreatic necrosis, pancreatic abscesses, pseudocysts, and collections of necrotic fat. These complications, all of which can be identified with diagnostic studies now available, require specific therapy and have different outcomes.

While there are many causes of acute pancreatitis, most are associated with gallstones, alcohol, hyperlipidemia, trauma, or operation.[43] Many large series document that the vast majority of these patients, about 80%, recover quickly after a 2- to 3-day illness requiring only minimal supportive treatment consisting of keeping the patient without oral intake and providing intravenous fluids.[21] Many patients may have a recurrent attack of pancreatitis if the causes are not removed or corrected.[23] In particular, if biliary tract disease is identified, operative correction should be carried out prior to hospital discharge.[23] On the basis of studies with computed tomography (CT), the pancreas may appear enlarged, presumably on the basis of edema and inflammation, and there may even be evidence of fluid collections about the pancreas that spontaneously resolve.[12] This is the classic edematous or interstitial pancreatitis, which is usually associated with at least some minimal evidence of fat necrosis, one of the earliest lesions of acute pancreatitis, if carefully sought.[33] Of those 20% of patients with a more protracted, severe illness who develop significant sequelae or complications of acute pancreatitis, the feature that seems to distinguish them from patients with less severe illness is the presence of significant pancreatic and/or peripancreatic necrosis, often associated with persistent fluid collections.

Pancreatic and peripancreatic necrosis may be focal or diffuse, but when extensive may be associated with life-threatening systemic manifestations, including a major capillary leak secondary to activation of the complement system, the clotting mechanism, prostaglandins, and kinins. Major fluid losses occur, characterized by hypovolemia, shock, hemoconcentration, and oliguric renal failure. Pulmonary insufficiency, hypocalcemia, clotting abnormalities, and endotoxemia may result. These pathophysiologic manifestations of necrosis have led various investigators to identify a constellation of such signs as manifesting "severe" pancreatitis, for example, Ranson's criteria, Imrie's criteria, Bank's criteria, and others.[3,18,31,42] When there is extensive pancreatic necrosis, the clinical presentation, aside from the systemic manifestations, varies with the location and extent of necrosis. Necrosis that involves a portion of the pancreatic ductal system results in a collection of pancreatic secretions or acute pseudocyst. Peripheral necrosis may extend through the capsule of the gland to surrounding tissues, producing peripancreatic necrotic collections of fat. Secondary infection may occur at any stage and present as infected pancreatic or peripancreatic necrosis, or as a walled-off collection of pus, that is, a pancreatic abscess or infected pseudocyst.

PANCREATIC PSEUDOCYST

When the necrosis involves surrounding parenchyma and a portion of the major or tributary pancreatic ducts responsible for transporting pancreatic exocrine secretions to the duodenum, a leakage of pancreatic secretion may occur into the parenchyma of the pancreas or surrounding tissues. These collections of pancreatic exocrine secretion in continuity with the pancreatic ductal system may resolve spontaneously, as occurs in about 40% of patients, or persist if there is proximal impediment to outflow from pancreatic ductal obstruction due to ampullary common duct stone, stricture, inflammation, edema, or necrosis.[12] A reactive fibrous wall forms about and contains these collections of pancreatic juice. After 4 to 6 weeks, the walls of these collections have matured to the point that they can hold sutures.

Peripancreatic Necrotic Fat Collections

Other collections of peripancreatic fat may liquify or form toothpaste-like collections of necrotic debris that also become surrounded by reactive fibrous walls and are indistinguishable by CT scan from pseudocysts filled with pancreatic juice. However, these collections, usually peripancreatic, are not in continuity with the pancreatic ductal system.

Infected Pancreatic Necrosis

Based on the studies of Beger et al.,[7] who operated on many patients with necrotizing pancreatitis, it is estimated that about 40% of patients with significant pancreatitis and peripancreatic necrosis become infected. This has been confirmed by others.[24,29] There seems to be some correlation between the extent of necrosis and the presence of infection. The mortality associated with infected pancreatic necrosis is influenced by the extent of the necrosis and the time of infection after onset of symptoms. The earlier the onset of infection, the graver the prognosis. Infected pancreatic and peripancreatic necrosis may be likened to a necrotizing fasciitis—the process is not walled off and may dissect extensively throughout the retroperitoneum. Anaerobic and gas-forming organisms may be present. These infections are not amenable to percutaneous drainage and often do not contain liquified pus but are accompanied by a thin grayish exudate. On conventional CT scan it is impossible to distinguish infected necrosis from sterile necrosis unless gas bubbles are detected. Gerzhof and Banks and others have demonstrated that thin needle aspiration of the pancreas and peripancreatic tissues with Gram staining and culture is an effective and highly reliable means for distinguishing infected pancreatic and peripancreatic necrosis from sterile necrosis.[27,29]

Pancreatic Abscess

Abscesses of the pancreas are by definition walled-off loculations of pus. They tend to occur later in the course of pancreatitis, 3 to 4 weeks after the onset of symptoms, and systemic manifestations are often less severe than in infected pancreatic necrosis. They are not distinguishable from pseudocysts on CT scan, and if there is any question as to the differential diagnosis, aspiration with Gram staining and culture should settle the issue. Whether these walled-off collections of pus result from liquification of localized areas of necrosis or represent infections of pseudocysts has no practical significance. They are treated by decompression either operatively or by percutaneous drainage with a pigtail catheter.

DIAGNOSIS

In defining criteria for diagnosing pancreatic and peripancreatic necrosis, abscesses, and cysts, the focus must be placed on factors that indicate a need for operative intervention. Standard clinical signs and symptoms, routine laboratory data, and severe prognostic signs have been evaluated by many authors.[3,15,39] Ranson's criteria include factors detectable on admission to the hospital, such as patient age over 55 years, hyperglycemia, leukocytosis, and transaminase level elevations, and subsequent risk factors detected during the early treatment of acute pancreatitis, such as a falling hematocrit, a rising blood urea nitrogen level, hypocalcemia, hypoxemia, a base deficit >4 mEq/L, and large fluid requirements (>6 L). These variables have been shown to be predictive of patient risk for serious morbidity or mortality.[5,42,43] In addition, a correlation exists between the number of positive early prognostic signs and the extent of pancreatic necrosis.[8] However, these criteria have several limitations. The signs and symptoms frequently cited are all nonspecific and can be found in high frequency in patients with acute interstitial pancreatitis, pancreatic or peripancreatic necrosis, infected necrosis, abscess, or pseudocyst. Since these signs do not distinguish between acute interstitial pancreatitis or its sequelae, the presence or absence of these findings does not provide surgical indications. A further limitation is the fact that 6 of the 11 signs of clinical severity require 48 hours to detect and rank patients. In our experience with 50 patients with necrotizing pancreatitis, we have found the Apache II score obtained the day of hospital admission to be an accurate predictor of death in all 7 patients who died. We had no survivors with Apache II scores over 27 and no deaths with Apache II scores under 25.[51] The Apache II score is not useful in predicting infectious complications of pancreatitis.

The diagnostic tests that are most useful are those that can detect the presence of pancreatic necrosis. There is continued interest in finding a laboratory test indicative of pancreatic necrosis. Both C-reactive protein and α_2-macroglobulin profiles in serum have been evaluated following acute pancreatitis. The levels in 23 patients with acute interstitial pancreatitis were compared to those in 27 patients with necrotizing pancreatitis in a study by Buchler et al.[14] The α_2-macroglobulin level was significantly decreased during the first 10 days of illness in the patients with necrotizing pancreatitis, with a calculated sensitivity of 85%. The C-reactive protein monitoring demonstrated persistent elevation throughout the 14-day study period in patients with necrotizing pancreatitis, with a 90% sensitivity. MacMahon et al. found similar results in 12 patients with severe pancreatitis, 9 of whom were later found to have an abscess or pseudocyst.[37] However, he found a delay in C-reactive protein rise to day 3 of illness and a delay in fall of α_2-macroglobulin to day 2 of illness in comparison to patients with mild pancreatitis. As a result, serial monitoring of these values may be more predictive of the presence of necrosis than a single measurement obtained on admission to the hospital. Schroder et al. reported on a series of patients monitored with serum phospholipase A_2 levels and found a correlation between serum levels and prognostic signs of severe pancreatitis.[46] Further, the serum phospholipase A_2 concentrations were significantly higher in patients requiring operative intervention compared with patients with acute pancreatitis who responded to supportive treatment alone.

Peritoneal lavage is a quick and simple test that may be performed in the emergency room to detect severe pancreatitis with necrosis.[38] The presence of

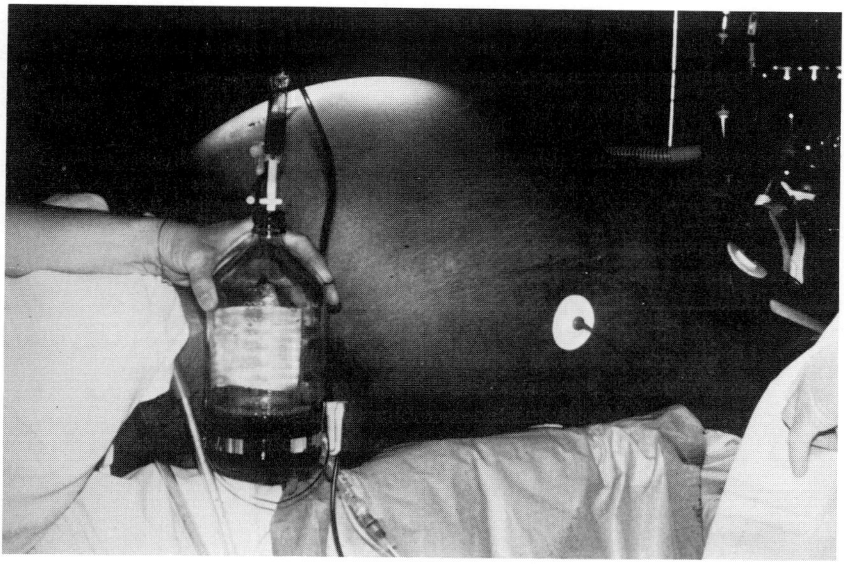

Figure 12-1. Available on hospital admission, diagnostic peritoneal lavage is useful in identifying pancreatic necrosis. Brownish or bloody fluid is characteristic of pancreatic necrosis.

free peritoneal fluid on insertion of the dialysis catheter (>10 mL) or dark fluid containing hemoglobin indicates the presence of pancreatic necrosis (Fig. 12-1). Serial lavages may be employed to follow the course of the inflammatory process or detect subsequent infection. The limitation of this test is that it may be falsely negative if the necrotic process is limited to the retroperitoneum at the time of the procedure.

Routine radiographic methods have been used previously to diagnose the presence of acute pancreatitis. These studies depend upon involvement or displacement of contiguous structures as demonstrated by plain films or gastrointestinal contrast studies.[54] In general, these examinations lack sensitivity and are not capable of demonstrating the full extent of the disease process. Gray-scale ultrasonography greatly increased our ability to visualize the pancreas, particularly in the diagnosis of pancreatic pseudocysts. However, in the presence of acute pancreatitis, paralytic ileus frequently prevents adequate evaluation of the pancreas. Williford et al. reported 20 inadequate studies in 54 patients undergoing ultrasonography to rule out pancreatic pseudocyst due to overlying bowel gas or visualization of only the head of the pancreas.[57] In addition, of the 18 ultrasound studies positive for pseudocyst, only 8 identified all the pathologic lesions present. Similar limitations for ultrasonography were described by Block et al. and Silverstein et al.[9,48] Diagnostic capabilities have been greatly enhanced with CT scanning of patients with acute pancreatitis. Abnormalities demonstrable by conventional CT include enlargement of the pancreas, either focal or diffuse; intrapancreatic gas or hemorrhage; pancreatic pseudocysts; extrapancreatic spread of the inflammatory process, such as to the lesser sac, pararenal spaces, and subdiaphragmatic region; or the presence of concurrent ascites or pleural effusions as well as pancreatico-pleural fistulas (Fig. 12-2).[36] Although conventional CT can provide information regarding the location and extent of intraabdominal pathologic lesions, it cannot predict accurately the nature of the collections detected.[44] The addition of intrave-

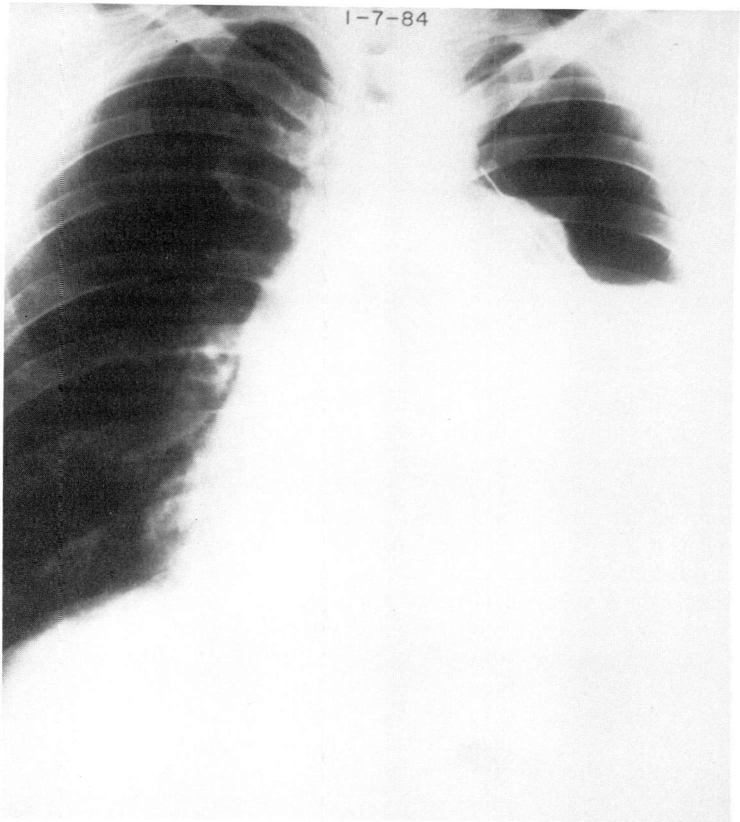

A

Figure 12-2. (A) Large pleural effusion secondary to pancreaticopleural fistula. (*Figure continues.*)

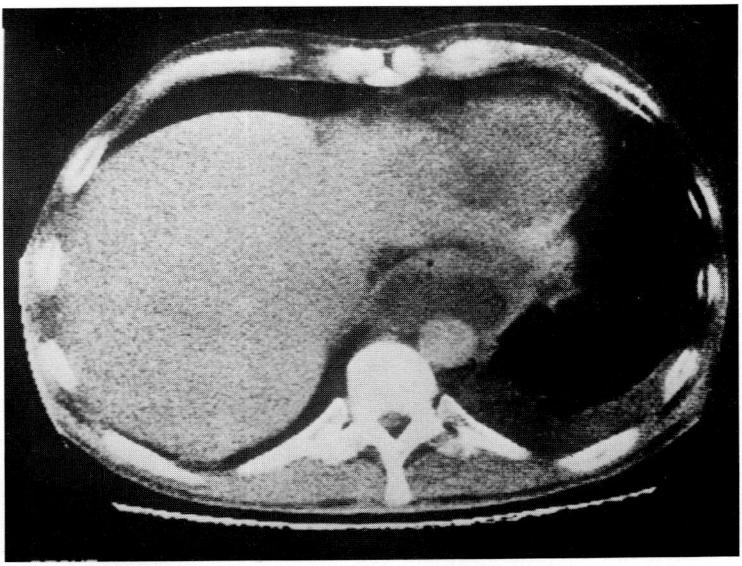

B

Figure 12-2 (*continued*). (B) CT scan demonstrates site of pancreaticopleural fistula traversing the diaphragm.

nous bolus contrast injection during CT scanning to obtain vascular enhancement can reliably distinguish between viable and nonviable pancreas (Fig. 12-3). The ability to identify and quantify pancreatic necrosis has great clinical significance. Kivisaari et al. followed 28 patients with acute pancreatitis undergoing intravenous contrast CT for subsequent outcome.[32] Eight scans revealed decreased enhancement of the pancreas, whereas in the remaining 20 scans, rapid enhancement of the pancreatic parenchyma occurred within 10 seconds. In the 8 patients with areas of decreased enhancement, these findings were shown to correlate with hemorrhage and necrosis at operation. There was one false-negative scan. In a similar study, 59 patients were compared by contrast CT findings, clinical grading, and intraoperative findings.[9] Clinical criteria were unreliable in predicting the presence of necrosis, whereas contrast CT accurately diagnosed pancreatic necrosis in 82% of cases. Acute interstitial pancreatitis is characterized by uniform enhancement of pancreatic tissue with an intravenous bolus of contrast material. In necrotizing pancreatitis, there is local or diffuse nonenhancement of involved tissue following intravenous contrast administration. We have found the CT scan with vascular enhancement in addition to identifying patients with pancreatic necrosis helpful in predicting infections, pseudocysts, and diabetes. The CT scan with vascular enhancement was not helpful in predicting mortality.

An acute pseudocyst demonstrates low tissue density and absence of enhancement in the region of the pseudocyst. A pancreatic abscess has decreased intensity in the region of the abscess (similar to a pseudocyst) with normal pancreatic parenchymal contrast enhancement. Contrast CT can thus predict the presence of nonviable pancreas and localize collections, but it cannot distinguish sterile versus infected necrosis or a pseudocyst versus an infected pseudocyst or abscess.

Along with pancreatic necrosis, infection following acute pancreatitis is a major determinant of morbidity and mortality. Beger et al. prospectively evaluated 114 patients with necrotizing pancreatitis for the presence of infected necrosis at operation and found a 39.4% incidence of positive cultures.[7] The only pathognomonic sign of infection by current diagnostic studies is the presence of gas bubbles seen on either plain radiographs or by CT scanning (Fig. 12-4). This finding may be present in only 9% to 29% of patients with subsequently documented infection.[19,20,53] In the absence of gas bubbles, the addition of ultrasound- or CT-directed needle aspiration is necessary to make a definitive diagnosis of infected versus sterile collections. Guided percutaneous aspiration with Gram

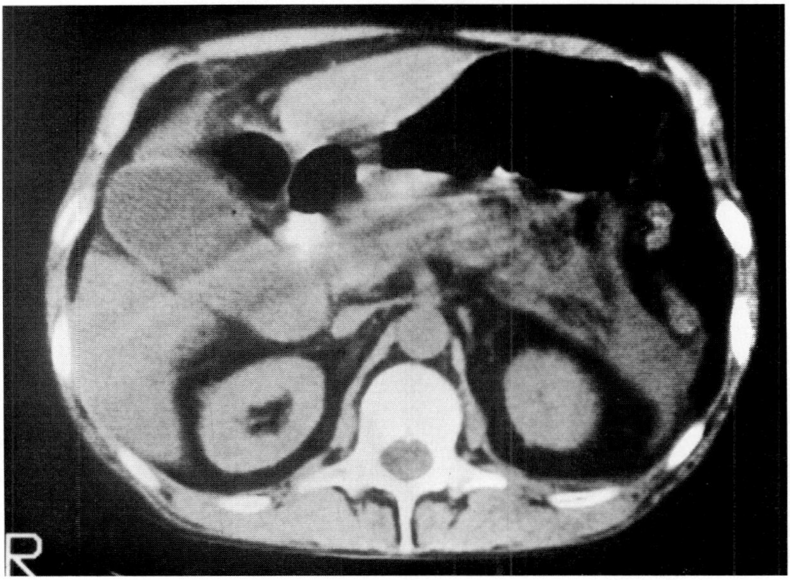

A

Figure 12-3. (A) CT scan showing inflammation and fluid collections in region of body and tail of the pancreas. (B) CT scan with vascular enhancement shows intact pancreas with surrounding fluid collections. (These films were made available by the courtesy of Hans Beger, chairman, Department of Surgery, Ulm University, Ulm, Germany.) (*Figure continues.*)

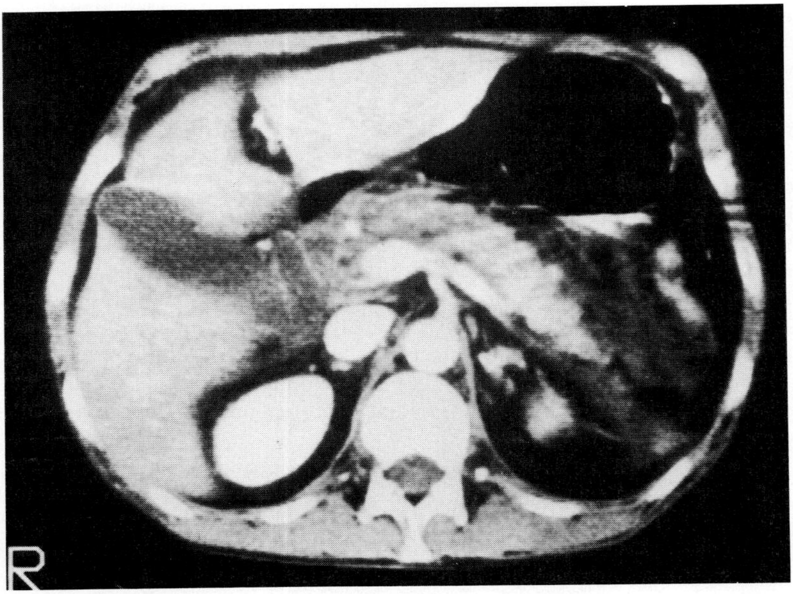

B

Figure 12-3. *(continued)*

staining and culture permits accurate detection of infection or abscess with no reported complications. Gerzof et al. performed guided percutaneous aspiration of pancreatic inflammatory processes in 42 patients with severe pancreatitis who were suspected of having an infective process based on clinical criteria.[27] Twenty patients with 41 sterile aspirates were managed medically with good result. The remaining patients were treated with antibiotics and drainage based upon the bacteriology of the aspirate. No complications of needle aspiration occurred. Similar success has been reported by Hiatt et al., Crass et al., Sostre et al.[17,29,49,56] Pseudocysts, abscesses, and fistulas may also be demonstrated by endoscopic retrograde cholangiopancreatography (ERCP), which should usually be performed as a preoperative study the day before surgery (Fig. 12-5).

TREATMENT

Pancreatic Necrosis

Acute interstitial pancreatitis that progresses to sterile necrosis is usually treated with vigorous supportive therapy. The presence of necrosis can be lethal because of severe associated systemic complications such as adult respiratory distress syndrome, acute renal failure, immunocompromise predisposing to systemic sepsis, and coagulopathy. Medical therapy included prompt fluid resuscitation, respiratory support with either supplemental oxygen or intubation as indicated by arterial blood-gas monitoring, nasogastric suction, frequent antacid therapy, or intravenous H_2-receptor blockers, and total parenteral nutrition. Minor sterile necrosis should resolve spontaneously. As the extent of glandular involvement increases, the incidence of morbidity and mortality rises. The presence of persistent tachycardia, fever, hemodynamic instability, deteriorating pulmonary function, or other signs of progressive systemic deterioration indicate extensive parenchymal or peripancreatic necrosis requiring operative intervention.

In addition to this acute presentation, we have found that some patients in whom the tail or a portion of the body and the tail of the pancreas has undergone necrosis and become a sequestrum surrounded by an intact capsule and reactive fibrosis, present months after their acute illness.

The operative approach in uninfected pancreatic necrosis limited to those patients evidencing progressive hemodynamic or pulmonary failure involves abdominal exploration to confirm the presence of pancreatic necrosis. The pancreas must be exposed to define the lesion and estimate the extent of parenchymal and/or peripancreatic necrosis. Neighboring viscera, including the biliary tree, stomach, duodenum, colon, and spleen, should be examined for pathologic lesions. If the preoperative assessment has been incorrect and acute interstitial pancreatitis without necrosis is found, anterior capsulectomy (performed to rule out necrosis)

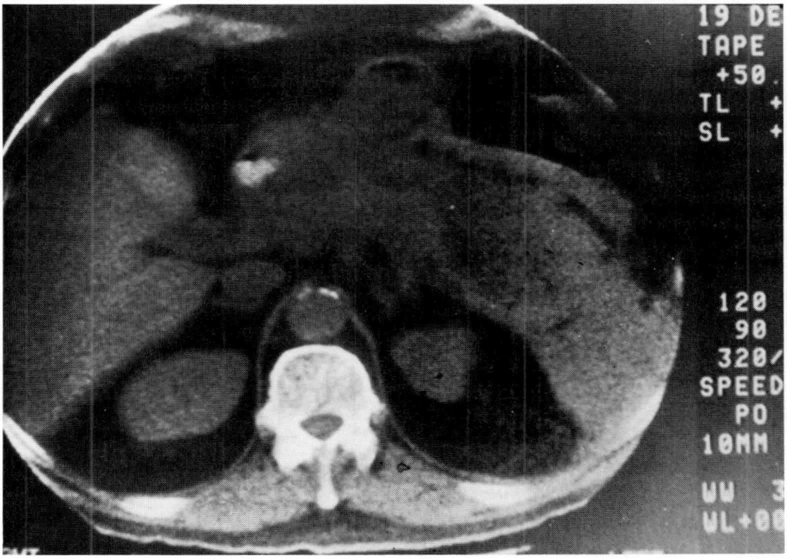

Figure 12-4. Marked enlargement of the body and tail of the pancreas are noted on CT scan, with suggestion of gas bubbles in the body of the pancreas.

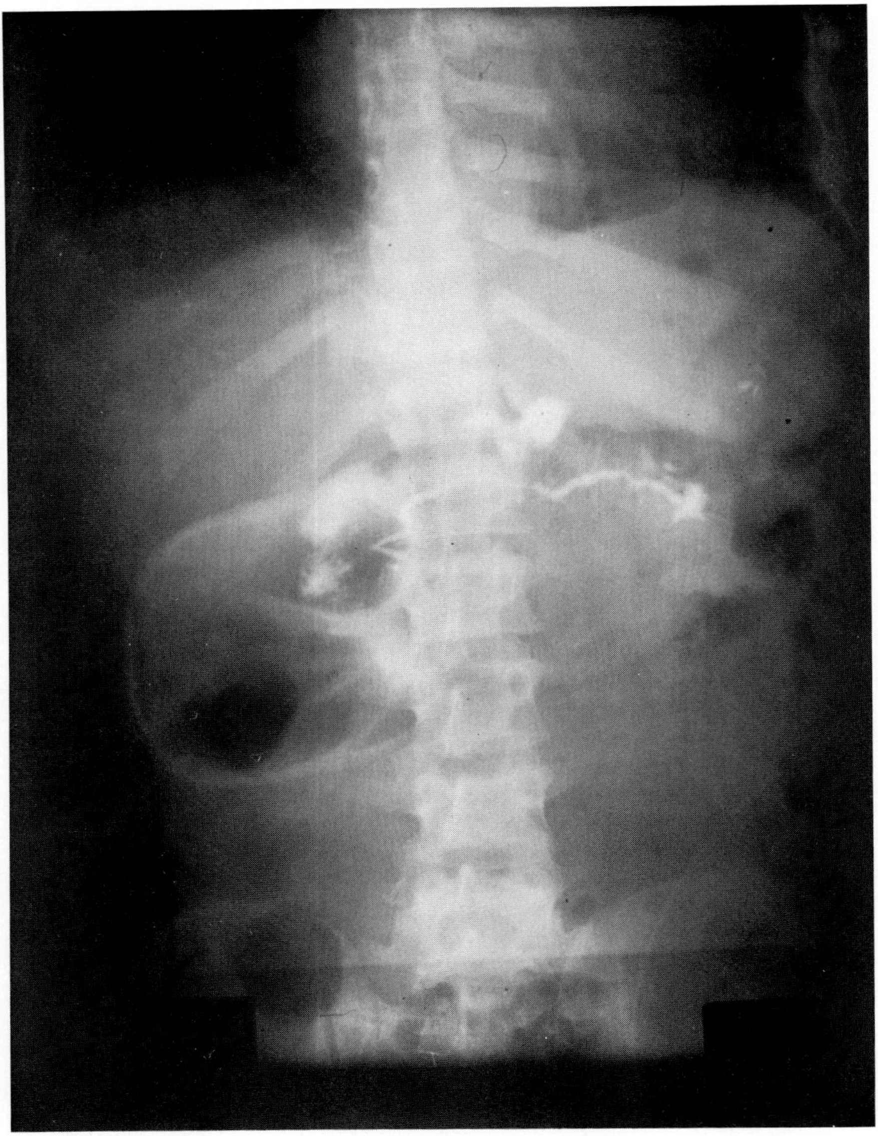

A

Figure 12-5. (A) On ERCP examination, a fistula directed superiorly is noted to arise from the main pancreatic duct in the body of the pancreas. (B) The fistula was found to enter the pericardial sac, and the patient presented with pericardial tamponade. (*Figure continues.*)

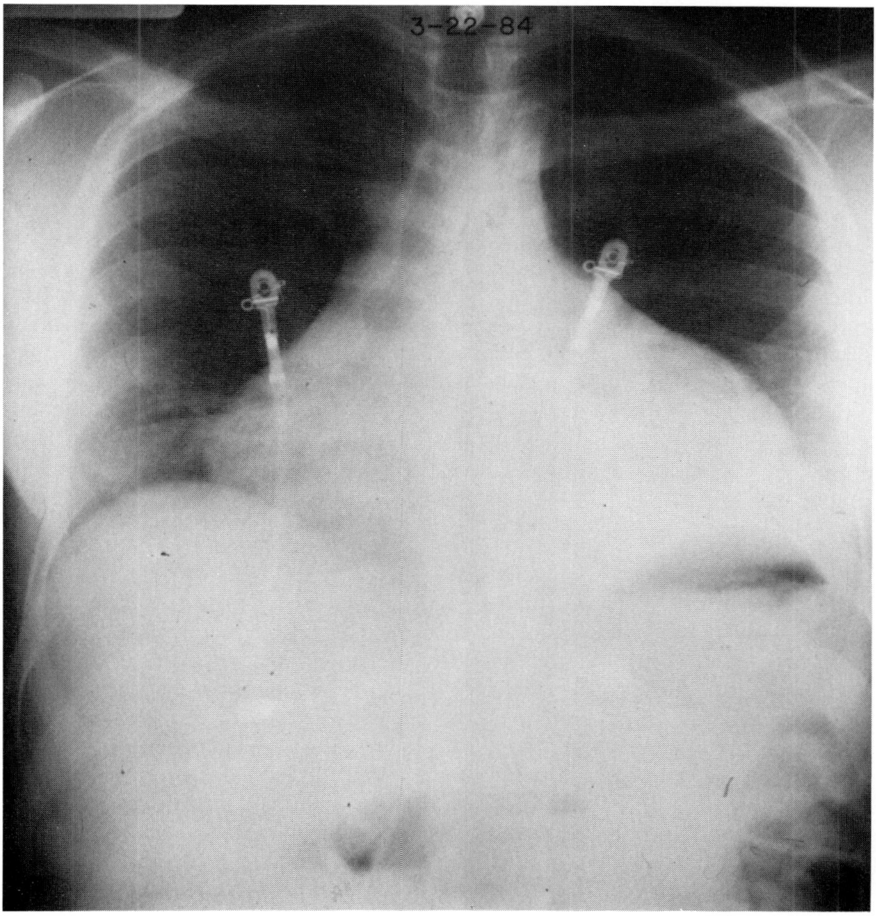

B

Figure 12-5. *(continued)*

with irrigation and drainage of the lesser sac is adequate. In the presence of pancreatic necrosis, simple drainage without excision of necrotic tissue has been associated with mortality rates of 59% to 93%.[26,35] Aggressive resection is not indicated when the area of demarcation between necrotic and viable pancreas is not clear and excessive removal of healthy tissue may result.[8,24] Focal areas of necrosis may be removed by necrosectomy, leaving any healthy pancreatic tissue behind. The addition of postoperative lavage and drainage is advocated to remove the products of ongoing necrosis following the initial exploration. Beger et al. reported the results of necrosectomy and postoperative lavage in 114 patients, including 40% with infected necrosis.[8] Abdominal lavage was associated with 26%

mortality, whereas local lavage of the lesser sac resulted in a 6% mortality. Gebhardt and Gall found a decrease in mortality from 43% to 33% when they compared necrosectomy alone to necrosectomy with lesser sac irrigation and drainage in 135 patients with necrotizing pancreatitis.[26] These authors reported a high mortality rate (52%–64%) associated with the presence of subtotal or total pancreatic necrosis, irrespective of the operative procedure employed. In these patients, there is often accompanying involvement of adjacent structures such as splenic vein thrombosis or necrosis of the duodenum or colon. These cases may require pancreatic resection along with splenectomy or resection of a portion of the colon with proximal colostomy. If the cause of pancreatic necrosis is biliary tract disease, this should be treated semielectively, that is, when the patient has recovered from the acute pancreatic inflammatory process, but prior to hospital discharge. The exception is the patient with jaundice or common bile duct dilatation at the time of initial exploration. In these patients, biliary decompression via T-tube placement with or without choledocholithotomy is indicated. The patient's overall condition dictates the extent and timing for performing these adjunctive procedures.

Pseudocyst

Approximately 40% of acute pseudocysts resolve spontaneously in 4 to 8 weeks following an acute attack of pancreatitis.[12,52] For pseudocysts that will ultimately require operative treatment, this delay permits maturation of the cyst wall. Initial size of the cyst may also be a contributing factor in choosing expectant management.[6] In general, the procedures available are excision, external drainage, or internal drainage, the choice of procedure depending upon the location of the pseudocyst within the gland.

Pseudocysts located in the pancreatic head, in continuity with and adherent to the duodenum, are usually treated by cyst-duodenostomy.[11] Pseudocysts adherent to the posterior gastric wall are easily drained through a cyst-gastrostomy. Pseudocyst adherence and fusion are important in performing anastomoses to the stomach or duodenum because an anastomotic leak is very difficult to correct following a cyst-duodenostomy or cyst-gastrostomy. A postoperative leak is less likely to occur if the anastomosis is performed between structures adherent to the pseudocyst wall. If the cyst is not adherent to the stomach or duodenum, a cyst-jejunostomy is formed using a defunctionalized Roux en Y jejunal loop. Once drained, the pseudocyst cavity rapidly shrinks and disappears over a few weeks, since it is not lined by a true epithelium. The major risk associated with internal drainage is hemorrhage from the cyst cavity, although it occurs in only about 3% to 10% of cases.[25,50] It is usually due to pseudoaneurysm formation of a visceral vessel and occurs within a few weeks of drainage. Preoperative angiography and embolization can prevent this complication.[25] Recurrence rates after internal drainage range from 3% to 8%, the lowest occurring with cyst-gastrostomy.[22] Excision can circumvent late hemorrhage and is associated with the lowest recurrence rates. Its greatest usefulness is in lesions of the tail of the pancreas. External drainage is usually reserved for infected pseudocysts or in patients requiring early intervention (prior to cyst wall maturation) for clinical deterioration. Percutaneous pseudocyst aspiration is an important diagnostic technique, but percutaneous drainage should be discouraged. The presence of an indwelling catheter may convert a sterile pseudocyst to an infected one. If the cyst is not well walled off, this may lead to contamination of the entire retroperitoneum. Furthermore, long-term resolution rates with this method remain less than 30%.[4,12]

Endoscopic methods have been employed to achieve internal drainage of pancreatic pseudocysts. There are many dangers associated with these methods. Bleeding may occur, either from the cyst wall or from visceral vessels. The latter is possible when a pseudocyst arises from the posterior aspect of the pancreas, stretching the intervening pancreas and splenic artery over its surface against the stomach. Contiguity of the cyst with the stomach or duodenum on CT does not imply fusion between these structures, and puncture through a nonfused area can produce a pancreatic leak or fistula. The cyst wall can be quite thick, making the procedure technically very demanding. A large (4 cm) incision is needed to prevent closure and recurrence, and a biopsy should be performed, both of which may be difficult endoscopically. Finally, the cyst may contain necrotic pancreas within it that cannot be removed by endoscopic drainage and may also lead to recurrence.

Infected Pancreatic Necrosis

Sterile necrosis progresses to infected necrosis in approximately 40% of cases. Nonoperative treatment is associated with nearly universal mortality.[1,24,40] Therefore, the detection of infected necrosis is an absolute indication for broad-spectrum antibiotics (until culture and sensitivity results are available), abdominal exploration, débridement of all necrotic tissue, and drainage. The current medical and surgical literature describing the management of infected necrosis is confusing, because no distinction is made between a localized abscess and infected, necrotizing pancreatitis. In interpreting the existing data and making treatment recommendations, we have examined the description of operative findings to classify these papers according to our definitions previously outlined. Altemeier and Alexander described the first large series of patients treated with anterior celiotomy, débridement of necrotic tissue, and external drainage through multiple flank stab wounds.[1] In this series, 86% of the patients recovered and 19% required reexploration for recurrent infection. Subsequently, several authors have reported mortality rates of 22.1% to 50% with closed external drainage.[2,16,30,40] All these series are notable for a high frequency of septic deaths. Shi et al. treated 34 cases of infected necrosis with external drainage, adding postoperative cavity irrigation.[47] Postoperative mortality remained 35% with over one half of the deaths due to sepsis. A contributing factor to the poor success of closed drainage is the nature of the necrotic debris associated with the infected process. Bolooki et al. and Miller et al. described the presence of large particulate debris that may occlude sump drains and lead to recurrent sepsis.[10,40] The only favorable literature report regarding closed drainage is the series by Warshaw and Jin in which catheter drainage was associated with a 95% survival rate.[53] The limitation of this series is that patients with true walled-off abscesses were included in their treatment group, which responded to percutaneous drainage when recurrent abscesses formed. Based upon these results, several authors advocate open packing of the abdomen following exploration and debridement and report survival rates of 82% to 100%.[13,19,34,41,54] Pemberton et al, compared closed drainage with open packing of the lesser sac[55] in 81 patients and found a decrease in mortality from 44% to 18% in the open-treated patients.[41] Davidson and Bradley and Knol et al. employed open packing in a total of 9 patients.[19,34] One patient required reoperation for persistent sepsis, and there were no deaths. In a series of 21 patients, Bradley and Fulenwider reported a 14% mortality rate with no sepsis-related deaths.[13]

The operative technique involves extensive debridement of all pancreatic and/or peripancreatic necrotic tissue through an anterior abdominal incision. We place several Davol sump drains in the lesser sac for postoperative irrigation, with saline or dialysate fluid. (A liter is given each hour while the other drains are on suction. Each hour, the drain through which the fluid is infused is rotated.) Following Davol drain placement, nonadherent gauze is placed over any exposed major vessels or viscera and roller gauze packing inserted. Large retention sutures of nonabsorbable material are placed and loosely tied over the packing to prevent evisceration. Dressings may then be changed every 2 to 4 days, initially under anesthesia, and later at the patient's bedside. This method permits continued debridement of necrotic tissue and any residual pockets of infection. The primary advantage of this technique is that it provides excellent drainage and enables the surgeon to treat the continued necrosis that occurs following initial debridement, and which would otherwise require another operation, without having to open and close the abdomen at each debridement.

The complications of infected pancreatic or peripancreatic necrosis are severe, regardless of the method of operative treatment. The earlier series employing closed drainage were followed by a high incidence of septic complications, ranging from 15% to 50%.[15,30] The use of open drainage has markedly diminished septic complications, but overall complication rates remain high, up to 95%.[13] Other frequently reported postoperative problems include pulmonary complications such as pneumonia, atelectasis, and pulmonary embolus, gastrointestinal and intraabdominal hemorrhage, colonic necrosis and fistula formation, and wound infection. After sepsis, intraabdominal or gastrointestinal hemorrhage was listed as the cause of death in several series.[24,25,30,47,53] The use of an intravenous H_2-receptor blocker, which was not routinely available in the earlier studies, diminished the occurrence of gastrointestinal bleeding. Visceral aneurysm formation also contributed to both intestinal and intraabdominal hemorrhage. Arteriography with embolization for temporary or permanent hemostasis has been reported with some success.[25,53] The incidence of postoperative fistulas ranges from 12% to 54%.[24,30,53] Pancreatic fistulas close spontaneously in nearly every case with bowel rest and hyperalimentation.[41,47,53] Enteric fistulas usually require additional operative treatment, such as proximal diversion with or without resection.[2,40,53] Colonic necrosis is a rare complication of acute interstitial pancreatitis, with only 39 reported cases in the literature.[45] It is not uncommon following infected pancreatic necrosis and may lead to progressive multisystem organ failure despite prompt resection.

Pancreatic Abscess

In contrast to the surgical treatment of infected necrosis, the treatment of pancreatic abscess by our strict definition is fairly simple. Whether an abscess results from infection of a pseudocyst or of a loculated collection of necrotic pancreatic or peripancreatic material, the approach to treatment is the same. Contributing factors in choosing the method of drainage include the presence of a unilocular versus a multilocular cavity and the location of the abscess(es). With the advent of CT-guided needle aspiration for diagnosis, a catheter may be placed percutaneously for a positive Gram stain, if a well-defined cavity in an accessible location is present. Gerzof et al. reported 11 infected pseudocysts treated in this manner.[28] Nine resolved with no recurrences at a mean follow-up of 24 months. Adequate treatment may be achieved with either percutaneous catheter drainage or operative exploration and placement of external drainage catheters, along with broad-spectrum intravenous antibiotics. For multilocular, complex, or inaccessible abscesses, or for persistent signs of untreated infection following percutaneous drainage, operative external drainage is the treatment of choice.

SUMMARY

To summarize our management approach, all patients with acute pancreatitis should have screening blood tests for C-reactive protein, α_2-macroglobulin and/or phospholipase A_2 levels. A case can be made for obtaining routine peritoneal lavage on hospital admission, as many patients with serious illness may not be identifiable clinically on presentation. In a prospective study, McMahon et al. found that severe pancreatitis was predicted correctly by diagnostic peritoneal lavage in 75% of cases, whereas clinical criteria were predictive in only 38% of severe attacks.[38] Early identification of pancreatic necrosis and prompt intervention is critical if long-term outcome is to be improved. A CT scan with vascular enhancement should be obtained in all patients with an Apache II score over 7 within 24 hours of admission. In the absence of signs of pancreatic or peripancreatic necrosis, supportive therapy alone is adequate. Sterile necrosis in a stable patient may also be treated expectantly. If hemodynamic or respiratory instability occur, then operative intervention is required, consisting of débridement of all necrotic tissue, lesser sac lavage, and open packing. An acute pseudocyst should be observed at least 6 weeks unless severe accompanying pancreatic necrosis and associated clinical deterioration demand early intervention. If signs of infection develop, CT or ultrasound-guided needle aspiration with Gram staining and culture should be performed. If a walled-off, well-loculated collection is the source, then either percutaneous or open drainage may be performed. All other infected collections should be treated with operative débridement and drainage.

Significant advances in our understanding of the pathophysiology and natural history of severe acute pancreatitis and the sequelae of pancreatic and peripancreatic necrosis, infected necrosis, pancreatic abscess, and pseudocyst have occurred. The precise definition of these clinical entities allows us to evaluate diagnostic tests, distinguish between treatment modalities, and assess more accurately their outcome. Utilizing this framework of knowledge, future studies comparing treatment methods may be compared more objectively, with ultimate improvement in patient care.

REFERENCES

1. Altemeier WA, Alexander JW. Pancreatic abscess. Arch Surg 87:96–105, 1963.
2. Aranha GV, Prinz RA, Greenlee HB. Pancreatic abscess: An unresolved surgical problem. Am J Surg 144:534–538, 1982.
3. Bank S, Wise L, Gersten M. Risk factors in acute pancreatitis. Am J Gastroenterol 78:637–690, 1983.
4. Barkin JS, Smith FR, Pereiras R, et al. Therapeutic percutaneous aspiration of pancreatic pseudocysts. Dig Dis Sci 26:585–586, 1981.
5. Becker JM, Pemberton JH, DiMagno EB, et al. Prognostic factors in pancreatic abscess. Surgery 96:455–461, 1984.
6. Beebe DS, Bubrick MP, Onstad GR, Hitchcock CR. Management of pancreatic pseudocysts. Surg Gynecol Obstet 159:562–564, 1984.
7. Beger HG, Bittner R, Block S, Buchler M. Bacterial contamination of pancreatic necrosis. Gastroenterology 91:433–438, 1986.
8. Beger HG, Krautzberger W, Bittner R, Block S, Buchler M. Results of surgical treatment of necrotizing pancreatitis. World J Surg 9:972–979, 1985.
9. Block S, Maier W, Buchler M, et al. Identification of pancreas necrosis in severe acute pancreatitis—Imaging procedures versus clinical staging. Abstract of the American Pancreatic Association. Dig Dis Sci 29:941, 1984.
10. Bolooki H, Jaffe B, Gliedman M. Pancreatic abscesses and lesser omental sac collections. Surg Gynecol Obstet 26:1301–1308, 1968.
11. Bradley EL. Cystoduodenostomy. Ann Surg 200:698–701, 1984.
12. Bradley EL, Clements JL, Gonzalez AC. The natural history of pancreatic pseudocysts: A unified concept of management. Am J Surg 137:135–141, 1979.
13. Bradley EL, Fulenwider T. Open treatment of pancreatic abscess. Surg Gynecol Obstet 159:509–513, 1984.
14. Buchler M, Malfertheiner P, Uhl W, Beger HG. Serum parameters to detect pancreatic necrosis. Abstract of the American Pancreatic Association. Dig Dis Sci 30:966, 1985.
15. Buggy BP, Nostrant TT. Lethal pancreatitis. Am J Gastroenterol 78:810–814, 1983.
16. Camer SJ, Tan EGC, Warren KW, Braasch JW. Pancreatic abscess. Am J Surg 129:426–431, 1975.
17. Crass RA, Meyer AA, Jeffrey RB, et al. Pancreatic abscess: Impact of computerized tomography on early diagnosis and surgery. Am J Surg 150:127–131, 1985.
18. Damman HG, Dreyer M, Walter TA, et al. Prognostic indications in acute pancreatitis: Clinical experience and limitations. In: Beger HG, Buchler M, eds. Acute Pancreatitis. Berlin, Springer-Verlag, 1987.
19. Davidson ED, Bradley EL. "Marsupialization" in treatment of pancreatic abscess. Surgery 89:252–256, 1981.
20. Federle MP, Jeffrey RB, Crass RA, Van Dalsem V. Computed tomography of pancreatic abscesses. AJR 136:879–882, 1981.
21. Frey CF. Hemorrhagic pancreatitis. Am J Surg 137:616–623, 1979.
22. Frey CF. Pancreatic pseudocyst—Operative strategy. Ann Surg 188:652–662, 1978.
23. Frey CF. A strategy for the surgical management of gallstone pancreatitis. In: Beger HG, Buchler M, eds. Acute Pancreatitis. Berlin, Springer-Verlag, 1987, pp 242–251.
24. Frey CF, Lindenauer SM, Miller TA. Pancreatic abscess. Surg Gynecol Obstet 149:722–726, 1979.
25. Frey CF, Stanley JC, Eckhauser F. Hemorrhage. In: Bradley EF, ed. Complications of Pancreatitis. Philadelphia, WB Saunders, 1982, pp 96–123.
26. Gebhardt C, Gall FP. Importance of peritoneal irrigation after surgical treatment of hemorrhagic, necrotizing pancreatitis. World J Surg 5:379–385, 1981.

27. Gerzof SG, Banks PA, Spechler SJ, et al. Role of guided percutaneous aspiration in early diagnosis of pancreatic sepsis. Abstract of the American Pancreatic Association. Dig Dis Sci 29:950, 1984.
28. Gerzof SG, Johnson WC, Robbins AH, et al. Percutaneous drainage of infected pancreatic pseudocysts. Arch Surg 119:888–893, 1984.
29. Hiatt JR, Fink AS, King W. Pitt HA. Percutaneous aspiration of peripancreatic fluid collections: A safe and effective diagnostic technique. Abstract of the American Pancreatic Association. Dig Dis Sci 30:974, 1985.
30. Holden JL, Berne TV, Rosoff L. Pancreatic abscess following acute pancreatitis. Arch Surg 111:858–861, 1976.
31. Imrie CW. Observations in acute pancreatitis. Br J Surg 61:539–544, 1974.
32. Kivisaari I, Somer K, Standertskjold-Nordenstam CG, et al. Early detection of acute fulminant pancreatitis by contrast-enhanced computed tomography. Scand J Gastroenterol 18:39–41, 1983.
33. Kloppel G, Dreyer T, Kern HF, Adler G. Human acute pancreatitis: Its pathogenesis in the light of immunocytochemical and ultrastructural findings in acinar cells. Virchows Arch Pathol Anat 409:791–803, 1986.
34. Knol JA, Eckhauser FE, Strodel WE. Surgical treatment of necrotizing pancreatitis by marsupialization. Am Surg 50:324–338, 1984.
35. Leger L, Chiche B, Louvel A. Pancreatic necrosis and acute pancreatitis. World J Surg 5:315–317, 1981.
36. Louie S, McGahan JP, Frey CF, Cross CE. Pancreatic pleuropericardial effusions: Fistulous tracts demonstrated by computed tomography. Arch Intern Med 145:1231–1234, 1985.
37. McMahon MJ, Bowen M, Mayer AD, Cooper EH. Relation of alpha-2-macroglobulin and other antiproteases to the clinical features of acute pancreatitis. Am J Surg 147:164–170, 1984.
38. McMahon MJ, Pickford IR, Playforth MJ. Early prediction of severity of acute pancreatitis using peritoneal lavage. Acta Chir Scand 146:171–175, 1980.
39. McMahon MJ, Playforth MJ, Pickford IR. A comparative study of methods for the prediction of severity of acute pancreatitis. Br J Surg 67:22–25, 1980.
40. Miller TA, Lindenauer SM, Frey CF, Stanley JC. Pancreatic abscess. Arch Surg 108:545–551, 1974.
41. Pemberton JH, Becker JM, Dozois RR, et al. Controlled open lesser sac drainage for pancreatic abscess. Ann Surg 203:600–604, 1986.
42. Ranson JHC, Rifkind KM, Roses DF, et al. Prognostic signs and the role of operative management in acute pancreatitis. Surg Gynecol Obstet 139:69–81, 1974.
43. Ranson JHC. Acute pancreatitis: Pathogenic outcome and treatment. Clin Gastroenterol 13:843–862, 1984.
44. Rotman N, Bonnet F, Larde D, Fagniez PL. Computerized tomography in the evaluation of the late complications of acute pancreatitis. Am J Surg 152:286–289, 1986.
45. Schein M, Saddia R, Decker G. Colonic necrosis in acute pancreatitis. Dis Colon Rectum 28:948–950, 1985.
46. Schroder T, Kivilaakso E, Kinnunen PKJ, Lempinen M. Serum phospholipase A_2 in human acute pancreatitis. Scand J Gastroenterol 15:633–636, 1980.
47. Shi ECP, Yeo BW, Ham JM. Pancreatic abscesses. Br J Surg 71:689–691, 1984.
48. Silverstein W, Isikoff MB, Hill MC, Barkin J. Diagnostic imaging of acute pancreatitis: Prospective study using CT and sonography. AJR 137:497–502, 1981.
49. Sostre CF, Flournoy JG, Bova JG, Goldstein HM, Schenker S. Pancreatic phlegmon. Dig Dis Sci 30:918–927, 1985.
50. Stanley JC, Frey CF, Miller TA. Major arterial hemorrhage: A complication of pseudocysts and chronic pancreatitis. Arch Surg 111:435–440, 1976.
51. Stanten R, Frey CF. Comprehensive review. Pancreatitis and pancreatic abscess. Arch Surg 126:1268–1275, 1990.
52. Warshaw AL. Inflammatory masses following acute pancreatitis. Surg Clin North Am 54:621–636, 1974.

53. Warshaw AL, Jin G. Improved survival in 45 patients with pancreatic abscess. Ann Surg 202:408–417, 1985.
54. Welch CE, Malt RA. Surgery of the stomach, duodenum, gallbladder, and bile ducts. N Engl J Med 316:999–1008, 1987.
55. Westheimer MD, Norris CS. Surgical management of necrotizing pancreatitis. Arch Surg 121:484–487, 1986.
56. Wetzner JM, Langevan SM, Robbins AH. Role of guided percutaneous aspiration in early diagnosis of pancreatic sepsis. Abstract of the American Pancreatic Association. Dig Dis Sci 29:950, 1984.
57. Williford ME, Foster WL, Halvorsen RA, Thompson WM. Pancreatic pseudocyst: Comparative evaluation by sonography and computed tomography. AJR 140:53–57, 1983.

CHAPTER

13

IMAGING OF PANCREATIC MASSES

Emil J. Balthazar and Martin Hirsch

EDITORIAL COMMENTS (Chapters 13 and 14)

The authors give a useful guideline regarding the value of sonography and CT scanning in pancreatic masses. It is evident that present-day ultrasonography is very dependent on the examiner. It is highly accurate in tumors of the head, of the pancreas and relatively poor in evaluating lesions of the body and tail. CT scanning has an accuracy in the region of 90%, but there are somewhat conflicting reports with regard to the accuracy of CT in staging pancreatic carcinoma for resectability, the predictive value for unresectability being almost double that for resectability—neither seem to have affected survival from cancer of the pancreas. Transendoscopic and intraoperative sonography may eventually detect lesions less than 2 cm, the lower limit for detection of lesions at the moment, especially apudomas and small insulinomas.

The authors do not discuss the importance of repeating CT scanning if the first scan is normal. The rapidity of growth of pancreatic carcinoma can obviously be remarkable, as evidenced by two recent cases of the editors in which investigation for abdominal pain in two middle-aged men resulted in entirely negative CT scans. One month later repeat CT scans showed obvious pancreatic masses and even hepatic metastases. It is important to remember that one may have to repeat expensive investigations at relatively short intervals in patients with persistent symptoms.

Angiography is advocated by the authors as an aid in equivocal cases of suspected carcinoma and to assist in the determination of resectability, an area in which CT scanning is less than ideal. We believe it is also helpful to the surgeon in demonstrating abnormal anatomic variation in blood supply, for example, right hepatic artery arising from the superior mesenteric; left hepatic artery arising from the left gastric.

In addition to providing imaging information and therapeutic access, endoscopy permits direct inspection of the stomach and duodenum, which may be involved by the pancreatic mass. Visualization and biopsy of duodenal wall and periampullary lesions is useful in selecting and planning surgical procedures. A lesion suspected of being malignant on a conventional upper GI contrast study or CT scan may in fact reveal itself as a papillary adenoma, an aberrant pancreas, or a pseudocyst.

CONTROVERSY

Sonography, CT scanning, and ERCP have unquestionably revolutionized the diagnosis follow-up of benign and malignant pancreatic masses. However, there are still many problems with the techniques, some authors claiming that a blinded evaluation of scans shows difference of opinion in almost 50%. ERCP undoubtedly poses a risk to the patient and cannot always be relied on to differentiate benign from malignant disease. The current status of the problems and resolutions are approached in this chapter.

Over the last decade, imaging of the pancreas has dramatically improved. The advent of high-resolution computed tomography (CT) and ultrasonography has enabled us to examine the gland directly. Today these modalities are the primary means of radiographic examination of the pancreas. Other modalities including upper gastrointestinal series (UGI), angiography, percutaneous transhepatic cholangiography (PTC), endoscopic retrograde cholangiopancreatography (ERCP), and transhepatic venous sampling are sometimes used to obtain additional information. Each has different indications and varying sensitivities and pitfalls.

The goals of imaging pancreatic masses include (1) rapid and accurate diagnosis with minimal morbidity and cost, (2) when indicated, confirmation of the radiologic diagnosis via fine needle aspiration biopsy under imaging guidance, (3) evaluation of the extent of disease and determination of resectability, and (4) patient management mainly by palliation, that is, biliary drainage and splanchnic nerve block.

The UGI barium examination is readily available; it is noninvasive and relatively inexpensive. It has, however, a limited role in the evaluation of suspected pancreatic masses because it is neither sensitive nor specific (Fig. 13-1). Only large tumors, compressing and displacing the adjacent duodenal loop and/or stomach, may be visualized, while the majority of pancreatic lesions are not seen. Unless there is evidence of bowel wall invasion, the gastrointestinal examination can not differentiate a cystic from a solid or a benign from a malignant mass. In addition, to establish the origin of the mass, whether pancreatic or peripancreatic, other imaging modalities are required.

Ultrasonography is generally used today as the initial examination in jaundiced patients and in patients with palpable upper abdominal masses. It is a noninvasive and fast examination, has no ionizing radiation, and allows imaging of the pancreas in multiple planes. The success of the examination is, however, greatly dependent on the skill of the operator. In addition, in obese individuals or when bowel gas overlies the pancreatic region, visualization of the gland is impaired. In a consecutive series of 500 patients, Arger et al. were able to see the head of the pancreas in 77%, while the tail of the pancreas was seen in only 37% of cases.[1] Other reports have stressed that incomplete or inadequate sonographic evaluation of the pancreas occurs in 13% to 38% of examinations.[16,21] Despite these limitations, ultrasonography is very useful as a preliminary screening test with its sensitivity and accuracy heavily dependent on the quality of the examina-

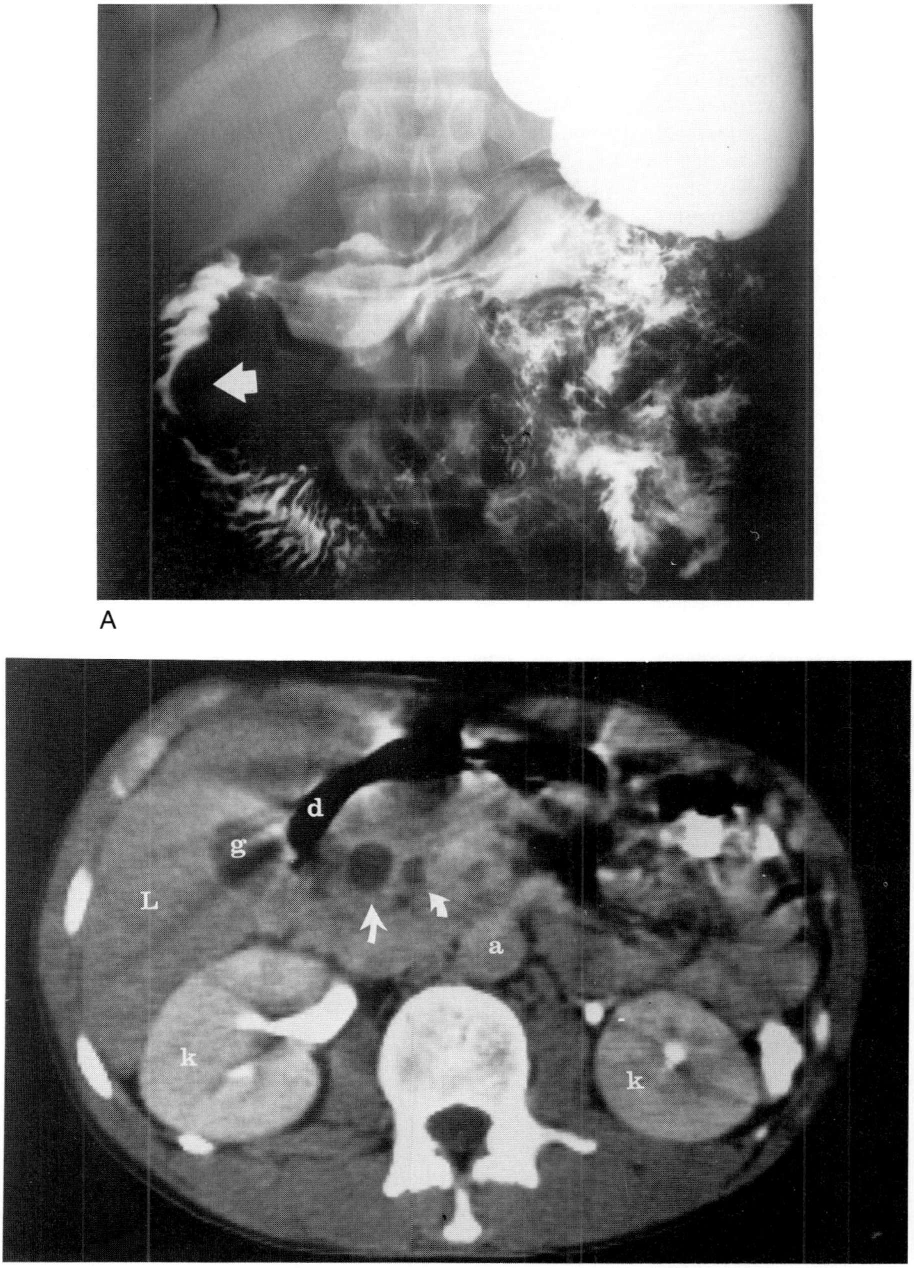

Figure 13-1. Chronic pancreatitis compressing the medial aspect of the second duodenal segment. (A) Upper GI examination shows the extrinsic compression (arrow) produced by an undetermined pancreatic mass. (B) CT examination shows a solid mass in the head of the pancreas with small cystic fluid collections (arrows) consistent with chronic pancreatitis. L = liver, d = duodenum, k = kidney, a = aorta, g = gallbladder.

tion. In most instances, valuable information regarding the liver, biliary tract, size of the pancreatic gland, and presence of lymphadenopathy can be obtained. In Lawson's series, ultrasonography was 87% accurate in differentiating the normal from the abnormal pancreas.[17]

More than any other imaging modality, CT has become the primary tool for evaluating the pancreas. Technically adequate examinations performed on fourth-generation scanners, using intravenous bolus administration of contrast material and rapid sequence imaging, result in a satisfactory visualization of the pancreas in virtually all patients. Depending on the location and density of the lesion, masses as small as 2 cm are seen. The CT diagnosis is based on the demonstration of a focal mass, its imaging characteristics (shape, contour, density), and the presence of secondary findings such as common duct and/or pancreatic duct dilatation, lymphadenopathy, vascular invasion, and liver metastasis. A history of allergic reaction, absence of retroperitoneal fat in cachectic individuals, or lack of cooperation with body or respiratory motion are limiting factors. Compared with the other imaging modalities, CT is by far the most sensitive and accurate in evaluating the pancreas.

With the recent increasing use of sonography and CT to diagnose pancreatic tumors and determine resectability, the role of angiography has greatly diminished. The procedure has a very low morbidity, but it is nevertheless invasive. Its primary indication remains in evaluation of patients with pancreatic neoplasms who appear to be resectable by CT criteria. Angiography provides a vascular roadmap for the surgeon and may document involvement of vessels missed by CT examination. It is also used in localizing small functioning islet cell tumors, sometimes in conjunction with percutaneous transhepatic venous sampling. Lastly, angiography has still a significant role in the diagnosis, evaluation, and treatment of pseudoaneurysms and bleeding pancreatic pseudocysts that develop as sequelae of pancreatitis.

Today PTC and ERCP are less commonly used in patients with pancreatic masses that are already documented by CT. These procedures, however, continue to play a very important role when noninvasive modalities are not diagnostic or equivocal. The level and cause of the biliary and/or pancreatic duct obstruction can be accurately assessed by these techniques. Both procedures are valuable, and both are greatly dependent on the skill and experience of the examiner. In our institution PTC is preferred in patients with intrahepatic biliary tract dilatation or in patients presenting clinically with jaundice and associated acute pancreatitis. It has a low morbidity, and successful visualization of the bile ducts can be accomplished in 80% to 95% of patients.[9] PTC is contraindicated in patients with ascites and/or elevated prothrombin time. When visualization of the pancreatic duct is necessary to establish the diagnosis or when the intrahepatic ducts are not distended, ERCP becomes the method of choice. The exact sensitivity of ultrasound still has to be evaluated.

PANCREATIC PSEUDOCYST

Pseudocysts are encapsulated pancreatic fluid collections that develop usually as a complication of pancreatitis. The wall of the cyst is formed by a fibrous capsule,

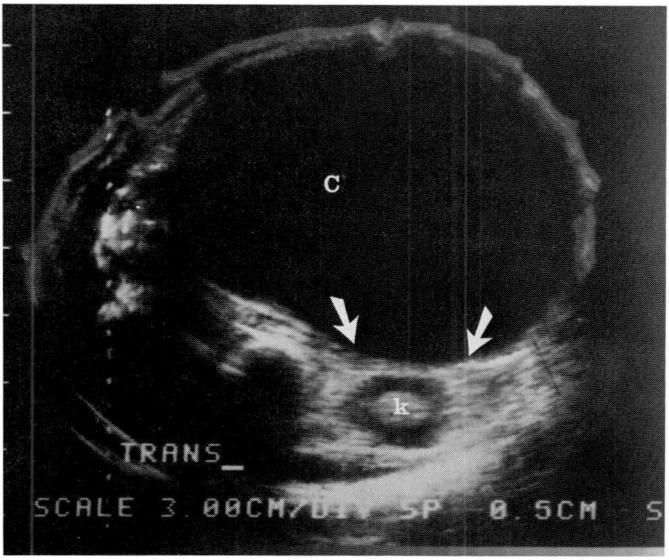

A

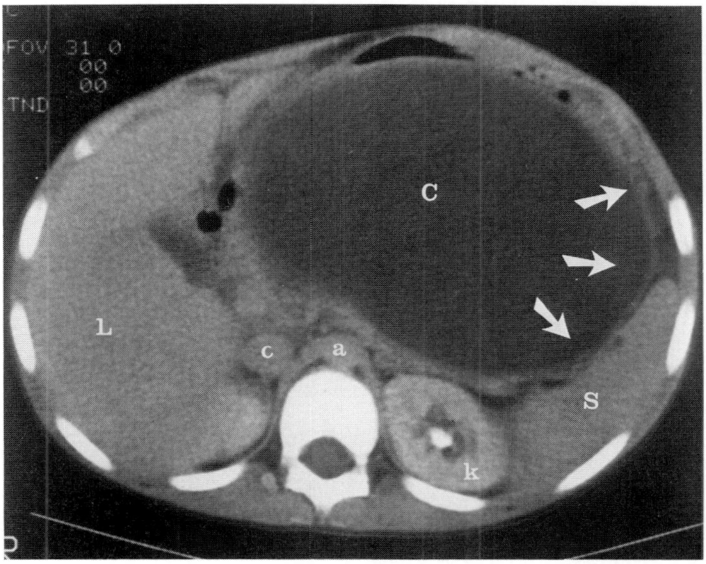

B

Figure 13-2. Large pancreatic pseudocyst secondary to pancreatitis. (A) Sonography shows a sonolucent large and well-encapsulated cystic structure. Note the strong posterior acoustic enhancement indicative of a fluid filled cyst (arrows). (B) CT at the same level shows the low-density fluid-filled pseudocyst and its well-defined peripheral capsule (arrows). C = cyst, k = kidney, L = liver, S = spleen, a = aorta, c = inferior vena cava.

and the absence of the epithelial lining differentiates a pseudocyst from a congenital pancreatic cyst.[3]

Pseudocysts vary in size from very small insignificant structures to very large cystic masses located usually in the peripancreatic space. They may be located in the gland, but not infrequently, they dissect fascial planes and occur at a distance in the abdomen, or even mediastinum. Their clinical significance is related to the size, the location, and the development of complications such as intraperitoneal rupture, infection, and bleeding.

Diagnosis

Ultrasonography can identify pseudocysts as small as 3 cm in 96% of patients.[8,10,18,19,22] They appear as isolated or multiple sonolucent, sharply marginated masses with strong posterior acoustic enhancement (Figs. 13-2 and 13-3). Internal septations are rarely seen. On CT, pseudocysts appear as round or oval cystic structures (Fig. 13-1B), marginated by a smooth, thin and well-defined capsule (Figs. 13-2 and 13-3). Their fluid contents (−5 to +20 Hounsfield units [HU]), benign cystic appearance, and location are very characteristic. They rarely calcify. The development of an infected pseudocyst or abscess is usually suspected on clinical grounds. In the proper clinical setting, the presence of internal echoes on ultrasonography or slightly higher density numbers on CT (+30

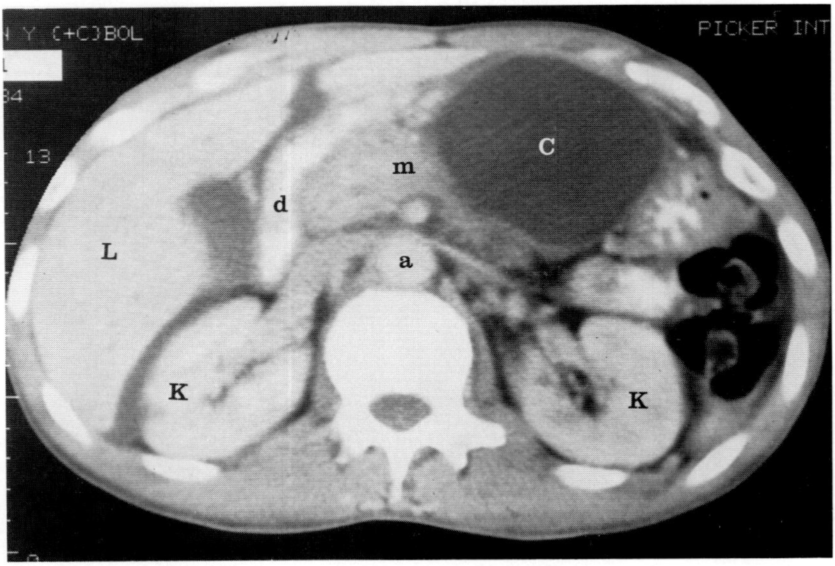

Figure 13-3. Pancreatic pseudocyst secondary to carcinoma of the pancreas. A well-defined encapsulated fluid collection is seen in the body and tail of the pancreas. A pancreatic mass is located anterior to the superior mesenteric artery. C = pseudocyst, m = mass in pancreas, K = kidney, d = duodenum, L = liver, a = aorta.

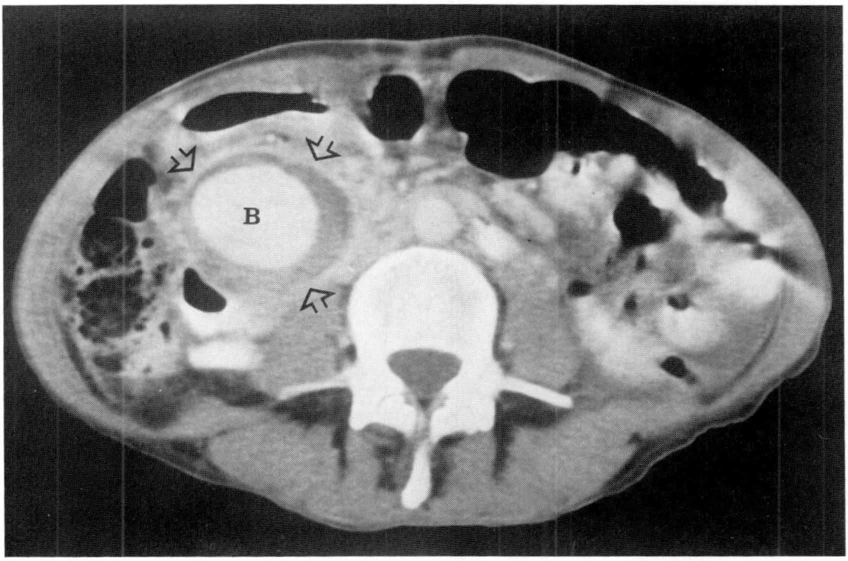

A

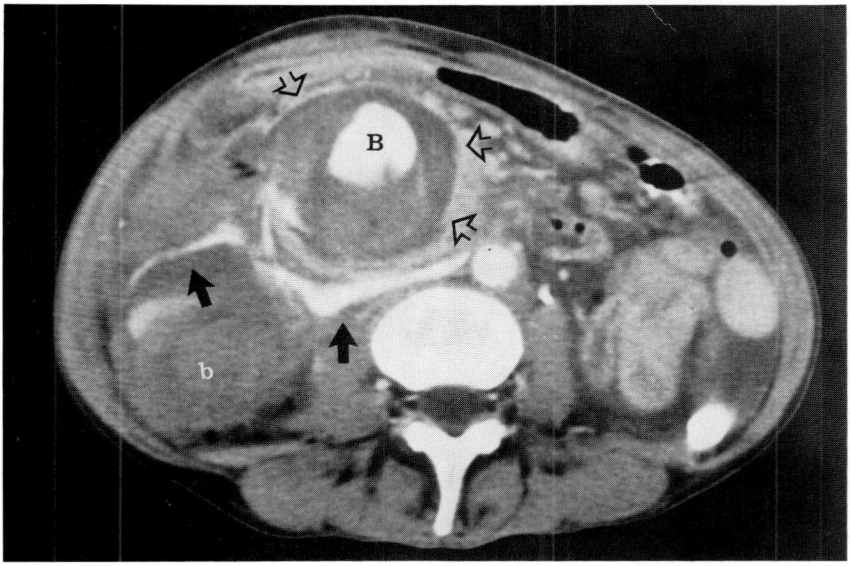

B

Figure 13-4. Bleeding pancreatic pseudocyst. (A) Initial CT examination reveals a high-density pseudocyst (open arrows) and contrast material extravasation indicative of intracystic bleeding (B). (B) Follow-up CT examination 24 hours later shows similar findings and in addition, evidence of cyst rupture with free spill of contrast material in peritoneal cavity (solid arrows), and large amounts of intraperitoneal blood (b) (*Figure continues.*)

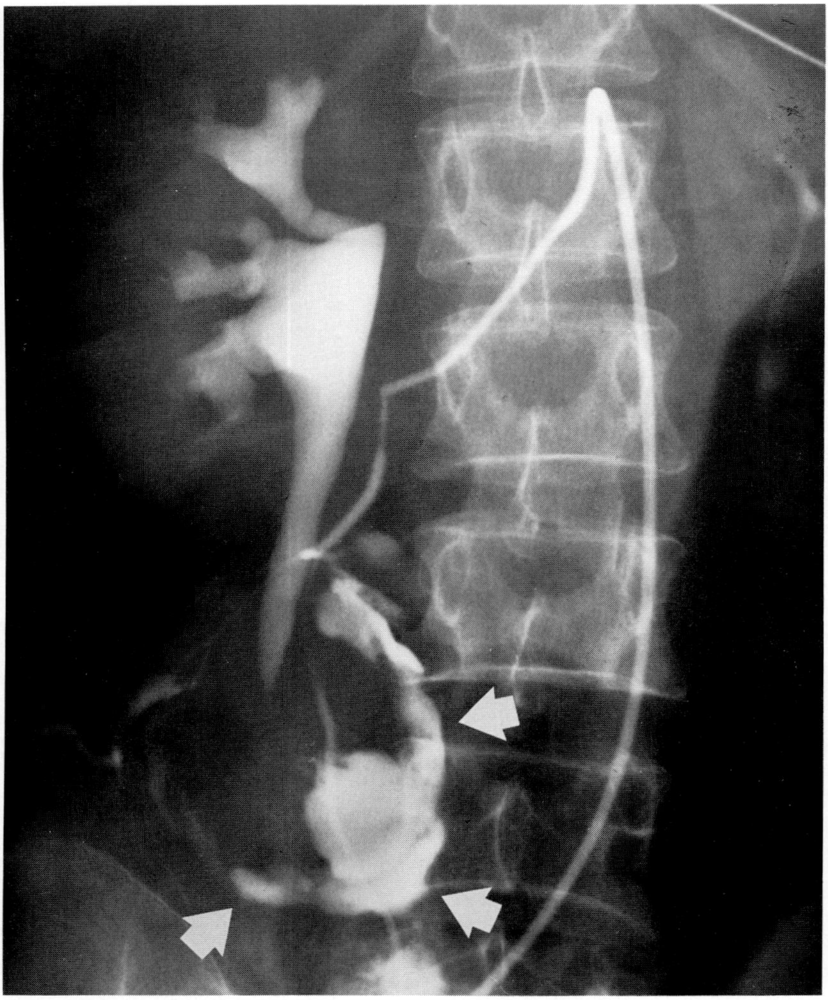

C

Figure 13-4 (*continued*). (C) Selective angiography of the pancreatic-duodenal artery documents the bleeding pseudocyst (arrows). Embolization of this vessel was immediately performed, and the bleeding stopped.

to +40 HU) should be considered suspicious. The presence of bubbles of gas in the cyst is diagnostic of an abscess; however, this sign is present in only about 20% of pancreatic abscesses.[23,26]

High-density CT numbers (+50 to +100 HU) in a pseudocyst are diagnostic of hemorrhage or pseudoaneurysm (Fig. 13-4). In these cases angiography is usually performed, often followed by selective embolization of the bleeding vessel (Fig. 13-4).

PANCREATIC CARCINOMA

Pancreatic ductal adenocarcinoma is one of the most common malignancies, and in the United States it is the fourth leading cause of tumor death in males. It accounts for 75% of neoplasms arising in the pancreas.[5,6] In a recent series of 159 cases, 62% of tumors were found in the pancreatic head, 26% in the body, and 12% in the tail.[14] Others series have reported similar figures.[7] Despite the recent advances in diagnostic imaging, the prognosis of pancreatic carcinoma remains poor. This is because at the time of the clinical presentation and radiologic diagnosis, most lesions are unresectable or show pathologic evidence of local spread or distant metastases.

Diagnosis

Depending on the size of the mass and quality of the examination, ultrasonography has a sensitivity and specificity in detecting pancreatic carcinoma reported as high as 80% to 90%.[1,17] The tumor appears usually as a hypoechoic, focal, or diffuse mass changing the contour and the configuration of the gland. Associated findings of pancreatic and/or common duct dilatation are often seen, and liver metastases have been reported in up to 47% of these patients.[12] Ultrasonography has a sensitivity in detecting liver metastases of about 75%;[24] it is useful in establishing the level of the biliary obstruction and sometimes in assessing vascular invasion and splenic vein obstruction.

Computed tomography has become the modality of choice in the diagnosis and evaluation of patients with pancreatic carcinoma. Fast scanners and good technique permit excellent visualization of the gland in almost 100% of patients and lead to detection rates of pancreatic carcinoma of over 90%.[13] In Freeny's series, a correct CT diagnosis was made in 91.4%, with 7.5% false-positive and 1% false-negative diagnoses. To avoid the false-positive interpretation, percutaneous needle aspiration biopsy of the mass for tissue confirmation can be performed.

The CT findings in a series of 100 consecutive patients with pancreatic carcinoma are shown in Table 13-1.[28] Visualization of a focal mass is the most common and the most reliable radiographic finding (Fig. 13-5). On contrast-enhanced images (bolus technique), pancreatic carcinoma appears as a hypodense, ill-defined mass, having a different texture than the rest of the gland (Fig. 13-6). Focal enlargement, asymmetry, and contour abnormalities related to the tumor are usually seen. When the lesion is located in the pancreatic head, there is evidence of common duct obstruction, dilatation of the gallbladder (Courvoisier gallbladder), and, often, atrophy of the body and tail of the pancreas with dilatation of the

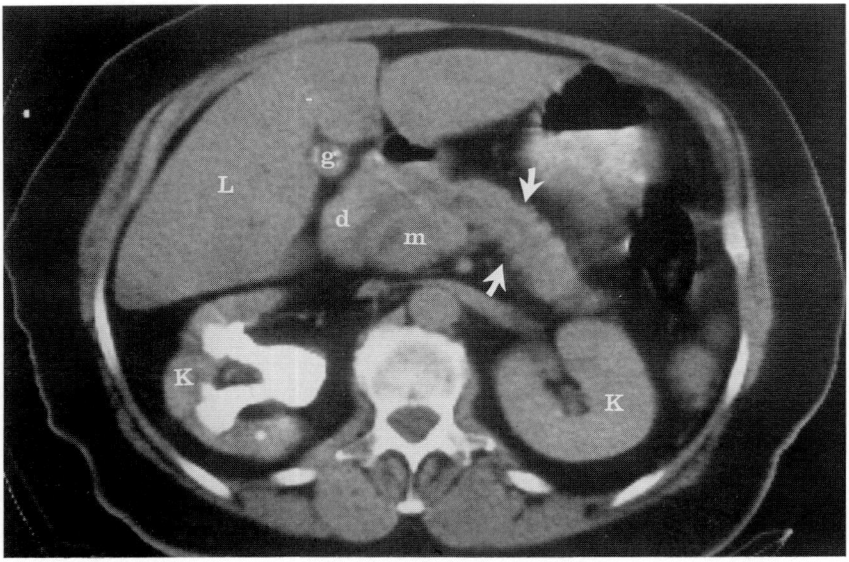

A

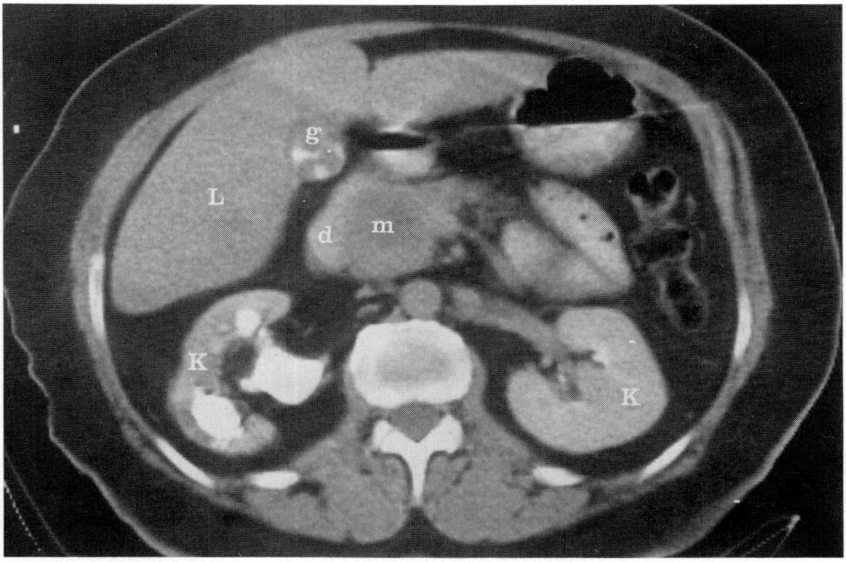

B

Figure 13-5. Carcinoma presenting as a focal mass in the head of the pancreas. (A) Normal pancreatic body and tail (arrows). Mass in head of pancreas (m) has a different texture and density compared with the normal gland. (B) Slightly lobulated tumor mass in the head of the pancreas (m). (*Figure continues.*)

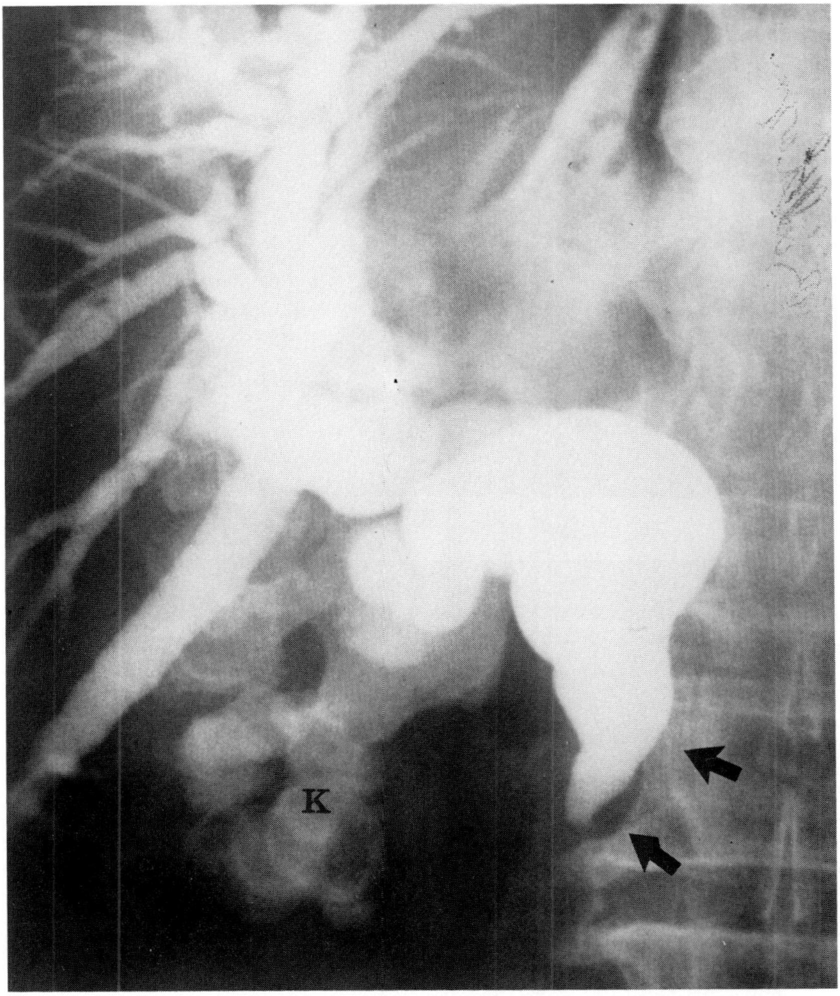

C

Figure 13-5 (*continued*). (C) Transhepatic cholangiogram shows massive dilatation of the bile ducts with total obstruction (arrows). Patient has a large staghorn calculus in the right kidney and gallstones. d = duodenum, L = liver, K = kidney, g = gallbladder.

pancreatic duct (Fig. 13-7). Diffuse involvement of the entire gland occurs in less than 5% of cases[28] (Fig. 13-8). Focal inflammatory masses that mimic the CT appearance of pancreatic carcinoma may be seen occasionally in patients with chronic pancreatitis (Fig. 13-1). In these patients ERCP examination and percutaneous needle biopsy help in the differential diagnosis.

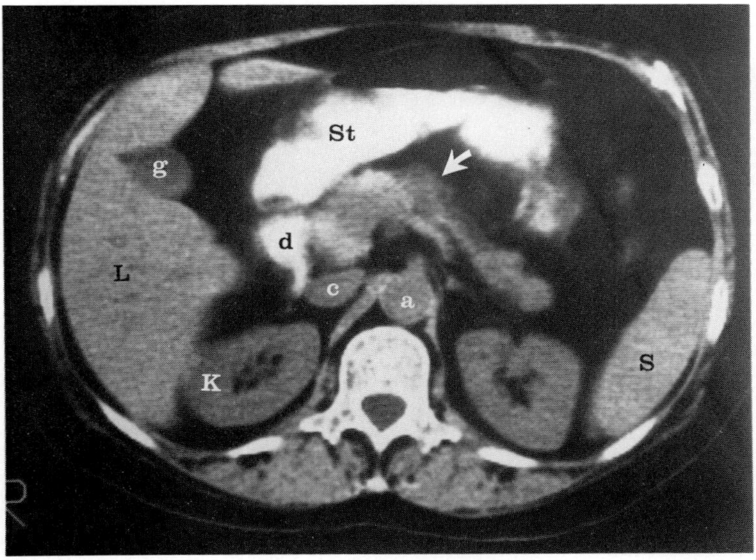

A

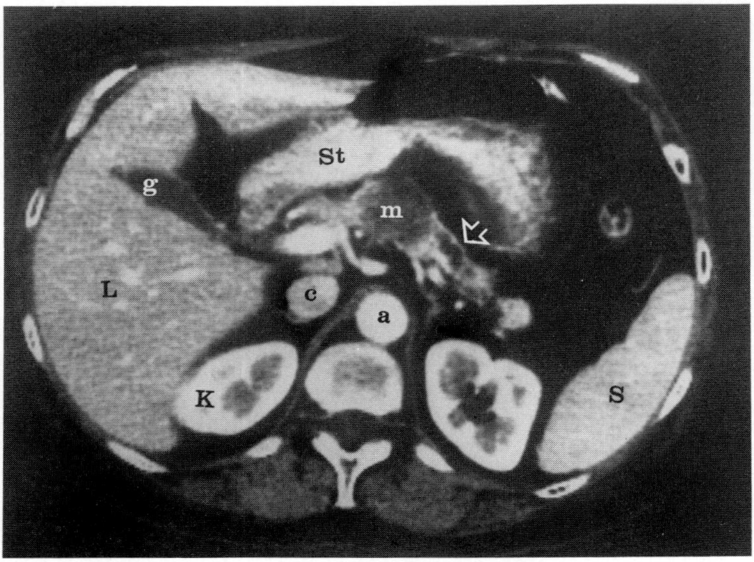

B

Figure 13-6. Bolus technique for diagnosis of pancreatic adenocarcinoma. (A) Initial CT performed without IV contrast material shows a slightly lobulated pancreatic body (arrow). Tumor is not well seen. (B) After rapid administration of IV contrast material, tumor mass of low attenuation measuring 3 cm in diameter is clearly visualized in the pancreatic body (m). Note distension of the proximal pancreatic duct (open arrow). L = liver, a = aorta, c = inferior vena cava, K = kidney, S = spleen, St = stomach, d = duodenum, g = gallbladder.

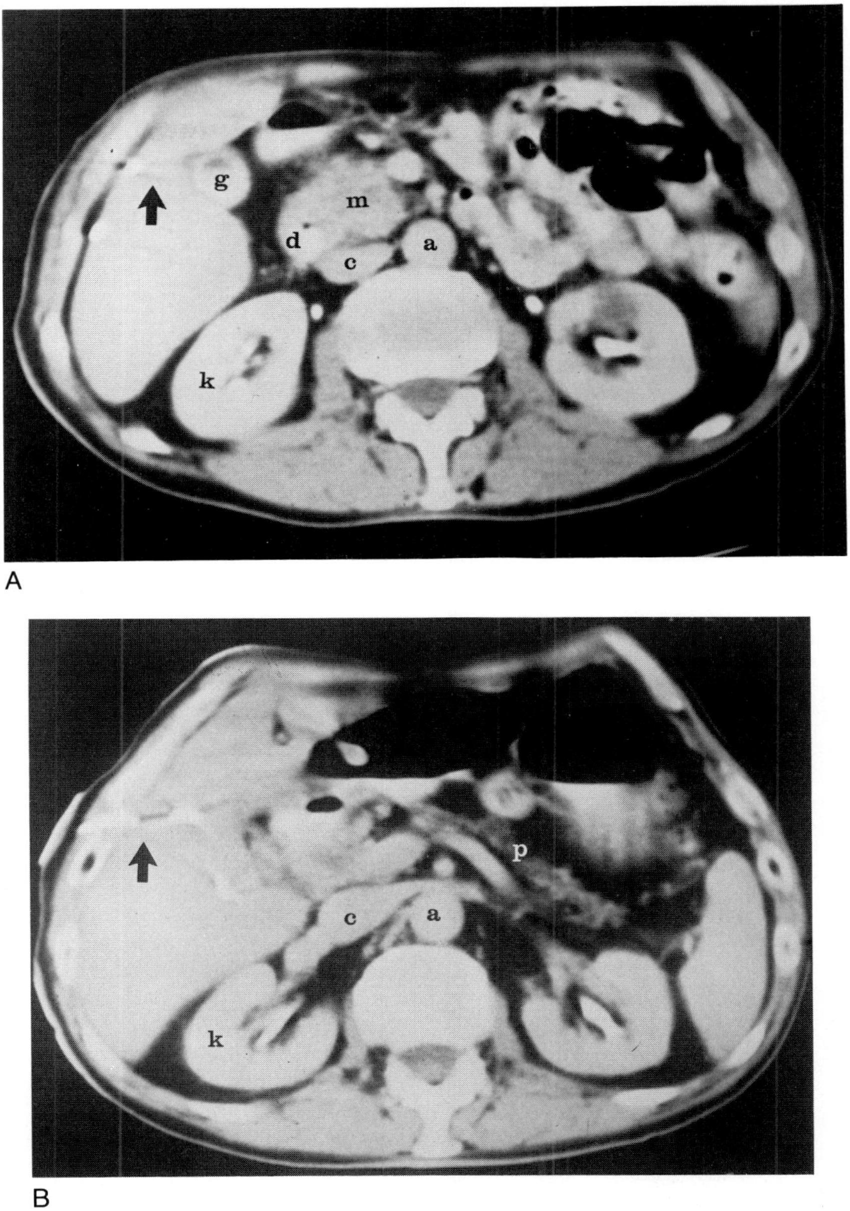

Figure 13-7. CT of carcinoma of the head of the pancreas. (A) Tumor mass (m) in the head of the pancreas compressing the duodenum (d). (B) Slightly cranial section shows atrophy of the body and tail of the pancreas (p). Patient has a draining percutaneous biliary catheter (arrow). a = aorta, c = vena cava, k = kidney, g = gallbladder.

TABLE 13-1. PANCREATIC CARCINOMA: CT CHARACTERISTICS OF 100 CASES*

	Frequency (%) (0 20 40 60 80 100)
Pancreatic mass	95
Low-density region within mass	75
Involvement of celiac or SMA	60
Dilated pancreatic duct	50
Dilated bile ducts	38
Hepatic metastases	30
Atrophy of tail of pancreas	20
Regional lymphadenopathy	15
Dilated collateral veins	12
Ascites	10
Thickened renal (Gerota's) fascia	5
Calcification in pancreas	2

* From Ward et al.[28]

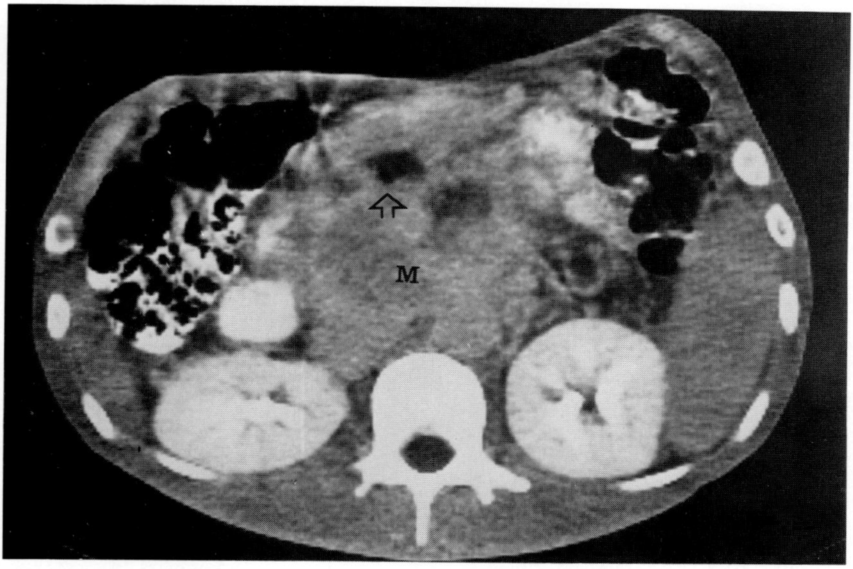

Figure 13-8. Massive carcinoma of the pancreas involving the entire gland and the retroperitoneal structures (M). Note obstruction of the dilated pancreatic duct (arrow).

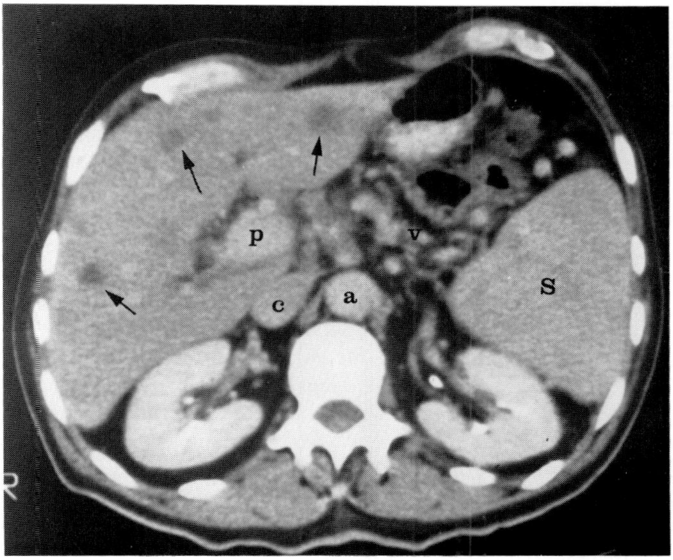

A

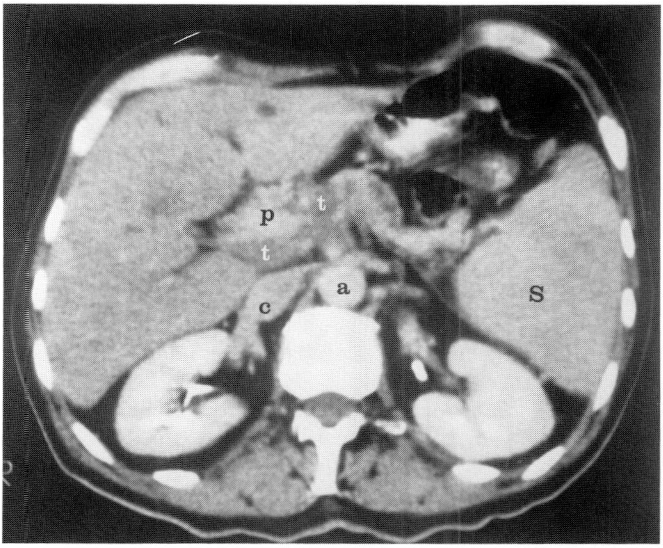

B

Figure 13-9. Unresectable carcinoma of the pancreas with CT evidence of metastatic disease. (A) Liver metastases (arrows), splenomegaly (S), and collateral veins (V) indicative of splenic vein obstruction. (B) Lower-density tumor around SMA and portal vein infiltrating the porta hepatis (t). a = aorta, c = vena cava, p = portal vein.

CT Staging

Pancreatic carcinoma is considered resectable if an isolated pancreatic mass with or without pancreatic or bile duct dilatation is seen. Patients are judged to have unresectable lesions if one or more of the following findings are demonstrated: local tumor extension outside the gland, contiguous organ invasion, vascular involvement, nodal and/or liver metastases, and ascites (Figs. 13-8 and 13-9). Based on these criteria, Freeny et al. concluded that in all patients in their series, CT correctly judged unresectability and did not overstage lesions.[14] However, while the positive predictive value for unresectable tumor was 100%, the negative predictive value of resectable tumor was only 55%, reflecting the limitation of CT imaging in the detection of small nodal metastases, microscopic local tumor extension, and small hepatic metastases. In assessing vascular involvement, CT compares favorably with angiography.[14] Angiography, however, may show arterial encasement and venous involvement sometimes missed by CT. For this reason it is still used in the preoperative assessment of these patients.

It should be stressed that the recent advances in radiologic detection and evaluation of patients with pancreatic cancer have had no impact on survival. In the series of Freeny et al., the average survival following resection was 14 months, following palliation (biliary or GI bypass) it was 8 months, and the average survival without any treatment was 5 months.[14] No patient survived 5 years.

CYSTIC NEOPLASMS OF THE PANCREAS

These are uncommon lesions consisting of about 1% of primary pancreatic tumors and about 10% to 15% of pancreatic cysts.[11] Their morphologic and histologic features distinguish them from benign simple cysts or pseudocysts and permit their classification into two distinct types: (1) serous cystadenoma and (2) mucinous cystadenoma and cystadenocarcinoma. Serous cystadenoma (microcystic or glycogen rich-cystadenoma) (Fig. 13-10) is composed of a multitude of small cysts in a honeycomb configuration, containing a serous fluid. The epithelial cells stain periodic acid–Schiff positive for glycogen. This tumor is benign, slow-growing, and without known endocrine function or malignant potential. Mucinous cystadenoma (macrocystic cystadenoma) is an encapsulated tumor composed usually of larger cystic cavities having thick walls and numerous papillary excrescences. The cysts contain mucin that may at times be hemorrhagic. These tumors may be benign but occasionally exhibit malignant features (cystadenocarcinoma), with rapid growth, local invasion, and distant metastases. Cystic pancreatic tumors are more commonly located in the body and tail of the gland.[4] When found in symptomatic individuals, they are usually large but have a much better prognosis than ductal adenocarcinoma.

Diagnosis

The radiologic diagnosis is based on the visualization of a sharply circumscribed and encapsulated tumor containing septations and multiple cystic cavities

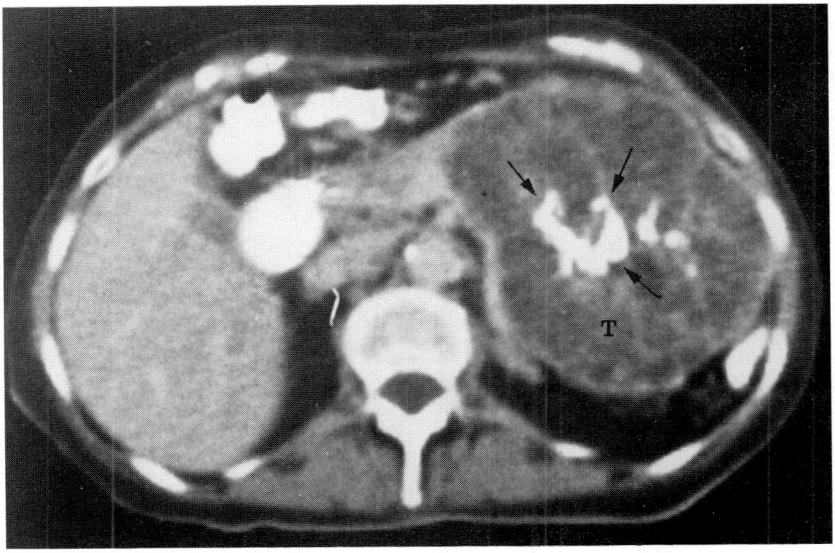

A

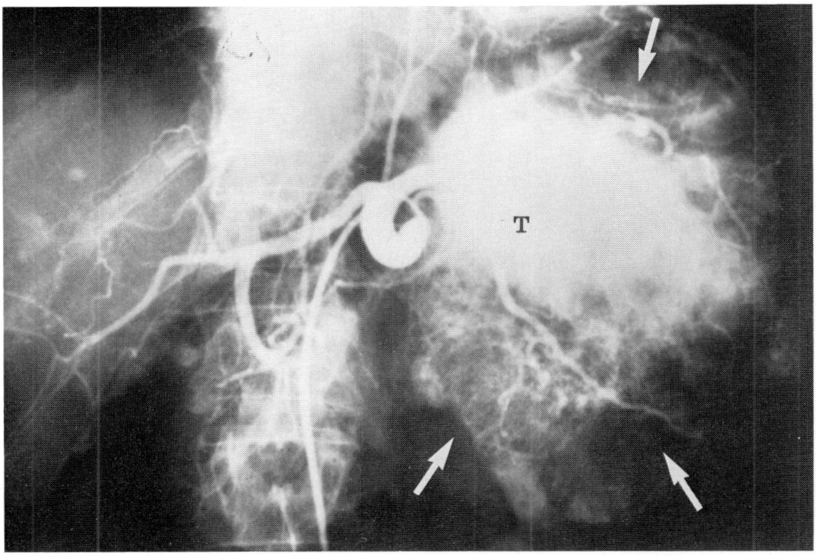

B

Figure 13-10. Serous cystadenoma of the tail of the pancreas. (A) CT shows a large encapsulated tumor (T) composed of multiple small, cystic structures and central calcifications (arrows). (B) Angiogram reveals a hypervascular tumor (T) with intense vascular blush (arrows).

filled with fluid. On sonography the cysts appear as mixed hypoechoic and echogenic structures. Few septations and occasionally larger cystic spaces may be seen, and calcifications are sometimes found either centrally or peripherally. On CT (Fig. 13-10), the tumor appears as a well-encapsulated cystic mass, containing multiple different-size cystic spaces. When a single dominant cyst is present, differentiation from a pseudocyst becomes difficult. The presence of central calcification having a stellate pattern and multiple tiny cysts suggests a benign serous cystadenoma, while peripheral calcifications and larger cysts are more commonly seen in mucinous cystadenoma. This differentiation, however, is often impossible to make radiographically, and patients need tissue confirmation or surgical resections. On angiography most of these tumors show irregular tumor vessels, hypervascularity (75%–85%), and arteriovenous shunting (40%).[4,11] The demonstration of local invasion or distal metastases indicates malignancy; however, these features are seldom seen in these patients.

Islet Cell Tumors

Pancreatic islet cell tumors belong to a group of endocrine neoplasms called apudomas (amine precursor uptake and decarboxylation). They occur either as solitary lesions or in association with other endocrine tumors. Based on the clinical presentation and laboratory findings, they are divided into functioning (80%) or nonfunctioning islet cell tumors. Radiologic studies alone can not differentiate these tumors, and the primary role of imaging modalities is in the finding, localization, and staging of these lesions.

Diagnosis

Nonfunctioning islet cell tumors tend to be larger at the time of the diagnosis but otherwise show similar imaging characteristics. The sensitivity of imaging modalities depends mainly on the size of the tumor and has been reported to be around 60% to 70%.[15] Tumors larger than 2 cm are commonly detected, while smaller tumors are only occasionally seen (Fig. 13-11). Sonography is less sensitive than CT but has been recently reported to yield excellent results in the intraoperative localization of small pancreatic insulinomas.[15] On CT, islet cell tumors present as homogeneous soft tissue masses, well circumscribed, having a different texture compared with the adjacent normal pancreatic parenchyma (Fig. 13-11). They can be easily differentiated from ductal cell adenocarcinoma because islet cell tumors show high enhancement with the bolus technique, reflecting their hypervascular nature (Fig. 13-12). This finding together with a dense and persistent blush and prominent draining veins on angiography are characteristic features (Fig. 13-13). On angiography or rapid sequence bolus CT, lesions as small as 5 mm have been diagnosed.[25] The sensitivity in detecting insulinomas is higher than in gastrinomas, in which multiple small tumors may be present in the pancreatic gland or duodenum. Radiographic staging of these tumors is based on visual-

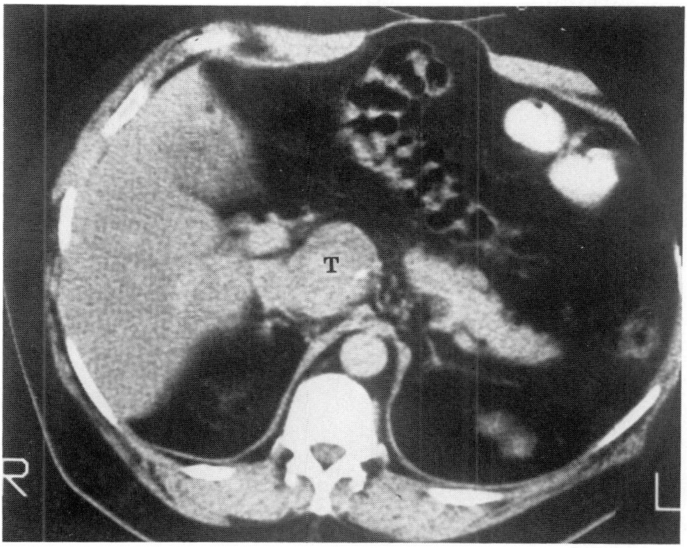

Figure 13-11. Nonfunctioning islet cell tumor of the head of the pancreas. CT shows a sharply defined mass of high attenuation (T).

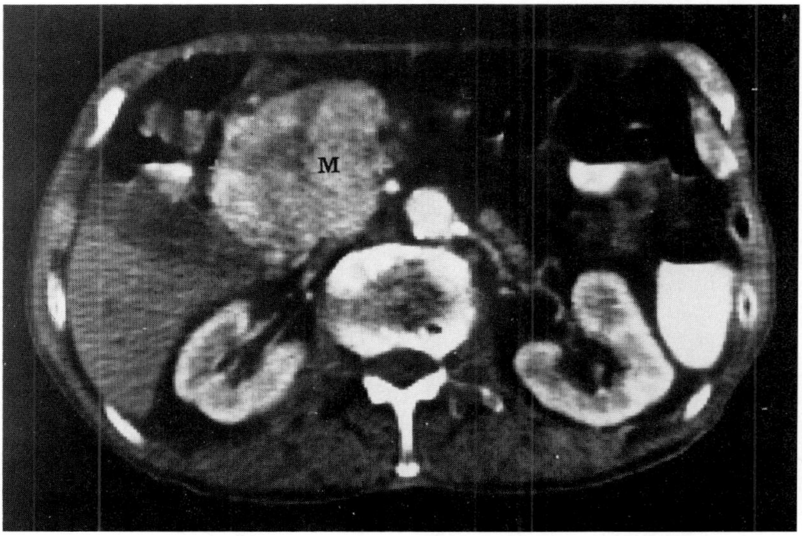

Figure 13-12. Nonfunctioning islet cell tumor diagnosed by CT with bolus technique. Pancreatic mass (M) is very dense, indicating a vascular tumor. This appearance is not compatible with pancreatic adenocarcinoma.

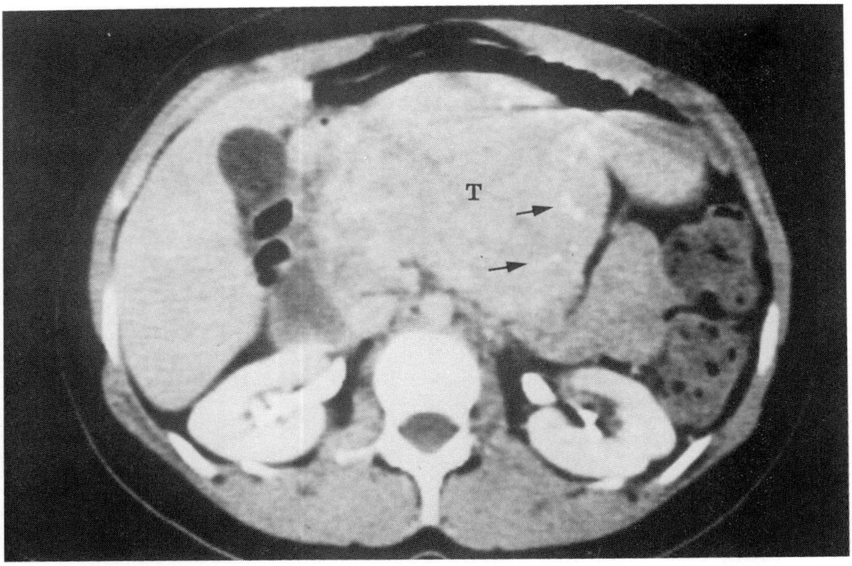

A

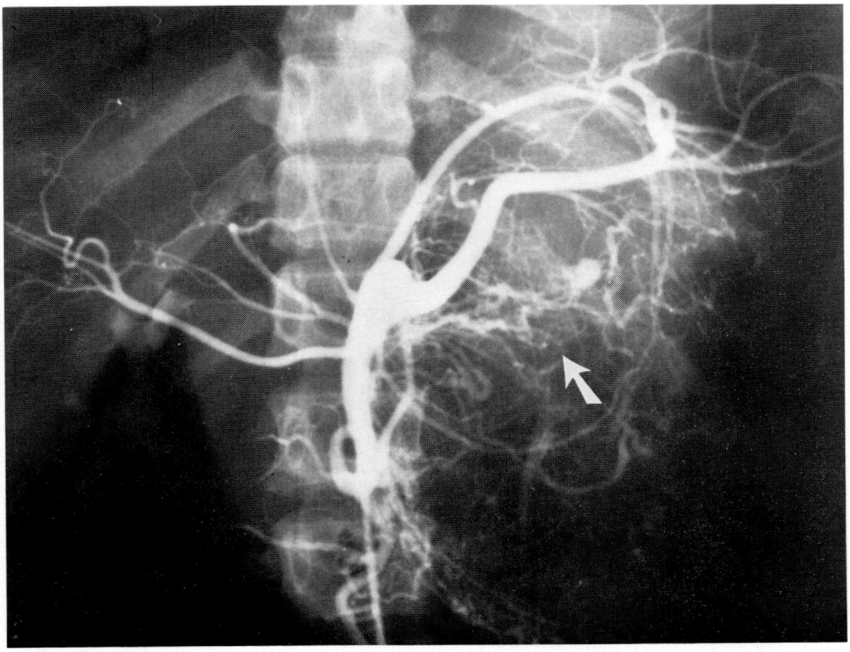

B

Figure 13-13. Pancreatic gastrinoma in a 30-year-old woman with Zollinger-Ellison syndrome. (A) CT examination shows a large, lobulated, and dense pancreatic tumor (T). A few speckles of calcification are seen in the tumor (arrows). (B) Angiography shows irregular abnormal vessels and a hypervascular tumor (arrow).

ization of vascular encasement or adjacent organ invasion, nodal disease, and liver metastases.

Percutaneous transhepatic venous sampling is a useful procedure performed usually when other noninvasive imaging modalities do not visualize focal pancreatic tumors. This technique developed by Lundenquist et al. involves the placement of a catheter in the main portal vein via a percutaneous transhepatic approach.[20] Venous samples for hormone assay are subsequently obtained from veins draining the head, body, and tail of the pancreas. The procedure is invasive but very useful in the diagnosis and localization of very small functioning islet cell tumors with reported success rates as high as 90%.[15] At operation endoscopic transillumination may help to delineate tumors in the duodenal wall.

PANCREATIC LYMPHOMA

Primary pancreatic lymphoma is a rare lesion accounting for 1.5% of pancreatic tumors.[27] Similarly, involvement of the pancreas occurs in less than 1% of patients suffering from systemic lymphoma. Lymphosarcoma can homogeneously infiltrate and replace the pancreas and is often associated with massive retroperitoneal adenopathy. Sonography shows a characteristic hypoechoic mass that may be confused with a pancreatic cyst. CT shows a homogeneous soft tissue mass with only minimal enhancement after intravenous contrast administration. Biliary and/or pancreatic duct dilatation may occur, but they are distinctly unusual.

PANCREATIC METASTASES

Among the more common primary tumors that metastasize to pancreas are melanoma, and carcinoma of the lung, breast, cervix, ovary, and prostate.[29] Solitary metastases are radiographically indistinguishable from pancreatic carcinoma. The diagnosis of metastatic disease is suspected if other metastatic deposits are recognized and if there is a history of a primary malignant tumor.

PAPILLARY EPITHELIAL NEOPLASM

This tumor has been recently described. It is usually seen in young asymptomatic women complaining of a slow-growing abdominal mass. The tumor is more commonly located in the tail of the pancreas, almost never metastasizes, and is believed to arise from primitive cells in the small ducts of the pancreas. Sonographic examination reveals a large echogenic, well-defined mass, and CT shows a heterogeneous soft tissue density mass with moderate enhancement after intravenous contrast administration[2] (Fig. 13-14). In a young asymptomatic woman, these features are considered suspicious; however, tissue confirmation is always indicated.

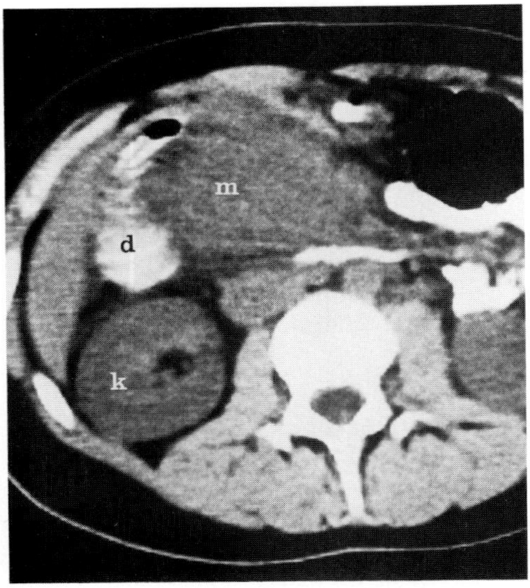

A

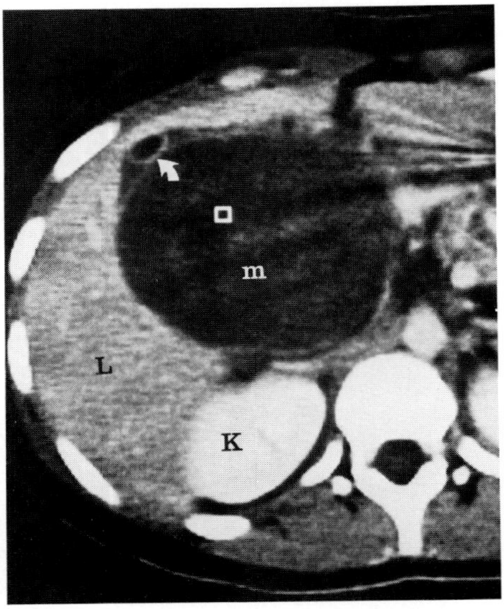

B

Figure 13-14. Papillary epithelial neoplasm of the pancreas in an 18-year-old woman presenting with upper abdominal pain, fever, and a palpable mass. (A) Noncontrast CT scan demonstrates a soft tissue mass in the head of the pancreas. (B) Contrast CT scan after an intravenous bolus shows the mass extending superiorly and compressing the gallbladder (arrow) against the undersurface of the liver. m = mass, L = liver, K and k = kidney, d = duodenum.

CONCLUSIONS

With the development of modern imaging equipment and continuous refinement of existing modalities and technology, the pancreas can be reliably evaluated. We do not advocate the use of algorithms and tend to select the proper imaging modality based on the clinical presentation and morphologic characteristics of the pancreatic lesions. Sonography because of its low cost, noninvasiveness, and availability is the initial screening test. Sonography is particularly useful in jaundiced patients to assess the status of the intrahepatic biliary tree, common duct, and gallbladder. CT is now the predominate means of evaluating pancreatic masses, and it is performed in almost all our patients. Angiography is used in equivocal cases and mainly to determine resectability. Newer modalities such as magnetic resonance imaging show promise but require further investigation and refinement to reliably evaluate the pancreas. Transhepatic cholangiography and ERCP continue to be used in special circumstances, particularly in determining the presence, nature, and location of obstructive lesions of the pancreatic and common bile ducts.

REFERENCES

1. Arger PH, Mulhern CB, Bonavita JA, Stauffer DM, Hale J. An analysis of pancreatic sonography in suspected pancreatic disease. J Clin Ultrasound 7:91–97, 1979.
2. Balthazar EJ, Subramanyam BR, Lefleur RS, Barone CM. Solid and papillary epithelial neoplasms of the pancreas: Radiographic, CT, sonographic and angiographic features. Radiology 150:39, 1984.
3. Bradley EL III, Gonzalez AC, Clements JC Jr. Acute pancreatic psueodcysts: Incidence and implications. Ann Surg 184:734–737, 1976.
4. Compagno J, Oertel JE. Mucinous cystic neoplasms of the pancreas with overt and latent malignancy (cystadenoma and cystadenocarcinoma). A clinicopathologic study of 41 cases. Am J Clin Pathol 69:573–580, 1978.
5. Cubilla AL, Fitzgerald PJ. Morphological patterns of primary nonendocrine human pancreas carcinoma. Cancer Res 35:2234–2248, 1975.
6. Cubilla AL, Fitzgerald PJ. Classification of pancreatic cancer (nonendocrine). Mayo Clin Proc 54:449–458, 1978.
7. Cubilla A, Fitzgerald PJ. Pancreatic cancer, I: Duct adenocarcinoma: A clinical pathologic study of 380 patients. Part 1. Pathol Ann 241–287, 1978.
8. Doust BD. Ultrasound examination of the pancreas. Radiol Clin North Am 13:467–478, 1975.
9. Ferrucci JT Jr, Wittenberg J. Refinement in chiba needle transhepatic cholangiography. AJR 129:11–16, 1977.
10. Filly R, Freimanis A. Echographic diagnosis of pancreatic lesions. Radiology 96:575–582, 1970.
11. Freeny PC, Weinstein CJ, Taft DA, Aller FH. Cystic neoplasms of the pancreas: New angiographic and ultrasonographic findings. AJR 131:759–802, 1978.
12. Freeny PC, Lawson TC. Adenocarcinoma of the pancreas. In: Radiology of the Pancreas. New York, Springer-Verlag, 1982, p 417.
13. Freeny PC, Marks WM, Ball TJ: Impact of high resolution computed tomography of the pancreas on utilization of ERCP and angiography. Radiology 142:35–39, 1982.
14. Freeny PC, Marks WM, Ryan J, et al: Pancreatic ductal adenocarcinoma: Diagnosis and staging with dynamic CT. Radiology 166:125–133, 1988.
15. Gunther RW, Klose KJ, Ruckert J, et al. Localization of small islet cell tumors. Gastrointest Radiol 10:145–152, 1985.

16. Kamin PD, Bernardino ME, Wallace S, et al. Comparison of ultrasound and computed tomography in the detection of pancreatic malignancy. Cancer 46:2410–2412, 1980.
17. Lawson TL. Sensitivity of pancreatic ultrasonography in the detection of pancreatic disease. Radiology 128:733–736, 1978.
18. Leopold GR. Pancreatic echography: A new dimension in the diagnosis of pseudocyst. Radiology 14:365–369, 1972.
19. Leopold GR. Ultrasound. In: Margulis AR, Burhenne HS, eds. Alimentry Tract Roentgenology. Abdominal Imaging. St. Louis, CV Mosby, 1979, vol 3. pp 275–290.
20. Lunderguist A, Eriksson M, Ingemansson S, et al. Selective pancreatic vein catheterization for hormonal assay in endocrine tumors of the pancreas. Cardiovasc Radiol 1:117–124, 1978.
21. Pollack D, Taylor KJW. Ultrasound scanning in patients with clinical suspicion of pancreatic cancer: A retrospective study. Cancer 47:1662–1665, 1981.
22. Sarti DA, King W. The ultrasonic findings in inflammatory pancreatic disease. Semin Ultrasound 1:178–191, 1980.
23. Siegelman SS, Copeland BE, Saba GP et al. CT of fluid collections associated with pancreatitis. AJR 134:1121–1132, 1980.
24. Snow JH Jr., Goldstein HM, Wallace S. Comparison of scintigraphy, sonography and computed tomography in the evaluation of hepatic neoplasms. AJR 132:915–918, 1979.
25. Stark DD, Moss AA, Goldberg H, Deveney CW. CT of pancreatic islet cell tumors. Radiology 150:491–493, 1984.
26. Stephens DH, Sheedy PF III. Computed tomography. In: Margulis AR, Burhenne HJ, eds. Alimentry Tract Roentgenology. Abdominal Imaging St. Louis, CV Mosby, 1979, pp 251–274.
27. Reed K, Vose PC, Jarstfer B. Pancreatic cancer: 30 year review (1947–1977). Am J Surg 138:929–938, 1979.
28. Ward EM, Stephens DH, Sheedy PF. Computed tomographic characteristics of pancreatic carcinoma: An analysis of 100 cases. Radiographics, 3(4), 19:547–565, 1983.
29. Wernecke K, Peters PE, Galanski M. Pancreatic metastases: Ultrasound evaluation. Radiology 160:399–402, 1986.

CHAPTER

14

ERCP IN PANCREATIC MASSES: MEDICAL ASPECTS

Simmy Bank, Bernard Stark, and Ronald Greenberg

ENDOSCOPY IN PANCREATIC MASSES

The relative safety of ultrasonography and CT scanning and skinny needle biopsy of masses in and around the pancreas has at times obviated the need for more invasive investigations. However, as with all techniques in medicine, these are not always diagnostic or accurate and often fail to reveal the true extent of carcinoma or involvement of surrounding structures, common bile duct, and pancreatic duct. Selective angiography is not infrequently required for diagnostic reasons as well as to delineate vessel encasement and to determine the vascular supply and arterial abnormalities if surgery is to be undertaken. It is also of diagnostic importance with regard to apudomas but of little help in the differential diagnosis between pancreatitis and carcinoma. Similarly, endoscopic retrograde cholangiopancreatography (ERCP) may assist in the differential diagnosis of pancreatic masses, delineate the extent of involvement of the biliary tree and pancreatic duct to obtain material for histologic and cytologic analysis, ascertain spread into adjacent organs, and lastly, relieve biliary or pancreatic obstruction.

INDICATIONS FOR ERCP IN THE DIAGNOSIS OF PANCREATIC MASSES

Suspicious Mass on Ultrasonography or CT Scanning

It is a relatively common occurrence for radiologists to report "fullness in the region of the head of the pancreas" or "slight enlargement of the head and body of the pancreas'' or ''increased echogenicity'' of one or other part of the gland. This type of report causes considerable consternation in the referring physician (and not infrequently the patient), resulting in uncertainty as to the significance of abdominal pain or other symptoms. As skinny needle aspiration is generally not indicated in this situation, the diagnostic options include (1) ERCP with visualization of the pancreatic and common bile ducts and their branches and (2) repeating the CT scan in 3 to 6 months to see whether the mass is more obvious or unchanged. This latter method has a tendency to have legal repercussions if a malignant condition is eventually diagnosed.

The Presence of a Pancreatic Mass on CT but Negative or Indefinite Skinny Needle Aspiration Cytologic Examination

Cytologic examination of pancreatic cancers obtained by skinny needle aspiration reveals carcinoma in 60% to 90% of cases.[24] This leaves between 10% and 40% in which a diagnostic problem between malignant, benign, or indeed an anatomic variant arises. There are three possible approaches: (1) repeat the skinny needle aspiration, (2) perform ERCP in an attempt to differentiate the various causes, and (3) subject the patient to surgery that may or may not provide absolute diagnostic proof (even with biopsy) at the time of laparotomy.

Obstructive Jaundice with Equivocal Findings at the Distal End of the Common Bile Duct on Ultrasonography or CT Scanning

Indications for ERCP in this situation are potentially both diagnostic and therapeutic, and because of this latter benefit, the test should be carried out only by endoscopists experienced in sphincterotomy, stent placement, and stone extraction and able to puncture the common bile duct above an area of distal obstruction at the lower end of the duct with a ''needle knife'' so as to allow access for therapeutic maneuvers. Clearly, the diagnosis may be obvious even before the ERCP is done, as it is not infrequent for carcinoma of the ampulla to present in this manner. In addition, the findings of an enlarged erythematous ampulla from a stone at the lower end of the common bile duct causing both jaundice and pancreatic edema or mild pancreatitis of the head of the pancreas is characteristic. In addition, the ERCP may reveal a number of unsuspected anatomic variants of the pancreatic or common bile duct as well as a normal pancreatic duct that would rule out a pancreatic cause of the jaundice in 95% of cases. Occasionally, a small peripheral carcinoma in the head or body of the pancreas may elude detection. The common bile duct may show compression in almost any area from the ampulla to the hilar portion of the duct and may reveal a variety of pathologic processes that may be associated with pancreatic enlargement. The following would require consideration: (1) carcinoma of the pancreas proximal to the ampulla, (2) bile duct carcinoma with pancreatic extension, (3) gallstone with adjacent pancreatic edema or subclinical pancreatitis, (4) sclerosing cholangitis affecting the main common bile duct and the pancreas, (5) lymphoma or secondary carcinoma of lymph nodes near the pancreatic head, (6) occasionally pancreatic cystadenoma or cystadenocarcinoma, (7) benign or malignant apudoma (e.g., gastrinoma, vipoma) (Fig. 14-1) (8) rare causes such as tuberculosis, *Ascaris,* or Crohn's disease, causing pancreatitis by obstructing the ampulla, and (9) large perivaterian diverticula, which can cause both jaundice and localized pancreati-

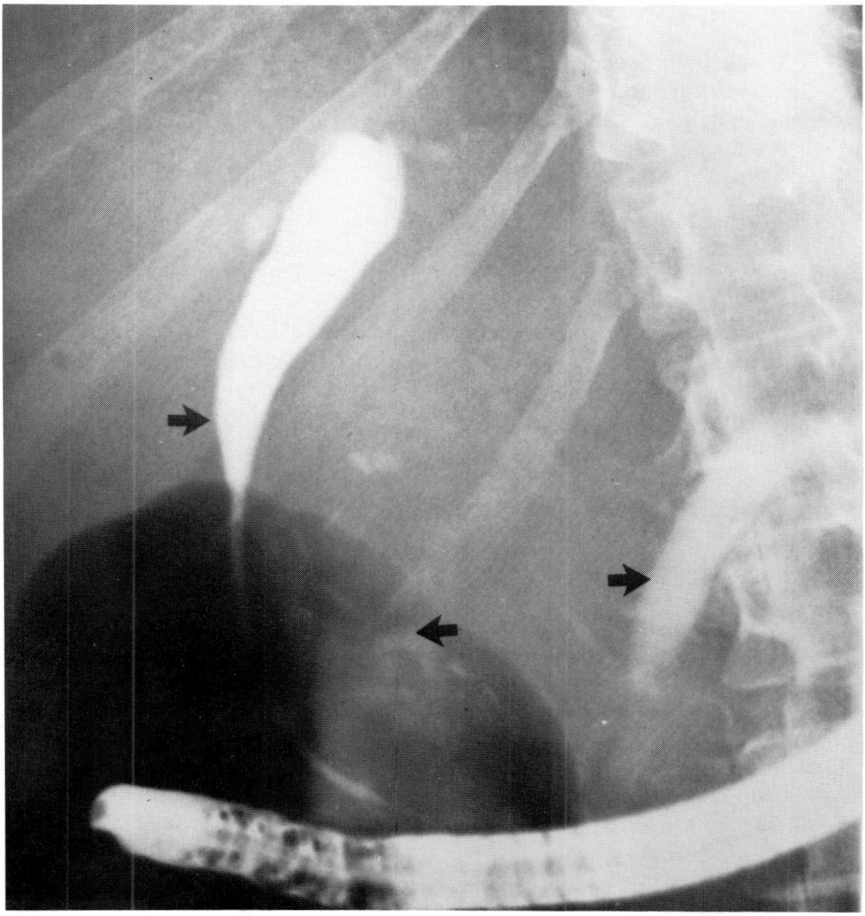

Figure 14-1. ERCP in 50-year-old woman with an abdominal mass, showing a smooth obstruction of the common duct and distortion of the pancreatic duct with interruption and disruption of the secondary ducts in the head of the pancreas (arrows). She had a sister with a leiomyosarcoma in the same area. Surgery in this patient revealed a nonfunctioning apudoma. On examination, the majority of cells appeared to contain vasoactive intestinal polypeptide.

tis.[1,22] All these may not show an obvious abnormality of the pancreatic duct. Clearly, if the duct is abnormal, carcinoma or pancreatitis is by far the most likely cause.

Obstructive Jaundice, Pancreatic Enlargement on CT, or Suspicious Enlargement of the Pancreatic Head and a Percutaneous Transhepatic Cholangiogram That Shows Common Bile Duct Obstruction But Does Not Define the Lesion

CT may fail to define the lesion other than to show common bile duct obstruction, and therefore the demonstration of a lesion may be best established from below, that is, by ERCP, to define whether it is an intrinsic biliary lesion or extrinsic bile duct compression. Biliary stenting may of course be accompanied in both techniques, but internal stenting at ERCP is preferable.

Diffuse Pancreatic Enlargement on Sonography and CT Scanning With or Without a Prominant Pancreatic Duct

Differential diagnosis in this situation includes (1) a normal anatomic variant of no consequence, (2) small ductal carcinoma with retrograde pancreatitis and edema, and (3) chronic pancreatitis related to a variety of etiologic factors, particularly chronic alcoholism. It is likely that ERCP will be able to differentiate these three conditions.

Pancreatic Mass in Patients With Known Acute or Chronic Pancreatitis

ERCP may be required to differentiate (1) pancreatic cyst, although sonography is usually quite diagnostic, (2) hypertrophic fibrosis of the pancreas, usually in the head of the gland, (3) necrosis with tumefaction after a recent acute attack, and (4) carcinomatous transformation in chronic pancreatitis.[6,10] Although skinny needle aspiration is probably the diagnostic procedure of choice in these conditions, it should be emphasized that cells derived from areas of ductal metaplasia in chronic pancreatitis may resemble those from carcinoma or cystadenoma.[5] Although ERCP may also not be diagnostic, it may assist in guiding the site for skinny needle biopsy.

Pancreatic Mass Associated with Ascites, Pleural Effusion, or Pericardial Effusion with High Amylase Content

Pancreatic effusions may be the one absolute indication for diagnostic ERCP in the presence of a pancreatic mass.[26] It is essential to ascertain the exact site of the leak of pancreatic juice if medical therapy has failed to improve the effusions. ERCP should be carried out as a preoperative measure under antibiotic cover to track the exact anatomic area of duct disruption into the peritoneal or pleural cavity or leak from a communicating pancreatic cyst.[23] Failure to demonstrate the leak may lead to surgical resection distal to the duct disruption with extravasation of pancreatic juice in the postoperative period, the commonest cause of postoperative mortality.

Hematopancrea (Hemosuccus Pancreaticus) or Upper Gastrointestinal Bleed in Patients with Pancreatic or Epigastric Mass

The occurrence of upper gastrointestinal bleeding in a patient with a pancreatic mass may be due to (1) bleeding from the short gastric vessels in the gastric fundus due to splenic vein obstruction (and more rarely the portal vein) or thrombosis, (2) erosion of a large vessel (e.g., pancreaticoduodenal, splenic, or gastroepiploic vessels) by an abscess or carcinoma, (3) bleeding into a cyst or carcinoma due to enzyme or tumor erosion of the blood vessels in the wall of the cyst or substance of the tumor, and (4) bleeding from pseudoaneurysm resulting from chronic pancreatitis.[11] If upper endoscopy is not diagnostic in these patients, urgent ERCP should be considered to facilitate diagnosis, followed by urgent angiography and embolization of the feeding blood vessels.[25] Surgical intervention is less likely to be successful.

Traumatic Pancreatitis with Enlargement of the Gland on Ultrasonography or CT

Recent studies have suggested a role for urgent ERCP in patients in whom pancreatic trauma is suspected, particularly if associated with an abdominal mass.[15] This is especially so with blunt trauma (for example, handlebar injury, truck backup injury). These injuries are particularly liable to cause a total break or disruption of the main pancreatic duct where it crosses the spinal column, either within the substance of the gland or in the extrapancreatic region, forming an intra- or peripancreatic communicating cyst. Experience with two such recent cases resulted in repeated surgical assaults on the cysts before the complete rupture of the duct was demonstrated at ERCP and resection to the distal disruption and internal drainage cured the pancreatic problem.

CONTROVERSIAL INDICATIONS FOR ERCP IN PANCREATIC MASSES

Acute Fulminating Pancreatitis

In patients with acute severe pancreatitis with multiple poor prognostic signs for survival (i.e., more than five of Ranson's early prognostic signs or one or more of Bank's clinical criteria) in whom CT scan shows evidence of multiple necrotic areas or gross surrounding necrotic masses, a number of European endoscopists are investigating the role of urgent ERCP to delineate the areas of necrotic material.[12] The indication for this is the probability that early removal of large areas of necrotic pancreas (necrosectomy) may improve the patients' prognosis, which in these patients carries a mortality in the region of 40% to 60%. This approach to the problem of fulminating pancreatitis will of course require a multicenter study before ERCP can be recommended in acute pancreatitis.

Known Pancreatic Cysts

Early reports of ERCP in patients with pancreatic cysts warned of the risk of bacterial infection, thus converting a sterile cyst into an abscess. With present attention to sterilization of the endoscopes, prophylactic antibiotics, monitoring fever and white blood cell counts, and most of all surgical backup should infection be expected, ERCP is now carried out with regularity in patients with cysts. In a series of 15 cysts investigated by endoscopy at our hospital, there were no deaths and only 4 required urgent percutaneous aspiration or surgery. Despite this, the question might be raised as to the necessity of doing ERCP in patients with cysts. By and large, ultrasonography is the most reliable diagnostic test for cysts and also the technique of choice for following the progression or regression of the cyst.[3] Perhaps the only point that can be made for a preoperative ERCP is to demonstrate whether or not the cyst is communicating with the pancreatic ductal system and, perhaps therapeutically more important, to define the morphology and number of cysts and to detect a grossly dilated pancreatic ductal system that may alter the therapeutic approach from percutaneous cyst drainage or cystogastrostomy to a Puestow-type longitudinal pancreaticojejunostomy.[2]

Preoperative ERCP for Chronic Pain and Pancreatic Enlargement

It is imperative that the morphology of the ductal system be known in patients with uncontrollable pain in whom a surgical procedure to relieve pain is contemplated. Those patients with grossly dilated ducts will benefit most from a longitudinal pancreaticojejunostomy, whereas disease confined to the distal portion will obtain best relief by distal pancreatectomy. Those with a grossly distorted and enlarged head of the pancreas will probably require a proximal pancreaticoduodenectomy,[19] or more limited resection of the head of the pancreas.

ERCP FINDINGS IN THE MAJOR DIAGNOSTIC PROBLEMS IN PANCREATIC MASSES

Enlargement of the Head of the Pancreas

This is perhaps the most frequent diagnostic problem for which an ERCP is requested. The differential diagnosis is between carcinoma and chronic pancreatitis or postacute pancreatitis with edema and necrosis. Other rare causes are apudomas, cysts in the head of the pancreas, cystadenoma, lymphoma, and tuberculosis (Fig. 14-1).

ERCP Findings in Carcinoma of the Head of the Pancreas

The most reliable sign of pancreatic carcinoma is the finding of a *double duct sign,* denoting compression and occasionally complete obstruction of both the pancreatic duct and the common bile duct.[16] This sign was thought until recently to be diagnostic of carcinoma, but there have been one or two recent disquieting reports of a positive double duct sign in pancreatitis, especially when maximally involving the angle between the common bile duct and the vertical portion of the proximal pancreatic duct, so-called groove pancreatitis, or in a proximal cyst (Fig. 14-2). The only other sign that is virtually diagnostic of carcinoma is a

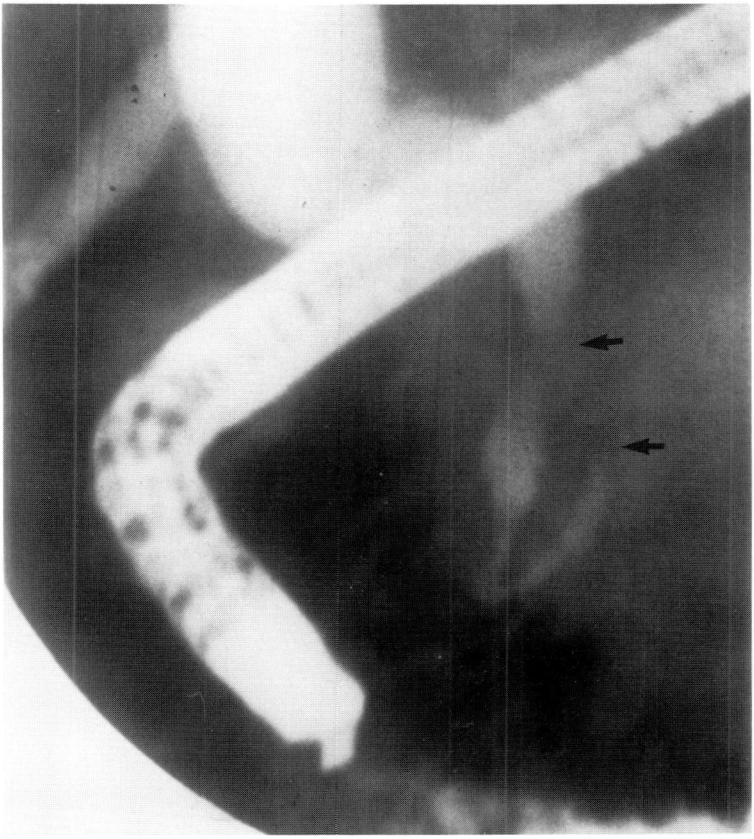

Figure 14-2. ERCP showing double duct sign, that is, compression of the bile duct and near complete obstruction of the pancreatic duct (arrows), in a patient with a prolonged attack of gallstone pancreatitis and pancreatic cyst.

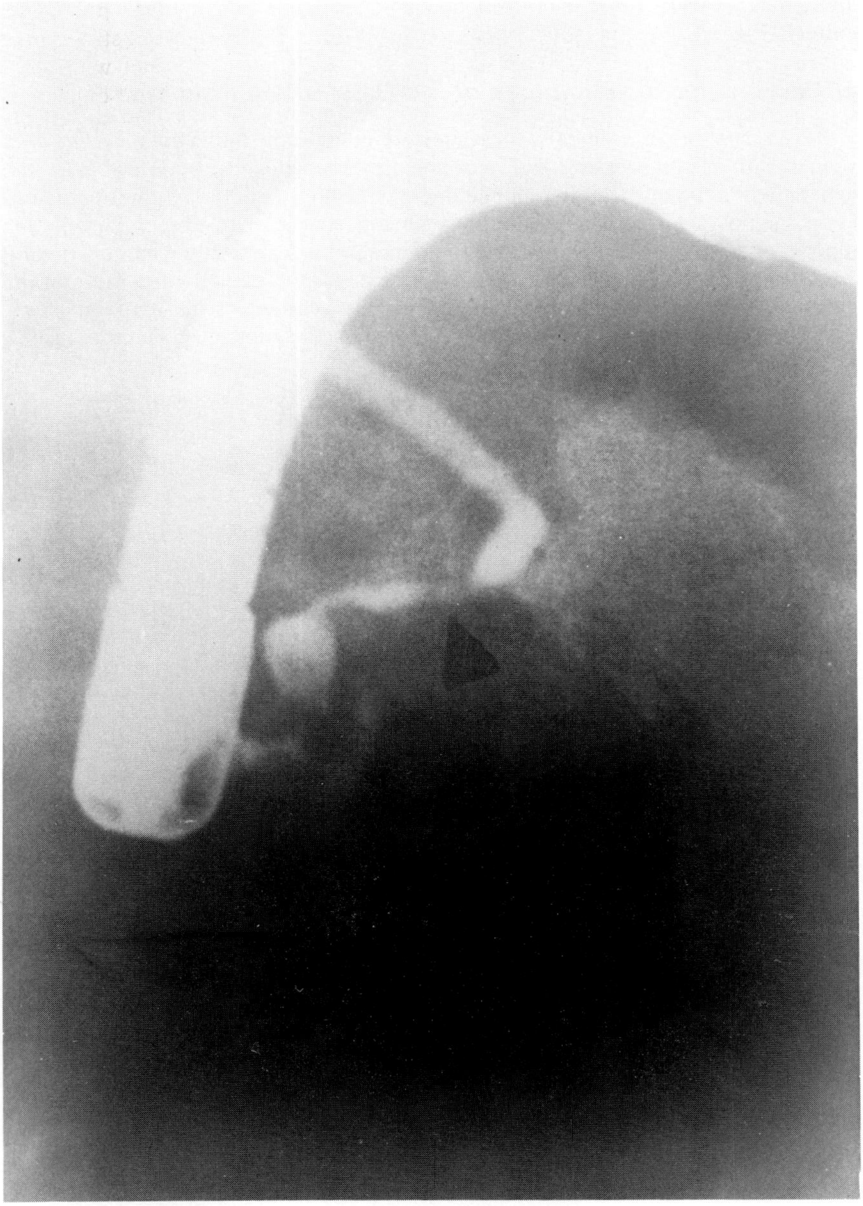

Figure 14-3. ERCP showing a localized apple core lesion (arrow) in the proximal pancreatic duct in a patient presenting with severe diarrhea and thought to have a Vipoma. Pathologic examination showed the features of adenocarcinoma.

relatively rare ERCP finding of an "apple core" filling defect in the pancreatic duct (Fig. 14-3). Usually carcinoma in the head results in complete obstruction of the duct or regular or irregular narrowing of a segment of the duct with gross dilatation of the duct beyond the narrowing. Other signs suggestive of carcinoma include dilated secondary ductules, acinar filling, or heterogeneous acinar staining, which might suggest a peripheral type of adenocarcinoma that is extremely difficult to diagnose.[17] Multiple irregular cystic areas in the head of the gland may denote areas of tumor necrosis and extravasation of necrotic material[14] (Fig. 14-4). Usually carcinoma tends to produce an irregular narrowing of the common bile duct in any area from the ampulla to near the porta hepatis. However, it is not

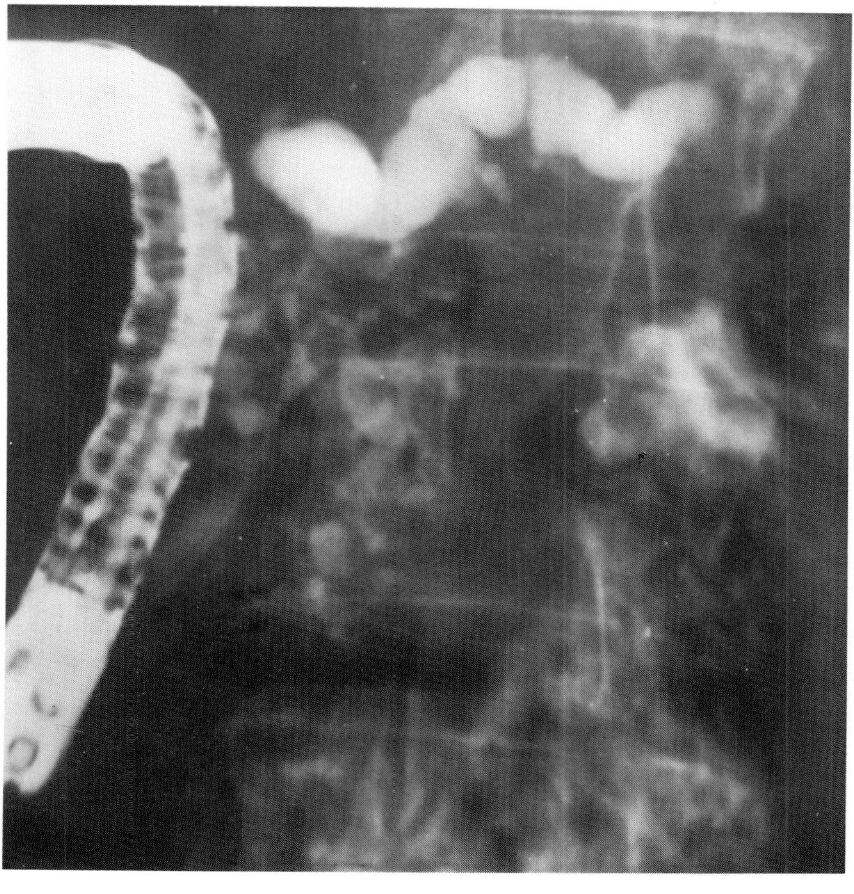

Figure 14-4. ERCP in a 55-year-old woman with abdominal pain and dilated pancreatic duct with chain-lake appearance, with grossly abnormal duct morphology in the head of the pancreas, originally thought to be chronic pancreatitis; surgery revealed a necrotic adenocarcinoma of the head of the pancreas with obstruction of the pancreatic duct.

infrequent for the duct to be smoothly narrowed and even tapered. As a rule, the intrahepatic ducts tend to be more dilated in malignant obstructive jaundice than in benign obstructive jaundice. Obstruction of the cystic duct in the absence of gallstones is of course highly suggestive of carcinoma but so rare as to be virtually unhelpful.

ERCP Findings in Chronic Pancreatitis

Chronic pancreatitis tends to produce generalized changes in the ductal system.[9] However, diseased areas localized to the head or tail of the gland are by no means uncommon. This can make differentiation from partial obstruction by carcinoma extremely difficult. The classic features are multiple strictures with a chain-of-lakes appearance, dilated or irregular side ducts, and intraductal filling defects due to protein plugs occurring in about 70% of the time with chronic pancreatitis.[18] The remaining 30% have a nondilated but irregularly stenosed ductal system that is less pathognomonic. Multiple cysts are of course very suggestive of chronic pancreatitis but are rare after acute attacks. Compression and marked attenuation of the common duct in its intrapancreatic portion is common and tends to be smooth and regular with mild to moderate dilatation of the suprapancreatic portion of the duct.[20] The ERCP may demonstrate common bile duct stones as the cause of the inflammatory process in the head of the pancreas.

ERCP Findings Common to Malignant and Benign Masses

In 20% of cases differentiation between malignant and benign disease may be virtually impossible or require further investigation (including laparotomy to be diagnostic).[17] The main areas of confusion that we have encountered are (1) proximal obstruction of the pancreatic duct with distal duct dilatation and appearance resembling the chain-of-lakes appearance of chronic pancreatitis (see Fig. 14-4), (2) tumor necrosis in the head of the pancreas causing cystic spaces resembling the multiple duct ectasia seen in chronic pancreatitis (see Fig. 14-4), (3) diffuse narrowing of the proximal pancreatic duct with sudden dilatation, cyst formation, and irregularity of the distal duct system in the body or tail, and (4) the double duct sign highly suggestive of malignancy, occasionally occurring in benign conditions. In this respect, it is necessary to remember that using the time factor as a diagnostic measure is fraught with danger (i.e., excluding carcinoma because of the patient's survival for 2–3 years afterward). The following case reports are illustrative and demonstrate the problem of presuming benign disease on the basis of time alone unless proof of carcinoma is obtained.

Case 1 Patient A. S. presented with abdominal pain and a mass in the head of the pancreas on CT scan. Skinny needle aspiration failed to confirm the presence of carcinoma. At operation a mass was felt in the head of the pancreas, and a diagnosis of carcinoma was made without biopsy. Two years later, the patient became jaundiced and ERCP showed a double duct sign. Because of the long history, a diagnosis of chronic pancreatitis was entertained. However, skinny needle aspiration now revealed adenocarcinoma.

Case 2 Patient B. M., a 50-year-old woman, presented with abdominal pain and jaundice. An operation showed a mass in the head of the pancreas, and a bypass was done. She had recurrent episodes of abdominal pain, and another operation was done 2 years later. A mass around the head of the pancreas was biopsied and showed granulomatous tissue. Because of the long duration of symptoms and history of tuberculosis, a diagnosis of tuberculosis or sarcoid was considered. One year later, after the patient had persistent abdominal pain, an ERCP showed complete obstruction of the pancreatic duct, and a third operation and deep biopsy now showed the presence of adenocarcinoma.

We have now seen at least four patients in the last 7 years who have survived 2 to 4 years without resection.

Total Pancreatic Duct Obstruction

Obstruction of the pancreatic duct whether in the head, body, or tail, with failure to fill the main duct beyond the obstruction, renders ERCP alone valueless as a diagnostic technique. The common causes of total duct obstructions are carcinoma and cyst; less common causes are sterile or infected necrotic mass, benign tumors, apudomas, and stricture following previous severe pancreatitis, an obstructing pancreatic stone or a large protein plug.[21] In this situation, it may be hazardous to venture a diagnosis on ERCP findings alone, and other means of diagnosing the cause of the obstruction are required. One important consideration in all these patients is to be quite sure that there has been adequate filling of the pancreatic duct, because partial filling of the duct may be erroneously diagnosed as representing an obstructive lesion.

Compression of the Pancreatic Duct or Common Bile Duct by Surrounding Lesions

Although the common bile duct is more likely to be compressed and even invaded by peripancreatic lymph nodes (e.g., secondary carcinoma, lymphoma, tuberculosis, etc.), the pancreatic duct is not immune from extrinsic distortion.[4] Large peripancreatic lesions such as lymphomatous glands, aortic aneurysm, and even retroperitoneal masses (e.g., hamartoma) may occasionally simulate intrapancreatic lesions.

ADDITIONAL INFORMATION OBTAINABLE AT ERCP

Indefinite findings at the time of ERCP warrant obtaining cytologic samples (either by flushing the pancreatic juice with secretin, brushing, or even biopsy) through the ERCP channel.[7] A positive result should be diagnostic of tumor. Pancreatic juice carcinoembryonic antigen content is rarely measured, and mapping of an area for directing the skinny needle is rarely feasible unless duct obstruction is present and the dye remains in the duct system for some time. Combination of ERCP, CT, and transhepatic cholangiography (THC) has also been carried out to better diagnose a mass. Placing of a nasobiliary or nasopancreatic stent to obtain cytologic samples and measure secretion is rarely carried out because in these situations, an internal stent is usually placed at the time of ERCP. As far as we are aware, a combined common bile duct (CBD) or pancreatic duct (PD) internal stent with a nasobiliary drain has not been carried out to obtain cytologic samples while internal drainage is proceeding. This may deserve a trial in difficult diagnostic problems. It is of course likely today that one or other therapeutic maneuver will be used in patients with pancreatic masses in the head to establish biliary drainage or, in particular and less commonly, stenting of the pancreatic duct or even transduodenoscopic cyst drainage.

THE PROS AND CONS OF ERCP IN ESTABLISHED OR SUSPECTED PANCREATIC MASSES ON CT OR ULTRASONOGRAPHY

The diagnostic value of ERCP in pancreatic masses clearly warrants its use as one of the first-line tests. Why, then, do so many experienced physicians, surgeons, and gastroenterologists agonize over the decision whether to refer their patients for ERCP as a diagnostic procedure? This hesitancy does not prevail if indications exist for therapeutic stenting, stone extraction, or sphincterotomy. The dilemma revolves around a general feeling among physicians and some gastroenterologists that the morbidity (and perhaps mortality) of ERCP, both diagnostic and therapeutic, is underreported. National statistics and surveys carried out by various societies have demonstrated a 0.3% to 0.5% mortality, 3% to 5% pancreatitis, and 40% hyperamylasemia rate.[13] Dr. Charles Frey (personal communication, American Pancreatic Association meeting, Chicago, 1988) has recently cared for 8 patients with severe pancreatitis, and 2 who died from seven centers in Sacramento and our own series constitute 0.25% deaths and 5.9% worrying cases in a series of 411 ERCPs carried out over 6 years. While it is true that the mortality probably does not exceed 0.5% in experienced groups, the data do not provide information with regard to the mortality or prolonged morbidity in nonpublished areas and in patients investigated for suspected masses and/or abdominal pain who are subsequently found to have either no pathologic lesions or benign disease in whom a complication is particularly distressing. It is thus correct that much soul searching occurs before the decision is taken to proceed with a diagnostic ERCP on the basis of a vague CT scan or ultrasound findings, particularly if the patient's history is not really that suggestive of pancreatic disease. Many variables such as the patient's age, the patient's demands to be sure of the relevance of the CT findings, and other factors need to be considered. Performing an ERCP in a patient in whom a diagnosis has been established by skinny needle aspiration or in whom a cyst is diagnosed by ultrasonography other than for therapeutic purposes may be regarded as unnecessary and possibly even meddlesome. Accepted that ERCP does constitute some risks, do these outweigh the benefits? Clearly, after an acute attack of pancreatitis, it may be very important to exclude a stone in a common bile duct, and in a patient with jaundice and dilated bile ducts, therapeutic endoscopic measures are desirable. However, the bulk of the difficult decisions relate to whether a mass is carcinomatous and whether this diagnosis changes therapeutic decisions. Physicians and surgeons differ with regard to the value of surgical resection or early radiotherapy or chemotherapy in cancer of the pancreas, and the literature contains diametrically opposing views ranging from increased longevity to no material advantage to decreased longevity if one includes those patients who died from partial or radical pancreatectomy. Thus, opinions may vary from optimism to pessimism, and in the former group ERCP would be carried out frequently, and in the latter it would often be delayed or shelved. Even the latter route requires careful consideration and discussion with the patient and relatives. As there are occasional papers in the literature that suggest that surgical resection of pancreatic tumors, especially if carried out early, prolongs survival, it has become reasonably commonplace for patients or their families to initiate legal action if the diagnosis has been delayed. In the present-day climate, there seems to be no possibility of not divulging to the patient the risks and benefits of ERCP. Interestingly enough, many elderly patients accept a decision to wait and see and repeat the CT scan at 3- or 6-month intervals rather than accept an invasive procedure.

REFERENCES

1. Altman HS, Phillips G, Bank S, Klotz H. Pancreatitis associated with duodenal Crohn's disease. Am J Gastroenterol 78:174–177, 1983.
2. Axon ATR, Classen M, Cotton PB, et al. Pancreatography in chronic pancreatitis—International definitions. Gut 25:1107–1112, 1984.
3. Bralley EL, Clements JL, Gonzalez AC. The natural history of pancreatic pseudocysts—A unified concept of management. Am J Surg 137:135–141, 1979.
4. Clark A, Peek JC, Forbes-Smith et al. Pancreatic pseudotumors associated with multifocal idiopathic fibrosclerosis. Gastrointest Radiol 13:30–32, 1988.
5. Compagno J, Oertel JE. Mucinous cystic neoplasm of the pancreas with overt and latent malignancy (cystadenocarcinoma and cystadenoma). A clinicopathologic study of 41 cases. Am J Clin Pathol 69:573–580, 1978.
6. DiMagno E. Early diagnosis of chronic pancreatitis and pancreatic cancer. Med Clin North Am 72:979–992, 1988.
7. Endo Y, Morii T, Tamura H, et al. Cytodiagnosis of pancreatic malignant tumors by aspiration under direct vision using a duodenal fiberscope. Gastroenterology 67:944–951, 1974.
8. Freeny PC, Ball TJ. Endoscopic retrograde cholangiopancreatography (ERCP) and percutaneous transhepatic cholangiography (PTC) in the evaluation of suspected pancreatic carcinoma, diagnostic limitations, and contemporary roles. Cancer 47:1666–1678, 1981.
9. Frey CF. Classification of pancreatitis. State of the art, 1986. Pancreas 1:62–68, 1986.
10. Foley WD, Stewart ET, Lawson TL, et al. Computed tomography, ultrasonography, and endoscopic retrograde cholangiopancreatography in the diagnosis of pancreatic disease: a comparative study. Gastrointest Radiol 5:29–35, 1980.
11. Hall RI, Lavelle MI, Venables CW. Chronic pancreatitis as a cause of gastrointestinal bleeding. Gut 23:250–255, 1982.
12. Hamilton I, Bradley P, Linott DJ, McMahon MJ, Axon ATR. Endoscopic retrograde cholangiopancreatography in the investigation and management of patients after acute pancreatitis. Br J Surg 69:504–506, 1982.
13. Ihre T, Hellens G. Complications and endoscopic retrograde cholangiopancreatography. Acta Chir Scand 143:167–171, 1977.
14. Kaplan JO, Isikoff MB, Barkin J, Livingston AJ. Necrotic carcinoma of the pancreas: "The pseudo-pseudocyst." J Comput Assist Tomogr 4:166–167, 1980.
15. McCarthy RL, Ward EM, Charboneau JW, Sheedy PF, May GR. Imaging of the

Pancreas. In: Go VLW, Gardner JD, Brooks FP, et al. The Exocrine Pancreas. New York, Raven Press, 1986, pp 841–872.
16. Moss AA, Federle M, Shapiro HA, et al. The combined use of computed tomography and endoscopic retrograde cholangiopancreatography in the assessment of suspected pancreatic neoplasm: A blind clinical evaluation. Radiology 134:159–163, 1980.
17. Nakajima M, Yamagichi Y, Akasaka Y. Endoscopic retrograde cholangiopancreatography (ERCP) in the diagnosis of pancreatic cancer. In: Kawai K, ed. Early Diagnosis of Pancreatic Cancer. Tokyo, New York, Igaku-Shoin, 1979, pp 140–145.
18. Niederau C, Grendell JH. Diagnosis of chronic pancreatitis. Gastroenterology 88:1973–1995, 1985.
19. O'Neill JA, Greene H, Gishan FK. Surgical implications of chronic pancreatitis. J Pediatr Surg 17:920–926, 1982.
20. Petrozza JA, Dutta SK, Latham PS, Iber FL, Gadaez TR. Prevalence and natural history of distal common bile duct stenosis in alcoholic pancreatitis. Dig Dis Sci 24:840–895, 1984.
21. Ralls PW, Halls J, Renner I, Juttner H. Endoscopic retrograde cholangiopancreatography (ERCP) in pancreatic disease. Radiology 134:347–352, 1980.
22. Rustgi AK, Saini S, Schapiro RH. Hepatic imaging and advanced endoscopic techniques. Med Clin North Am 73:895–909, 1989.
23. Sankaran S, Sugawa C, Walt AJ. Value of endoscopic retrograde pancreatography in pancreatic ascites. Surg Gynecol Obstet 148:185–192, 1979.
24. Taavitsainen M, Koivuniemi A, Bondestam S, Kivsgari L, Tierla E. Ultrasonically guided fine-needle aspiration biopsy in focal pancreatic lesions. Acta Radiolog 28:541–543, 1987.
25. Waltman AC, Luers PR, Athanasoulis CA, Warshaw AL. Massive arterial hemorrhage in patients with pancreatitis. Arch Surg 121:439–443, 1986.
26. Weaver DW, Walt AJ, Sugawa C, Boawman DL. A continuing appraisal of pancreatic ascites. Surg Gynecol Obstet 154:845–848, 1982.

CHAPTER

15

PANCREATIC REGENERATION: FACT OR FANTASY?

David A. Dreiling, John Robert, and Aholeab E. Toleldano

EDITORIAL COMMENT

The authors review the historical data from animal work showing that under circumstances in which ductal continuity is restored and obstruction relieved, pancreatic acinar regeneration does appear to occur. The evidence presented for regeneration in humans is not entirely persuasive to us, although it seems clear that pancreatitis can resolve, particularly some cases of acute necrotizing disease with restoration of normal pancreatic secretion. With regard to chronic pancreatitis, the DuVal procedure, rarely done nowadays, was followed by demonstrable increases in pancreatic secretory capacity, whereas the more commonly utilized Puestow operation, although followed by clinical improvement in digestion, has not been shown to increase pancreatic secretion. In patients with chronic pancreatitis who cease drinking alcohol, the observed restoration of exocrine secretory capacity may represent a return of normal function to damaged tissue rather than true hypertrophy or hyperplasia. The important conclusion to be drawn is that pancreatic exocrine secretory function can be improved after injury, necrosis, acute and chronic inflammation, and ductal decompression even if cellular regeneration remains unproved.

CONTROVERSY

There is experimental evidence that certain hormones (cholecystokinin, caerulein) and various antitrypsins will produce pancreatic growth as judged by pancreatic weight, enzyme enhancement, and DNA increase. However, only functional status is measurable in humans after pancreatic damage, usually by means of a formal intubated pancreatic function test. In many instances, it is difficult to differentiate the healing process of the injury (which may be occurring at a variable time) from acinar or ductal regeneration. Perhaps the arbitrary difference is unimportant. Clearly, the pancreas does not have a remarkable ability to regenerate, but there does seem to be an improvement in function in some patients after acute and chronic damage. Does this functional improvement represent regeneration of new tissue or recovery of function in diseased or damaged tissue?

Hepatic regeneration by a process of ductular reduplication and differentiation following hepatic injury and/or resection is a relatively well understood and accepted phenomenon.[19] It is surprising that the pancreas, arising from the same anlage possessing a duct system with characteristics similar to the hepatic ducts, has not been generally accepted as possessing similar potential, more so since there exists extensive literature implying a regenerative capacity.

Martinotti in 1892 was the first to report pancreatic ductal proliferation after partial pancreatectomy.[5] Sobolew, in 1902, attempting to produce atrophy of the pancreas by ligation of its ducts in cats, rabbits, and dogs, noted pancreatic atrophy commencing 6 to 12 days after ligation.[14] In half the animals, this atrophy progressed to fibrous replacement of the parenchyma. In the other half, there was a regression of the pathologic lesions and a restoration of normal histologic findings. Sobolew interpreted the latter observations as due to reestablishment of duct patency followed by regeneration.

Laguesse and de la Roche, following guinea pig pancreatic segments isolated between two ligatures, reported microscopic parenchymal alterations at 3, 7, and 14 days as well as 1, 2, and 6 months after ligation.[16] By the third day the acini appeared markedly reduced in numbers and their lumina greatly dilated. At the seventh day after ligation the acini had completely disappeared, but excretory ducts and islet tissue persisted. By the 14th day the duct system had been disorganized and surrounded by proliferating connective tissue. At the end of a month following ligation, the ducts appeared as cords of embryonic cells from which, in time, as documented by further sequential histologic study, pseudoacini were formed. Tiberti, in 1907, repeated these investigations in the rabbit pancreas, observing the histologic alterations 1, 2, 3, and 4 months after ductal ligation.[25] Tiberti reported the appearance of small epithelial masses that lacked the capillary plexuses characteristic of islets. Tiberti considered these cell nests to be the result of proliferation of acinar cells that had not succumbed to the primary injury of duct obstruction. He conceived the phenomenon as a proliferative attempt to produce new acini.

Kyrle, in 1908, reported studies of regeneration in the canine pancreas after partial resections and also after segmental transplantations into the spleen.[15] He described active proliferation of the duct epithelium, resulting in the formation of branching adenomatous structures, some of which took on the appearance of acini and actually developed zymogen granules. In the same year, Weichselbaum, cited by Graver, reported his search for evidence of pancreatic regeneration in postmortem pancreases of diabetics patients.[12] In 19 of 151 cases, Weichselbaum found proliferation of the epithelium of smaller and moderate-sized ducts, formations of solid cell processes from the ducts, and also formations of hollow evaginations from the ducts. These three histologic findings were interpreted as the first stages in the new formation of islet tissue.

Carraro, in 1909, studied regeneration in the pancreas of goats and rabbits injured by ethyl chloride freezing.[4] Two days after freezing, Carraro found large numbers of mitoses in the acinar and ductal, but not the islet, cells. Mitoses continued until the fourth day after ethyl chloride injury, after which the histologic picture was dominated by proliferating connective tissue and strands of solid and hollow regenerating epithelial cells. The islets and acini did not appear to participate in this regeneration; rather, the regenerating epithelial cells appeared to derive from the ducts. During the second week following injury, the regenerating epithelial cords and tubes gave rise to small excrescences or buttonlike structures composed of globose cells within a pale cytoplasm free of zymogen granules and surrounding a centrally placed nucleus. These cell clusters, so different in morphology from mature acinar cells, were called pseudoacini by Carraro. By the third week following freezing the pseudoacini were gradually replaced by proliferating connective tissue, resulting finally in a scarred, atrophic parenchyma containing only occasional nests of epithelial cells.

Bensley, in 1911, summarized the phenomenon of pancreatic regeneration of rabbits and guinea pigs in a Harvey lecture.[3] He described a rabbit in which the pancreatic duct was ligated near the bowel. When the animal was sacrificed 21 months later, the short segment of duct between the bowel and the ligature had regenerated histologically normal pancreatic tissue. Bensley described the regenerative process in the duct-ligated pancreases of the rabbit and guinea pig as follows:

> Towards the end of the first month, regenerative processes become prominent, resulting in the formation of new acini and new islets from the remains of the duct system. Thus, both primary tissues are present in the pancreas for a certain period, and throughout this period, acini are being constantly formed, pass through a series of development states and, to some extent, undergo atrophy or become de-differentiated. At the same time, islet tissue is being progressively increased by the addition of new islets developed from the duct system with which they remain in continuity.

Bensley also reported the postmortem findings in the pancreas of a rabbit that had, 15 months previously, been subjected to ligation and section of its duct in two places. The excluded, doubly ligated duct had effected a new communication with the bowel at a distance of about 2 cm from the main pancreatic duct. This new duct was larger than normal, and the pancreatic tissue that it drained, though somewhat reduced in size and richer in connective tissue, was in other respects normal. Bensley accepted these findings as indirect evidence that if duct continuity be reestablished at a sufficiently early period, the pancreas might be entirely restored.

Parker, in 1919, studied the regenerative efforts of the guinea pig pancreas after injury by bacterial toxins, chloroform, arsenicals, and so forth.[18] He described polymorphonuclear and endothelial invasion of the necrotic parenchymal lesions induced by these toxins, rapid phagocytosis of necrotic material, and cellular débridement, followed by active parenchymal regeneration. Allen in 1922,[1] Fisher in 1924,[10] and Shaw and Latimer in 1926[21] all studied pancreatic regeneration from stump or duct remnants in dogs. Fisher demonstrated the regeneration of 0.5 g of pancreatic tissue from such a stump in a totally pancreatectomized dog kept alive with insulin for 8 months. This capacity of ductal tissue for regeneration of pancreatic parenchyma persisted even after autotransplantation of ducts to different body sites and after homotransplantation to different hosts. In other experiments, Fisher showed the morbid tendency of pancreatic ducts to proliferate new ductal tissue and to reestablish continuity whenever these ducts were ligated or severed.[10]

Shaw and Latimer, in 1926, implanted isolated pancreatic ductal segments 1 to 2 cm in length under the serosa of the duodenum in partially or completely pancreatectomized dogs.[21] After prolonged intervals, a minimal period of 8 weeks being stressed by this group, these ductal autografts became vascularized and underwent varying degrees of cellular differentiation, with the regeneration of parenchymal tissue, that is, ductules, pancreatic acini, and islets. The transplanted regenerating duct system often reestablished continuity with the gut lumen; when continuity was not achieved, regeneration appeared to be arrested and secretory detritus accumulated and distended the transplanted tissue.

Graver, intrigued by Bensley's statement that "there is indirect evidence, also, that if duct continuity be established at a sufficiently early period (after ligation), the pancreas might be entirely restored," reinforced the concept that duct-to-lumen continuity was all-important by an experimental protocol in the rabbit.[12] In this protocol the pancreatic duct was ligated, the animal was observed until the pancreatic parenchyma was completely destroyed (as proved by biopsy), and finally the dilated pancreatic duct, transected distal to the point of ligation, was directly introduced and sutured through a slit in the bowel wall. Although the technique was crude, successful reimplantation was achieved in 6 rabbits out of 69 animals in the series. Graver concluded from his results that the rabbit pancreas was a highly plastic organ capable of undergoing structural changes with astonishing rapidity.

Ireneus, in 1941, studied pancreatic regeneration in dogs after experimental pancreatitis was induced by the intrapancreatic ductal injection of 10 mL of sterile bile.[14] Sequential biopsies of the pancreas taken up to 8 weeks after injury disclosed that, following acute pancreatitis, the acinar cells tended to recover both histologically and functionally.

Recent investigations[5,30,32] of experimental pancreatic regeneration have been oriented toward quantitation of the regenerative process[5] and toward precise delineation of secretory recovery.[30,32] Condorelli et al. resected 30% to 50% of the pancreas in 20 dogs.[5] The animals were sacrificed at 5, 15, 30, 60, and 90 days afterward. For the first 2 months no significant changes were noted, but thereafter these investigators observed a progressive increase in the volume of the gland. On microscopic examination regenerative changes were apparent in all portions of the gland, indicating that partial extirpation could stimulate generalized regeneration.

White and Magee studied the effect of varying periods of obstruction upon the exocrine functional capacity, using as parameters the volume, protein output, protease, and amylase content of a 24-hour collection of pancreatic juice from fistulized dogs.[32] Their studies indicated that recovery of pancreatic secretory capacity could occur following pancreatic ductal obstruction for periods up to 10 days. This reversal of obstructive pancreopathy and functional recovery was more precisely described and quantitated by the investigations of Tiscornia et al., who correlated histologic regeneration and recovery of functional capacity in dogs in which the pancreatic ducts had been ligated and transected for periods varying from 1 to 7 weeks, following which ductal continuity had been restored by direct end-to-end microsurgical ductal anastomoses.[30] Sequential biopsies and repeated testings of the maximal exocrine secretory capacity of the pancreas with secretin and pancreozymin indicated that secretory functional return paralleled histologic recovery, that return of exocrine secretion occurred even in glands that had been reduced to disorganized ductal tissue (i.e., even after complete disappearance of acinar tissue), and that in some instances not only was complete maximal secretion attained but regeneration resulted in a statistically significant secretion of fluid, electrolyte, and enzymes greater than that observed prior to ductal obstruction and ductal reconstruction. Complete recovery of secretion was seen only in animals in which pancreatic ductal continuity, as indicated by pancreatography, had been completely successful. In those instances of technical failure, the percentage recovery of secretory capacity could be quantitated with the histologic and anatomic findings.

Widespread application of various ductal decompression procedures, for example, sphincterotomy, caudal pancreaticojejunostomy, and split pancreaticojejunostomy, as therapy for chronic pancreatitis has brought a number of statements without supporting data from various investigators upholding the opinion of Doubilet and Mulholland that relief of pancreatic duct obstruction in humans resulted in histologic regeneration and secretory recovery.[6,13,20,22,24]

Puestow and Gillesby, in 1958, stressed that adequate surgical drainage of the pancreas resulted in pancreatic regeneration to "a degree" and that even the "severe burned-out pancreas" might partially recover.[20]

Thal, in 1959, concluded that early ductal decompression was important and that relief of obstruction protected both islet and acinar tissue. Even in advanced disease, Thal believed that partial return of exocrine secretion might follow a drainage procedure.[24]

Hepp et al. recommended pancreaticointestinal anastomoses without sacrifice of parenchyma to permit as much pancreatic regeneration as possible and stressed early and complete ductal decompression by splitting the main pancreatic duct longitudinally in order to provide adequate drainage of the gland.[13]

In 1963, Silen et al., commenting on their results with longitudinal pancreaticojejunostomy, cited two patients in whom steatorrhea disappeared following ductal decompression.[22] These investigators accepted this observation as evidence of pancreatic secretory recovery. Elmslie (cited by Silen et al.[22]), commenting on these results, described a patient in whom a gradual improvement in the pancreatic response to secretin and pancreozymin was noted in tests done up to 8 weeks after a pancreatic ductal drainage.

Experimental studies of the effect of pancreatic denervation,[6,20] exclusion of pancreatic juice from the duodenum, and/or feeding of trypsin inhibitors to animals have provided additional evidence of pancreatic regeneration. Tiscornia et al. found that there were nervous trophic and antitrophic circuits controlling the weight of the pancreas.[26,27] Interruption of an antitrophic circuit, that is, truncal vagotomy, resulted in significant increase in weight of the pancreas due to parenchymal hypertrophy and hyperplasia. Wormsley et al. reported that the ingestion of a soybean diet containing potent trypsin inhibitors resulted in a twofold increase in pancreatic weight associated with parenchymal hypertrophy, hyperplasia, and frequent mitotic figures.[11,17] There was even significant increase in acinar cell zymogen granules. These observations have been translated into a clinical trial of feeding appropriate trypsin inhibitors to patients following pancreatic resection or pancreatic secretory deficiency due to chronic alcoholic pancreatitis.

More direct evidence of pancreatic regeneration in humans is scattered in the literature, for example,

1. Sequential secretin tests annually over a 10-year period in alcoholics with chronic pancreatitis showed that patients who ceased drinking had a gradual

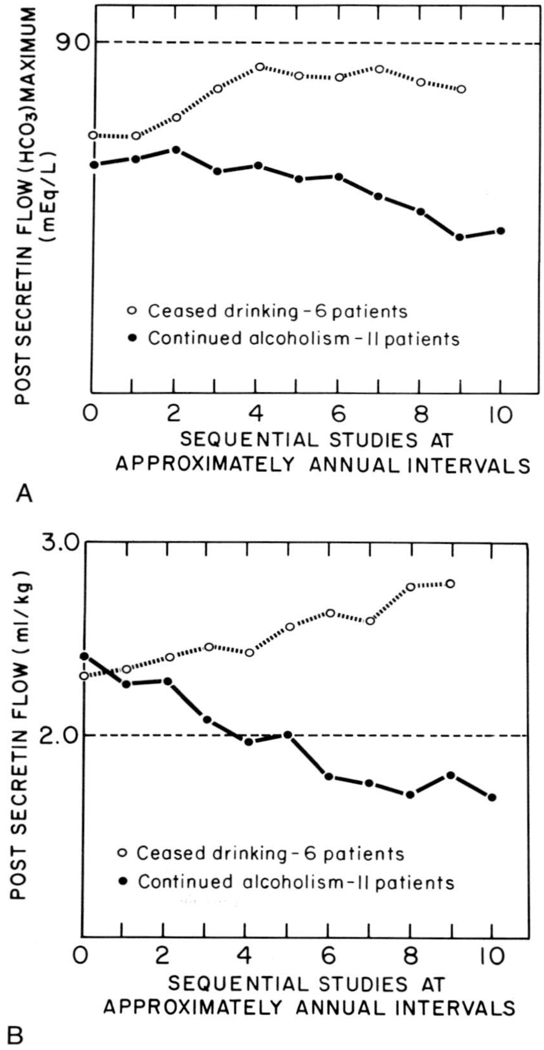

Figure 15-1. Sequential (A) bicarbonate responses and (B) secretin flow of chronic alcoholic patients who did or did not cease drinking.

restoration of secretion while those who did not displayed an inexorable decline in secretion (Fig. 15-1).[7]

2. Sequential secretin tests done before and after an extended DuVal procedure (i.e., resection of the body and tail of the pancreas with retrograde pancreatojejunostomy Roux en Y), and at approximately trimonthly intervals for a period of 2 years, revealed a remarkable restoration of pancreatic secretory capacity in those who ceased drinking. The parameters of secretion, that is, flow and bicarbonate and enzyme secretion, not only returned to preoperative levels but overshot these values and achieved normal ranges (Fig. 15-2).[8] Moreover in those patients in whom sequential endoscopic pancreatography was done, there was an elongation of the main pancreatic duct, often a doubling in length.

3. Surgeons and gastroenterologists have repeatedly observed clinically that 1 year following the discovery at surgery of a hemorrhagic pancreatic necrosis the patient has no steatorrhea or any other symptom of pancreatitis, and pancreatic secretion study shows normal secretory capacity. One remarkable illustration of this phenomenon was observed by one author. A patient was explored for a perforated duodenal ulcer. At surgery, no ulcer was found. Instead the entire pancreas appeared necrotic, and hemorrhage was extensive. The pancreas was palpated by the first assistant. As he withdrew his hand, the entire

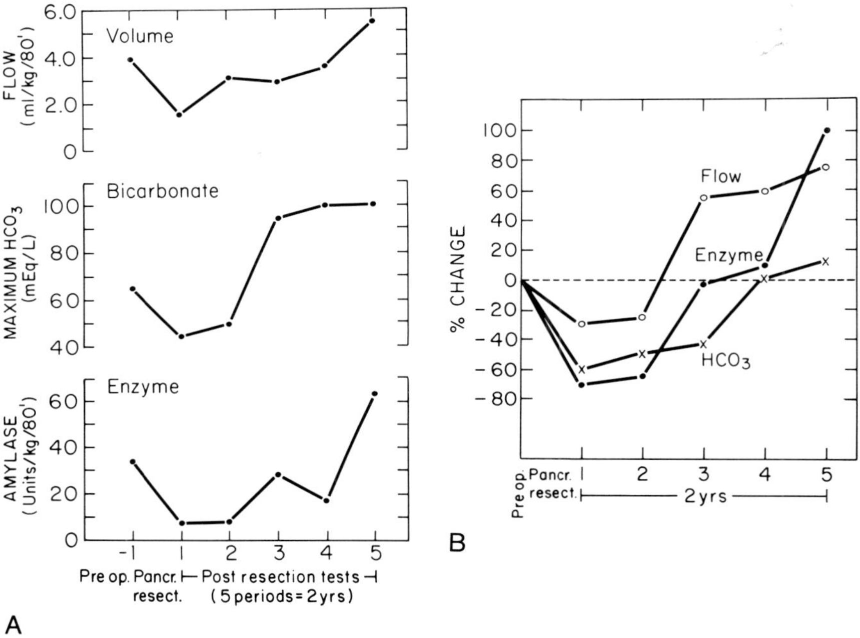

Figure 15-2. Sequential trimonthly secretin test responses of flow, maximum bicarbonate levels, and enzyme levels following extended DuVal distal resection with pancreaticojejunostomy. (A) Absolute data. (B) Percentage change.

TABLE 15-1. SEQUENTIAL SECRETIN TEST STUDIES (1 u/kg i.v.) PANCREATIC FISTULA AND DUODENUM

	Fistula			Duodenum			Combined		
	Flow, cm^3/kg	$[HCO_3]$, meq/L	Amylase, U/kg	Flow, cm^3/kg	$[HCO_3]$, meq/L	Amylase, U/kg	Flow, cm^3/kg	$[HCO_3]$, meq/L	Amylase, U/kg
3 mo	0.2	32	1.0	—	—	—			
6 mo	0.3	54	1.9	—	—	—			
1 yr	0.5	64	2.1	—	—	—			
18 mo	0.6	88	2.5	1.2	90	4.6	1.8	90	7.1
2 yr	—	—	—	—	—	—	2.7	101	19.9
Lower limit normal range							2.0	90	6.0

pancreas appeared to have been evulsed. The duodenal curve and all the major vessels were clearly seen. No pancreatic parenchyma could be identified in the abdomen. Drains were placed to the pancreatic bed and the wound closed. After a stormy course, the patient was discharged with an abdominal tube draining pancreatic juice. The patient returned every 3 months for a period of 2 years for secretin tests on secretion obtained from the pancreatic fistula. The results are given in Table 15-1. For the first year the fistula secretion increased in quality and quantity. At the end of that period a lipiodol fistulogram was done through the tube prior to an attempt to surgically eradicate the pancreaticocutaneous fistula. This revealed the distal duct from which there was an irregular sinus entering the duodenum. Thereupon another secretin test was done with duodenal intubation. After intravenous secretin administration, pancreatic juice was obtained not only from the cutaneous fistula but also from the duodenum. If one added the two responses, the total approached normal ranges. Shortly, thereafter, the cutaneous fistula closed spontaneously. By the end of the second postoperative year the standard secretin test was in normal range and the patient was completely asymptomatic and remained so until lost to follow-up.

Review of the experimental literature appears to support without contradiction that (1) the pancreas has a remarkable ability to regenerate its parenchyma and to recover its exocrine secretory capacity, (2) restoration of duct-to-intestinal continuity or relief of ductal obstruction is important in this regeneration, and (3) regeneration appears to derive from the ductular system and progresses to restoration of acinar tissue and islets.

These data have been taken as the physiologic justification of pancreatic ductal decompression operations in the therapy of chronic pancreatitis, a surgical approach to this disorder that is not only generally practiced but widely accepted. All that remains to absolutely prove the capacity of the pancreas to regenerate under certain conditions is to add sequential pancreatic biopsy to the overwhelming clinical and secretory evidence. It seems clear, however, that pancreatic regeneration is fact not fantasy.

REFERENCES

1. Allen FM. Experimental studies in diabetes. J Metab Res 1:5–41, 1922.
2. Almeida AL, Grossman MI. Experimental production of pancreatitis with ethionine. Gastroenterology 20:554–577, 1952.
3. Bensley RR. Studies on the pancreas of the guinea pig. Am J Anat 12:297–388, 1910.
4. Carraro A. Sulla rigenerazione del pancreas. Sperimentale 64:937–949, 1910.
5. Condorelli A, Mancuso M, Ricceri R. Experimental study of the regenerative capacity of the pancreas after partial resection of the gland. Policlinico (Chir) 70:163–180, 1963.
6. Doubilet H, Mulholland JH. Eight year study of pancreatitis and sphincterotomy. JAMA 160:521–528, 1956.
7. Dreiling DA, Bordalo O. Secretory patterns in minimal pancreatic pathologies. Am J Gastroenterol 60:60–69, 1973.
8. Dreiling DA, Bordalo O. A toxic metabolic hypothesis of pathogenesis of alcoholic pancreatitis. Alcoholism 1:293–299, 1977.
9. Feldman M, Dreiling DA, Paulino A III, Schaffner F, Janowitz HD. Effect of D-L-ethionine on electrolyte secretion of the pancreas. Am J Physiol 205:878–884, 1963.

10. Fisher NF. Regeneration of pancreas from pancreatic duct. JAMA 83:502–503, 1924.
11. Folsch UR, Winckler K, Wormsley KG. Effect of a soybean diet on enzyme content and ultrastructure of the rat exocrine pancreas. Digestion 11:161–171, 1974.
12. Graver TP. Regeneration in the pancreas of the rabbit. Proc Inst Med Chig 6:80–82, 1926.
13. Hepp J, Mercadier M, Moreaux J. Operative methods in surgical treatment of chronic pancreatitis. Acta Gastroenterol Belg 23:471–510, 1960.
14. Ireneus C Jr. Experimental bile pancreatitis (with special reference to recovery and to the toxicity of the hemorrhagic exudate). Arch Surg 42:126–140, 1941.
15. Kyrle J. Uber die Regenerationsvorgange im tierischen Pankreas. Arch Mikrosk Anat 725:141–160, 1908.
16. Laguesse MME, Gontier de la Roche A. Les ilots de Langerhans dans pancreas du cobaye apres ligature. C R Soc Biol (Paris) 54:854–856, 1902.
17. McGuinness EE, Morgan CH, Levison DA, et al. The effects of long-term feeding of soya flour on the rat pancreas. Scand J Gastroenterol 15:497–502, 1980.
18. Parker F Jr. Toxic necrosis and regeneration of the acinar cells of the pancreas. J Med Res 40:471–476, 1919.
19. Popper H, Schaffner F. Liver Structure and Function. Blakiston Division, New York, McGraw-Hill, 1957.
20. Puestow CB, Gillesby WJ. Retrograde surgical drainage of the pancreas for chronic relapsing pancreatitis. AMA Arch Surg 76:898–907, 1958.
21. Shaw JW, Latimer EO. Regeneration of pancreatic tissue from the transplanted pancreatic duct in the dog. Am J Physiol 76:49–53, 1926.
22. Silen W, Baldwin J, Goldman L. Treatment of chronic pancreatitis by longitudinal pancreaticojejunostomy. Am J Surg 106:243–258, 1963.
23. Sobolew LW. Zur normalen und pathologischen Morphologie der innerer Sekretin Bauchspeicheldruse. Virchows Arch Pathol Anat 168:191–194, 1902.
24. Thal AP. Surgery of the pancreatic ducts. Minn Med 42:119–122, 1959.
25. Tiberti N. Intorno alla rigenerazione del pancreas. Arch Fisiol 5:258–260, 1907.
26. Tiscornia OM, Dreiling DA. Chronic truncal vagotomy: Its effect on weight and function of the rat pancreas. Mt Sinai J Med 48:295–305, 1981.
27. Tiscornia OM, Celener D, Cresta MA, et al. Trophic and antitrophic circuits controlling pancreatic weight in the rat. Mt Sinai J Med 53:343–355, 1986.
28. Tiscornia OM, Dreiling DA, Kark AE. The effect of hypophysectomy on canine pancreatic secretion. Surgery 60:883–890, 1966.
29. Tiscornia OM, Hansky J, Janowitz HD, Dreiling DA. The adrenal cortex and external pancreatic secretion in the dog. Mt Sinai J Med 32:551–555, 1965.
30. Tiscornia OM, Jacobson JH II, Dreiling DA. Microsurgery of the canine pancreatic duct; experimental study and review of previous approaches to the management of pancreatic duct pathology. Surgery 58:58–72, 1964.
31. Tiscornia OM, Janowitz HD, Dreiling DA. The effect of alloxan upon canine exocrine pancreatic secretion. Am J Gastroenterol 49:328–340, 1968.
32. White TT, Magee DF. Recovery of pancreatic exocrine function after controlled duct obstruction. Surg Gynecol Obstet 114:463–466, 1962.

CHAPTER

16

ALCOHOL- AND NON-ALCOHOL-INDUCED PANCREATITIS: CLINICAL ASPECTS

Rudolf W. Ammann

EDITORIAL COMMENTS (Chapters 16 and 17)

Dr. Ammann stresses the difficulties with the current pathologic classification of pancreatitis in that it can be almost impossible to decide between acute and chronic in the early stages of the disease. Only long-term follow-up may eventually allow differentiation. The author somewhat confuses the terminology by using such terms as *acute (reversible) pancreatitis* and *chronic (progressive) pancreatitis*. Furthermore, it is claimed that pathologists are unable to determine postacute from chronic progressive changes and that this may explain the discrepancy in incidence of chronic pancreatitis at autopsy compared with the low clinical rate. There are three new concepts proposed by the author in advance of the main crux of the paper (i.e., the difference in natural history between alcohol-induced and non-alcohol-induced chronic pancreatitis): (1) two peaks of idiopathic pancreatitis, a juvenile peak and the more senile peak, idiopathic senile chronic pancreatitis, (2) the relationship of chronic pancreatitis to analgesic abuse, and (3) the disappearance of calcification in long-standing chronic pancreatitis, which might decrease the incidence of calcific pancreatitis, that is, postcalcific pancreatitis.

The major differences between alcohol-induced and non-alcohol-induced chronic pancreatitis in the author's series are:

1. The less rapid progression to exocrine insufficiency in non-alcohol-induced chronic pancreatitis.

2. A greater disassociation between exocrine and endocrine insufficiency.

3. Different patterns of correlation of calcification to the length of disease. Most of the non-alcohol-induced chronic pancreatitis group had no pain, and we do not really know when the disease started.

4. Differences in the incidences of pain and pain relief with the progression of the disease between the two groups.

5. Differences in complications, surgery, and extrapancreatic carcinoma rates between the two groups.

All these might indeed suggest that there may be morphologic, genetic, and ultrastructural differences between the two groups, and indeed it is probably true that in alcohol-induced chronic pancreatitis there are more inflammatory cells and perineural fibrosis. However, most of the studies appear to be similar, and it remains to be seen whether any differences in any of these factors will be found in the various groups (particularly alcohol-induced, idiopathic, and tropical chronic pancreatitis). One of the problems with the author's definitions is that diabetes is regarded only as overt diabetes rather than abnormal glucose tolerance or abnormalities in insulin secretion and exocrine insufficiency by decreased chymotrypsin in the stool and not by pancreatic function studies. Lastly, the author appears to have challenged the concept that the mortality from chronic pancreatitis may be related to socioeconomic differences and that there is an almost uniform 50% or more mortality within 10 to 12 years after diagnosis in different series from various parts of the world.

The masterly pathophysiologic studies over the years by Dr. Sarles and his group have included the demonstration of pancreatic protein hypersecretion in chronic alcoholic patients, the concept of intraductal protein deposition, the demonstration of the stabilizer of calcium precipitation either in the ducts or around the protein plugs, and more recently, the demonstration of a number of pancreatic stone protein glycoproteins that may prevent calcium deposition. The studies have been instrumental in our understanding of the various forms of pancreatitis, in particular alcohol-induced calcifying pancreatitis. More recently, the protein precipitates and stones have come under some beautiful scanning electron microscopic and stereoscopic structural studies by various Japanese groups and Dr. C.S. Pitchumoni in New York. In all these studies, scant reference is made to the effect of volume of flow of pancreatic juice, which may also be important in stone formation.

There are a few interesting factors related to the whole concept of calcifying pancreatitis: (1) Although a high level of alcohol consumption is usual in these patients, there is increasing evidence that individual sensitivity to alcohol may be important (genetic? level of pancreatic stone protein? flow rates?) leading to the interesting statement in Dr. Sarles's paper that "definition by some arbitrary alcohol consumption is impossible." If this is so, then the categorization of patients into alcoholic or nonalcoholic groups would require that even patients with seemingly little alcohol intake, that is, from 1 to 20 g/day, might have to be considered to have alcohol-induced pancreatitis, and even "social" drinkers might not be protected from alcohol pancreatitis. (2) With regard to dietary factors in alcohol-induced pancreatitis, we now have a wide spectrum of hypotheses from increased fat and protein consumption in affluent countries to low intakes in poorer countries, thus again suggesting that some dietary influence on genetic factors and pancreatic stone proteins, and so forth, may increase susceptibility to the disease. (3) These studies still leave unanswered the vexing problem in all alcoholic disease, namely, disease expression between groups or individuals drinking equal quantities of alcohol. Is this related to acquired damage to cells producing pancreatic stone protein or a genetic low level of pancreatic stone protein in certain individuals who respond with calcifying chronic pancreatitis to a variety of etiologic factors? These may include alcohol or other genetic factors, for example, HLA type, blood groups, abnormalities in transcription genes in the ability to form fibrosis, and so forth. (4) Lastly, to date, it does appear as though the histologic pattern, pancreatic stone protein levels, chemical abnormalities, and intraductal changes are similar in all groups of calcifying chronic pancreatitis. However, Dr. Sarles concedes that this may need further study, especially in the light of the differences in disease patterns shown by Dr. Ammann. At present, however, these abnormalities appear to be the same whether the disease is alcohol-induced, nutritional, or a tropical pancreatitis (NATP, idiopathic calcifying chronic pancreatitis), or even has one of the metabolic causes.

CONTROVERSY

The pathology of calcific pancreatitis has generally been regarded as similar whether the cause is alcohol, idiopathic, familial, or nonalcoholic tropical. Clinically, the various types have also been considered to be similar in their expression. With rapid advances in pathogenesis and improved methods of assessing function, it was thought timely to reexamine the possible differences that may exist in the various etiologic forms of chronic pancreatitis.

Definitions play a major role in the controversies about pancreatitis. According to the new classification, two types of pancreatitis are distinguished: acute and chronic pancreatitis.[24] The chief dilemma in clinical practice is the inability to discriminate acute and chronic pancreatitis in the early course of the disease because (1) there is broad overlap in the clinical spectrum of acute and chronic pancreatitis in the early years after onset and (2) no reliable morphologic routine method is available (comparable to liver biopsy) for direct evaluation of the structural changes of the pancreas.[5,19,29,35] The modern imaging and function tests have so far not solved this major diagnostic problem.

Acute and chronic pancreatitis can be distinguished, however, based upon the typical long-term profile into acute (reversible) pancreatitis and chronic (progressive) pancreatitis (CP) (Fig. 16-1).[5] The typical markers of chronic pancreati-

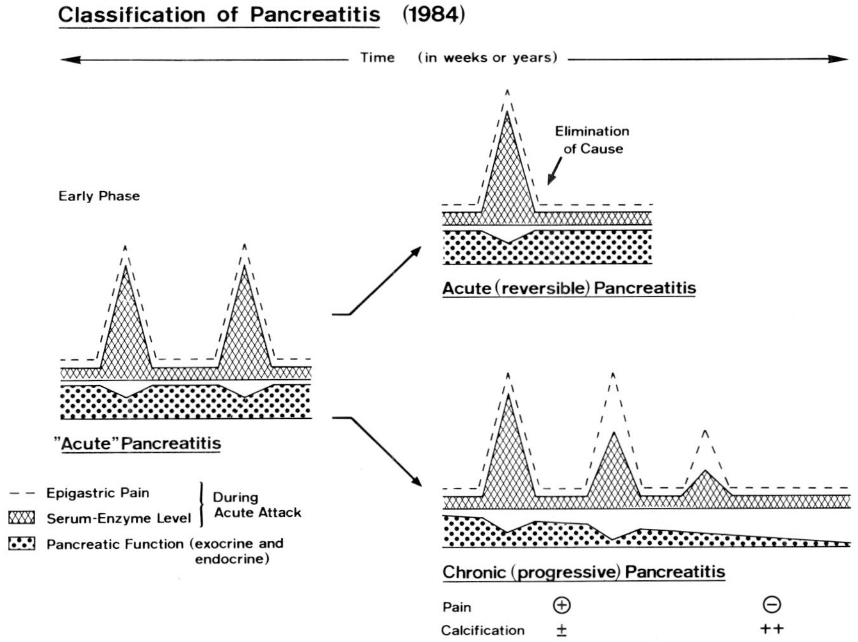

Figure 16-1. Clinical classification of pancreatitis based upon the new definitions of Marseilles.[23] Acute (reversible) and chronic (progressive) pancreatitis are characterized by identical episodes of "acute" pancreatitis in the early phase; they differ, however, by a distinct long-term profile. In chronic (progressive) pancreatitis, progressive pancreatic dysfunction with or without pancreatic calcification develops about 5.5 years after onset, and with advancing disease CP becomes "secondarily" painless. Primary painless CP lacks the early phase of recurrent "acute" pancreatitis.

tis, e.g., pancreatic calcification and/or progressive exocrine and endocrine insufficiency, become apparent on the average 5.5 years after onset of pancreatitis.[3,5,6] In clinical practice, the long-term monitoring of both pancreatic function and structure from onset of pancreatitis is the only reliable method for a definite classification (or exclusion) of chronic pancreatitis (CP) (except in advanced CP, which can be diagnosed at once).

Differences in the terminology of pancreatitis between clinicians and pathologists are responsible for many controversies in the literature. The clinical interpretation of "acute" pancreatitis (based primarily upon clinical and laboratory evidences) (Fig. 16-1) should not be confounded with acute pancreatitis according to the clinical-morphologic definition of Marseilles, since identical episodes of "acute" pancreatitis are commonly observed in early phases of acute (reversible) and chronic (progressive) pancreatitis (Fig. 16-1). Similarly, the term *chronic pancreatitis* as used by the pathologist (or by endoscopists) does not necessarily correspond to the clinical entity of chronic (progressive) pancreatitis, particularly because postacute morphologic changes, for example, fibrosis, pseudocysts, and ductal alterations, may persist following severe acute (reversible) pancreatitis.[3,19,23,24] Postacute morphologic changes remain stationary (like scars), while pancreatic function recovers. That is in contrast to the dynamic progressive evolution of dysfunction and morphology typically observed in CP, as documented by long-term studies of CP.[1,3,6] Thus morphologic alterations in pancreatography must be interpreted with caution in terms of CP as long as pancreatic function is not impaired permanently.[3] The same holds true for histopathologic findings. The inability of the pathologist to discriminate postacute and chronic (progressive) pancreatitis[14] (except in advanced CP) explains in part the marked discrepancy in the prevalence of chronic pancreatitis, which is 0.2% to 15% in unselected autopsy series[5,14,17] compared with 0.01% to 0.12% in clinical series.[5,29,39,40] The special type of "obstructive chronic pancreatitis"[24] with a typical morphologic pattern as seen in patients with outflow obstruction (mainly secondary to periampullary tumors) will not be considered here for the same reason. The patients with "obstructive CP" should be classified clinically according to the cause of obstruction (e.g., mainly tumors), particularly because the clinical-biological long-term evolution of "obstructive pancreatitis" corresponds as a rule to acute (reversible) pancreatitis following surgical relief of the obstruction.[24,35]

Etiologically, CP (in the temporate zone) can be divided into two main groups: alcoholic and nonalcoholic CP. The nonalcoholic type comprises a large group of cases of unknown origin (idiopathic CP) and a rather small group due to rare causes. In Table 16-1, the etiology in our personal series of 287 cases with CP is summarized. In tropical countries of Africa and Asia, nutritional CP is a special entity of the nonalcoholic type as reviewed recently.[33] It will not be considered here.

No sharp line of demarcation exists between alcoholic and nonalcoholic CP. The incidence of nonalcoholic CP in large series ranges between 10% and 30%, the lower figures being found in countries where alcohol intake is ubiquitous and vice versa.[12,40] According to Sarles et al., the risk of CP increases logarithmically with the mean daily intake of alcohol, and no statistical threshold for minimal alcohol toxicity seems to exist.[35] In previous studies, Sarles et al. noted a mean

TABLE 16-1. ETIOLOGY OF CHRONIC PANCREATITIS*

Alcoholic CP (AICP)		205	(71%)
Non-alcoholic CP (NAICP)		82	(29%)
Idiopathic-juvenile CP (IJCP)	15		
Idiopathic-senile CP (ISCP)	49		
Heredity	3		
Hyperparathyroidism	5		
Trauma	2		
Chronic analgesic abuse	6		
Miscellaneous	2		
Total		287	

* From Ammann et al.[1]

intake of 158 (50–450) g of alcohol in CP compared with 76 (0–208) g in acute (reversible) pancreatitis (38 of 70 due to gallstones) and with 65 (0–285) g in a control population of Marseilles.[37] Thus it is evident that in a place like Marseilles, most patients with acute (reversible) pancreatitis fulfill theoretically the criteria of alcoholic pancreatitis (alcohol intake above zero). However, in most series of alcoholic CP, the mean daily alcohol intake is above 50 to 80 g.[5,12,21,22,28,31,34]

ETIOLOGY AND OUTCOME OF PANCREATITIS

Gallstones and chronic alcohol abuse are the two leading etiologic factors of pancreatitis. In the comments to the classification of Marseilles[24] it was stated that it was not then possible to attribute a special clinical and morphologic entity to a distinct cause (except for "obstructive CP"). Most experts will, however, agree that cholelithiasis is a major factor for acute (reversible) pancreatitis and that gallstone pancreatitis virtually never progresses to CP.[21,38]

Alcoholic CP may be associated with gallstones on the average in 6% (0%–17%) of patients,[5,34] particularly because (1) the high prevalence of cholelithiasis in the general population enhances the chance of coincidence and (2) secondary gallstone formation is a common phenomenon in CP associated with long-standing extrahepatic cholestasis.[5]

The role of alcohol abuse on the evolution of pancreatitis is less well defined. Most experts believe that "acute" alcoholic pancreatitis occurs regularly on the basis of preexisting clinically latent CP.[3] This hypothesis is based mainly on indirect evidence, particularly the facts that (1) CP in industrialized countries is predominantly due to alcohol abuse, (2) alcoholic "acute" pancreatitis occurs with a background of heavy alcohol intake over an average period of 10 years or longer,[37] and (3) marked functional and/or morphologic changes in the pancreas are found in a high percentage of asymptomatic patients with chronic alcoholism.[3,5]

Increasing evidence has been presented recently indicating that alcoholic pancreatitis in some instance does not progress to CP. Over the last 10 years, in a prospective study of 144 patients with alcoholic "acute" pancreatitis, it has been shown that two thirds of the cases progressed to CP, whereas about one third of the cases did not.[3] This latter group showed the typical long-term course of acute (reversible) pancreatitis.[3] Interestingly nonprogression of alcoholic pancreatitis occurred in 16 of 49 cases despite continued severe alcohol abuse, which is at variance with observations from South Africa.[12] However, the fact that alcohol is not the only causative factor in CP and that only a small proportion of chronic alcoholic patients develops CP is consistent with our observations. Furthermore in a recent large autopsy study of acute pancreatitis, histopathologic evidence of CP was absent in the alcoholic group in 131 of 247 cases (54%).[34] Thus the predictive value of the alcohol cause on the evolution of pancreatitis is challenged in the recent literature and has to be clarified by additional studies. In the following discussion only CP will be considered.

EPIDEMIOLOGY OF CP

The incidence of CP varies in different geographic regions, but no precise data on epidemiology are available. In a recent review of epidemiologic data of more than 40 publications (comprising over 7000 cases of CP from Europe or America), Worning found a nearly 10-fold increase in CP over the last 25 years (increase of incidence from 1.5 to 12.5 cases per 100,000 inhabitants per year).[39] For Japan, Sato calculated in 1974 an incidence of 1.45 per 100,000 per year,[39] a figure that corresponds very closely to the incidence in Zurich (1971–1982) of 1.64,[4] but which is markedly lower than that at the Mayo Clinic, with an incidence of 3.5 (1950–1969).[29]

In accordance with the data of Worning,[39] the incidence of CP in Zurich has increased about 10-fold over the last 25 years, particularly CP due to alcohol abuse.[4] In the same period the ratio of male to female patients with alcoholic CP remained constant (10 : 1) and the mean age (at onset) slightly decreased from 42.7 ± 13.9 (1953–1962) to 39.9 ± 7.2 years (1973–1982). The percentage of calcific CP cases in the series increased from 67% (1953–1962) to 85% (1973–1982).[4]

A close correlation between the average alcohol consumption and the incidence of CP has been postulated.[35,36,39,40] No close linear relationship between alcohol consumption and the incidence of CP is found in Switzerland. The highest consumption of alcohol occurred around 1900, with 40 g of pure alcohol per day and per person (over 15 years); it dropped to about 20 g/day at the end of World War II and increased steadily since 1950 to about 30 g/day in 1980.[4] Additional factors, particularly improvement in diagnosis, seem to be responsible for the 10-fold increase in incidence of CP in Switzerland over the last 25 years. Interestingly, alcoholic liver cirrhosis in Switzerland is about 30 times more frequent than alcoholic CP.[4] As noted by many experts with large series, CP is associated with liver cirrhosis in less than 10% (2%–9.9%) of chronic alcoholic patients.[5]

Alcoholic noncirrhotic liver disease, particularly alcoholic hepatitis, is, however, observed in over 20% of cases in the course of alcoholic CP.[16]

THE NATURAL HISTORY OF NONALCOHOLIC (IDIOPATHIC) AND ALCOHOLIC CHRONIC PANCREATITIS

Alcohol-induced CP (AICP) and non-alcohol-induced CP (NAICP) have many features in common, particularly the progressive exocrine and endocrine insufficiency and the high incidence of pancreatic calcification.[1] However, marked differences seem to exist between AICP and NAICP, in particular in regard to age distribution and clinical features (e.g., high incidence of primary painless forms in NAICP). In addition a disproportionate and delayed progression of pancreatic dysfunction and pancreatic morphology in NAICP compared with AICP seems to exist.[1] Many of the controversies in the literature about definition, diagnosis, and therapy of CP may be related in part to differences in the natural history of AICP and NAICP, which have not been appreciated in the past.

Clinical Features

The relevant clinical data in our series of AICP and NAICP are summarized in Table 16-2.

Nonalcoholic CP comprises a rather heterogenous group of patients (Tables 16-1 and 16-2). A small number of patients have CP due to various (rare) causes like heredity, trauma, hyperparathyroidism, and so forth (Table 16-1). Based upon the age distribution, the large group of idiopathic CP seems to be composed of two different populations, one with a peak around 25 years (termed accordingly idiopathic juvenile CP, IJCP)[11] and the other with a peak around 65 years (termed accordingly idiopathic senile CP, ISCP)[7,10] (Fig. 16-2) as reported previously.[1,4,6,7,10,11] A relationship between the latter form and pancreatic lithiasis observed with increasing frequency in autopsy series of very old people (4.2% at age 70 and 16.9% at 90 years) appears probable.[7,31] The age distribution of AICP in our series shows a peak around 35 (Fig. 16-3).

Primary painless forms are very common in ISCP in contrast to IJCP (Table 16-2). Common to both forms of idiopathic CP is the prevalence of male patients

TABLE 16-2. PERTINENT CLINICAL DATA ON AICP AND NAICP

	n	Calcific CP, %	Sex, % M	Sex, % F	Age at Diagnosis (Range) Median	ppCP,* %
AICP	205	85	91	9	42.5 (26–72)	4.9
NAICP	82	77	80	20		53.7
Subgroups*						
IJCP	15	93	87	13	32.0 (9–50)	0
ISCP	49	69	88	12	65.8 (44–75)	69.4
Rare causes	18	83	56	44	46.0 (16–78)	55.6

* IJCP = idiopathic juvenile CP; ISCP = idiopathic senile CP; ppCP = primary painless CP.

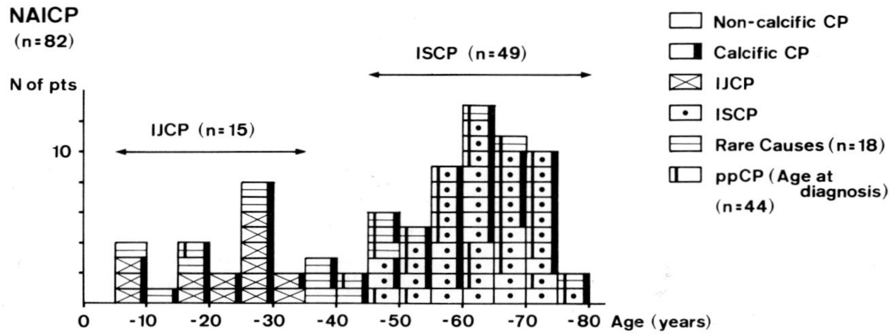

Figure 16-2. Idiopathic CP shows a typical age distribution with two peaks suggesting two cohorts of patients. One, IJCP ($n = 15$), has a peak around 25 years compared with ISCP ($n = 49$), with a peak around 65 years. The age distribution of CP due to rare causes ($n = 18$) is also indicated.

and the high incidence of calcification (Table 16-2). Chronic renal failure associated with CP has been discussed repeatedly in the past.[25] In recent studies evidence has been presented for a relationship between CP and chronic analgesic abuse (associated with analgesic nephropathy). In a prospective study of 95 cases with chronic renal failure, 53 had a history of chronic analgesic abuse and 42 had a

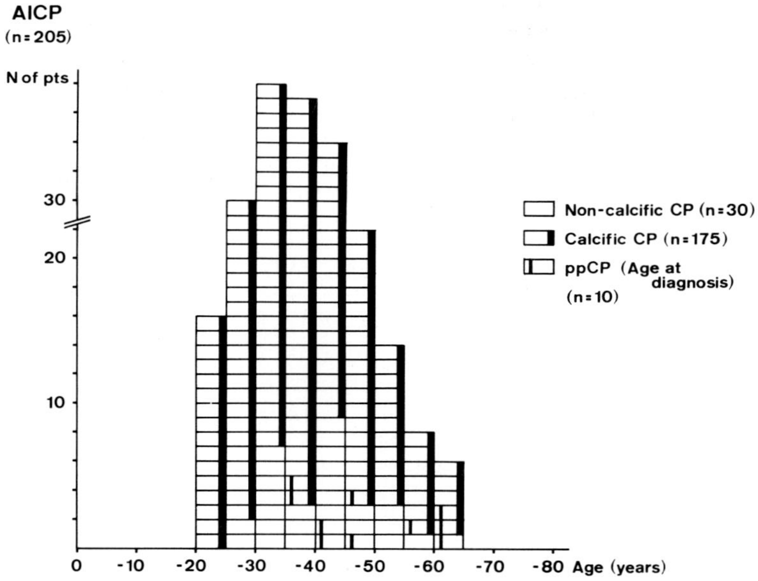

Figure 16-3. Alcoholic CP ($n = 205$) shows an age peak (at onset) of around 35 years.

nephropathy of other origin (control group). Evidence of CP, in particular pancreatic calcification, was present in 6 of the 53 cases with analgesic abuse (11%), but in none of the control group.[24]

The high incidence of primary painless CP is a very characteristic clinical feature of NAICP compared with AICP (Table 16-2), particularly in the two subgroups of ISCP (69.4%) and CP due to rare causes (55.6%). Gross pancreatic insufficiency, for example, diarrhea or steatorrhea, weight loss, and/or diabetes, are the leading clinical symptoms of primary painless CP. The first classic description of painless CP was published in 1956 by Bartholomew LG and Comfort MW, and the problem was reviewed in 1972[18] and 1976.[10] Primary painless CP has many features in common with ISCP, particularly onset at an age over 50 years, prevalence in males, high incidence of calcification, and the rare association with alcohol abuse.[10,18] We have therefore postulated that painless CP is not a nosologic entity but a syndrome that is commonly seen in ISCP but that may rarely occur in AICP and also in CP due to other causes.[10]

Exocrine and Endocrine Function in AICP and NAICP

Chronic pancreatitis is a dynamic process with progressive evolution of morphologic changes and exocrine dysfunction in relation to duration of CP. Therefore, for the evaluation of the natural history of CP, the time course from onset (or from diagnosis) has to be taken into account. In a recent study the natural history of AICP has been analyzed in relation to duration of pancreatitis from onset.[6] For evaluation and comparison of the natural history of AICP and NAICP, duration of CP from the time of diagnosis was considered because of the high incidence of patients with primary painless CP in the group of NAICP (with unknown onset of pancreatitis).[1]

Both AICP and NAICP showed a progressive deterioration of pancreatic function with duration of CP (Fig. 16-4). However, marked differences in the natural history of NAICP compared with AICP exist particularly in four aspects: (1) less rapid progression of dysfunction in NAICP, (2) dissociation in the covariation of exocrine and endocrine dysfunction, (3) differences in the correlation between onset of calcification and pancreatic exocrine insufficiency, and (4) differences in the relationship between lasting pain relief and pancreatic dysfunction.

Most experts agree that progressive pancreatic dysfunction is a characteristic feature of CP, especially in AICP,[5,6,12,15,23,29,30,36] but there is no general agreement on this issue.[26,40] Differences in the tempos of progression of exocrine insufficiency from diagnosis in AICP and NAICP were noted[1] (Fig. 16-4). The frequency of marked exocrine insufficiency (fecal chymotrypsin < 40 μg/g) was, for instance, 80% at 4 years in AICP compared with 10 years in NAICP (Fig. 16-4). A slower rate in progression of exocrine insufficiency in NAICP (compared with AICP) has also been observed in other series.[29,32] Thus it seems likely that in series comprising a high percentage of patients with NAICP (followed over a short period), no marked progression of pancreatic dysfunction in relation to duration of CP becomes evident. The high percentage of patients with NAICP

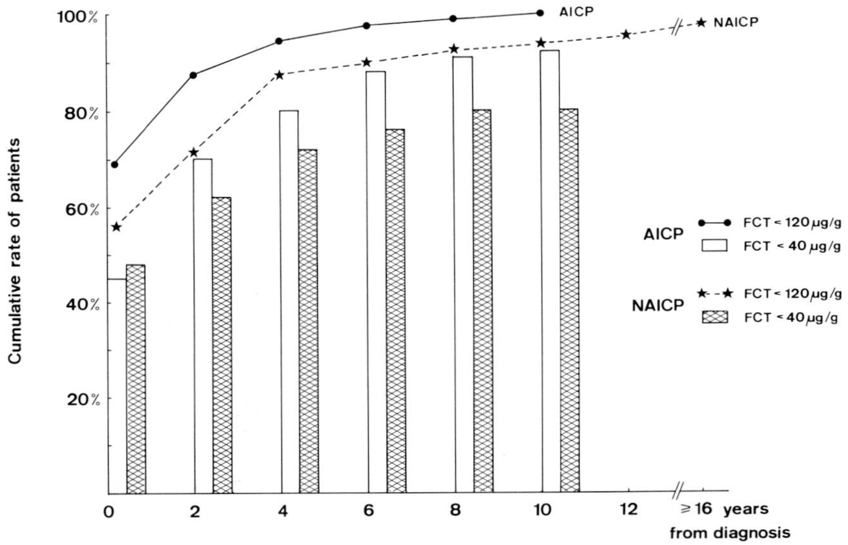

Figure 16-4. The rate of progression of exocrine insufficiency in relation to duration of CP (from diagnosis) differs in AICP and NAICP. FCT = fecal chymotrypsin test (pathological < 120 μg/g). The bars indicate the percentage of cases with marked exocrine insufficiency (FCT < 40 μg/g). The frequency of marked exocrine insufficiency was 80% at 4 years in AICP compared with 10 years in NAICP.

(45% of 127 patients) in the series of Kondo et al.[26] and the rather short follow-up (less than 5 years in 46% of cases) seem to confirm this assumption.

Interaction of Exocrine and Endocrine Insufficiency

A progressive increase in endocrine insufficiency in close association with both (1) progressive exocrine insufficiency and (2) duration of CP is typically found in AICP.[3,5,6,9,13] Onset of diabetes in NAICP is markedly delayed compared with AICP (Fig. 16-5). In AICP less than 50% of patients with marked exocrine insufficiency (fecal chymotrypsin < 40 μg/g) for ≥2 years are nondiabetic. On the contrary in NAICP, over 50% of patients with marked exocrine insufficiency for 8 to 10 years are still nondiabetic.[1]

Marks et al. have stated that overt diabetes usually precedes steatorrhea by 2 to 10 years in alcoholic CP.[30] This observation is at variance with our experience. In patients without diabetes, steatorrhea has been documented in 56.5% (AICP) (u = 65; 38 of them severe) and 80.4% (NAICP) (u = 37; 33 of them severe), respectively (Table 16-3). Particularly interesting is the high percentage of nondiabetic patients (67%–77%) in NAICP with mild to severe steatorrhea (while in AICP only 42% of patients with severe steatorrhea were nondiabetic) (Table 16-3). Other investigators have noted a more marked islet cell dysfunction in

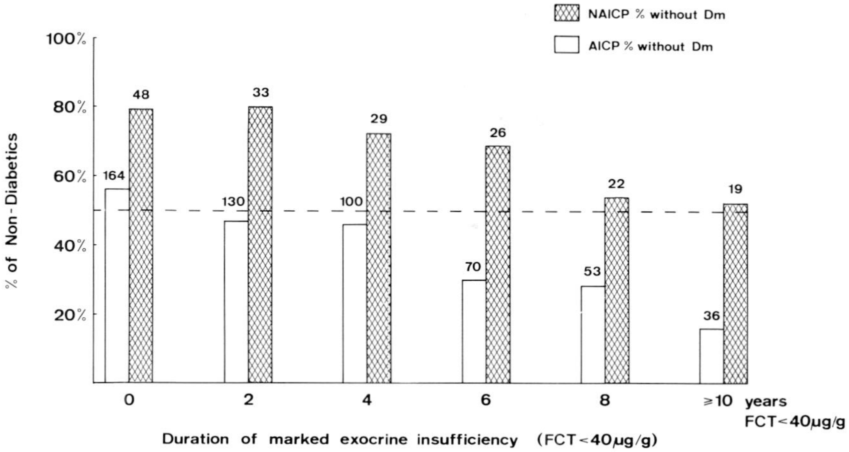

Figure 16-5. Covariation of exocrine and endocrine insufficiency; percentage of nondiabetic patients in relation to duration of marked exocrine insufficiency (FCT < 40 µg/g). (The number of cases at risk is indicated on the top of the bars.) In AICP, less than 50% of the patients were nondiabetic within 2 years of marked exocrine insufficiency. In NAICP over 50% of the patients were still nondiabetic with marked exocrine insufficiency for 10 years or longer. (From Ammann et al.[1] with permission.)

AICP than in NAICP.[21,29] The disproportionate progression of exocrine and endocrine dysfunction in NAICP is at present unexplained. As pointed out by Bank, studies performed to date do not appear to show marked differences in morphology, pancreatic secretion, and/or pancreatic stone protein (PSP) levels between AICP and NAICP.[12] Morphometric studies of the relationship between exocrine

TABLE 16-3. RELATIONSHIP BETWEEN STEATORRHEA AND DIABETES

	Total	Diabetes			
		Present		Absent	
	n	*n*	%	*n*	%
Group A: AICP (no. of cases: 137)					
Steatorrhea					
Absent (0–7 g)	64	14	21.9	50	78.1
Mild (8–15 g)	50	23	46.0	27	54.0
Severe (>16 g)	91	53	58.2	38	41.8
Total number of estimations	205	90		115	
Group B: NAICP (no. of cases: 58)					
Steatorrhea					
Absent (0–7 g)	12	3	25	9	75
Mild (8–15 g)	6	2	33	4	67
Severe (>16 g)	43	10	23.3	33	76.7
Total number of estimations	61	15		46	

and endocrine tissue in NAICP compared with AICP would be very interesting. It should be noted that the "disproportionate steatorrhea" commonly observed in NAICP is comparable to the well-known clinical situation in cystic fibrosis that is characterized by the rare occurrence of diabetes despite severe pancreatic steatorrhea.[1]

Evolution and Regression of Pancreatic Calcification in Relation to Exocrine Insufficiency

The relationship between pancreatic calcification and pancreatic dysfunction is debated,[6,13,27] and a recent publication emphasized that pancreatic calcifications are not indicative of severe exocrine insufficiency.[27] As shown in Fig. 16-6, there is a steep increase in exocrine insufficiency from about 23% before to over 90% within 2 years of onset of calcification in AICP.[1] These figures together with previous results[6] and observations reported by others[13,30] indicate a rather close correlation between exocrine insufficiency and pancreatic calcification in AICP. In NAICP the correlation of the two features is less marked, since onset of calcification preceded exocrine insufficiency in 40% of patients by 13 years or longer (Fig. 16-6). These data suggest that the evolution of exocrine insufficiency and pancreatic calcifications is less closely correlated in NAICP. In the series of Lankisch et al.,[27] 27 of 79 cases (34.2%) had NAICP, and this fact may explain in part the discrepancy of results. On the other hand in a series of the Mayo Clinic, only 27% of patients with NAICP showed pancreatic calcifications and onset of calcification was significantly delayed in NAICP compared with AICP,[29] which is at variance with our experience.

Some very recent results complicate the issue of pancreatic calcification. It is generally believed that pancreatic calcifications increase progressively with

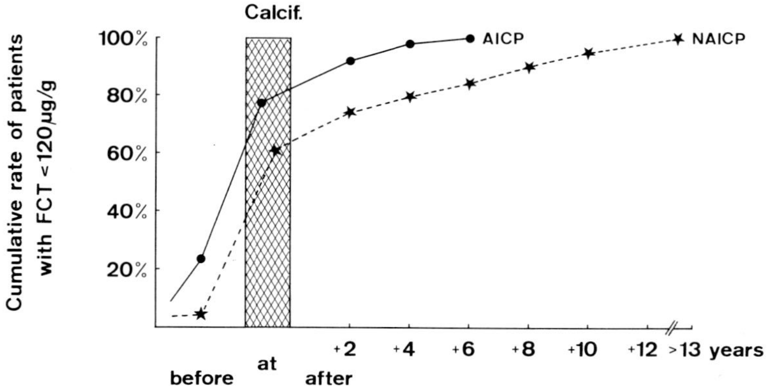

Figure 16-6. Onset of calcification (time 0) in relation to exocrine insufficiency (FCT < 120 μg/g). In AICP, around 90% of cases had exocrine insufficiency within 2 years from onset of calcification. In NAICP, pancreatic calcification preceded exocrine insufficiency in about 40% of cases for up to 13 years or longer. (From Ammann et al.[1] with permission.)

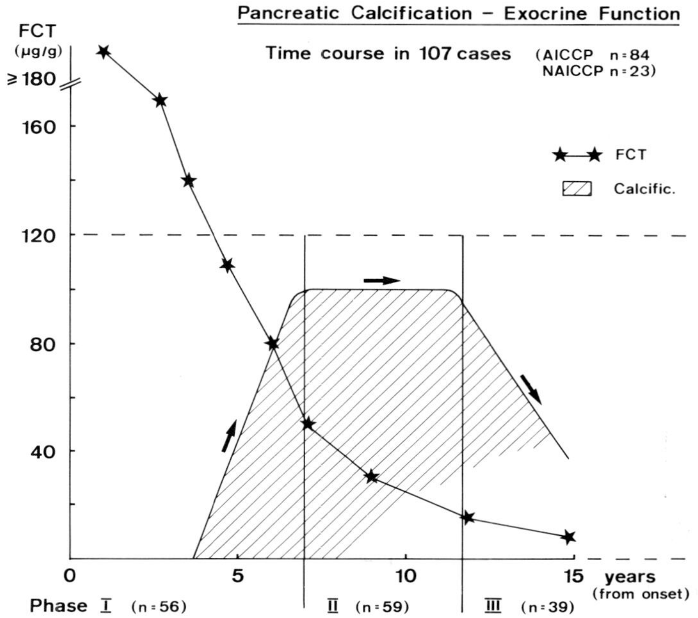

Figure 16-7. Scheme of evolution of pancreatic calcification in relation to duration of CP from onset (107 cases with AICP or NAICP with documented calcification in three or more film series over ≥4 years). In about 50% of cases an initial increase of calcification (phase I) was documented, and about 50% of cases showed stationary calcification (phase II). Dissolution of pancreatic calcification was observed in around 35% of cases in the late phase of CP (phase III) in association with progressive exocrine insufficiency. (From Ammann et al.[1] with permission.)

advancing CP. However, in both AICP and NAICP, regression of pancreatic calcification has been observed in about 30% to 40% of patients, particularly in advanced CP and in patients after longitudinal pancreaticojejunostomy, despite severe and progressive pancreatic dysfunction[2] (Fig. 16-7). Thus some patients with long-standing CP without calcification may have reached a stage of "post-calcific" CP.[2] Lithogenesis in CP is most probably a multifactorial process that is related primarily to two antagonizing mechanisms: promoting and inhibiting factors of stone formation (and dissolution). Deficiency of pancreatic stone protein in pancreatic juice is probably a major stone-promoting factor according to Sarles.[35] Physicochemical changes in pancreatic secretion (e.g., changes in pH and others) may enhance dissolution of stones.[2] It may well be that the factors responsible for stone formation differ in AICP compared with NAICP.

Complications in CP and Surgical Therapy

Pancreatic surgery was performed in our series about twice as commonly in AICP as in NAICP (Table 16-4) (48% vs. 26%). This is not surprising in view of

TABLE 16-4. PANCREATIC SURGERY: INDICATION AND PROCEDURES*

	Indication		Procedures			Total No. of Cases		
	PPZ ⊕	PPZ ⊖	WJ	LP	D			
	n	*n*	*n*	*n*	*n*	*n*	Op ⊕	Op ⊖
AICP	76	22	37	28	33	205	98 (48%)	107 (52%)
NAICP								
IJCP	4	6	5	1	4	15	10	5
ISCP	6	—	1	2	3	49	6	43
Rare causes	2	3	3	1	1	18	5	13
NAICP total	12	9	9	4	8	82	21 (26%)	61 (74%)

* PPZ = pancreatic pseudocyst; WJ = wirsungojejunostomy; LP = left hemipancreatectomy; D = drainage of cysts, either by cystojejunostomy or external drainage.

the high incidence of primary painless forms in NAICP. The main indication for surgery was persistent pain, primarily due to pseudocysts (74% of 119 pancreatic operations). In the remaining 31 patients (without pseudocysts) a pancreaticojejunostomy or left hemipancreatectomy was performed either for severe pain (n = 16), during exploratory laparotomy for suspected pseudocyst or cancer (n = 8) (before modern imaging techniques were available, 1963–1978), or simultaneously (e.g., prophylactically) with a bilidigestive anastomosis in patients with extrahepatic cholestasis (n = 7).

Various extrapancreatic complications commonly encountered in CP are listed in Table 16-5. Most of these complications were markedly more frequent in AICP than in NAICP (e.g., extrahepatic cholestasis, splenic vein thrombosis, peptic ulcer, gastrointestinal bleeding of nonulcer origin—probably related to pseudocysts, portal hypertension, erosive gastritis, Mallory-Weiss syndrome—and pulmonary tuberculosis). In AICP, cholestasis is a rather frequent complication that may be due to alcoholic liver disease or to extrahepatic stenosis of the common bile duct. In our experience the ratio of AST to ALT is of great help for discriminating primary alcoholic liver disease (ratio > 1.5) and extrahepatic cholestasis (ratio < 1.5) (except in cases complicated by cholangitis or in cholestasis associated with normal transaminases).[16]

According to the literature, peptic ulcer disease may be increased in CP (up

TABLE 16-5. EXTRAPANCREATIC COMPLICATIONS

	AICP (n = 205)			NAICP (n = 82)		
	n		%	n		%
Extrahepatic cholestasis	38		18.5	5		6.1
Splenic vein thrombosis	11		5.4	1		1.2
Pancreatic ascites	4		2.0	2		2.4
Duodenal stenosis	3		2.4	2		3.7
Colon stenosis	2			1		
Gallstones	20		9.8	10		12.2
Peptic ulcer	18		8.8	4		4.9
Gastric surgery before CP	17		8.3	3		3.7
GI bleeding, nonulcer	10		4.9	2		2.4
Liver cirrhosis	16		7.3	3		3.7
Pulmonary tuberculosis	14		6.8	0		
Carcinoma						
Oral cavity, larynx	9	23	11.2	1	10	12.2
Lung	9			5		
Stomach or colon	3			3		
Urogenital	1			1		
Leukemia	1			—		
Pancreas	1	4	1.9	5	5	6.1
Adenometastasis of liver; primary site in pancreas?	3			—		
Total number of patients with cancer	25			15		
Total carcinomas	27			15		

to 38%).[38] However, much lower figures (2%–10%) were found in our series (Table 16-5) and have been reported from other centers.[12,29–31,36] There is no explanation for these differences. It is noteworthy that gastric surgery for peptic ulcer had been performed before onset of pancreatitis in over 8% of patients with AICP in our series (Table 16-5). The decreased bicarbonate secretion by the diseased pancreas has been postulated as a factor for the high ulcer diathesis. The rather low incidence of peptic ulcers in NAICP is at variance with this hypothesis (Table 16-5).

There is some controversy about the coexistence of AICP and alcoholic cirrhosis. In some large series from South Africa, France, Italy, and Switzerland, liver cirrhosis was found in only 63 of 1263 cases with AICP (5%)[5] (Table 16-5). It has been postulated that patients with AICP die before they reach the stage of cirrhosis. This hypothesis has not been validated and would imply that most patients with liver cirrhosis have unequivocal evidence of AICP. Although abnormal pancreatic function and pancreatic fibrosis are found in about 50% of cases with cirrhosis (alcoholic or nonalcoholic),[5] the typical markers of AICP are absent in liver cirrhosis in most instances (e.g., pancreatic calcification, progressive exocrine insufficiency).

As reported previously, there is an increased incidence of extrapancreatic cancer in AICP (11.2%) and in NAICP (12.2%)[6] (Table 16-5). The relationship between CP and extrapancreatic cancer is probably multifactorial.[6] Cancers probably originating from the pancreas were more frequent in NAICP (6.1%) compared with AICP (2%) (Table 16-5). Pancreatic cancer occurred predominantly in calcific CP (7 of 9 cases). The risk of pancreatic cancer compared with a control population is elevated by a factor of about 15 to 30.[8]

Pathogenesis of Pain and Pain Management

The pathogenesis of pain is ill-defined. It is likely that different mechanisms of pain exist in CP. Primarily three mechanisms of pain in CP have to be considered: (1) "acute" pancreatitis, (2) pancreatic pseudocysts and perifocal inflammation, and (3) high intraductal pressure. With progressive destruction of glandular tissue, the morphologic substrate (e.g., mass of intact glandular tissue) for acinar necrosis and for maintenance of high secretory pressure vanishes. The formation of pseudocysts is probably also related primarily to the mass of intact glandular tissue (e.g., pseudocysts form as a result of acinar necrosis or disruption of ducts due to high pressure). Thus theoretically the likelihood of pain due to one of the three different pain mechanisms should decrease in association with progressive destruction and atrophy of glandular tissue. Our experience in AICP supports this assumption.[5,6,9]

Clinically, AICP is characterized by (1) an early phase of recurrent short episodes of "acute" pancreatitis (up to 5 years from onset),[15] and (2) a late phase with severe pancreatic dysfunction, calcification, and absence of pain ("secondary" painless CP) (Fig. 16-1).[5,6] Therapy of episodic pancreatitis is conservative as in acute pancreatitis. Alcohol abstinence usually prevents recurrence of pancreatitis. The typical pain pattern may be interrupted in about 50% of cases by short periods of persistent severe pain, particularly in early phases of CP.[5,15]

Severe persistent pain is usually due either to pseudocysts or to high ductal pressure. With the help of modern imaging technics these local complications are easily recognized, and relief of persistent pain can be achieved as a rule by a drainage procedure. Recurrent episodes of pancreatitis postoperatively are, however, very common in AICP, particularly in combination with continued alcohol abuse in patients who have not yet reached the late phase of "secondary painless CP."[5,6,9] Surgery for severe, persistent pain secondary to local complications is not debated (Table 16-4) (~50%), but surgery is palliative and does not markedly shorten the early phase with recurrent pancreatitis. Thus in our experience the duration of painful episodes up to the stage of "secondary" painless CP is about identical in patients with or without pancreatic surgery.[6] Girdwood et al. have confirmed our results and have shown that lasting pain relief is found in association with advanced pancreatic dysfunction even in patients with marked abnormalities of the ductal system and despite continued alcohol abuse.[20]

In NAICP, lasting pain relief (± surgery), although occurring in the majority of cases in association with marked exocrine dysfunction, was noted in 8 of 27 cases (30%) despite normally preserved exocrine function for 6 years or longer after the last pain episode.[1] Thus it appears that the covariation between lasting pain relief and severe exocrine dysfunction is not as close in NAICP, suggesting that there are differences in the pathogenesis of pain in NAICP and in AICP. Some of the controversies in the literature about the relationship between pain and pancreatic function may be due to these differences in the natural history of AICP and NAICP.[26,31,40]

Mortality and Survival in CP

Mortality in CP is related to a number of different factors as shown in Table 16-6 for the present series. It is obvious that the mortality directly due to CP and its complications is rather low (<20%), as noted by others,[28,31] although great variation exists from one study to the other.[40] Interestingly no marked difference was noted regarding frequency of CP-related deaths in AICP and NAICP (Table 16-6) and the overall mortality in both groups (42% in AICP vs. 52% in NAICP). It

TABLE 16-6. CAUSES OF DEATHS

	AICP	(n = 87)	NAICP	(n = 43)	Total	(n = 130)
CP-related	12	(13.8%)	7	(16.3%)	19	(14.6%)
Cyst or abscess	4		1		5	
Pancreatic operation	2		4		6	
Diabetes	6		2		8	
CP-unrelated	75	(86.2%)	36	(83.7%)	111	(85.4%)
Malignancy	17		7		24	
Cardiovascular	11		10		21	
Severe infection	18		4		22	
Postop. (nonpancreatic)	5		6		11	
Cirrhosis	10		3		13	
GI bleeding	6		1		7	
Miscellaneous	8		5		13	

should be noted, however, that in NAICP over 75% of deaths occurred in patients with ISCP (e.g., CP of the old-age group, 33 of 43 deaths). The mean age at death was 54 years in AICP compared with 67 years in NAICP.[6]

According to Bank, prognosis of CP is markedly related to socioeconomic conditions, intellectual capacity, alcohol or narcotic addiction, and adequacy of medical care.[12] The mortality rate in AICP of about 50% at 12 years in South Africa and Brazil[12] is quite similar to our figures in AICP and NAICP (Table 16-6). This appears rather surprising in view of the marked differences in populations and environmental factors (e.g., high percentage of nonwhite and chronic alcoholic patients in South Africa and Brazil). It should be noted that narcotic addiction is negligible in our series, while continued alcohol abuse in AICP is the rule (about 50%–60% of patients).[3,6]

In Fig. 16-8 the cumulative survival in our series for alcoholic and nonalcoholic CP is outlined. In contrast to the figures published previously,[6] time zero in the present series corresponds to the time of diagnosis (compared with the time of onset of pancreatitis),[6] and in addition all patients with NAICP are considered in Fig. 16-8 (e.g., including the patients with primary painless CP who were not registered in the previous publication).[6] It is evident that the 50% survival is about identical in alcoholic and nonalcoholic CP (e.g., 12–14 years) and corresponds very closely to the data of alcoholic CP from South Africa and Brazil.[12] In a series from Denmark, the calculated cumulative survival of 50% was only about 7 years.[40] Surprisingly, the influence of alcohol consumption on the survival compared with nondrinkers is not evident, either in our series or in the experience of other experts.[40]

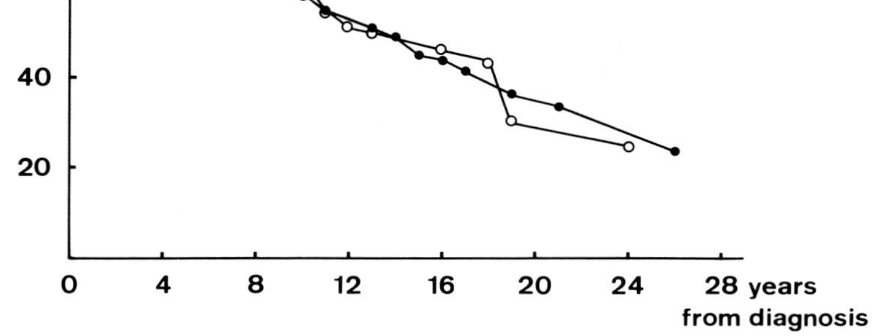

Figure 16-8. Cumulative survival of patients with AICP and NAICP (from diagnosis, $n = 287$) (BMDP1L, live tables and survival functions).

REFERENCES

1. Ammann R, Buehler H, Muench R, Freiburghaus AH, Siegenthaler W. Differences in the natural history of idiopathic (non-alcoholic) and alcoholic chronic pancreatitis. Pancreas 2:368–377, 1987.
2. Ammann R, Muench R, Otto R, et al. Evolution and regression of pancreatic calcification in chronic pancreatitis. Gastroenterology 95:1018–1028, 1988.
3. Ammann RW, Buehler H, Bruehlmann W, et al. Acute (non-progressive) alcoholic pancreatitis: Prospective longitudinal study of 144 patients with recurrent alcoholic pancreatitis. Pancreas 1:195–203, 1986.
4. Ammann R. Epidemiology and etiology of chronic pancreatitis in Zurich. In: Sato T, and Yamauchi H, eds. Pancreatitis, Its Pathophysiology and Clinical Aspects. Tokyo, University of Tokyo Press, 1985, pp 65–69.
5. Ammann R. Klinik, Spontan-verlauf und Therapie der chronischen Pankreatitis. Schweiz Med Wochenschr 119:696–706, 1989.
6. Ammann R, Akovbiantz A, Largiadér F, Schueler G. Course and outcome of chronic pancreatitis. Gastroenterology 86:820–828, 1984.
7. Ammann R. Chronic pancreatitis in the elderly. Gastroenterology Clinics of North America. 19:905–914, 1990.
8. Ammann R, Schueler G. Chronic pancreatitis, pancreatic cancer, alcohol and smoking. Gastroenterology 87:744–745, 1984.
9. Ammann R, Largiadér F, Akovbiantz A. Pain relief by surgery in chronic pancreatitis? Scand J Gastroenterol 14:209–215, 1979.
10. Ammann R, Sulser H. Die "senile" chronische Pankreatitis—Eine neue nosologische Einheit? Schweiz Med Wochenschr 106:429–437, 1976.
11. Ammann R. Die idiopathische "juvenile" chronische Pankreatitis. Dtsch Med Wochenschr 101:1789–1794, 1976.
12. Bank S. Chronic pancreatitis: Clinical features and medical management. Am J Gastroenterol 81:153–167, 1986.
13. Bank S, Marks IN, Lurie B, Novis BH, Barbezat GO. Precalcific pancreatitis. S Afr Med J 46:2093–2097, 1972.
14. Becker V. Chronische Pankreatitis; Klinische Morphologie. Stuttgart, G Thieme Verlag, 1984.
15. Bernades P, Belghiti J, Athouel M, et al. Histoire naturelle de la pancréatite chronique. Gastroenterol Clin Biol 7:8–13, 1983.
16. Buehler H, Muench R, Schmid M, Ammann R. Cholestasis in alcoholic chronic pancreatitis. Diagnostic value of the transaminase ratio for differentiation between extrahepatic and intrahepatic cholestasis. Scand J Gastroenterol 20:851–856, 1985.
17. Doerr W. Pathogenese der akuten und chronischen Pankreatitis. Verh Dtsch Ges Inn Med 70:718–758, 1964.
18. Fitzgerald O. Painless pancreatitis and other painless pancreatic disorders. Clin Gastroenterol 1:195–218, 1972.
19. Frey ChF. Classification of pancreatitis: State-of-the-art 1986. Pancreas 1:62–68, 1986.
20. Girdwood AH, Marks IN, Bornman PC, Kottler RE, Cohen M. Does progressive pancreatic insufficiency limit pain in calcific pancreatitis with duct stricture or continued alcohol insult? J Clin Gastroenterol 3:241–245, 1981.
21. Gullo L, Durbec JP. Epidemiology and etiology of pancreatitis. In: Gyr K, Singer MV, Sarles H., eds. Pancreatitis: Concepts and Classification. Amsterdam, Excerpta Medica, 1984, pp 371–376.
22. Gullo L, Barbara L, Labo G. Effect of cessation of alcohol use on the course of pancreatic dysfunction in alcoholic pancreatitis. Gastroenterology 95:1063–1068, 1988.
23. Gyr K, Toskes P. Pancreatic function testing. In: Gyr K, Singer MV, Sarles H., eds. Pancreatitis: Concepts and Classification. Amsterdam, Excerpta Medica, 1984, pp 329–335.
24. Gyr K, Singer MV, Sarles H. Reviewed classification of pancreatitis. Gastroenterology 89:683–685, 1985.

25. Hangartner PJ, Buehler H, Muench R, et al. Chronische Pankreatitis als wahrscheinliche Folge eines Analgetikaabusus. Schweiz Med Wochenschr 117:638–642, 1987.
26. Kondo T, Hayakawa T, Noda A, et al. Follow-up study of chronic pancreatitis. Gastroenterol Jpn 16:46–53, 1981.
27. Lankisch PG, Otto J, Erkelenz I, Lembcke B. Pancreatic calcifications: No indicator of severe exocrine insufficiency. Gastroenterology 90:617–621, 1986.
28. Levy P, Milan C, Pignon JP, Baetz A, Bernades P. Mortality factors associated with chronic pancreatitis. Gastroenterology 96:1165–1172, 1989.
29. Di Magno EP, Clain JE. Chronic pancreatitis. In: Go VL, Gardner JD, Brooks FP, et al., eds. The Endocrine Pancreas. New York, Raven Press, 1986, pp 541–575.
30. Marks IN, Bank S. Chronic pancreatitis. In: Berk JJ, Haubrich WS, Kalser MH, Roth JLA, Schaffner F, eds. Bockus Gastroenterology. Philadelphia, WB Saunders, 1985, vol 6, pp 4020–4040.
31. Miysake H, Harada H, Kunichika K, Ochi K, Kimura I. Clinical course and prognosis of chronic pancreatitis. Pancreas 2:378–385, 1987.
32. Nagata A, Homma T, Oguchi H, Furuta S. Serial observation of chronic pancreatitis by ERP and PS-test. In: Sato T, Yamauchi H, eds. Pancreatitis. Tokyo, University of Tokyo Press, 1985, pp 295–302.
33. Pitchumoni CS. Special problems of tropical pancreatitis. Clin Gastroenterol 13:941–959, 1984.
34. Renner IG, Savage WT, Pantoja JL, Renner VJ. Death due to acute pancreatitis. Dig Dis Sci 30:1005–1018, 1985.
35. Sarles H. Epidemiology and physiopathology of chronic pancreatitis and the role of the pancreatic stone protein. Clin Gastroenterol 13:895–912, 1984.
36. Sarles H, Gerolami A. Chronic pancreatitis. Clin Gastroenterol 1:167–193, 1972.
37. Sarles H, Muratore R, Sarles JC, et al. Aetiology and pathology of chronic pancreatitis. Bibl Gastroenterol 7:75–120, 1965.
38. Sarner M, Cotton PB. Definitions of acute and chronic pancreatitis. Clin Gastroenterol 13:865–870, 1984.
39. Worning H. Epidemiologic studies on chronic pancreatitis. In: Sato T, Yamauchi H, eds. Pancreatitis, Its Pathophysiology and Clinical Aspects. Tokyo, University of Tokyo Press, 1985, pp 79–88.
40. Worning H. Chronic pancreatitis: Pathogenesis, natural history and conservative treatment. Clin Gastroenterol 13:871–894, 1984.

CHAPTER

17

ALCOHOLIC PANCREATITIS

Henri Sarles

DEFINITION OF ACUTE AND CHRONIC PANCREATITIS

In a number of papers dealing with diseases of the exocrine pancreas, words such as acute, chronic, relapsing, cysts, pseudocysts are used with different meanings by different authors. This has introduced a considerable difficulty, in the comparison of different series and frequently makes it impossible to understand these papers clearly. The concept of relapsing pancreatitis proposed by Comfort, Gambill, and Baggenstos[9] is still used by many English speaking groups who assume that all transitions exist between the most acute necrotic pancreatitis and the most progressive calcified pancreatitis. These workers appear to believe that these two extreme conditions and the intermediate cases supposed to exist between them represent variations of the same disease.[7] This does not stand objective examination. One argument against this concept is that acute pancreatitis, which is proposed as the cause of chronic lesions, is found in patients with a mean age 13 years greater than the average age of onset of clinical chronic pancreatitis.[17]

This confusion between acute and chronic lesions led to the first effort to define precisely and clearly acute and chronic pancreatitis in the first Marseille Classification[32] in 1963. This defined acute pancreatitis as characterized by reversible lesions when the patients survived and chronic pancreatitis as a persistent and progressive destruction of the parenchyma which was replaced by fibrosis. It was also proposed to use the term acute relapsing pancreatitis when acute, reversible lesions recurred, due to the persistence of the extrapancreatic causes (gallstones for instance) and chronic relapsing pancreatitis when the clinical evolution of chronic pancreatitis was marked by repeated episodes of pain. The first Marseille Classification has been largely accepted but the absence of a clear distinction between different pancreatic diseases persists in some papers. Twenty-one years later, a meeting at Cambridge[37] and the second Symposium on the Classification of Pancreatitis held in Marseille in 1984[38] maintained the same distinction between acute and chronic pancreatitis.

One difficulty, even with such a simple classification is that the words "acute pancreatitis" correspond to different lesions which are a nonspecific response of the pancreas to different causes, either extrapancreatic (gallstones, hyperlipoproteinemia, drugs, and so forth), or intrapancreatic (acute exacerbation of chronic pancreatitis, acute pancreatitis secondary to pancreatic cancer). In contrast, chronic pancreatitis is a group of diseases with characteristic features corresponding to specific aetiologies.

The following definitions will be used in this chapter.

1. Acute pancreatitis is a group of different lesions: edema, necrosis, or hemorrhagic necrosis of the pancreas and fat necrosis, which is often extrapancreatic. These lesions may be isolated or associated with each other. They are a nonspecific response of the pancreas to intra or extrapancreatic insults.

2. Chronic pancreatitis is a group of diseases characterized by a persistent loss of exocrine parenchyma, that is replaced by fibrosis.

DIFFERENT FORMS OF CHRONIC PANCREATITIS

A computer study of the histologic features of 98 cases of chronic pancreatitis had shown that chronic pancreatitis cases could be easily classified according to their features into at least two clearly different populations. The largest group has been called calcifying chronic pancreatitis; it is characterized by lobular distribution of the lesions; alterations of the intralobular ducts (dilatation of the ducts and epithelial atrophy); frequent protein plugs (sometimes calcified) in the duct lumen; perineural inflammatory infiltration, and nerve changes. A study utilizing a three-dimensional reconstruction of pancreatic ducts and serial sections reached the same conclusion.[26] The lesions of calcifying pancreatitis demonstrated by this method showed characteristically: (1) a patchy distribution of the lesions that were related to the ducts; (2) a frequent finding in the ducts of plugs of precipitated protein, that tended to evolve into calculi by deposition of calcium on their surface (these plugs rarely contained mucopolysaccharides); (3) all sizes of duct were involved and showed irregular dilatation, loss of lining epithelium, encroachment of periductal connective tissue to form stenosis, and the formation of pancreatic cysts or the complete disappearance of acini and ducts in the territory drained by a blocked duct. In chronic pancreatitis secondary to an obstruction in the main pancreatic duct, the lesions were different in almost every respect from those described above.

More recently, a multicenter pathologic study has been done on 359 cases of chronic pancreatitis from five different centers in France, Italy, South Africa, and Brazil (2 centers).[31] This study has confirmed that obstructive pancreatitis which occurs distally to an obstruction of the pancreatic ducts, and in which the obstruction precedes the pancreatitis (tumors, scars), can easily be distinguished from the larger group of patients who presented with features of chronic calcifying pancreatitis.

In the study of Payan et al.,[28] patients classified as calcifying pancreatitis by their pathologic features included those with and those without pancreatic stones (calcifications) visible on plain x-ray films of the abdomen. The distribution of sex, age at the onset of pain and consumption of alcohol, fat, and protein were independent of the presence of pancreatic stones. Three studies[3,14,34] on the natural history of chronic pancreatitis (excluding patients presenting with obstructive pancreatitis) have shown that the probability for a patient to present with visible stones on films of the abdomen increased hyperbolically with the duration of symptoms and tended to a percentage well above 90%. Therefore, for this large group of patients, the name calcifying chronic pancreatitis will be adopted with precalcified and calcified stages.

Chronic Calcifying Pancreatitis

CCP is characterized by the features described above. Tasso et al.[39] in the morphometric study of the ultrastructural features of pancreases from CCP patients found that the first visible lesion of the disease which appeared before lesions of ducts and acini was the formation in the lumen of the ducts and acini of protein precipitates or plugs. Harada et al.[15,16] were the first authors to study protein plugs by scanning electron microscopy. These plugs consist of interlacing networks with amorphous material filling the networks. Protein plug formation starts in the form of random and loose interlacing networks of fibrils. These enlarge by adherence of smaller aggregates and stratiform deposition of reticular substances and amorphous material. Kern et al.[20] confirmed this study and found that intraluminal plugs are formed by a network of densely packed fibers which vary in diameter from 10 to 25 or 30 nm. The fibrils do not reveal a substructure such as regular spacing or cross-striation. In many cases, fibrils are contained in the central part of the precipitates which form a homogenous electron-dense material enclosing several fibrils into a homogenous mass. The authors suggest that such condensations represent focal points of calcium carbonate crystallization within the protein matrix.

Phan Kieu Dong et al.[13] conducted the first ultrastructural study of pancreatic stones; they showed that the stones were formed of calcite crystals deposited in successive lamina. These were covered by an organic material that was destroyed by immersion in hydrogen peroxide for 3 hours at 80°C. Harada et al.[15,16] studied stones with a scanning electron microscope and x-ray probe microanalyzer. They found a central core and surrounding shells. Some stones had core composed of a calcium-rich amorphous substance and interlacing fibrils that were probably protein. Others had a core consisting of multiple cavities with smooth walls, composed of a calcium-deficient amorphous substance. These shells show a common structure: zones or layers or bands of a calcium-rich amorphous substance, a network of fibrils filled with a calcium-rich substance, and laminated parallel or polygonal plates of calcite, parallel to the surface in one layer and perpendicular or oblique in the next one. Calcium is in the cryptocrystalline state as well as in the crystalline state of calcite. Crystalline calcite shows spirals of epitaxial growth along with findings suggestive of dissolution. Comparisons of stones and protein plugs confirm that protein plugs can become stones as a result of calcite deposition accompanied by precipitation of a network of fibrils and an amorphous substance. In recent papers,[4,19] pancreatic stones were decalcified so the organic matrix could be studied by scanning and transmission electron microscopy. After the calcium carbonate was removed, the stones consisted of multiple partitions arranged like a sponge. They were embedded in a gel-like matrix. The organic partitions frequently were composed of dense surface layers and sparse central reticular accumulations which had surrounded and bound calcium carbonate crystals. The organic matrix was heterogeneous in texture. Some areas had dense, regular proteinaceous fibrous material. Some deposits resembling fibrin were observed. Altered cellular constituents appeared to make up minor portions of the matrix. Calcium carbonate which was precipitated in vitro from pancreatic juice resembled the morphology of pancreatic stones more than that of pure calcium carbonate crystals. These results are consistent with the co-formation of pancreatic stones from constituents in the pancreatic juice and precipitated calcium carbonate.

The basal membrane of the small ducts disappears and duct cells atrophy[28] where they are in contact with plugs and stones. This explains the importance and the severity of duct lesions in CCP compared to obstructive pancreatitis. There is loss of epithelium and fibrotic stricture formation of small ducts. This leads to the exclusion of a growing number of territories of exocrine parenchyma drained by diseased ducts. Another consequence of duct obstruction is the dilatation of ducts leading to the formation of intrapancreatic retention cysts which, at least in some places retain an epithelial (true cysts). When these enlarge, they can breach the surface of the pancreas. If this occurs fluid collections progress in peripancreatic spaces where they form large retention pseudocysts. These start as intrapancreatic retention cysts and extend outside the pancreas where they are limited by neighboring organs and fibrosis.

Pancreatic plugs and stones are built up of calcium carbonate in the form of calcite and of protein in different proportions.[2,12] The protein composition of pancreatic stones and plugs is dominated by a family of molecules discovered in our laboratory: the pancreatic stone protein (PSP). These are small proteins (14,000 to 19,000 kd) with different degrees of phosphorylation and glycosylation. The first molecule to be discovered was isolated from pancreatic calculi.[10,11,21,23] It is rich in aspartate and glutamate. Its molecular weight is 14,000. It is phosphorylated (2 phosphoserines, 1 phosphothreonine) and poorly glycosylated. It prevents the formation of calcium carbonate crystals in a metastable solution of calcium.[24] This could be important as pancreatic juice is always supersaturated in calcium in the same way as many other secretions.[25] Therefore, it is reasonable to assume the existence of a stabilizer of calcium in solution. As PSP is decreased in the pancreatic juice of patients presenting with CCP,[29] it is probable that PSP is the stabilizer of calcium in pancreatic juice and that its decrease plays a role in CCP. This explains why PSP is bound to calcite in pancreatic stones: this group of substances binds to the growth sites of crystals and stop their growth. When the stabilizer is not present in sufficient quantity, crystals grow irregularly that trap those molecules of stabilizer which have bound to the calcite.

However PSP is also responsible for the precipitation of protein in plugs and stones. This could be explained by the fact that different molecular forms of PSP have been extracted from pancreatic juice.[22] PSP S2-5 are four glycoproteins of higher molecular weight than PSP. Active trypsin transforms them into PSP S1 of molecular weight 14,000 by the release of a peptide carrying the sugars.[29]

The 133 N-terminal amino acid sequence of PSP S1 is known.[5] It is probably similar to the sequence of PSP extracted from stones. PSP S1-5 have been extracted from pancreatic juice by immunologic techniques at acid pH. These molecules are not phosphorylated. It is possible that dephosphorylation was an artefact due to acid pH. It is probable that the molecule which is insoluble at pH 7 and which is found in the x-ray transparent stones could be different from the stabilizer by its content in phosphoric acid or its glycosylation.

Nevertheless, different molecular forms of PSP are responsible for:

1. The stabilization of pancreatic juice that is supersaturated in calcium. The decrease of this form is responsible for the calcified part of pancreatic stones.

2. The formation of protein precipitates in ducts and acini. These two phenomena are found in different proportions in pancreatic stones: one case of giant stones composed of pure calcium carbonate in the absence of PSP has been described.[35] The more usual calcified stones contain 0.5% of PSP.[35] Some rare x-ray transparent stones contain only PSP.

Obstructive Pancreatitis

Obstructive pancreatitis is due to an obstruction of the duct preceding the pancreatitis (scars, tumors). In contrast to CCP, the discriminant features of obstructive pancreatitis are the regular distribution of the lesions distal to the obstruction, the low frequency and intensity of duct lesions and the rarity of protein plugs. If CCP and obstructive pancreatitis are easy to differentiate at the level of the optical microscope, the ultrastructural lesions of the advanced stages are identical. This is easily explained by the fact that the lesions of acini in CCP are secondary to obstruction of the ducts. However, in CCP, obstruction is a consequence of the disease and not its original cause.

MODIFICATIONS OF PANCREATIC JUICE INDUCED BY CHRONIC ALCOHOL CONSUMPTION[20]

The biochemical modifications of pancreatic juice as opposed to duodenal collections observed in alcoholic pancreatitis have been classified as described below:[12]

1. A decrease of PSP and increase in lactoferrin concentrations occur independently of the consumption of alcohol. They are also observed in other types of chronic calcifying pancreatitis and possibly precede the first symptoms.

2. Modifications related to alcohol consumption are found in the pancreatic juice of all alcoholics, irrespective of whether or not they present with chronic pancreatitis. These changes are increased concentration of total protein in pancreatic juice, decreased concentration of secretory trypsin inhibitor, and decreased pH and concentration of bicarbonate and of citrate.

Increased concentration of serum proteins and calcium are observed in any type of pancreatic lesion and probably secondary to transudation of interstitial fluid.

The increased secretion of enzymes and calcium in chronic pancreatitis has been confirmed by Clain et al.[8] Renner et al.[30] have recently compared the pure pancreatic juice collected after secretin and CCK stimulation in chronic alcoholic patients without liver cirrhosis (CA), chronic alcoholics with liver cirrhosis (CC), and nonalcoholic volunteers (V). In CA, volumes increased after both hormones, protein concentration and output increased after CCK, but chymotrypsin output decreased when compared to both other groups. In contrast, trypsin output was markedly increased in both groups of alcoholics when compared to controls.

An increased synthesis of protein has recently been shown in chronic pancreatitis patients by measuring the incorporation of selenium-75-labeled methionine into the protein of duodenal aspirates during stimulation with secretin and CCK.[6]

The increased concentration and output in pure pancreatic juice and the increased biosynthesis of secretory proteins is now sufficiently well documented in chronic alcoholics and chronic pancreatitis patients to be accepted. As it is also observed during hypercalcemia, which is another cause of chronic pancreatitis, it could play a part in the formation of lesions, especially the intraductal plugs which seem to be at the origin of stones.

THE MORPHOLOGY OF ALCOHOLIC PANCREATITIS

Chronic Calcifying Pancreatitis

Most authors consider that alcoholic pancreatitis is characterized clinically by recurrent attacks of pain, followed after a number of years, by exocrine and endocrine pancreatic insufficiency and the formation of pancreatic stones visible on plain films of the abdomen: the usual form of alcoholic pancreatitis is CCP. The mean daily alcohol consumption of these patients is 150–175 ml of pure alcohol per day for a mean of 17 years in males, and 13 years in females in most European countries.[36] There is a linear correlation between the log of the relative risk for CCP and the mean daily consumption of alcohol. There is a difference in the risk between total abstainers and patients drinking such small quantities as 1–20 g alcohol per day.[33] This proves that there is no statistical threshold of toxicity but a continuous spectrum of individual thresholds between patients who will spontaneously develop the disease (idiopathic cases, patients sensitive to very low alcohol doses) and people who will drink huge quantities of alcohol without developing pancreatic lesions. Therefore, the definition of alcoholic pancreatitis by some arbitrary level of alcohol consumption is impossible: is a patient drinking 10 g alcohol per day an idiopathic case or a patient sensitive to low alcohol doses who would not have developed the disease if he had never drunk any alcohol?

Alcohol is not the only etiologic factor for CCP. There is also a linear correlation between the log of the risk and the mean daily consumption of protein, but average fat diets (80–100 g fat per day) are associated with the lowest risk, low fat diets with higher risk and high fat diets with the highest risk.[14] Hypercalcemia is also a cause of CCP. There are hereditary dominant forms and possibly other nondominant hereditary form.[12] Finally, CCP is also found in young subjects living in tropical countries associated with low protein, low fat diets.[12]

The biochemical composition of pancreatic calculi from alcoholic, idiopathic and tropical forms is similar.[35] Two exceptional stones were observed in our series. A case of pure calcium carbonate stones without PSP and a case of a transparent stone without calcium were found in non-alcoholic young women. Alcoholic patients have calcified stones with a small percentage of PSP. Therefore, it is probable that CCP is in reality a family of diseases due to the formation of stones and plugs with different chemical compositions.

We have compared the lesions of pancreases from alcoholic patients and from idiopathic pancreatitis. The lesions were not significantly different. Therefore, there is actually no reason to think that alcoholic CCP is in any way different from CCP of other origin, though this requires further study before we can be certain of this.

Acute Pancreatitis

Acute alcoholic pancreatitis is generally observed in chronic alcohol drinkers[36] and probably represents the first episode of CCP. Therefore, it is probable that most acute alcoholic pancreatitis is associated with or is a complication of CCP. Acute alcoholic, i.e., alcoholic pancreatitis is mostly observed in people drinking huge quantities of alcohol at the weekend and not in those who have a regular daily consumption of ethanol.[18] At the present moment, there is no convincing proof that alcoholic pancreatitis could occur without chronic lesions, but neither is there any argument to the contrary. Isolated acute alcoholic pancreatitis is a possibility. Amman et al.[1,2] have assumed that approximately one third of patients presenting with acute alcoholic pancreatitis will not develop chronic pancreatitis. They found that 12 to 14 years after the presenting bout of pancreatitis, some patients still had not developed pancreatic insufficiency. However, this was diagnosed on changes in fecal chymotrypsinogen which is not a sensitive test. Apparently all patients presented with moderate or severe changes of pancreatic ducts showed by endoscopic retrograde pancreatography. Histologic examination was performed in 7 cases. Four presented with pseudocysts, 0.5 to 7 years after the clinical onset. Three were postmortem specimens of patients who died 1 and 2 years after the onset of symptoms. Only mild interstitial fibrosis was found in five of the seven specimens. This favors the assumption that isolated acute alcoholic pancreatitis may exist but does not provide conclusive proof. In the seven patients, the delay between pathologic study and onset of symptoms is small and it is not said how many slides were made. We have previously shown that the lesions of CCP are patchy and may be present in one area of the pancreas but not in others. Nevertheless, the work of Amman et al. does at least show that after the first attack of alcoholic acute pancreatitis, chronic lesions develop at variable rates in different patients.

Adaptative Modifications to Chronic Alcohol Consumption

Noronha et al.[27] among others have described the ultrastructural modifications in the pancreas of patients consuming more than 80 g alcohol a day but who were free of pancreatic disorders. They found an increased accumulation of fat droplets, a decreased number of zymogen granules, mostly in the form of prozymogens, a dilatation of the endoplasmic reticulum and, less frequently, mitochondrial abnormalities and increased numbers of lysosomes. With the exception of fat droplets, these modifications are similar to those previous found in alcoholic pancreatitis patients by Tasso et al.[39] who examined those areas of the exocrine pancreas from which appeared normal at the optical level. Most of these modifications and especially fat accumulation, are found in various tissues in alcoholics (such as liver) and are not specific of the pancreas. Fat accumulation and mitochondrial modifications are a reversible phenomenon when the toxic agent is withdrawn. Tasso et al.[39] described other modifications of acinar cells: increased size of the cell and of the nucleus, increased length of endoplasmic reticulum and Golgi apparatus which appear to be dilated, increased number of residual bodies, and modifications of mitochondria. These were interpreted as due to an increased synthesis and transport of secretory protein which is in agreement with the changes seen in pancreatic juice in alcoholics.[12] Therefore, these modifications appear to be adaptative, reversible modifications due to alcohol consumption rather than having a role in the pathogenesis of alcoholic pancreatitis.

CONCLUSION

Most cases of alcoholic pancreatitis belong to the group of chronic calcifying pancreatitis. This family of diseases has different etiologies, including alcohol, high protein, low and high fat diets, hypercalcemia, heredity, and the unknown cause of tropical pancreatitis. There is no evidence that the lesions arising in these different etiological forms are different. CCP is not an inflammatory disease like alcoholic hepatitis or alcoholic liver cirrhosis but is a diffuse microlithiasis characterized by the precipitation of calcium carbonate and one molecular form of a newly discovered family of molecules (PSP). PSP is a stabilizer of calcium that prevents calcium carbonate crystallization in the supersaturated pancreatic juice. It is decreased in all forms of CCP. This decrease probably plays a part in the pancreatic lithogenesis characteristic of CCP and is probably not dependent on alcohol consumption. Nevertheless, alcoholism modifies pancreatic secretion particularly by increasing the secretion of protein (enzymes), in the same way as hypercalcemia, and this could play an accessory part.

Acute alcoholic pancreatitis frequently corresponds to an exacerbation of calcifying chronic pancreatitis. The same is observed in idiopathic, hereditary and hypercalcemic CCP. It is possible but not proven that in some cases, acute lesions are not associated with incipient chronic lesions and that in these cases, patients heal completely when they stop drinking.

Acute lesions could be due to the same mechanism as chronic lesions: i.e., precipitation of calcium carbonate and PSP forming plugs and stones, but another mechanism for acute lesions cannot be excluded.

REFERENCES

1. Ammann RW, Akovbiantz A, Largiader F, Schueler G. Course and outcome of chronic pancreatitis, longitudinal study of a mixed medical-surgical series of 245 patients. Gastroenterology 86:820–828, 1984.
2. Ammann RW, Buehler H, Bruehlmann W, Kehl O, Muench R, Stamm B. Acute (nonprogressive) alcoholic pancreatitis: Prospective longitudinal study of 114 patients with recurrent alcoholic pancreatitis. Pancreas 1:195–203, 1986.
3. Bernades P, Belghiti J, Athouel M, Mallardo N, Breil P, Fekete F. Histoire naturelle de la pancreatite chronique. Etude de 120 cas. Gastroenterol Clin Biol 7:8–13, 1983.
4. Bockman DE, Kennedy RH, Multigner L, De Caro A, Sarles H. Fine structure of the organic matrix of human pancreatic stones. Pancreas 1:204–210, 1986.
5. Bonicel J, Rovery M, De Caro A, Rouimi P. Cleavage of the ARG-ILE bond in the native polypeptide chain of human pancreatic stone protein. FEBS LETT 216:195–199, 1987.
6. Boyd EJS, Clark G, Dunbar J, Wormsley KG. Pancreatic enzyme synthesis in pancreatic disease. Scand J Gastroenterol 20:734–740, 1985.
7. Cattel RB, Warren KW. Surgery of the pancreas, London, W.B. Saunders, 1953.
8. Clain JE, Barbezat GO, Marks IN. Exocrine pancreatic enzyme and calcium secretion in health and pancreatitis. Gut 22:355–358, 1981.
9. Comfort MW, Gambill EE, Baggenstoss AH. Chronic relapsing pancreatitis: A study of 29 cases without associated disease of the biliary or gastrointestinal tract. Gastroenterology 6:239–285, 1946.
10. De Caro A, Bonicel J, Rouimi R, De Caro J, Sarles H, Rovery M. Complete amino acids sequence of immunoreactive form of pancreatic stone protein isolated from pancreatic juice. Eur J Biochem 168:201–207, 1987.
11. De Caro A, Lohse J, Sarles H. Characterization of a protein isolated from pancreatic calculi of men suffering from chronic calcifying pancreatitis. Biochem Biophys Res Commun 87:1176–1182, 1979.
12. De Caro A, Multigner L, Pitchumoni CS, Geevarghese PJ, Sarles H. Identification of the pancreatic stone protein in stones from tropical Indian pancreatitis. Gastroenterology 88:1360, 1985.
13. Dong PK, Bellanger G, Leger L. Mecanisme de formation des calculs pancreatiques. J Chir 103:(2)119–126, 1972.
14. Durbec JP, Sarles H. Multicenter survey of the etiology of pancreatic diseases. Relationship between the relative risk of developing chronic pancreatitis and alcohol protein and lipid consumption. Digestion 18:337–350, 1978.
15. Harada H, Takeda M, Tanaka J, Miki H, Ochi K, Kimura I. The fine structure of pancreatic stones as shown by scanning electron microscopy and x-ray probe microanalyser. Gastroent Japonica 18:530–537, 1983.
16. Harada H, Ueda O, Yasuoka M, Nakamura T, Hayashi T, Kobayashi T, Kimura I. Scanning electron microscopic studies on protein plugs obtained from patients with chronic pancreatitis. Gastroent Japonica 17:98–101, 1982.
17. Ink O, Labayle D, Buffet C, Chaput JC, Etienne JP. Pancreatite chronique alcoolique: relations de la douleur avec le sevrage et la chirurgie pancreatique. Gastroenterol Clin Biol 8:419–425, 1984.
18. Kager L, Lindberg S, Agren G. Alcohol consumption and acute pancreatitis in men. Scand J Gastroenterol 7:(suppl)15, 1972.

19. Kennedy RH, Bockman DE, Uscanga L, Choux R, Grimaud JA, Sarles H. Pancreatic extracellular matrix alterations in chronic pancreatitis. Pancreas 2:61–72, 1987.
20. Kern HF, Warshaw AL, Scheele GA. Fine structure of protein precipitation in acinar lumina of the normal human pancreas and in chronic pancreatitis. In Gyr KE, Singer MV, Sarles H, eds. Pancreatitis. Concepts and Classification, Amerstdam, Excerpta Medicine, 1984, pp 101–105.
21. Montalto G, Bonicel J, Multigner L, Rovery M, Sarles H, De Caro A. Partial amino-acid sequence of human pancreatic stone protein. A novel pancreatic secretory protein. Biochem J 238:227–232, 1986.
22. Montalto G, Lusher M, De Caro A, Multigner L, Sarles H, Delaage M. Analyse au moyen d'un anticorps monoclonal des composants du suc pancreatique humain apparentes a la proteine des calculs pancreatiques. C R Acad Sci Ser D 300:199–202, 1985.
23. Moore EW, Verine HJ. Pancreatic calcification and stone formation: a thermodynamic model of calcium in pancreatic juice. Am J Physiol 252:707–718, 1987.
24. Multigner L, De Caro A, Lombardo D, Campese D, Sarles H. Pancreatic stone protein. A phosphoprotein which inhibits calcium carbonate precipitation from human pancreatic juice. Biochem Biophys Res Commun 110:69–74, 1983.
25. Multigner L, Sarles H, Lombardo D, De Caro A. Pancreatic stone protein. II. Implication in stone formation during the course of chronic calcifying pancreatitis. Gastroenterology 89:387–391, 1985.
26. Nakamura K, Sarles H, Payan H. Three-dimensional reconstruction of the pancreatic ducts in chronic pancreatitis. Gastroenterology 62:942–949, 1972.
27. Noronha M, Salgadinho A, Ferrieira De Almedia MJ, Dreiling DA, Bordalo O. Alcohol and the pancreas. I. Clinical associations and histopathology of minimal pancreatic inflammation. Am J Gastroenterol 76:114–119, 1981.
28. Payan H, Sarles H, Demirdjian M, Gauthier AP, Cros RC, Durbec JP. Study of the histologic features of chronic pancreatitis by correspondance analysis. Identification . . . Entity. Biomedicine 18:663–670, 1972.
29. Provansal-Cheylan M, Rouzidi D, Mariani A, Sarles H, PSP quantification in human pancreatic juice: Comparison of 3 methods. Digestion 38:53, 1987.
30. Renner IG, Rinderknecht H, Russell Wisner J. Pancreatic secretion after secretin and cholecystokinin stimulation in chronic alcoholics with and without cirrhosis. Dig Dis Sci 28:1089–1093, 1983.
31. Sahel J, Cros RC, Durbec JP, Sarles H, Bank S. et al. Multicenter pathological study of chronic pancreatitis. Morphological regional variations and differences between chronic calcifying pancreatitis and obstructive pancreatitis. Pancreas 1:471–477, 1986.
32. Sarles H. Pancreatitis. Symposium in Marseille 1963. Basel, Karger, 1965.
33. Sarles H. Etiopathogenesis and definition of chronic pancreatitis. Dig Dis Sci 31:91S–107S, 1986.
34. Sarles H. An international survey on nutrition and pancreatitis. Digestion 9:389–403, 1973.
35. Sarles H, De Caro A, Multigner L, Martin E. Giant pancreatic stones in teetotal women due to absence of the "stone protein"? Lancet II:714–715, 1982.
36. Sarles H, Sarles JC, Camatte R, Moratore R, Gaini M, Guien G, Pastor J. Observations on 205 confirmed cases of acute pancreatitis, recurring pancreatitis, and chronic pancreatitis. Gur 6:545–559, 1965.
37. Sarner M, Cotton PB. Classification of pancreatitis. Gut 25:756–759, 1984.
38. Singer MV, Gyr K, Sarles H. Revised classification of pancreatitis. Report of the second international symposium on the classification of pancreatitis in Marseille, France, March 28–30, 1984. Gastroenterology 89:683–690, 1985.
39. Tasso F, Stemmelin N, Sarles H, Clop J. Comparative morphometric study of the human pancreas in its normal state and in primary chronic calcifying pancreatitis. Biomedicine 18:134–144, 1973.

CHAPTER

18

THE ASSESSMENT OF CHRONIC PANCREATITIS

Eric J. S. Boyd and Kenneth G. Wormsley

EDITORIAL COMMENTS

As the authors indicate, there does not appear to be one test that has the specificity and sensitivity to be diagnostically accurate in all patients for the diagnosis of early chronic pancreatitis. One question the authors do not address is whether the clinical history is as accurate as most tests. They suggest that either (1) a number of tests have to be taken in conjunction or (2) the abnormality has to be gross enough, for example, 95% confidence level or two times the standard deviation below or above the normal value. However, this will of course fail to diagnose many of the milder forms of the disease. Thus, we are again left with a classification already suggested by Marks and Bank of three categories, namely, definite chronic pancreatitis, probable chronic pancreatitis, and possible chronic pancreatitis. As Ammann has outlined in chapter 16, the grading from possible to definite may only be solved by time, either symptomatically or by serial monitoring with one or another of the tests outlined in the present chapter. One is left with the impression that morphologic changes on ERCP are perhaps the most specific and accurate of all the tests outlined. However, this should be tempered by the not inconsequential morbidity of ERCP, especially if nothing is to be gained at that stage by making the diagnosis. It may of course help make an etiologic diagnosis in a few patients. We do at least now have a number of noninvasive tests that could be used to follow up possible pancreatitis for progression of the disease, namely, stool chymotrypsinogen levels, isoamylase P level in serum and urine, radioimmunoassay trypsinogen levels, and the Bentiromide and fluorescein tests, and on the endocrine side, glucose tolerance, serum PP, serum insulin levels, and C-peptide levels, both with and without provocation. It is also clear that CT scanning may elucidate early calcification before it is detectable on straight or lateral x-ray views of the abdomen.

The differentiation from carcinoma of the pancreas, particularly if it is superimposed on chronic pancreatitis, is an even greater difficulty. The authors have outlined the many tests available to date, including measuring levels of enzymes, fetoproteins, and so forth. Although helpful, none are absolute, and false-positive and false-negative results are common. Clearly, CT scanning, skinny needle cytologic examination, and ERCP will remain the dominant tests until a more specific procedure is found. Whether a delay in diagnosis materially influences the outcome is a point of some discordance between gastroenterologists, surgeons, and oncologists.

CONTROVERSY

Despite the recent advances in technology, there are still considerable difficulties in the early diagnosis of chronic pancreatitis and in differentiating chronic pancreatitis from carcinoma. Other chapters in this book have demonstrated a high incidence of nondiagnosis or misdiagnosis by CT, sonography, and pancreatic function testing early on in the disease and lack of definition by ERCP between chronic pancreatitis and carcinoma. Recently, a series of serologic and tolerance tests have become available, but all tend to be abnormal, mainly in clinically obvious disease. The purpose of this chapter is an attempt to put all these tests into perspective.

WHAT IS CHRONIC PANCREATITIS?

Two recent international meetings, the first in Cambridge in 1983[187] and the second in Marseilles in 1984,[197] have sought to classify, and have suggested diagnostic criteria for, chronic pancreatitis (CP).[67] A subsequent report of the meetings proposed a plan for the complete evaluation (operational classification) of patients suspected of suffering from CP.[14] Suggested diagnostic criteria, compiled from reports of both meetings, are presented in Table 18-1.

Clearly there are three current bases for making a diagnosis of CP—morphologic, histopathologic, and pathophysiologic. In other words, "typical" CP is characterized by morphologic abnormalities of the pancreatic ductal system, often together with intraductal lithiasis and calcification, and by acinar destruction, fibrosis, and calcification and is associated with pancreatic exocrine insufficiency.

Curiously, etiologic criteria play a negligible role in the definition of the disease. Yet the etiologic determinants are obviously those aspects of CP that, if identifiable, permit prognostic assessment, and that enable appropriate preventive or supportive therapy to be provided.

At present only a few predisposing circumstances have been identified, including alcoholism, some metabolic disorders (for example, hypercalcemia and hyperlipidemia), familial or hereditary factors, and some anatomic abnormalities. Why, for example, alcohol consumption produces chronic pancreatitis in a small proportion of individuals is not known. It is not known when the link between alcohol intake and pancreatic damage starts, because apparently the disease presents in some patients with repeated attacks of pain in the form of acute pancreatitis, while in other parts of the world the alcohol-associated CP presents with exocrine or endocrine insufficiency, often in the absence of pain, at least during a substantial part of the natural history of that form of the disease.[5]

In order to assess CP it is therefore necessary to identify the cause(s), plus the factors that are responsible for the development of the pancreatic disease in some individuals but not in others. This is not yet possible, so that the detection of CP is, at present, totally unsatisfactory. Let us, instead, briefly consider the current criteria that have been used in the definition and assessment of chronic pancreatitis.

TABLE 18-1. PROPOSED CRITERIA FOR THE DIAGNOSIS OF CHRONIC PANCREATITIS*

HISTOPATHOLOGIC	Irregular sclerosis with destruction and permanent loss of exocrine parenchyma, which may be focal, segmental, or diffuse. There are segmental duct dilation and stenosis. Pancreatic islets are unaffected. Hemochromatosis and cystic fibrosis are not included in the definition.	
FUNCTIONAL	Progressive or permanent impairment of the pancreatic secretion of bicarbonate and enzymes in the duodenal aspirate in response to direct stimulation of the gland with exogenous secretagogues.	
MORPHOLOGIC		
Pancreatography	Equivocal	Fewer than 3 abnormal side branches
	Mild	More than 3 abnormal branches
	Moderate	Abnormal main duct and branches
	Marked	As above plus one or more of the following: Large cavities (>10 mm) Gross gland enlargement (>2 × normal) Intraductal filling defects or calculi Duct obstruction, stricture, or gross irregularity
Ultrasonography and CT	Equivocal	Only one of the following: Main duct enlargement (<4 mm) Gland enlargement (up to 2 × normal) Cavities (<10 mm) Irregular ducts Focal acute pancreatitis Parenchymal heterogeneity Duct wall echo increase Irregular head or body contour
	Mild	Any two of the above
	Moderate	Any two of the above
	Marked	As above plus one or more of the following: Large cavities (>10 mm) Gross gland enlargement (>2 × normal) Intraduct filling defects or calculi Duct obstruction, stricture, or gross irregularity Contiguous organ invasion

* From Sarner and Cotton[187] and Singer et al.[197]

In the present state of knowledge, the only permissible criterion for establishing the presence of CP is histologic evidence of destruction of the acinar pancreas. Unfortunately, it is rarely possible to obtain histologic confirmation of the disease in order to establish the diagnosis and to provide a yardstick for other "diagnostic" procedures. Since operative pancreatic biopsy results in complications, including hemorrhage, pancreatitis, and fistula formation in 5% to 20% of patients, together with a mortality rate of 1.5% to 3.7%, it is considered that open biopsy is never justified merely to exclude the diagnosis of CP (that is, to confirm normal pancreatic morphology).[73,122,171] In any case, too little information is available, not only about the early lesions of CP but even about the likelihood of obtaining a representative sample of pancreatic tissue from advanced disease, to permit interpretation of surgically obtained tissue.[73,122,171] In this connection, we know that alcohol-associated acute pancreatitis is a manifestation of chronic pancreatitis in northern Europe and in the United States, yet virtually nothing is known about the morphologic and histologic changes in the pancreas of patients who have recovered from their first attack of acute pancreatitis. Of course, less complicated techniques such as fine needle aspiration biopsy of the pancreas provide even less representative samples of tissue and are therefore even less suitable for confirming or refuting the presence of chronic pancreatic disease.[1,76,109,137]

As a result of the technical difficulties of obtaining satisfactory representative pancreatic histologic samples, the majority of the pancreatic histologic material that is available for comparative diagnostic purposes comprises tissue from individuals with severe or complicated disease, or from individuals with coexistent pancreatic cancer. There are therefore no histopathologic criteria to use as background standards against which to set the results of biochemical and morphologic (imaging) investigations. To all intents, it is impossible to confirm a diagnosis of CP or to evaluate the real extent of pancreatic damage except in patients with end-stage pancreatic disease. The lack of firm diagnostic criteria not only has resulted in failure to provide definitive clinical indices for assessing confirmatory investigations, but also has led to considerable semantic confusion. ''Early,'' ''mild,'' or ''minimal'' radiologic (morphologic) appearances or exocrine functional changes, as defined by investigational results, have never been correlated with histopathologic findings and do not, therefore, indicate early or mild CP. The common tendency to extrapolate from investigational findings to (assumed) severity of pancreatic disease is therefore both misleading and invalid.

A further problem in making an unequivocal diagnosis of chronic pancreatitis is that many of the criteria shown in Table 18-1 only illustrate the presence of severe pancreatic disease and often do not permit satisfactory differentiation between CP and pancreatic cancer. Histologically proven CP or pancreatic cancer may be present despite the absence of the tabulated (or any other) morphologic or functional criteria.

Clinical study of patients suspected of suffering from CP therefore provides

TABLE 18-2. SUGGESTED OPERATIONAL CLASSIFICATION OF INDIVIDUAL PATIENTS SUFFERING FROM CP*

1. Histologic assessment (whenever possible)
2. Exocrine functional assessment
3. Morphologic assessment
   Endoscopic pancreatography
   Ultrasonography
   CT
4. Endocrine functional assessment
5. Etiologic assessment
6. Evaluation of complications

It was also suggested by the authors that the frequency and severity (Ranson or Imrie score) of acute relapses be documented, and that the treatment and therapeutic response be recorded.

* Modified from Banks et al.[14]

primarily evidence about the severity of pancreatic destruction and, possibly, the presence or absence of pancreatic cancer. In addition, information becomes available about the function and morphologic status of the gland and, in some instances, about etiology and complications (Table 18-2).

DIFFERENTIATION OF CP FROM PANCREATIC CANCER

The criteria presented in Table 18-1 do not permit definitive differentiation between CP and pancreatic cancer. This diagnostic problem is aggravated by the coexistence of the two conditions, since pancreatic cancer is frequently accompanied by surrounding and "upstream" changes of CP ("obstructive CP").[69,70,111] Conversely, it has also been proposed that there is an increased risk of the development of pancreatic cancer in CP since the latter is potentially a premalignant condition.[174]

Sometimes, the differentiation between CP and pancreatic cancer is made easy since the clinical investigation provides unequivocal evidence for pancreatic cancer. For example, the presence of metastases confirms the diagnosis of pancreatic cancer. Similarly, endoscopic retrograde cholangiopancreatography (ERCP) may reveal appearances that are considered to be diagnostic of pancreatic cancer (Table 18-3), or computerized tomography (CT) may demonstrate isodense enlargement of the pancreas with negative enhancement after intravenous injection of contrast material, a finding that is considered to be a reliable sign of pancreatic malignancy.[111,223] Less frequently, CT may show invasion of vessels or contiguous tissues.[132] However, in the majority of patients in whom preliminary investigations point to the presence of some pancreatic disease, it is not possible to differentiate between pancreatic cancer and CP without further studies. The techniques that have been used for differential diagnosis are summarized in Table 18-4.

Cytologic Examination of Duodenal Aspirate or of Pure Pancreatic Juice

It is possible to obtain material for cytologic examination from duodenal aspirate or during endoscopic retrograde pancreatography (ERP). Reported results of the cytologic examination of duodenal aspirate indicate that satisfactory

TABLE 18-3. ENDOSCOPIC PANCREATOGRAPHIC SIGNS OF PANCREATIC CANCER

1. Abrupt complete obstruction of an otherwise normal main pancreatic duct
2. Encasement of a long segment of main pancreatic duct with normal ductal appearances on either side
3. Parenchymal filling of necrotic tumor areas
4. *Double-duct* sign of invasion of main pancreatic duct and common bile duct by periampullary cancer

TABLE 18-4. DIFFERENTIATION OF PANCREATIC CANCER FROM CP

1. Cytology
   - Duodenal aspirate
   - Pure pancreatic juice
   - Fine needle aspiration cytology
2. Lactoferrin concentrations
   - Pure pancreatic juice
   - Duodenal aspirate
3. Tumor antigens and markers
   - Carcinoembryonic antigen (CEA)
   - Pancreatic oncofetal antigen (POA)
   - Tissue polypeptide antigen (TPA)
   - Carbohydrate antigen 19-9 (CA19-9)
   - Carbohydrate antigen 50 (CA-50)
   - Carbohydrate antigen 125 (CA-125)
   - DU-PAN 2
   - Serum galactosyltransferase isoenzyme 2
   - Serum elastase 1
   - α-fetoprotein (αFP)
   - Serum ribonuclease
   - Serum ferritin

material for examination is obtained in from 39% to 83%.[58,148] Diagnostic sensitivity ranged from 14% to 60%,[63,125,148] depending in part on the site of the tumor, with positive results more likely in carcinomas of the head of the pancreas. False-positive cytologic results were found in as many as 10% of patients with CP, particularly if there had been a recent acute relapse.

Cytologic material may be obtained at ERP in about 90% of patients either by brushing, by lavage and aspiration, or after stimulation of pancreatic secretion by secretin.[53,77] Results have varied widely, with sensitivity ranging from 33% to 97% and false-positive rates ranging from 0 to 10%.[53,126,137] It has been concluded that the diagnostic value of cytologic examination of pure pancreatic juice is similar to that of duodenal drainage studies.[125] While positive cytologic results have a high predictive value, a negative study does not exclude pancreatic cancer.

Measurement of Lactoferrin in Pure Pancreatic Juice or Duodenal Aspirate

Lactoferrin is an iron-binding protein found in many secretions. Early reports indicated that lactoferrin concentrations in pure pancreatic juice were consistently increased in patients with CP and that measurement of lactoferrin concentrations could completely differentiate between patients with CP and those with pancreatic cancer.[60,61,142] For example, in one reported study, a single patient with CP and a coexistent pancreatic cancer had increased concentrations of lactoferrin in the pure pancreatic juice and was the only patient with pancreatic cancer not satisfactorily differentiated from CP on the basis of pancreatic juice lactoferrin concentrations.[60]

Subsequent reports indicated that even though there was some overlap between concentrations of lactoferrin in the duodenal aspirate of patients with CP and those suffering from pancreatic cancer, the ratio of lactoferrin to lipase in the duodenal aspirate permitted complete discrimination between the two diseases.[143] However, more recent reports have cast doubt on the significance of lactoferrin measurements as a marker for CP since there has been complete overlap in values among patients with CP, those with pancreatic cancer, and patients with no pancreatic disease.[6,78,146]

Measurement of Tumor Antigens

A range of tumor antigens has been reported as being of value in the differentiation between pancreatic cancer and CP (Table 18-4).

Carcinoembryonic Antigen (CEA)

Increases in serum concentrations of CEA have been reported in from 34% to 83% of patients with pancreatic cancer.[56,63,125,164,181,195,229] However, the specificity of an abnormally increased concentration is low, since increased concentrations may also be found in as many as 70% of patients with CP and 28% of patients with acute pancreatitis. In addition, it seems that serum concentrations of CEA are usually only raised in the presence of advanced and inoperable cancer.[56,229] Similarly, values of CEA concentrations in the duodenal aspirate of patients with pancreatic cancer overlap significantly with those of patients with nonmalignant disease of the pancreas.[58,175,181,211]

Pancreatic Oncofetal Antigen (POA)

POA concentrations in the serum are increased in 40% to 91% of patients with pancreatic cancer.[72,125,229] However, since raised concentrations have also been reported in from 17% to 21% of patients with CP measurement of serum POA concentration is insufficiently specific to be of discriminative value.[125,194]

Tissue Polypeptide Antigen (TPA)

This protein is produced by rapidly growing tissues and has 93% to 96% sensitivity for pancreatic cancer, while apparently positive in only about 5% of patients with CP.[157,158] Thus, although raised serum concentrations may occur in patients who have extrapancreatic disease, measurement of serum concentration of TPA may be of value in the discrimination between CP and pancreatic cancer in patients with unequivocal evidence of chronic pancreatic disease.

Carbohydrate Antigen 19-9 (CA19-9)

The sensitivity of serum CA19-9 concentrations has ranged from 69% to 91% in patients with pancreatic cancer.[42,87,180,181] Circulating concentrations are dependent on the size of the tumor,[55] but the tissue expression of the antigen (which is present also in normal pancreatic tissue) may be poor in very anaplastic tumors.[86] Very high concentrations of CA19-9 (>600 U/l) have a specificity of 99% for pancreatic cancer.[207] In patients with CP, increased serum concentrations of CA19-9 are found in from 4% to 22% of patients.[179,181,194,195] Increased concentrations of CA19-9 are more common in patients with relapsing CP than in patients with burnt-out calcific pancreatitis.[194] Increased concentrations of CA19-9 also occur in 4% to 31% of patients with acute pancreatitis,[158,194] while measurement is unreliable in the presence of obstructive jaundice.[87] Measurement of serum CA19-9 concentrations is more diagnostically discriminating than concentrations of CA19-9 in pancreatic juice.[150,196] In conclusion, it seems that serum concentrations of CA19-9 are only of diagnostic value if they are greatly raised, while moderate increases are poorly specific.

Carbohydrate Antigen 50 (CA-50)

Early reports indicate that the sensitivity of this antigen for pancreatic cancer is 92%, with a specificity of 89%, but numbers of patients have been small, and the studies require confirmation.[85]

Carbohydrate Antigen 125 (CA-125)

Elevated concentrations of CA-125 occur in a range of gastrointestinal malignancies, and false-positive results occur in patients with acute pancreatitis. However, no false-positive results were observed in patients suffering from CP.[181]

DU-PAN 2

Although serum concentrations of this glycoprotein were raised in 94% of patients with pancreatic cancer, increased concentrations were also detected in patients with biliary obstruction from benign causes,[128] so that the specificity may be unsatisfactory for discriminative purposes (although the matter has not been directly assessed in published reports).

Serum Galactosyltransferase Isoenzyme 2

Serum concentrations of this enzyme are increased in 67% of patients with pancreatic cancer and also in 71% of patients with nonpancreatic malignancies.[164] However, since the false-positive rate for nonmalignant disease was only 2%, it has been suggested that measurement of serum galactosyltransferase 2 may be useful in the differentiation of pancreatic cancer from CP.

Serum Elastase 1

The sensitivity, specificity, and efficiency of serum elastase 1 measurements in the diagnosis of pancreatic cancer, compared with CP were 72%, 60%, and 64%, respectively.[89] Since serum concentrations are also increased during attacks of acute pancreatitis, measurement of serum elastase 1 levels is not useful for clinical diagnostic purposes.[121]

α-Fetoprotein (αFP)

Raised serum concentrations of αFP are found in only 3% to 33% of patients with pancreatic cancer and are not of diagnostic value.[63,164,194,229]

Serum Ribonuclease

Recent reports about the diagnostic value of concentrations of serum ribonuclease indicate that increased concentrations occur in from 30% to 42% of patients with pancreatic cancer[63,164] and that false-positive results occur in 14% to 36% of patients. This tumor marker is therefore unsuitable for differentiating CP from pancreatic cancer.

Serum Ferritin

Serum ferritin concentrations are increased in from 50% to 78% of patients with pancreatic cancer,[149,151,164] but raised concentrations may also be found in 35% of patients with CP and in all patients with recurrent acute pancreatitis. Measurement of serum ferritin levels cannot be used to differentiate pancreatic cancer from CP.

Summary

No single tumor marker is sufficiently sensitive or specific for satisfactory differentiation between CP and pancreatic cancer. Combinations of tumor markers, used to produce diagnostic "profiles," have similarly been unsatisfactory.[121,149] At present, reliable differentiation of CP from pancreatic cancer can only be made by cytologic criteria, demonstration of metastases, or at laparotomy after histologic examination of the pancreas.

OPERATIONAL CLASSIFICATION OF PATIENTS WITH CP

Functional Assessment

In the original Marseilles classification, a persistently or progressively impaired pancreatic secretory response to exogenous secretagogues was recommended as a criterion that was diagnostic of CP.[185] However, the criteria for performance of the secretory studies and interpretation of the results were not defined. In addition, tests of pancreatic exocrine secretion are not capable of differentiating CP from pancreatic cancer (because secretory capacity may be impaired in both types of pancreatic disease), nor of providing information on the etiology or prognosis of the pancreatic disease. Although studies using exogenous secretagogues with direct aspiration of pancreatic secretion are the most satisfactory tests for confirming the presence of severe pancreatic damage and, therefore, pancreatic disease, other less invasive methods have been used to assess exocrine pancreatic function and may be employed as part of the operational classification of the CP; to assess the progress of exocrine function with time; and to evaluate the requirement for, and effects of, therapeutic intervention. Tests of pancreatic function remain diagnostically valuable because patients with CP may have abnormal exocrine function in the absence of any clinical morphologic abnormality. The converse is also occasionally true.

Duodenal Drainage Studies Using Exogenous Secretagogues

Unfortunately the test protocols used in various centers differ enormously in terms of secretagogues employed, dosages and modes of administration of secretagogues (infusion or bolus injection), duration of stimulation, analytic measurements performed on the duodenal aspirate, and indices that provide the best diagnostic discrimination. Valid comparisons of data from various centers are therefore not possible.[23] However, it is possible to conclude that when studies involving the aspiration of pancreatic secretion in response to exogenous secretagogues are performed, secretagogues should be administered by constant-rate intravenous infusion, at doses that produce maximal (or near maximal) outputs of bicarbonate and enzymes, for periods that permit a secretory plateau to be achieved. Secretion of bicarbonate and enzymes should be expressed as peak outputs per unit time since these provide the best diagnostic discrimination.[23]

When correctly performed, direct duodenal drainage studies have a sensitivity ranging from 83% to 95% and a specificity ranging from 89% to 95%.[24] Abnormal results may be found in patients with diabetes mellitus, 15% of whom have decreased bicarbonate outputs, and one third of whom have impaired secretion of at least one enzyme in response to secretin and cholecystokinin (CCK).[118] Patients who have undergone truncal or selective gastric vagotomy (but not highly selective vagotomy) have a reduction of about 25% to 33% secretory response to exogenous hormones.[18,19,230] The reduction in the secretory response to exogenous hormones is greater for bicarbonate than for enzymes. When pancreatic exocrine hypofunction is detected, it is necessary to demonstrate that this is persistent. Thus, patients with long-standing malnutrition, particularly in association with celiac disease, may suffer from reversible pancreatic hypofunction.[152,166] Impaired secretory responses may also occur during recovery from acute pancreatitis.[82,216]

That the results of pancreatic stimulation with secretin and CCK correlate with histologic abnormalities of the pancreas has been confirmed by a study in which secretory results were compared with histologic appearances of the pancreases that had been resected surgically.[93] Statistically significant correlation was found between abnormalities of the secretion of bicarbonate and dilatation of the small, as well as the main, pancreatic ducts. There was also significant correlation between impaired bicarbonate secretion and acinar atrophy.

The sensitivity and specificity of the commonly performed variants of the secretin (± CCK) test in detecting exocrine pancreatic disease are less than 100%, so that attempts have been made to increase the diagnostic performance of the secretory tests that involve direct measurement of the pancreatic secretory response to exogenous secretagogues.

"Extended" Pancreatic Function Tests Discrimination between patients with CP and patients without pancreatic disease increases with the duration of secretory stimulation. In one study, although there was marked overlap of secretory outputs of normal individuals and patients with CP after 30 minutes of stimulation, there was nearly complete discrimination after stimulation for 90 minutes.[81] A different approach involved an attempt to "exhaust" the pancreas in patients with CP by two consecutive periods of secretory stimulation, but the secretory responses of bicarbonate and enzymes during the second period of stimulation were similar to those during the first period, so that the diagnostic discrimination was not improved.[74]

Dose–Response Studies Following a "standard" secretin test in which secretin (1 Crick Harper Raper Units (CHRU)/kg) is administered by intravenous injection and duodenal aspirate is collected for 80 minutes, an increased dose of secretin (4 CHRU/kg) is administered and duodenal aspirate collected for a further 80-minute period.[46] It seems that this sequence of administration of secretagogue increases the sensitivity of the test, since the normal subjects both volume and bicarbonate concentration increase by about 100% and 15%, respectively, while in CP the secretory rate may increase but the bicarbonate concentration remains unchanged. A more elaborate technique, in which stepwise increases in the dose of secretin were administered by intravenous infusion, demonstrated an increased sensitivity to secretin in the early phase (first 2 years) of CP.[161] However, calculated maximal secretory rates did not provide any greater discrimination than did observed outputs at the maximal dose of secretin (2 CHRU/kg per hour).

Tests of Enzyme Synthetic Capacity The rate of incorporation of ^{75}Se-methionine administered by constant intravenous infusion into the TCA-insoluble fraction of the duodenal aspirate during stimulation of pancreatic secretion with secretin 1 Clinical Units CU/kg per hour plus CCK 1 Ivy Dog Units IDU/kg per hour was used as an index of pancreatic enzyme synthesis. In a prospective study using independent criteria for the diagnosis of CP, it was found that the enzyme synthetic capacity was a more sensitive index of the presence of CP (88%) than bicarbonate output (75%) but was less specific (73% compared with 92%).[25] When both enzyme synthesis and bicarbonate output were either both abnormal or both normal, the sensitivity and specificity were 100% and 95%, respectively.

Analysis of Pure Pancreatic Juice Pure pancreatic juice can be collected during ERP, but stimulation with secretin (± CCK) is necessary to allow collection of sufficient quantities for analysis. Discrimination between patients with and without CP is poor because there is a marked overlap in bicarbonate and enzyme concentrations between the two groups.[43,60,79] In one study only 2 of 14 patients with CP had bicarbonate concentrations below 90 mmol/L.[43] Unfortunately only data on electrolyte and enzyme concentrations (rather than outputs) in pure pancreatic juice are available because there are unavoidable and unquantifiable losses of pancreatic juice around the intraductal catheter and possibly also through the accessory pancreatic duct. In general it appears that secretory studies of pure pancreatic juice do not provide any information that is not more easily available from duodenal drainage studies, and indeed the latter are diagnostically more discriminating.

It has, however, recently been suggested that information derived from the components of pure pancreatic juice may provide a useful discriminant between patients with and without pancreatic disease. Thus, it has been reported that electrophoresis of the proteins of pure pancreatic juice shows significant abnormalities of glycoprotein content in patients with CP.[106,226]

Studies of Duodenal Aspirate Using Endogenous Stimulation of Pancreatic Secretion

Tests involving direct stimulation of pancreatic secretion using exogenous secretagogues are technically demanding, poorly standardized, and expensive, so that many investigators prefer to use the Lundh test to assess exocrine pancreatic function. The Lundh test provides a measure of the functional integrity of the digestive process, of which pancreatic exocrine secretion is the most important part. The standard Lundh test lasts 2 hours and involves measurement of the tryptic activity of sampled duodenal aspirate following a standard liquid meal.[104] However, a 30-minute collection of duodenal aspirate provides similar diagnostic information.[159] It is also preferable to measure more than one enzymic activity in the duodenal aspirate since there is sometimes selective reduction in the concentration of one enzyme during the course of pancreatic disease.[102] The complete aspiration of duodenal contents following a meal is not possible, so that the Lundh test provides information solely about enzymic "concentrations" but not about enzyme outputs. In addition, the Lundh test provides no information on bicarbonate secretion by the pancreas, although the pH of the duodenal aspirate may give an indication of whether there is likely to be inactivation of endogenous and exogenous digestive enzymes in the duodenum and may be used to assess the effects of enzyme replacement therapy.[189] The specificity of the Lundh test is less than that of the secretin (± CCK) test. False-positive results occur in the disorders listed in Table 18-5. Although some reports have claimed that the Lundh test is more sensitive than the secretin (± CCK) test, the majority of comparative studies have indicated that the secretin-CCK test is more sensitive, particularly in the early or less severe forms of CP.[84,124,176]

Tubeless Pancreatic Function Tests

In some patients duodenal intubation is impossible for anatomic reasons (pyloric stenosis or previous gastric surgery) or because the patient is too young

TABLE 18-5. NONPANCREATIC DISEASES ASSOCIATED WITH ABNORMAL LUNDH TESTS*

	Patients with Abnormal Lundh Tests, %
Obstructive jaundice	38
Celiac disease	18
Partial gastrectomy	44
Vagotomy	13
Diabetes	18
Miscellaneous	18

* From Lurie et al.,[124] Mottaleb et al.,[140] Zeitlin and Sircus.[231]

or cannot tolerate the procedure. In addition, tests involving intubation are less acceptable to patients who are undergoing repeated studies to assess the progress of pancreatic disease or the effects of therapy. Attempts have therefore been made to evaluate pancreatic function indirectly by the use of orally administered substrates (the digestion of which is studied) and also by the measurement of pancreatic enzymes in serum or in the stool.

The *N*-benzoyl-l-tyrosyl-*p*-aminobenzoic acid (Bentiromide) Test *N*-benzoyl-l-tyrosyl-*p*-aminobenzoic acid (NBT-PABA) is a peptide substrate for pancreatic chymotrypsin. The test is based on the recovery of *p*-aminobenzoic acid (PABA) in the urine after oral administration of the peptide. The test, as reported in the literature, has not been standardized, but the optimal dose appears to be 500 mg, followed by a urine collection for 6 hours.[213] Lower doses of the peptide result in difficulties measuring urinary aromatic amine concentrations and increase the proportional interference from amines in food and drugs as, for example, prunes, paracetamol, thiazides, sulphonylureas, and sulphonamides. On the other hand, higher doses of the peptide may cause nausea, while urinary PABA excretion becomes more dependent on hepatic conjugation than on pancreatic function. Prolonging the urine collection beyond 6 hours does not increase the diagnostic value of the test. The reported sensitivity of the NBT-PABA test has ranged from 65% to 96%,[10,92,103] but these values reflect the severity of the pancreatic disease in the study population. For example, the sensitivity of the PABA test was only 42% in patients with mild impairment of bicarbonate or enzyme secretion in response to pancreatic stimulation with secretin and CCK.[119] However, when pancreatic exocrine insufficiency was so severe that steatorrhoea resulted, the sensitivity of the test was 97%. Correlation with morphologic studies has shown that abnormal results are observed when more than half of the pancreas has been resected or when the main pancreatic duct is obstructed within 6 cm of the ampulla of Vater.[92]

The specificity of the test is also low. Since the test depends on the secretion of chymotrypsin and therefore reflects the stimulation of pancreatic secretion by the release of endogenous secretin and CCK, as in the Lundh test, false-positive results occur under similar circumstances (as those listed in Table 18-5). In addition, false-positive results may occur in patients with intestinal disease, as a result of impaired absorption of PABA; in hepatic disease, as a result of impaired conjugation of PABA; and in renal disease, as a result of impaired excretion of the PABA conjugate. False-positive results have ranged from 18% to 37% in different studies.[119,136] False-positive results that return to normal after treatment with metronidazole have been reported from patients with giardiasis.[154]

Attempts have been made to improve to specificity of the PABA test, by including administration of unesterified PABA under similar conditions on a separate day,[136] or by giving [^{14}C]PABA with the peptide, in order to control for abnormalities of absorption, conjugation, or excretion of PABA.[135,212] A PABA excretion index is calculated from the proportions of ingested PABA excreted on each day. Alternatively, *p*-aminosalicylic acid (which has similar absorptive, metabolic, and excretory pathways to PABA) may be administered together with the NBT-PABA to avoid the necessity for repeated testing or the use of radioisotopes.[99] The use of the PABA excretion index has increased the specificity of the one day by 9% to 20%.

Serum PABA measurements from 90 to 150 minutes after oral administration of NBT-PABA have been reported as being diagnostically superior to the single-day (urinary) PABA test, and to provide as good, or better, discrimination than calculation of the PABA excretion index derived from the modified PABA tests.[35,115,116,210] However, in one study, serum PABA concentrations were less sensitive (10%) than urine collections (30%) in the diagnosis of mild pancreatic insufficiency.[35] The NBT-PABA test with either urine collections or serum PABA measurements was less sensitive (63%) than the Lundh test (80%) in patients with CP.[41]

A variant of the NBT-PABA test, using a slightly different substrate (*N*-acetyltyrosyl-*p*-aminobenzoic acid) has been employed to assess the adequacy of pancreatic enzyme replacement therapy.[68] Pancreatic enzyme supplements were shown to increase the excretion of PABA in children with cystic fibrosis.

Fluorescein Dilaurate (Pancreolauryl) Test Fluorescein dilaurate (FDL) is a substrate for pancreatic cholesterol ester hydrolase. FDL is administered orally in a manner similar to NBT-PABA, and the fluorescein that is liberated by hydrolysis of the substrate is absorbed, conjugated, and excreted in the urine, which is collected for 10 hours. Fluorescein conjugates are more easily measured and are less susceptible to drug and dietary interference than are the urinary aromatic amines measured in the NBT-PABA test. Unesterified fluorescein is administered on a separate day to calculate an excretion index analogous to the PABA excretion index. The sensitivity and specificity of the FDL test have been marginally superior to those of the PABA test in the majority of studies in which there has been a direct comparison in the same patients.[35,108,116,119,220] Sensitivity of the FDL test is also dependent on the degree of pancreatic exocrine insufficiency as assessed by the secretin-CCK test. With mild impairment of pancreatic exocrine secretion, the sensitivity of the FDL test was 59%. When the exocrine insufficiency was sufficiently severe to result in steatorrhea, the sensitivity of the FDL test was 100%.[119]

Serum fluorescein concentrations at 3½ or 4 hours after oral administration of FDL have also been used instead of urine collections to assess pancreatic exocrine function. The sensitivity of the serum fluorescein concentrations was greater than that of urinary fluorescein excretion.[35,116]

It appears that oral tests of pancreatic function are only reliably abnormal in the presence of pancreatic exocrine insufficiency that is so severe (less than 10% of normal) that steatorrhea is produced. In addition, the tests give a high proportion of falsely positive results, particularly after gastric surgery.[95] This type of test is therefore unsuitable for the diagnosis of pancreatic exocrine insufficiency but may be useful for following the progress of patients with established pancreatic disease and for assessing the efficacy of replacement therapy.

Measurement of Pancreatic Enzymes in Body Fluids

In the basal state and after stimulation of pancreatic secretion, pancreatic enzymes can be detected in the serum and in the stool. Attempts have been made to correlate the activities (denoting concentrations) of these enzymes with pancreatic exocrine function.

Serum Amylase Measurement of the activity of total serum amylase activity either in the basal state or after stimulation of pancreatic secretion by food or exogenously administered seretagogues (evocative testing) is of no value in the detection of chronic pancreatic disease.[120,209] On the other hand, pancreatic isoamylase (iso-P) concentrations do bear some relationship to the severity of CP.[120,209] The isoenzymic activity is measured using a wheat inhibitor assay or by monoclonal antibodies. Serum concentrations of iso-P rise with increasing age, and increased concentrations are found in normal individuals and in patients with chronic liver disease, chronic renal failure, or acute pancreatitis.[51,57,144] Low concentrations may be found in patients with alcoholic cirrhosis even in the presence of normal pancreatic exocrine function. Abnormally low concentrations of iso-P are found in the serum of 15% to 43% of patients with exocrine pancreatic insufficiency and in 2% to 4% of healthy controls or patients with nonpancreatic gastrointestinal disease.[105,110,117,201]

Low serum iso-P concentrations are related to the degree of exocrine pancreatic insufficiency and are usually found only in patients with severe pancreatic disease. Low concentrations of iso-P are found in about two thirds of insulin-dependent diabetic patients.[118] However, approximately 40% of insulin-dependent diabetic patients who have low serum iso-P concentrations have normal pancreatic exocrine secretion in response to stimulation with secretin and CCK. Low concentrations of iso-P are, therefore, not sufficiently sensitive to be useful for the diagnosis of CP. Increased concentrations of iso-P occur in about 30% of patients with CP.[110] Increased concentrations of iso-P may be related to ductal obstruction or to episodes of acute inflammation, and under these circumstances the serum iso-P concentrations do not correspond with the severity of the CP disease.

Serum Immunoreactive Trypsin (IRT) Trypsinogen can be measured in the circulation by a radioimmunoassay that detects both cationic and anionic trypsinogen, in addition to trypsinogen complexed with α_1-antitrypsin and α_2-macroglobulin.[130] However, trypsinogen bound to protease inhibitors is not fully immunopotent.

Low concentrations of serum IRT are found in 13% to 27% of patients with CP.[131,178,206] When basal concentrations of serum IRT were compared with the pancreatic enzyme and bicarbonate secretory response to secretin and CCK, low basal concentrations of IRT were found in only 20% of patients with mild impairment of bicarbonate secretion but were abnormally low in 94% of patients with severe impairment of exocrine secretion as shown by steatorrhea and diabetes (Table 18-6). Basal concentrations of IRT are also sometimes low in insulin-dependent diabetic patients and do not always reflect the presence of impaired exocrine pancreatic secretion in these patients.[39,118] Low concentrations of serum IRT have been claimed to have a specificity greater than 98%, and a sensitivity of 85% in patients with CP with steatorrhea, although in the absence of steatorrhea the sensitivity is 30%.[205] However, it has been pointed out that the sensitivity of serum IRT measurements in CP patients without steatorrhea is virtually zero.[64] Measurement of serum IRT is therefore only of value in patients whose CP is sufficiently severe to result in steatorrhea. The diagnostic value of serum IRT and serum iso-P concentrations is similar.[139]

TABLE 18-6. CORRELATION BETWEEN EXOCRINE PANCREATIC FUNCTION AND SERUM IMMUNOREACTIVE TRYPSIN CONCENTRATIONS*

Pancreatic Exocrine Function in Response to Secretin-CCK	Patients with Abnormally Low Concentrations of IRT, %
↓ HCO_3 output only	20
↓ HCO_3 output, ↓ enzyme output (−1 SD)	47
↓ HCO_3 output, ↓ ↓ enzyme output (−2 SD)	60
Plus diabetes	74
Plus steatorrhea	79
Diabetes and steatorrhea	94

* From Andriulli et al.[7]

Increased circulating concentrations of IRT occur in acute pancreatitis and in 27% to 52% of patients with CP.[131,178] In the latter patients the increased concentrations of IRT do not reflect (impaired) exocrine function but denote either ductal obstruction or acute pancreatitis.

Serum Lipase, Serum Elastase 1, and Serum Phospholipase A_2 These enzymes are detected in the circulation as proenzymes. They appear to be useful markers for acute pancreatic inflammation but do not correlate well with exocrine pancreatic function, for which purpose serum iso-P and IRT concentrations are superior. Raised concentrations of each of these three enzymes are may be found in patients with CP.[30,100,138,219]

Summary The role of serum enzyme measurements in the evaluation of exocrine pancreatic function is limited. Low concentrations of iso-P or IRT are found only in patients with severe exocrine insufficiency, in whom the predictive power of abnormally low concentrations of iso-P and IRT is high for the impaired exocrine function. However, many patients with CP have normal or increased concentrations of serum pancreatic enzymes as a result of ductal obstruction or acute inflammation. Under these circumstances normal or increased concentrations of serum pancreatic enzymes do not, of course, represent normal or exaggerated pancreatic exocrine secretory responses.

Pancreatic Polypeptide

Pancreatic polypeptide (PP) is found solely in the pancreas, where it is localized to the islets and the intervening tissue. Plasma concentrations of PP increase in parallel with the secretion of pancreatic enzymes in response to exogenous and endogenous stimulation of pancreatic secretion, but there seems to be no direct correlation with exocrine pancreatic function. Changes in plasma concentrations of PP during the administration of secretagogues have also been denied.[123,156,167] Serum concentrations of PP increase with age.[17] Increased plasma PP concentrations are also found in up to 40% of alcoholics, even though 40% of these patients suffer from exocrine pancreatic insufficiency.[62,134]

Low plasma concentrations of PP are found in as many as 88% of patients with CP disease and exocrine insufficiency but are also found in 35% of apparently healthy controls, so that the specificity of low concentrations of PP in basal blood samples is poorly specific for the presence of exocrine pancreatic insufficiency.[113]

In order to improve the diagnostic value of plasma PP measurements, attempts have been made to stimulate the release of PP into the circulation by the administration of secretagogues. In one study the integrated plasma PP response to CCK correlated well with the degree of exocrine pancreatic insufficiency in 20 patients with CP, and only one patient had results in the control range.[156] An infusion of secretin plus cerulein caused an increase in plasma PP concentrations in healthy subjects, while in patients with CP and steatorrhea there was impaired release of PP into the circulation and there was good diagnostic discrimination from normal.[6] However, in patients with only mild pancreatic exocrine insufficiency there was marked overlap in plasma PP concentrations between patients and controls. Thus, abnormally low basal PP concentrations are not sufficiently specific to provide a marker for patients other than those with severe exocrine pancreatic insufficiency. The plasma PP response to secretagogues is only consistently abnormal in patients with exocrine pancreatic insufficiency so severe as to result in steatorrhea.

Measurement of Pancreatic Enzymes in the Stool

Trypsin and chymotrypsin can be measured in feces, either as activities in random samples or as output in timed collections.[3,141] However, chymotrypsin is more resistant to degradation during passage through the gut and is therefore preferable to trypsin for the assessment of exocrine pancreatic function.

Stool concentrations of chymotrypsin are correlated with exocrine pancreatic secretion in response to secretin and CCK. When the secretory response to secretin and CCK is only mildly or moderately impaired, the fecal chymotrypsin concentrations are abnormal in 8% to 60% of patients.[119,193] However, when there is severe exocrine impairment with steatorrhea, abnormal fecal chymotrypsin concentrations are found in 72% to 96% of patients.[49]

False-positive results have been reported in from 8% to 20% of patients, including those with partial gastrectomy, small intestinal disease, or nonspecific diarrhea (as a result of dilution of intestinal contents). Measurement of fecal chymotrypsin concentrations appears to be of value only in the detection of severe exocrine pancreatic insufficiency so severe as to result in steatorrhea. Measurement of fecal chymotrypsin concentrations has been used for the long-term follow-up of pancreatic function in patients with established CP.[4]

Morphologic Evaluation

ERP

The technique of ERP is well established and in the majority of patients is well tolerated and safe. However, in a few patients technical problems vitiate the test. For example, in one large series of 3444 examinations, it proved impossible to cannulate the pancreatic duct in 13% of patients, and in 11% the radiographs obtained were unsatisfactory for diagnostic purposes because of poor ductal filling, movement artifact, or the superimposition of the endoscope on the area of interest.[37] These problems may be minimized by careful attention to detail. Although more difficult, it is possible to perform ERP successfully in about two thirds of patients who have undergone previous gastric surgery, including Biliroth II partial gastrectomy.[66]

ERP demonstrates unequivocal abnormalities in from 53% to 85% of patients with CP diagnosed by independent criteria.[27,33,177,217,225] In addition to confirming the diagnosis of CP, ERP may also permit a confident diagnosis of pancreatic cancer (Table 18-3); allow the detection of etiologically important abnormalities contributing to obstructive CP; or demonstrate evidence of complications, for example, common bile duct stenosis,[186] pseudocysts,[114,208] or the site of leakage in pancreatic ascites.[184]

Although moderate to severe ERP changes provide satisfactory diagnostic confirmation in most patients with CP, controversy surrounds the significance of "equivocal" and "mild" changes on the endoscopic pancreatogram. In the first case there is usually considerable observer variation in the reporting of these abnormalities.[155] Moreover, it has been shown that these appearances do not always indicate CP. Similar appearances are attributable to the aging process in the pancreas,[20,145,198] with dilatation of the peripheral ducts in 40% of autopsy pancreases.[203] Reversible appearances, compatible with mild CP, can be observed when ERP is performed shortly after an attack of acute pancreatitis.[90] When histologic information has been available in patients who have had mild pancreatographic abnormalities, only about 50% have had histologic evidence of CP.[112,199,214] Similarly, about 50% of patients with mild ERP changes who have also had duodenal drainage studies of pancreatic exocrine function have had secretory impairment.[11,52,75,182,190] It seems, therefore, that "mild" changes on ERP do not provide evidence for the diagnosis of CP, with the low specificity (less than 65%) attributable to the problem of interpreting the "minimal" changes.[78] Although one recent study found "fairly good correlation" between functional and anatomic assessments, marked discrepancies occurred, so that it was impossible to predict the exocrine functional status of individual patients from the ductal morphology or to make the converse extrapolation.[26]

Ultrasonography

Ultrasonographic examination of the pancreas is noninvasive, cheap, and widely available. It is considered to be the most satisfactory imaging technique for the purpose of screening patients with suspected chronic pancreatic disease. The diagnostic performance of ultrasonography is, however, dependent on both the quality of the scanning equipment and the experience of the operator. Acoustic access to the pancreas may be unsatisfactory in obese patients, in the presence of bowel gas, or because of the anatomic configuration of the ribs, so that satisfactory examination of the pancreas is obtained in about 75% to 80% of patients studied.

There have been few prospective studies of ultrasonography in the evaluation of CP in which the final diagnosis was confirmed or refuted by reliable independent criteria. However, ultrasonography has been claimed to be more specific than ERP (because "mild" ERP abnormalities are of little diagnostic value),[168] but probably less sensitive than either ERP or CT in the diagnosis of CP.[38,65,97] For example, it has proved impossible to predict exocrine function from ultrasonographic morphologic findings, since the latter appearances may be quite normal in patients with severe pancreatic secretory impairment.[21]

Ultrasonography may provide evidence of etiologic factors, such as biliary calculi or of complications such as stenosis of the bile duct or pseudocysts and can confirm the diagnosis of pancreatic cancer by demonstrating the presence of metastases.[2] Ultrasonography may also be used to guide fine needle biopsy of the pancreas.

In view of the subjective nature of ultrasonographic diagnostic criteria, ultrasonographic abnormalities should be confirmed whenever possible by alternative imaging techniques.

CT

For the pancreatic parenchyma, CT is the most satisfactory imaging technique. CT is less operator-dependent than ultrasonography and produces images that allow more objective assessment. The quality of the scans is dependent on the age and sophistication of the machine employed. Pancreatic scans can be obtained in all patients, and, in contrast to ultrasonography, CT in obese patients provides satisfactory images because fat enhances the demarcation of tissue planes. Most recent studies have shown that CT scanning is more sensitive and specific in the diagnosis of CP than is ultrasonography.[65,97] CT may demonstrate unequivocal evidence of CP in the form of pancreatic calcification that is not visible on plain abdominal radiographs.[129] CT may permit the detection of pancreatic cancer by demonstration of metastases, by demonstration of a pancreatic mass with negative enhancement after intravenous contrast injection, and by demonstration of invasion of neighboring organs or blood vessels.[111,132,223] Biliary tract disease can also be identified, as can complications of CP, such as pseudocysts,[32,155] hemorrhage into cysts from pseudoaneurysms,[32] splenic vein thrombosis,[127] and bile duct stenosis.[16]

Assessment of Endocrine Function

Pancreatic islet cells are relatively well preserved in the initial stages of CP, and there may even be histologic evidence of islet cell hyperplasia.[222,233] As the disease progresses, insulin-secreting β cells and glucagon-secreting α cells disappear, not necessarily at the same rate.[15] Transient hyperglycemia may follow acute relapses of CP with resolution and normoglycemia being restored as the attack subsides. Abnormal glucose tolerance is found in 14% to 65% of patients with early CP and is present in as many as 90% of patients when calcification is present.[204] In European patients, steatorrhea precedes diabetes in about half of the patients with alcoholic CP and about 80% of patients with nonalcoholic CP.

To some extent, the impaired secretion of insulin depends on functional, rather than pathologic, abnormalities of the pancreas, since the insulin secretion and impaired glucose tolerance can be improved by satisfactory treatment of the steatorrhea, with resulting reversal of the impaired secretion of gastric inhibitory peptide.[50]

Symptomatic hyperglycemia should be treated, even if only for a short time. Concentrations of glycosylated hemoglobin should be measured at regular intervals. Elevated concentrations indicate significant elevation of blood glucose concentrations during the preceding 3 months, and if concentrations of glycosylated hemoglobin are greater than 10%, hypoglycemic therapy is probably required. When glycosylated hemoglobin concentrations are used to monitor therapy of diabetes in CP, it is probably inadvisable to attempt to reduce concentrations to the normal range (4.5% to 6%), since patients with diabetes secondary to pancreatitis are reported to develop hypoglycemia very easily and to have a relatively low risk of developing microvascular complications,[47,191] although this has recently been contested.[36]

Etiologic Evaluation

Alcohol

The history of alcohol intake should be assessed using independent witnesses if necessary. In addition, evidence should be sought for alcohol-related damage of other organs, particularly the liver, by the appropriate blood tests, imaging techniques, and biopsy. It has been hypothesized that clinical CP is rare in patients with established alcoholic cirrhosis.[168] However, autopsy studies indicate that the incidence of histologic CP in patients dying of alcohol-induced liver disease is 40% to 50%.[8,163,170] Conversely, about three quarters of patients suffering from alcohol-induced pancreatitis have alcohol-induced liver disease, with established cirrhosis in from 13% to 25%.[8,169]

Anatomic Abnormalities

Several anatomic abnormalities appear to be associated with an increased incidence of CP (Table 18-7). Anatomic abnormalities may be associated with the specific entity of obstructive CP, which is characterized by dilatation of the ductal system with diffuse atrophy of the acinar parenchyma and uniform diffuse fibrosis, usually without calcification or the formation of calculi. In obstructive CP the structural changes may regress and function can improve when the obstruction is removed.

TABLE 18-7. ANATOMIC ABNORMALITIES ASSOCIATED WITH OBSTRUCTIVE CP

1. Pancreas divisum[171]
2. Annular pancreas[44]
3. Periampullary diverticulum[107]
4. Ampullary carcinoma
5. Posttraumatic or postinflammatory stricture
6. Familial anomalous pancreatic ducts[215]

Biliary Disease

Calculous biliary disease commonly causes acute pancreatitis. It seems possible that in a few individuals gallstones result in the development of CP.[12] Gallstones should be sought by cholecystography or ultrasonography and may be demonstrated at endoscopic retrograde cholangiography (ERC). Primary and secondary sclerosing cholangitis, and primary biliary cirrhosis, are associated with pancreatographic abnormalities of mild to moderate degree,[54,91,224] and with impairment of exocrine pancreatic function.[54]

Hereditary and Metabolic Disease

It may be necessary to investigate the family history in patients with unexplained pancreatitis[9,200] and to evaluate nutritional status in patients with nonalcoholic tropical pancreatitis.[153] CP may be associated with primary hypertriglyceridemias[96] or with hypertriglyceridemia secondary to alcohol abuse.[34] Conversely, hyperlipidemia in patients with pancreatitis may be secondary to an acute attack of pancreatitis, in which case the disturbance of serum lipid concentrations is transient.[29] In a small proportion of patients, CP is apparently caused by hypercalcemia secondary to hyperparathyroidism.[98,165] In all patients, fasting plasma lipid and serum calcium concentrations should be monitored in order to rectify potential causes of chronic pancreatic disease.

It has been reported that α_1-antitrypsin concentrations in serum are significantly lower than normal in some patients with CP.[133] In some patients with CP, it seems that linkage with HLA antigens (HLA-B5 or B13) may indicate that genetic factors are involved in the development of idiopathic CP,[83,101] while association with HLA-Bw39 may indicate a genetic predisposition to alcoholic CP.[228]

In view of the finding of sweat electrolyte concentrations of sodium above 90 mmol/L in one third of patients with CP, it has been proposed that some patients with CP suffer from a heterozygous form of cystic fibrosis.[13]

Connective Tissue Disease

Up to one third of patients with progressive systemic sclerosis (PSS) have impaired exocrine pancreatic function as demonstrated by an abnormal Lundh or secretin-CCK test.[94] This has been considered to be caused by pancreatic fibrosis,[162] although an increased incidence of pancreatic fibrosis in PSS has also been denied.[40]

EVALUATION OF COMPLICATIONS OF CP

The most significant complications that occur in patients with CP and that should be sought in all patients are local complications involving the pancreas itself, and the neighboring blood vessels and viscera. Stenosis of the bile duct is present in from 2% to 49% of patients.[31,48,71,160,186] It is best demonstrated by ERC, which reveals a long tapering, smooth stricture.[186] Complete biliary obstruction is uncommon but may occur temporarily as a result of edema during an acute exacerbation.[133] Progression to secondary biliary cirrhosis is uncommon even though liver function tests may remain abnormal for years.[45,202,227] No satisfactory policy has yet been defined for surgical intervention.

Patients with CP have an increased incidence of duodenal ulcer.[160,192,218] Endoscopy should always be performed to exclude or confirm the presence of a duodenal ulcer, since scarring of the duodenal bulb on radiologic examination may be attributable either to duodenal ulceration or to contiguous pancreatitis.[59] Acid secretory studies are worth performing since many patients with non-alcohol-related CP have gastric hypersecretion.[80,188] The resultant excessive acidity of the contents of the upper small intestine,[22] as well as the increased amounts of acid in the stomach, should be treated with histamine H_2-receptor antagonists to prevent inactivation of endogenous and exogenous pancreatic enzymes[189] and to reverse the pH-dependent precipitation of bile acids.[232] In addition, gastric hypersecretion aggravates the malassimilation of vitamin B_{12} that occurs in patients with CP.[147,221]

Evidence for gastrointestinal blood loss should always be sought in patients with CP, and if it is found, specific investigations should be undertaken to determine whether duodenal ulceration, esophageal varices (resulting from splenic vein thrombosis), or pseudoaneurysms caused by disruption of medium-sized blood vessels in the walls of pancreatic cysts are present.[88,183]

SUMMARY AND CONCLUSIONS

The most satisfactory diagnostic criterion for CP is histologic examination of pancreatic tissue, but it is seldom justifiable to perform pancreatic biopsy. Other proposed criteria are less satisfactory because they may not be specific for CP but may also occur in pancreatic cancer. While it may be possible to confirm the presence of pancreatic cancer in patients being evaluated for CP, it may be impossible completely to exclude cancer since tumor markers are unsatisfactory for the differentiation of cancer from chronic inflammatory disease, negative fine needle aspiration cytology does not exclude cancer, and even open biopsy may give an incorrect diagnosis in a proportion of patients.

Noninvasive tests of pancreatic exocrine function are too insensitive to provide satisfactory criteria of impaired exocrine secretion for diagnostic purposes but may be of value in monitoring the progress of CP that has been diagnosed by other criteria. Endoscopic pancreatography should be attempted in all patients, but mild changes are insufficient evidence on which to base a diagnosis of CP. Ultrasonography is an excellent screening test of pancreatic morphology, but ultrasonography abnormalities should always be confirmed by further investigations.

Attempts should always be made fully to evaluate all aspects of CP in order to provide a rational basis for therapy, to define treatable causes of obstructive CP, and to demonstrate complications that require specific treatment. In addition, a comprehensive operational approach to the evaluation of CP may improve the current inadequate status of the classification, etiology, diagnosis, and prognosis of this disease.

REFERENCES

1. Alpern GA, Dekker A. Fine needle aspiration of the pancreas. An analysis of its use in 52 cases. Acta Cytol 29:873–874, 1985.
2. Alpern MB, Sandler MA, Kellman GM, Madrazo DC. Chronic pancreatitis: Ultrasonic features. Radiology 155:215–219, 1985.
3. Ammann RW, Akovbiantz A, Häcki W, Largiader F, Schmid M. Diagnostic value of the faecal chymotrypsin test in diagnosis of pancreatic insufficiency, particularly chronic pancreatitis: Correlation with the pancreozymin-secretin test, faecal fat excretion and final clinical diagnosis. Digestion 21:281–289, 1981.
4. Ammann RW, Akovbiantz A, Largiader F, Scheuler G. Course and outcome of chronic pancreatitis. Gastroenterology 86:820–828, 1984.
5. Ammann RW, Buehler H, Muench R, Freiburghaus AW, Siegenthaler W. Differences in the natural history of idiopathic (nonalcoholic) and alcoholic chronic pancreatitis. A comparative long-term study of 287 patients. Pancreas 2:368–377, 1987.
6. Anagnostides AA, Cox TM, Adrian TE. Pancreatic exocrine and endocrine responses in chronic pancreatitis. Am J Gastroenterol 79:206–212, 1984.
7. Andriulli A, Masoero G, Felder M, et al. Circulating trypsin-like immunoreactivity in chronic pancreatitis. Dig Dis Sci 26:532–537, 1981.
8. Angelini G, Merigo F, Degani G, et al. Association of chronic alcoholic liver and pancreatic disease: A prospective study. Am J Gastroenterol 80:998–1003, 1985.
9. Appel MF. Hereditary pancreatitis: Review and presentation of an additional kindred. Arch Surg 108:63–65, 1974.
10. Arvanitakis C, Greenberger N. Diagnosis of pancreatic disease by a synthetic peptide: A new test of pancreatic function. Lancet 1:663–666, 1976.
11. Ashton MG, Axon ATR, Lintott DJ. Lundh test and ERCP in pancreatic disease. Gut 19:910–915, 1978.
12. Axon ATR, Ashton MG, Lintott DJ. Pancreatogram changes in patients with calculous biliary disease. Br J Surg 66:466–470, 1979.
13. Bank S, Marks IN, Novis B. Sweat electrolytes in chronic pancreatitis. Dig Dis Sci 23:178–181, 1978.
14. Banks PA, Bradley EL, Dreiling DA, et al. Classification of pancreatitis—Cambridge and Marseille. Gastroenterology 89:928–930, 1985.
15. Banks S, Marks IN. Clinical and hormonal aspects of pancreatic diabetes. Am J Gastroenterol 64:13–32, 1975.
16. Baron RL, Stanley RJ, Lee JKT, Koehler RE, Levitt RG. Computed tomographic features of biliary obstruction. Am J Roentgenol 140:1173–1178, 1983.
17. Berger D, Crowther RC, Flayel JC, Pek S, Fajans SS. Effects of age on fasting plasma levels of pancreatic polypeptide. J Clin Endocrinol 47:1183–1187, 1978.
18. Berstad A, Roland M, Petersen H, Liavag I. Altered pancreatic function after proximal gastric vagotomy in man. Gastroenterology 71:958–960, 1976.
19. Berstad A, Roland M, Petersen H, Liavag I. Effect of vagotomy on exocrine pancreatic and biliary secretion in man. Am J Surg 141:40–47, 1981.
20. Bockman DE, Boydston WR, Parsa I. Architecture of the human pancreas: Implications for early changes in pancreatic disease. Gastroenterology 85:55–61, 1983.
21. Bolondi L, Priori P, Gullo L, et al. Relationship between changes detected by ultrasonography and pancreatic exocrine function in chronic pancreatitis. Pancreas 2:222–229, 1987.
22. Bommelaer G, Benque A, Tuvignon P, Moreau J, Ribet A. 24hrs continuous duodenal pH recording in chronic pancreatitis. Gastroenterology 82:1022, 1982.
23. Boyd EJS, Wormsley KG. Laboratory tests in the diagnosis of the chronic pancreatic diseases, Part I: Secretagogues used in tests of pancreatic secretion. Int J Pancreatol 2:137–148, 1987.
24. Boyd EJS, Wormsley KG. Laboratory tests in the diagnosis of the chronic pancreatic diseases, Part II: Tests of pancreatic secretion. Int J Pancreatol 2:211–221, 1987.
25. Boyd EJS, Clark G, Dunbar J, Wormsley KG. Pancreatic enzyme synthesis in pancreatic disease. Scand J Gastroenterol 20:734–740, 1985.

26. Braganza JM. The Pancreas. In: Pounder RE, ed. Recent Advances in Gastroenterology. London, Churchill Livingstone, 1985, pp 251–280.
27. Braganza JM, Hunt LP, Warwick F. Relationship between pancreatic exocrine function and ductal morphology in chronic pancreatitis. Gastroenterology 82:1341–1347, 1982.
28. Brugge WR, Burke CA. Lactoferrin secretion in alcoholic pancreatic disease. Dig Dis Sci 33:178–184, 1988.
29. Buch A, Buch J, Carlsen A, Schmidt A. Hyperlipaemia and pancreatitis. World J Surg 4:307–314, 1980.
30. Malfertheimer P, Büchler M, Stanesca A, Uhl W, Ditschuneit H. Serum elastase-1 in inflammatory pancreatic and gastrointestinal diseases and in renal insufficiency. Int J Pancreatol 1987; 2:159–170.
31. Buehler H, Muench R, Schmid M, Ammann R. Cholestasis in alcoholic chronic pancreatitis. Scand J Gastroenterol 20:851–856, 1985.
32. Burke JW, Erikson SJ, Kellum CD, et al. Pseudoaneurysms complicating pancreatitis: Detection by CT. Radiology 161:447–450, 1986.
33. Caletti G, Brocchi E, Agostini D, et al. Sensitivity of endoscopic retrograde pancreatography in chronic pancreatitis. Br J Surg 69:507–509, 1982.
34. Cameron JL, Zuidema GD, Margolis S. A pathogenesis for alcoholic pancreatitis. Surgery 77:754–763, 1975.
35. Cavallini G, Piubello W, Brocco G, et al. Serum PABA and fluorescein in the course of Bz-Ty-PABA and Pancreolauryl tests as an index of exocrine pancreatic insufficiency. Dig Dis Sci 30:655–663, 1985.
36. Couet C, Genton P, Pointel JP, et al. The prevalence of retinopathy is similar in diabetes mellitus secondary to chronic pancreatitis with or without pancreatectomy and in idiopathic diabetes mellitus. Diabetes Care 8:323–328, 1985.
37. Cotton PB, Frost RG, Shorvon PJ. Computer analysis of a decade of ERCP. Gut 23:432, 1982.
38. Cotton PB, Lees WR, Vallon AG, et al. Grey-scale ultrasonography and endoscopic pancreatography in pancreatic diagnosis. Radiology 134:453–459, 1980.
39. Dandona P, Elias E, Beckett AG. Serum trypsin concentrations in diabetes mellitus. Br Med J 2:1125, 1978.
40. D'Angelo WA, Fries JF, Masi AT, Shulman LE. Pathologic observations in systemic sclerosis (scleroderma). Am J Med 46:428–440, 1969.
41. Delchier J-C, Soule J-C. BT-PABA test with plasma PABA measurements: evaluation of sensitivity and specificity. Gut 24:318–325, 1983.
42. Del Favero G, Fabris C, Plebani M, et al. CA19-9 and carcinoembryonic antigen in pancreatic cancer diagnosis. Cancer 57:1576–1579, 1986.
43. Denyer ME, Cotton PB. Pure pancreatic juice studies in normal subjects and patients with chronic pancreatitis. Gut 20:89–97, 1979.
44. Dharmsathaphorn K, Burrell M, Dobbins J. Diagnosis of annular pancreas with ERCP. Gastroenterology 77:1109–1114, 1979.
45. Di Bisceglie AM, Paterson AC, Segal I. The liver in biliary obstruction due to chronic pancreatitis. Liver 5:189–195, 1985.
46. Dreiling DA, Greenstein AJ, Bordalo O. Comparison of standard and augmented secretin test responses in patients with and without pancreatic disease. Am J Gastroenterol 61:433–442, 1974.
47. Duncan LPJ, McFarlane A, Robson JS. Diabetic retinopathy and nephropathy in pancreatic diabetes. Lancet 1:822–826, 1958.
48. Durbec JP, Sarles H. Multicentre survey of the etiology of pancreatic diseases. Relationship between the relative risk of developing chronic pancreatitis and alcohol, protein and lipid consumption. Digestion 18:337–350, 1978.
49. Dürr HK, Otte M, Forrell MM, Bode JC. Faecal chymotrypsin: A study on its diagnostic value by comparison with the secretin-cholecystokinin test. Digestion 17:404–409, 1978.
50. Ebert R, Creutzfeld W. Reversal of impaired GIP and insulin secretion in patients with pancreatogenic steatorrhoea following enzyme substitution. Diabetologia 19:198–204, 1980.

51. Ellis C, Koehler DF, Eckfeldt JH, Levitt MD. Evaluation of an inhibitor assay to determine serum amylase distribution. Dig Dis Sci 27:897–890, 1982.
52. Elsborg L, Bruusgaard A, Strandgaard L, Reinicke V. Endoscopic retrograde pancreatography and the exocrine pancreatic function in alcoholism. Scand J Gastroenterol 16:941–944, 1981.
53. Endo Y, Morii T, Tamura H, Okuda S. Cytodiagnosis of malignant tumours by aspiration under direct vision using a duodenal fibrescope. Gastroenterology 67:944–951, 1974.
54. Epstein O, Chapman RWG, Lake-Bakaar G, et al. The pancreas in primary billiary cirrhosis and primary sclerosing cholangitis. Gastroenterology 83:1177–1182, 1982.
55. Fabris C, Del Favero G, Basso D, et al. Serum markers and clinical data in diagnosing pancreatic cancer: A contrastive approach. Am J Gastroenterol 83:549–553, 1988.
56. Fabris C, Farini R, Piccoli A, et al. CEA and ferritin in chronic pancreatic disease: A comparative evaluation. Hepatogastroenterology 32:146–148, 1985.
57. Fahrenkrug J, Staun-Olsen P, Magid E. Immunoreactive trypsin and pancreatic isoamylase activity in serum of patients with chronic renal failure or hepatic cirrhosis. Clin Chem 27:1655–1657, 1981.
58. Farini R, Nitti D, Del Favero G, et al. CEA concentration and cytology in duodenal fluid during the secretin-pancreozymin test. Hepatogastroenterology 27:213–216, 1980.
59. Farman J, Werbeloff L, Marks IN, et al. Proximal duodenal deformities due to pancreatitis. Br J Radiol 39:662–668, 1966.
60. Fedail SS, Harvey RF, Salmon P, Brown P, Read AE. Trypsin and lactoferrin levels in pure pancreatic juice in patients with pancreatic disease. Gut 20:983–986, 1979.
61. Fedail SS, Harvey RF, Salmon P, Read AE. Radioimmunoassay of lactoferrin in pancreatic juice as a test for pancreatic disease. Lancet 1:181–182, 1978.
62. Fink RS, Adrian TE, Margot DH, Bloom SR. Increased plasma pancreatic polypeptide in alcohol abuse. Clin Endocrinol 18:417–421, 1983.
63. Fitzgerald PJ, Firther JG, Watson RC, et al. The value of diagnostic aids in detecting pancreas cancer. Cancer 73:457–461, 1978.
64. Flamion B, Delhaye M, Horanyi Z, et al. Comparison of elastase-1 with amylase, lipase, and trypsin-like immunoreactivity in the diagnosis of acute pancreatitis. Am J Gastroenterol 82:532–535, 1987.
65. Foley WD, Stewart ET, Lawson TL, et al. Computed tomography, ultrasonography and endoscopic retrograde pancreatography in diagnosis of pancreatic disease: A comparative study. Gastrointest Radiol 5:29–35, 1980.
66. Forbes A, Cotton PB. ERCP and sphincterotomy after Billroth-II gastrectomy. Gut 25:471–474, 1984.
67. Frey CF. Classification of pancreatitis: State-of-the-art, 1986. Pancreas 1:62–68, 1986.
68. Fric P, Malis F, Kasafirek E, Slaby J. A new method of testing pancreatin therapy in vivo by the use of a peroral chymotrypsin substrate 4(*N*-acetyl-1-tyrosyl) amino benzoic acid. Hepatogastroenterology 27:220–223, 1980.
69. Frick MP, O'Leary JF, Walker HC, Goodale RL. Accuracy of endoscopic retrograde cholangiopancreatography (ERCP) in differentiating benign from malignant pancreatic disease. Gastrointestinal Radiol 7:241–244, 1982.
70. Gambill EE. Pancreatitis associated with pancreatic carcinoma: A study of 26 cases. Mayo Clin Proc 46:174–177, 1971.
71. Gastard J, Joubaud F, Farbos T, et al. Etiology and course of primary pancreatitis in Western France. Digestion 9:416–428, 1973.
72. Gelder FB, Reese CJ, Moosa AR, Hall T, Hunter R. Purification, partial characterisation, and clinical evaluation of a pancreatic oncofoetal antigen. Cancer Res 38:313–324, 1978.
73. George P, Brown C, Gilchrist J. Operative biopsy of the pancreas. Br J Surg 62:280–283, 1975.
74. Gilinsky NH, Mee AS, Marks IN. Evaluation of an extended pancreatic function test in normal subjects and patients with chronic pancreatitis. S Afr Med J 63:118–120, 1983.

75. Girdwood AH, Hatfield ARW, Bornman PC, et al. Structure and function in noncalcific pancreatitis. Am J Dig Dis 29:721–726, 1984.
76. Goldstein HM, Zornoza J, Wallace S, et al. Percutaneous fine-needle aspiration biopsy of pancreatic and other abdominal masses. Radiology 123:319–322, 1977.
77. Goodale RL, Gajl-Peczalska K, Dressel T, Samuelson J. Cytologic studies for the diagnosis of pancreatic cancer. Cancer 47:1652–1655, 1981.
78. Gowland M, Warwick F, Kalantzis N, Braganza JM. Relative efficiency and predictive value of ultrasonography and endoscopic pancreatography in diagnosis of pancreatic disease. Lancet 2:190–193, 1981.
79. Gregg JA, Sharma MM. Endoscopic measurement of pancreatic juice secretory flow rate and pancreatic secretory pressures after secretin administration in human controls and in patients with acute relapsing pancreatitis, chronic pancreatitis and pancreatic cancer. Am J Surg 136:569–574, 1978.
80. Gullo L, Corinaldesi R, Casadio R, et al. Gastric acid secretion in chronic pancreatitis. Hepatogastroenterology 30:60–62, 1983.
81. Gullo L, Costa PL, Fontana G, Labo G. Investigation of exocrine pancreatic function by continuous infusion of caerulein and secretin in normal subjects and in chronic pancreatitis. Digestion 14:97–107, 1976.
82. Gullo L, Sarles H, Mott C. Functional investigation of the exocrine pancreas following acute pancreatitis. Rendic Gastroenterol 4:18–21, 1972.
83. Gullo L, Tabacchi PL, Corazza GR, et al. HLA-B13 and chronic calcific pancreatitis. Dig Dis Sci 27:214–216, 1982.
84. Gyr K, Agrawal NM, Felsenfeld O, Font RG. Comparative study of secretin and Lundh test. Am J Dig Dis 20:506–512, 1975.
85. Habib NA, Hershman MJ, Haberland F, et al. The use of CA-50 radioimmunoassay in differentiating benign and malignant pancreatic disease. Br J Cancer 53:697–699, 1986.
86. Haglund C, Lindgren J, Roberts PJ, Nordling S. Gastrointestinal cancer-associated antigen CA19-9 in histological specimens of pancreatic tumours and pancreatitis. Br J Cancer 53:189–195, 1986.
87. Haglund C, Roberts PJ, Kuusela P, et al. Evaluation of CA19-9 as a serum tumour marker in pancreatic cancer. Br J Cancer 53:197–202, 1986.
88. Hall RI, Lavelle MI, Venables CW. Chronic pancreatitis as a cause of gastrointestinal bleeding. Gut 23:250–255, 1982.
89. Hamano H, Hayakawa T, Kondo T. Serum immunoreactive elastase in diagnosis of pancreatic cancer. A sensitive marker for pancreatic cancer. Dig Dis Sci 32:50–56, 1987.
90. Hamilton I, Bradley P, Lintot DJ, McMahon MJ, Axon ATR. Endoscopic retrograde cholangiopancreatography in the management of patients with acute pancreatitis. Br J Surg 69:504–506, 1982.
91. Hamilton I, Lintott DJ, Ruddell WSJ, Axon ATR. The endoscopic retrograde cholangiogram in chronic liver disease. Clin Radiol 34:417–422, 1983.
92. Harada H, Mishima K, Shundo T, et al. Exocrine pancreatic function test by a synthetic peptide. Am J Gastroenterol 71:45–52, 1979.
93. Heij HA, Obertop H, Van Blankenstein M, Ten Kate FW, Westerbroek DL. Relationship between functional and histological changes in chronic pancreatitis. Dig Dis Sci 31:1009–1013, 1986.
94. Hendel L, Worning H. Exocrine pancreatic function in patients with progressive systemic sclerosis. Scand J Gastroenterol 24:461–466, 1989.
95. Heptner G, Domschke S, Domschke W. Exocrine pancreatic function after gastrectomy: Specificity of indirect tests. Gastroenterology 97:147–153, 1989.
96. Herefort K, Sobra J, Fric P, et al. Familial hyperlipoproteinaemia and the exocrine pancreas. Scand J Gastroenterol 6:139–143, 1971.
97. Hessel SJ, Siegelman SS, McNeil BJ, et al. A prospective evaluation of computed tomography and ultrasound of pancreas. Radiology 143:129–133, 1982.
98. Hirskovic T, Keating FR, Gross JB. Coexistent pancreatitis and hyperparathyroidism. Observations in 15 cases. Gastroenterology 52:1093, 1967.

99. Hoek FJ, Van den Bergh FAJTM, Klein Elhorst JT, et al. Improved specificity of the positive PABA test with *p*-aminosalicylic acid (PAS). Gut 28:468–473, 1987.
100. Hoffman GE, Schmidt D, Bastian B. Bestimmung der Phospholipase A in der Serum bei akuter Pankreatitis. J Clin Chem Clin Biochem 23:582–583, 1985.
101. Homma T, Aizawa T, Nagata A, Oguchi H. HLA antigens in chronic idiopathic pancreatitis compared with chronic alcoholic pancreatitis. Dig Dis Sci 26:449–452, 1981.
102. Ihse I, Arnsejo B, Kugelberg C, Lilja P. Intestinal activities of trypsin, lipase and phospholipase after a test meal: An evaluation of 474 examinations. Scand J Gastroenterol 12:663–668, 1977.
103. Imamura K, Nakamura T, Miyazawa T, et al. Oral administration of chymotrypsin labile peptide for a new test of exocrine pancreatic function (PFT) in comparison with the pancreozymin-secretin test. Am J Gastroenterol 69:572–578, 1978.
104. James O. Progress report: The Lundh test. Gut 14:582–591, 1973.
105. Johnson SG, Levitt MD. Relation between serum pancreatic isoamylase concentration and pancreatic exocrine function. Dig Dis Sci 23:914–918, 1978.
106. Jutley JK, Denyer ME, Kelleher J, Mitchell CJ. Composition of pure pancreatic juice in normal human subjects and pancreatic disease. Digestion 38:96–102, 1987.
107. Kalvaria I, Bornman PC, Girdwood AH, Marks IN. Periampullary cyst: A surgically remediable cause of pancreatitis. Gut 28:358–362, 1987.
108. Kay G, Hine P, Braganza JM. The pancreolauryl test: A method of assessing the combined functional efficiency of pancreatic esterase and bile salts in vivo? Digestion 24:241–245, 1982.
109. Keighley MRB, Moore J, Thompson H. The place of fine-needle aspiration cytology for the intra-operative diagnosis of pancreatic malignancy. Ann R Coll Surg Engl 66:405–408, 1984.
110. Kelleher J, Lowsowsky MS, Ruddel WSJ, et al. Assessment of rapid pancreatic isoamylase assay as a screening test for pancreatic disease. Br Med J 18:791–795, 1983.
111. Kilmanskog F, Schrumpf E, Bergan A, Larsen S. Diagnostic value of computed tomography in pancreatic carcinoma. Acta Radiol 23:131–141, 1982.
112. Kizu M, Newmann J, Cotton PB, Kasugi T. Histological correlation with pancreatography in necropsy specimens. Gut 18:399–400, 1977.
113. Koch MB, Go VLW, DiMagno EP. Can plasma human pancreatic polypeptide be used to detect disease of the exocrine pancreas? Mayo Clin Proc 60:259–265, 1985.
114. Kolars JC, Allen M O'C, Ansel H, Silvis SE, Vennes JA. Pancreatic pseudocysts: Clinical and endoscopic experience, Am J Gastroenterol 84:259–264, 1989.
115. Lang C, Gyr K, Conene D, Stalder GA. Value of serum PABA as a pancreatic function test. Gut 25:508–512, 1984.
116. Lankisch PG, Brauneis J, Otte J, Göke B. Pancreolauryl and NBT-PABA tests: Are serum tests more practicable alternatives to urine tests in the diagnosis of exocrine pancreatic insufficiency? Gastroenterology 90:350–354, 1986.
117. Lankisch PG, Koop H, Otto J. Estimation of serum pancreatic amylase: Its role in the diagnosis of exocrine pancreatic insufficiency. Am J Gastroenterology 81:365–368, 1986.
118. Lankisch PG, Manthey G, Otto J, et al. Exocrine pancreatic function in insulin-dependent diabetes mellitus. Digestion 25:211–216, 1982.
119. Lankisch PG, Schruber A, Cho J. Pancreolauryl test—Evaluation of a tubeless pancreatic function test in comparison with other indirect and direct tests for pancreatic exocrine function. Dig Dis Sci 28:490–493, 1983.
120. Lesi C Melzi D'Eril GV, Paresi F, et al. Clinical significance of serum pancreatic enzymes in the quiescent phase of chronic pancreatitis. Clin Biochem 19:235–238, 1985.
121. Lesi C, Ruffilli E, DeMutiis R, et al. Usefulness of serum elastase-1 in clinical practice. Digestion. 35:37, 1986.
122. Lightwood R, Reber HA, Way LW. The risk and accuracy of pancreatic biospy. Am J Surg 132:189–193, 1976.

123. Linnestad P, Schrumpf E. Pancreatic polypeptide release stimulated by food, secretin and cholecystokinin in chronic pancreatitis. Scand J Gastroenterol 18:385–389, 1983.
124. Lurie B, Brom B, Bank S, Novis B, Marks IN. Comparative response of exocrine pancreatic secretion following a test meal and secretin-pancreozymin stimulation. Scand J Gastroenterol 8:27–32, 1973.
125. MacKie CR, Cooper MJ, Lewis MH, Moosa AR. Non-operative differentiation between pancreatic cancer and chronic pancreatitis. Ann Surg 198:480–487, 1979.
126. MacKie CR, Dhorajiwala J, Blackstone MO, Bowie J, Moosa AR. Value of new diagnostic aids in relation to the disease process in pancreatic cancer. Lancet 2:385–388, 1979.
127. Madsen MS, Petersen TH, Sommer H. Segmental portal hypertension. Ann Surg 204:72–77, 1986.
128. Mahvi DM, Meyers WC, Bast RC, Siegler HF, Metzgar RS. Carcinoma of the pancreas. Therapeutic efficacy as defined by a serodiagnostic test utilizing a monocloncal antibody. Ann Surg 202:440–444, 1985.
129. Malfertheiner P, Maier W, Walliser A, Büchler M, Ditschuneit H. CT-Morphologie und exocrine Funktion bei chronischer Pankreatitis. Z Gastroenterol 21:729–735, 1983.
130. Malvano R, Marchisio M, Massaglia A, et al. Radioimmunoassay of trypsin-like substance in human plasma. Scand J Gastroenterol 15 (suppl 60):3–10, 1980.
131. Masoero G, Andriulli A, Bianco A, et al. Diagnostic accuracy of serum cationic trypsin estimation for pancreatic disease. Dig Dis Sci 27:1089–1094, 1982.
132. Megibow AJ, Bosniak MA, Ambos MA, Beranbaum ER. Thickening of the coeliac axis and/or superior mesenteric artery: A sign of pancreatic carcinoma on computed tomography. Radiology 141:449–453, 1981.
133. Mikas AA, Hirschowitz B. Alpha$_1$-antitrypsin and chronic pancreatitis. Lancet 2:1032–1033, 1972.
134. Mirey E, Jow E, Slavin RE, Tobin F. Pancreatic function and intestinal absorption in chronic alcoholism. Gastroenterology 59:657–664, 1970.
135. Mitchell CJ, Field HP, Simpson FG, et al. Preliminary evaluation of a single-day tubeless test of pancreatic function. Br Med J 1:1751–1753, 1981.
136. Mitchell CJ, Humphrey CS, Bullin AW, Kelleher J, Losowsky MS. Improved diagnostic accuracy of a modified oral pancreatic function test. Scand J Gastroenterol 14:737–741, 1979.
137. Mitchell ML, Carney CN. Cytologic criteria for the diagnosis of pancreatic carcinoma. Am J Clin Pathol 83:171–176, 1985.
138. Møller-Petersen J, Klaerke M, Dati F. Evaluation and comparison of cathodic trypsin-like immunoreactivity, pancreatic lipase and pancreatic isoamylase in the diagnosis of acute pancreatitis in 849 consecutive patients with acute abdominal pain. Clin Chim Acta 157:151–166, 1986.
139. Moller Petersen J, Pedersen JO, Thorsgaard Pedersen N, Nyboe Andersen B. Serum cathodic trypsin-like immunoreactivity, pancreatic lipase, and pancreatic iso amylase as diagnostic tests of chronic pancreatitis or pancreatic steatorrhoea. Scand J Gastroenterol 23:287–296, 1988.
140. Mottaleb A, Rapp F, Noguera ELA, et al. The Lundh test in the diagnosis of pancreatic disease: A review of five years' experience. Gut 14:835–841, 1973.
141. Muller L, Wisniewski ZS, Hansky J. The measurement of faecal chymotrypsin: A screening test for pancreatic exocrine insufficiency. Aust Ann Med 19:47–49, 1970.
142. Multigner L, Figarella C, Sahel J, Sarles H. Lactoferrin and albumin in human pancreatic juice: A valuable test for diagnosis of pancreatic disease. Dig Dis Sci 25:173–178, 1980.
143. Multigner L, Figarella C, Sarles H. Diagnosis of chronic pancreatitis by measurement of lactoferrin in duodenal juice. Gut 22:350–351, 1981.
144. Münch R, Kehl O, Bühler H, Medici T, Ammann R. Änderung der Serum-Pankreasenzyme nach i.-v.-Stimulation mit Sekretin bei pankreasgesunden Probanden. Schweiz Med Wochenschr 117:756–760, 1987.

145. Nagai H, Ohtsubo K. Pancreatic lithiasis in the aged: Its clinicopathology and pathogenesis. Gastroenterol 86:331–338, 1984.
146. Nicolai JJ, Teunen A, Zuyderhout F, Hoek F, Tytgat GNJ. Lactoferrin in pure pancreatic juice. Scand J Gastroenterol 19:765–769, 1984.
147. Nicolas J-P. Guéant JL, Gaucher P. Malabsorption de la vitamine B_{12} et insuffisance pancréatique exocrine. Gastroenterol Clin Biol 7:307–314, 1983.
148. Nieburgs HE, Drailing DA, Rubio C, Rusman H. The morphology of cells in duodenal drainage smears. Histological origin and pathological significance. Am J Dig Dis 7:489–505, 1967.
149. Nittsu Y, Kohgo Y, Yokata M, Urushizaki I. Radioimmunoassay of serum ferritin in the diagnosis of pancreatic cancer. Ann NY Acad Sci 259:450–452, 1975.
150. Nishida K, Tasaki N, Miyagawa H, Yoshikawa T, Kondo M. Estimation of carbohydrate antigen (CA 19-9) levels in pure pancreatic juice of patients with pancreatic cancer. Am J Gastroenterol 83:126–129, 1988.
151. Nitti D, Fabris C, Del Favero G, et al. Serum ferritin in pancreatic disease. An accurate test of malignancy? Digestion 25:258–262, 1982.
152. Novis BH, Bank S, Marks IN. Exocrine pancreatic function in intestinal malabsorption and small bowel disease. Am J Dig Dis 17:489–494, 1972.
153. Nwokolo C, Oli J. Pathogenesis of juvenile tropical pancreatitis syndrome. Lancet 1:456–458, 1980.
154. Okada M, Fuchigami T, Ri S, Kohrogi N, Omar T. The BT-PABA pancreatic function test in giardiasis. Postgrad Med J 59:79–82, 1983.
155. O'Malley VP, Cannon JP, Postier RG. Pancreatic pseudocysts: Cause, therapy and results. Am J Surg 150:680–682, 1985.
156. Owyang C, Scarpello JH, Vinik AI. Correlation between pancreatic enzyme secretion and plasma concentration of human pancreatic polypeptide in health and chronic pancreatitis. Gastroenterology 83:55–62, 1982.
157. Panucci A, Fabris C, Del Favero G, et al. Tissue polypeptide antigen (TPA) in pancreatic cancer diagnosis. Br J Cancer 52:801–803, 1985.
158. Panucci A, Fabris C, Del Favero G, et al. Is tissue polypeptide antigen more accurate than serum CEA in diagnosing pancreatic cancer? J Clin Pathol 39:75–77, 1986.
159. Pap A, Berger Z, Varro. Trophic effect of cholecystokinin-octapeptide in man: A new way in the treatment of chronic pancreatitis. Digestion 21:163–168, 1981.
160. Pedersen NT, Andersen BN, Pedersen G, Worning H. Chronic pancreatitis in Copenhagen. Scand J Gastroenterol 17:925–931, 1982.
161. Peteresen H, Myren J. Secretin dose-response in health and chronic pancreatic inflammatory disease. Scand J Gastroenterol 10:851–861, 1975.
162. Piper WN, Helwig BB. Progressive systemic sclerosis. Arch Dermatol 72:535–546, 1955.
163. Pitchoumoni CS, Glasser M, Saran RM, Panchacharam P, Thelmo W. Pancreatic fibrosis in chronic alcoholics and nonalcoholics without clinical pancreatitis. Am J Gastroenterol 79:382–389, 1984.
164. Podolsky DK, McPhee MS, Alpert E, Warshaw AL, Isselbacher KJ. Galactosyltransferase isoenzyme II in the detection of pancreatic cancer: Comparison with radiologic, endoscopic and serologic tests. N Engl J Med 304:1313–1318, 1981.
165. Prinz RA, Aranha GV. The association of primary hyperparathyroidism and pancreatitis. Am Surg 51:325–329, 1985.
166. Regan PT, DiMagno EP. Exocrine pancreatic insufficiency in coeliac sprue: A cause of treatment failure. Gastroenterology 78:484–487, 1980.
167. Regan PT, Go VLW, DiMagno EP. Comparison of the effects of cholecystokinin and cholecystokinin-octapeptide on pancreatic secretion, gall bladder contraction and plasma pancreatic polypeptide in man. J Lab Clin Med 96:743–748, 1980.
168. Renner IG, Rinderknecht H, Wisner JR. Pancreatic secretion after secretin and cholecystokinin stimulation in chronic alcoholics with and without cirrhosis. Dig Dis Sci 28:1084–1093, 1983.
169. Renner IG, Savage WT, Pontija JL, Renner VJ. Death due to acute pancreatitis: A retrospective analysis of 405 autopsy cases. Dig Dis Sci 30:1005–1018, 1985.

170. Renner IG, Savage WT, Stace NH, et al. Pancreatitis associated with alcoholic liver disease: A review of 1022 autopsy cases. Dig Dis Sci 29:593–599, 1984.
171. Reshef R, Shtamler B, Novis B. Recurrent acute pancreatitis associated with pancreas divisum. Am J Gastroenterol 83:86–88, 1988.
172. Reuben A, Cotton PB. Operative pancreatic biopsy: A survey of current practice. Ann R Coll Surg Engl 60:53–57, 1978.
173. Rinderknecht H, Renner IG, Stace NH. Abnormalities in pancreatic secretory profiles of patients with cancer of the pancreas. Dig Dis Sci 28:103–110, 1983.
174. Rocca G, Gaia E, Iuliano R, et al. Increased incidence of cancer in chronic pancreatitis. J Clin Gastroenterol 9:175–179, 1987.
175. Rolny P, Elwing H, Nilsson L-A. The CEA concentration in duodenal fluid in patients with pancreatic disease. Scand J Gastroenterol 12:759–763, 1977.
176. Rolny P, Jagenburg R. The secretin-CCK test and a modified Lundh test: A comparative study. Scand J Gastroenterol 13:927–931, 1978.
177. Rolny P, Lukes PJ, Gamklon R, et al. A comparative evaluation of endoscopic retrograde pancreatography and secretin-CCK test in the diagnosis of pancreatic disease. Scand J Gastroenterol 13:777–781, 1978.
178. Ruddel WSJ, Mitchel CJ, Hamilton I, Leck JP, Kelleher J. Clinical value of serum immunoreactive trypsin concentration. Br Med J 1:1429–1432, 1981.
179. Safi F, Büchler M, Schenkluhn B, Berger HG. Diagnostic significance of the tumour marker CA19-9 in carcinoma of the pancreas. Dtsch Med Wochenschr 109:1869–1873, 1984.
180. Sakahara H, Endo K, Nakajima K, et al. Serum CA19-9 concentrations and computed tomography findings in patients with pancreatic carcinoma. Cancer 57:1324–1326, 1986.
181. Sakamoto K, Haga Y, Yoshimura R, et al. Comparative effectiveness of the tumour diagnostics CA19-9, CA125 and carcinoembryonic antigen in patients with diseases of the digestive system. Gut 28:323–329, 1987.
182. Salmon PR, Baddley H, Machado G, et al. Endoscopic pancreatography, scintigraphy and exocrine function in pancreatitis: A comparative study. Gut 16:830, 1975.
183. Sandblom P. Gastrointestinal haemorrhage through the pancreatic duct. Ann Surg 171:61–66, 1970.
184. Sankaran S, Sugawa C, Walt AJ. Value of endoscopic retrograde pancreatography in pancreatic ascites. Surg Gynecol Obstet 148:185–192, 1979.
185. Sarles H, ed. Pancreatitis Symposium, Marseilles 1963. Bibl Gastroenterol 7:7–8, 1965.
186. Sarles H, Sahel J. Progress report: Cholestasis and lesions of the biliary tract in chronic pancreatitis. Gut 19:851–857, 1978.
187. Sarner M, Cotton PB. Classification of pancreatitis. Gut 25:756–759, 1984.
188. Saunders JHB, Gargill JM, Wormsley KG. Gastric secretion of acid in patients with pancreatic disease. Digestion 17:365–369, 1977.
189. Saunders JHB, Drummond S, Wormsley KG. Inhibition of gastric secretion in treatment of pancreatic insufficiency. Br Med J 1:418–419, 1977.
190. Seligson L, Che JW, Ihre T, Lundh G, Pyk E. Evaluation of the diagnosis pancreatitis. Scand J Gastroenterol 17:905–911, 1982.
191. Sevel D, Bristow JH, Bank S, et al. Diabetic retinopathy in chronic pancreatitis. Arch Ophthalmol 86:245–250, 1971.
192. Schulze S, Pedersen NT, Jørgensen MJ, Mølmann KM, Rune SJ. Association between duodenal bulb ulceration and reduced exocrine pancreatic function. Gut 24:781–783, 1983.
193. Scotta MS, Marzani MD, Maggiore G, et al. Faecal chymotrypsin: A new diagnostic test for exocrine insufficiency in children with cystic fibrosis. Clin Biochem 18:233–234, 1985.
194. Schmiegel WH, Eberl W, Kreiker C, et al. Multiparametric tumour marker (CA19-9, CEA, AFP, POA) analyses of pancreatic juices and sera in pancreatic disease. Hepatogastroenterology 32:141–145, 1985.

195. Schmiegel WH, Krieker C, Eberl S, et al. Values of serum carcinoembryonic antigen and elastase-1 in diagnosis of pancreatic carcinoma. Gut 25:1347–1351, 1984.
196. Schmiegel WH, Kreiker C, Eberl W, et al. Monoclonal antibody defines CA19-9 in pancreatic juices and sera. Gut 456–460, 1986.
197. Singer M, Gyr K, Sarles H. Revised classification of pancreatitis. Gastroenterology 89:683–685, 1985.
198. Schmitz-Moormann P, Himmelmann GW, Brandes J-W, et al. Comparative radiological and morphological study of human pancreas. Pancreatitis-like changes in postmortem ductograms and their morphological pattern. Implications for ERCP. Gut 26:406–414, 1985.
199. Schmitz-Morrman P, Riedel R, Ihm P. Morphometrische Untersuchungen der Kaliberschwankungen am normaler Ductus pancreaticus major. Z Gastroenterol 19:299–308, 1981.
200. Sibert JR, Hereditary pancreatitis in England and Wales. J Med Genet 15:189–201, 1978.
201. Skude G, Ihse I. Isoamylases in pancreatic carcinoma and chronic pancreatitis. Scand J Gastroenterol 12:53–57, 1977.
202. Snape WJ, Long WN, Trotman BW, Marin GA, Czaja AJ. Marked alkaline phosphatase elevation in partial common bile duct obstruction due to calcific pancreatitis. Gastroenterology 70:70–73, 1986.
203. Stamm BH. Incidence and diagnostic significance of minor pathologic changes in the adult pancreas at autopsy: A systematic study of 112 autopsies in patients without known pancreatic disease. Hum Pathol 15:677–683, 1984.
204. Stasiewicz J, Adler M, Delcourt A. Pancreatic and gastrointestinal hormones in chronic pancreatitis. Hepatogastroenterology 27:152–160, 1980.
205. Steinberg WM. Diagnosis of chronic pancreatitis. Gastroenterology 89:1449–1452, 1985.
206. Steinberg WM, Anderson KK. Serum trypsinogen in diagnosis of chronic pancreatitis. Dig Dis Sci 29:988–993, 1984.
207. Steinberg WM, Gelfand R, Anderson KK. Comparison of the sensitivity and specificity of the CA19-9 and carcinoembryonic antigen in detecting cancer of the pancreas. Gastroenterology 90:343–349, 1986.
208. Sugawa C, Walt AJ. Endoscopic retrograde pancreatography in the surgery of pancreatic pseudocysts. Surgery 86:639–647, 1979.
209. Tait AD, Maniolos K, Duncombe VM, Davis AE. Serum pancreatic isoamylase estimation by the inhibitor method as a diagnostic test for chronic pancreatitis. Aust NZ J Med 14:600–605, 1984.
210. Tanner AR, Robinson DP. Pancreatic function testing: Serum PABA measurement is a reliable and accurate measurement of exocrine function. Gut 29:1736–1740, 1988.
211. Tatsuta M, Yamamura H, Yamumoto R, et al. Carcinoembryonic antigen in the bile in patients with pancreatic and biliary cancer. Correlation with cytology and percutaneous transhepatic cholangiography. Cancer 50:2903–2909, 1982.
212. Tetlow VA, Lobley RW, Herman K, Braganza JM. A one-day oral pancreatic function test using a chymotrypsin-labile peptide and radioactive marker. Clin Trials J 17:121–130, 1980.
213. Toskes PP. Bentiromide as a test of exocrine pancreatic function in adult patients with pancreatic exocrine insufficiency: Determination of appropriate dose and urinary collection interval. Gastroenterology 85:585–598, 1983.
214. Trapnell JE, Chronic relapsing pancreatitis: A review of 64 cases. Br J Surg 66:471–475, 1979.
215. Turner LJ. Chronic pancreatitis and congenital strictures of the pancreatic duct. Am J Surg 145:582–584, 1983.
216. Tympner F, Domschke W, Rösch W, Koch H, Demling L. Course of electrolyte and enzymic pancreatic function after acute pancreatitis. Z Gastroenterol 14:684–687, 1976.
217. Valentini M, Cavallini G, Vantini I, et al. A comparative evaluation of endoscopic

retrograde pancreatography and the secretin-cholecystokinin test in the diagnosis of chronic pancreatitis: A multi-centre study in 124 patients. Endoscopy 13:64–67, 1981.
218. Vantini I, Piubello S, Scuro LA, et al. Duodenal ulcer in chronic relapsing pancreatitis. Digestion 23:23–28, 1982.
219. Ventrucci M, Gullo L, Daniele C, et al. Comparative study of serum pancreatic isoamylase, lipase and trypsin-like immunoreactivity in pancreatic disease. Digestion 28:114–121, 1983.
220. Ventrucci M, Gullo L, Daniele C, Priori P, Labo G. Pancreolauryl test for pancreatic exocrine insufficiency. Am J Gastroenterol 78:806–809, 1983.
221. Von der Lippe E. The absorption of vitamin B_{12} in chronic pancreatic insufficiency. Scand J Gastroenterol 12:257–259, 1977.
222. Wacjner G. Adenomatous hyperplasia of the islets of Langerhans in chronic pancreatitis. Bibl Gastroenterol 7:179, 1967.
223. Ward EM, Stephens DH, Sheedy PF II. CT characteristics of pancreatic carcinoma: An analysis of 100 cases. Radiography 3:547–565, 1983.
224. Warwick F, Anderson RJL, Braganza JM. Sclerosing-cholangitis-like changes in pancreatic disease. Clin Radiol 36:51–56, 1985.
225. Waye JD, Adler M, Dreiling DA. The pancreas: A correlation of function and structure. Am J Gastroenterol 69:176–181, 1978.
226. White TT, Allan BJ, Schilling JJ, Miyashata H. Human pancreatic secretory protein profiles in pancreas cancer and chronic pancreatitis. Dig Dis Sci 30:200–203, 1985.
227. Wilson C, Auld CD, Schlinkert R, et al. Hepatobiliary complications in chronic pancreatitis. Gut 30:520–527, 1989.
228. Wilson JS, Gossat D, Tait A, et al. Evidence for an inherited predisposition to alcoholic pancreatitis. Dig Dis Sci 29:727–730, 1984.
229. Wood RAB, Moosa AR. The prospective evaluation of tumour associated antigens for the early diagnosis of pancreatic cancer. Br J Surg 64:718–720, 1977.
230. Wormsley KG. The effect of vagotomy on the human pancreatic response to direct and indirect stimulation. Scand J Gastroenterol 7:85–91, 1972.
231. Zeitlin IJ, Sircus W. Factors influencing duodenal trypsin levels following a standard test meal as a test of pancreatic function. Gut 15:173–179, 1974.
232. Zentler-Munro PL, Fine DR, Batten JL. Northfield TC. Role of pH-dependent bile acid precipitation in fat maldigestion due to pancreatic steatorrhoea. Ann R Coll Surg Engl 64:51–52, 1982.
233. Zollinger RM, Elliott DW, Endahl GL, et al. Origin of the ulcerogenic hormone in endocrine-induced ulcer. Ann Surg 156:570–576, 1962.

CHAPTER

19

MANAGEMENT OF PAIN IN CHRONIC PANCREATITIS

Donald R. Campbell and
Norton J. Greenberger

EDITORIAL COMMENT (Chapters 19 and 20)

Drs. Campbell and Greenberger stress the enigma of the whole understanding of pancreatic pain. The observation that pain diminishes with time and with the development of pancreatic insufficiency is of particular interest. This suggests that pain is in some way related to acinar preservation and decreases with the decrease in the pancreatic acinar cell mass, despite the fact that pain does not seem to be correlated with attacks of inflammatory pancreatitis as evidenced of by the frequent lack of serum enzyme elevation during such attacks. Follow-up for 5 years in patients with calcific pancreatitis in Cape Town did not show a reduction in pain, and it seems that it is patients with early attacks of pancreatitis in whom pain "burn-out" is more evident. The authors stress the importance of excluding cysts as a major cause of pain and treating them either by percutaneous aspiration or by operation. In this regard, the whole controversy about duct pressure and pain appears somewhat irrelevant. As with most hollow organ symptomatology, the presence or absence of pain seems to be more related to the individual patient sensitivity than to certain pressure changes. Hence the fact that there is little difference in duct size and morphology in patients with chronic pancreatitis with and without pain and the fact that operation tends to relieve the pain, albeit temporarily, tend to suggest that certain patients are more liable to pain from duct distension or increase in duct pressure changes than others. In addition, the question of pain becomes all the more difficult to understand when Ammann's findings are considered (chapter 16), namely nonalcoholic, senile, chronic pancreatitis and perhaps nonalcoholic tropical pancreatitis often seem to be relatively painless diseases despite similar histologic and morphologic appearances.

With regard to medical treatment, the authors include the fascinating studies of stimulating secretion with secretin to wash out early protein plugs (in accord with the editor's finding of hyperconcentration of protein due to volume deficiency at ERCP in patients with early disease). One would have to guard against concomitant cholecystokinin therapy as this may aggravate the protein precipitation. Another point of great interest is that high-dose pancreatic protease replacement therapy helps best for pain in nonalcoholic female patients before overt calcification. However, as the authors state, it should at least be given a trial in all patients for 6 or 8 weeks before surgery is contemplated. The authors have explicitly not gone into detail with regard to a variety of therapeutic measures such as citrate administration and endoscopic obliteration of the ductal system by prolamine, acrynocyalate, and so forth. However, the use of judicious narcotics may convert an invalid to one who can hold down a job.

The surgical approaches to pancreatic pain in chronic pancreatitis and in other pancreatic diseases are discussed in detail by Dr. White. He gives us an elaborate description of the innervation of the pancreas and the pathophysiology of pain. Clearly, the most suitable candidates for relief are those with pseudocysts, which are not infrequently multiple. For patients with diffuse ductal dilatation, the lateral pancreaticojejunostomy (modified Puestow procedure) achieves complete or significant relief of pain in 80%. It appears that there will be an increasing role for pancreaticoduodenectomy (Whipple procedure) for intractable pain with disease confined to the head of gland as the mortality of this operation decreases. It seems likely that subtotal or total pancreatectomy will continue to fall into disfavor particularly if further data accrue to support the concept that chronic pancreatitis frequently "burns out" and pain disappears after 3 to 5 years. The technique of blocking the celiac ganglia with a long-acting local anesthetic (bupivacaine hydrochloride) as a trial before surgical excision of the ganglia is intriguing. However, this procedure, perhaps because of technical difficulties, has not become widely used.

CONTROVERSY

The pain of chronic pancreatitis presents challenging problems to the clinician. What is the mechanism? Can the mechanism of the pain be altered to provide relief? What is the natural history? Is there any rational basis for the various surgical approaches to this intractable symptom? What is value of proteinase feedback therapy? These questions and other perplexing aspects are addressed in the following two chapters.

Management of abdominal pain, the sine qua non of chronic pancreatitis (CP), regularly frustrates the internist and surgeon. This pain is often disabling and may be associated with continued alcohol abuse, narcotic abuse, and frequent interactions with physicians. Due to an incomplete understanding of the factors responsible for the pain associated with this disorder, a universally accepted approach to this problem has not been developed. The appropriate management of pain in patients with CP is controversial, and numerous approaches exist. The approaches to pain management (Table 19-1) are discussed in detail below and include the following:

1. Pancreatic enzyme supplementation. This is based on the concept of negative-feedback regulation of pancreatic exocrine secretion (the presence of intraduodenal trypsin inhibits pancreatic exocrine secretion).

2. Surgical procedures. Some of these are based on the importance of ductal decompression while others involve resection of the diseased organ.

3. Interruption of neural pathways. This is based on decreasing sensory input from the visceral afferent fibers of the autonomic nervous system.

4. Miscellaneous. This includes unique therapeutic modalities that have not been studied extensively, or in a controlled fashion.

Before discussing management in detail, it is important to review current concepts of pain in CP and the natural history of this disabling symptom.

TABLE 19-1. PAIN MANAGEMENT IN CP

Pancreatic Extract	
Non-enteric-coated pancreatic enzymes	
(H_2 antagonists, antacids, sodium bicarbonate, and H^+-K^+ pump inhibitors may improve efficacy)	
Surgical Procedures	
Pancreaticoduodenectomy (Whipple)	Denervated splenopancreatic flap
Lateral pancreaticojejunostomy	Sphincteroplasty
Caudal pancreaticojejunostomy	Pseudocyst drainage
Pancreatic ductal ligation	Pancreaticogastrostomy
Pancreatolithotomy	
Subtotal pancreatectomy (Distal pancreatectomy)	
Interruption of Neural Pathways	
Celiac ganglia blockade or ganglionectomy	
Left splanchnicectomy	
Complete denervation of the pancreas	
Miscellaneous	
Ductal injection or obstruction with acrylate glue	
Electric stimulation of the celiac plexus	
Depot secretin injections	
Acupuncture	
Transcutaneous electric nerve stimulation	

THE PAIN OF CP

The mechanisms responsible for pain in patients with CP are unknown, but some combination of the five factors listed in Table 19-2 appear to be operative in these patients. Although the pathophysiology of this pain is poorly understood, several studies have provided important clinical information that must be considered when formulating a rational approach for managing these patients.

Natural History

Several investigators have reported that spontaneous relief of pain occurs in untreated patients with CP when they are followed for extended periods.[1,11,20,24,30,33] Hayakawa and Kondo reported that with conservative management pain disappeared or decreased in 83% of 66 patients with CP.[11] Similarly, Ammann et al. found that the proportion of patients experiencing lasting pain

TABLE 19-2. POSSIBLE MECHANISMS OF PAIN IN PANCREATIC DISEASES

Pseudocysts and perifocal inflammation
Parenchymal (acinar) inflammatory process
Dilation of pancreatic duct (elevated ductal pressure)
Infiltration or entrapment of sensory nerves
Pressure of enlarged or inflamed gland on retroperitoneal structures

relief was similar in 67 patients undergoing a surgical procedure compared with 87 patients who were treated conservatively (approximately 85% in both groups).[1] Miyake et al. also found that 70% of the 106 patients they followed experienced improvement or disappearance of pain when followed for 1 to 20 years.[25] Scuro et al. found no significant difference in the probability of experiencing pain relief between two groups of patients who were followed for 10 years; 68% of the 95 patients who underwent side-to-side pancreaticojejunostomy experienced pain relief and 43% of 98 nonoperated patients experienced pain relief.[33] Thus, these studies indicate that in many patients the pain associated with CP resolves spontaneously.

Two of the most important factors associated with pain relief in patients with CP are (1) duration of CP and (2) continued abstinence from alcohol. The large series of Ammann et al. of 145 patients with alcohol-induced chronic calcific pancreatitis, studied over a 20-year period,[1] confirmed their earlier work and that of other investigators[8] that suggested that relief of pancreatic pain occurs as the underlying disease progresses to the stage of pancreatic calcification and exocrine insufficiency. These investigators found that an average of 4.5 years elapsed from the onset of pain to lasting pain relief. Their observation that the development of frank exocrine dysfunction is temporally related to the remission of chronic abdominal pain demonstrates that the natural history of this disorder is not one of chronic abdominal pain, but rather progression to pancreatic insufficiency with concurrent resolution of painful symptoms. Similarly, Ink et al. found that an average of 3.5 years elapsed from the onset of pain until its disappearance.[13] In addition to confirming a close relationship between pain relief and duration of disease, the Ink et al. study of patients undergoing surgical procedures for relief of pain associated with CP also found that the mean number of years of pain was lower among the patients who became abstinent early and that pain relief was more frequent if alcohol abstinence occurred before surgery. In addition, Scuro et al. found that complete alcohol withdrawal and/or progression to pancreatic insufficiency (presence of steatorrhea) were associated with a more favorable result in the patients undergoing surgery.[33] These studies demonstrate that continued abstinence increases the likelihood of pain relief in patients managed conservatively as well as those managed with surgical procedures for relief of abdominal pain associated with CP. The natural history of this disorder has been clarified by these studies. It appears that the pain of CP will "burn out" and remit when the disease progresses to the stage of pancreatic calcification and steatorrhea, and that an average of 3 to 4 years elapses between the onset of pain and its resolution.

Importance of Pancreatic Ductal Anatomy and Intraductal Pressures

As previously mentioned, the pathophysiology of pain in CP is poorly understood, but the predominant theory is that pain stems from intraductal hypertension and that ductal obstruction is the most frequent cause of intraductal hypertension. This hypothesis was originally proposed because those with the most severe pain tended to be chronic alcoholic patients with significant dilatation and stricture formation of the pancreatic duct. However, when Bornman et al. studied

39 patients with CP in a controlled manner, they found no correlation between pain and the presence of strictured or dilated ducts.[3] Kugelberg et al. performed endoscopic retrograde cholangiopancreatography (ERCP) on 13 patients who experienced pain relief after pancreaticojejunostomy for CP.[17] Although all patients experienced pain relief, only four had patent shunts. Similarly, Jensen et al. also found no correlation between duct morphology and severity of pain.[15] They did, however, find that patients with pancreatic pseudocysts seemed to be concentrated in the groups with severe pain. In fact, over 50% of the patients with pseudocysts in the series of Ammann et al. had complete pain relief by simple pseudocyst drainage.[1] These studies indicate that there is no correlation between duct morphology (dilation and/or stricture formation) and severity of pain. However, persistent pseudocysts are generally associated with significant pain, and this pain can be relieved with surgery. Thus, in patients with CP and pain the ductal morphology does not appear to be correlated with severity of pain unless a pancreatic pseudocyst is present; in such cases pain appears to be more severe and responds well to decompression of the pseudocyst.

Although the occurrence of pain relief following surgical procedures designed to decompress the pancreatic duct suggests that ductal pressures might be an important factor in the pathophysiology of pain, this area remains controversial. Novis et al. performed endoscopic manometry of the pancreatic duct and sphincter zone in patients with CP and found no significant difference in the mean pressures in the pancreatic duct, sphincter of Oddi (basal and phasic), and frequency of papillary contraction when comparing patients with alcoholic pancreatitis and controls.[26] Ebbehoj et al. evaluated pancreatic tissue pressure (PTP) and pain in 14 patients with CP. They found that long-term pain relief was not related to PTP decrease after surgery, PTP per se after the operation, the type of operation, or the patency of the anastomosis. However, Bradley found that pancreatic duct pressures are significantly higher in patients with CP than in controls.[5]

In summary, the pathophysiology and mechanisms responsible for the pain of CP are uncertain. Therefore, management of pain is not directed at a known cause, but rather to various potential mechanisms, and this probably accounts for the inconsistent response to current therapeutic modalities.

MEDICAL THERAPY FOR PAIN ASSOCIATED WITH CP

Table 19-3 emphasizes that *standard* medical therapy for CP should include (1) removal of causative factors (e.g., alcohol), (2) management of exocrine and endocrine insufficiency, and (3) symptomatic treatment of pain. Supplemental medical therapy is directed at regulating pancreatic exocrine secretion and includes both agents that stimulate pancreatic exocrine secretion and those that inhibit it.

Stimulation of Pancreatic Secretion

Tympner and Rosch proposed using depot secretin therapy as an alternative approach to the management of pain in patients with advanced recurrent CP who

TABLE 19-3. MEDICAL THERAPY FOR CP

Standard Therapy
Removal of causative factor (e.g., alcohol)
Management of exocrine insufficiency (diarrhea)
Management of endocrine insufficiency (diabetes)
Symptomatic treatment of pain
Supplemental Therapy
Pharmacologic therapy to increase exocrine secretion (e.g., depot secretin)
Pharmacologic therapy to decrease exocrine secretion (e.g., anticholinergics, pancreatic enzymes, hormonal antagonists)

do not have pancreatic duct obstruction or pseudocysts.[37] Their rationale for the use of depot secretin was that it might "wash out" the sticky, protein-rich secretions in the pancreatic duct and therefore decrease intraductal pressures with subsequent pain relief. Several of their previous publications described patients with CP who experienced pain relief following multiple stimulation studies to evaluate pancreatic exocrine secretion.[37] They also found that the viscosity of pancreatic secretions was higher in patients with CP compared with controls. After 6 to 7 days of therapy there was a significant decrease in the pain score of patients who were treated with depot secretin compared with placebo-treated controls. Pap et al. have also studied the use of hormonal stimulants in treating CP.[29] They studied cholecystokinin (CCK) octapeptide and soy flour singularly and in combination for the treatment of CP. They found amelioration of symptoms during and after the treatments in almost all patients. Although these studies utilizing agents that stimulate pancreatic exocrine secretion are very provocative, they remain preliminary.

Inhibition of Pancreatic Secretion

A more traditional approach to the medical management of pain associated with CP involves pharmacologic inhibition of pancreatic exocrine secretion. Since pancreatic exocrine secretion is modulated through both neural and humoral mechanisms, medical therapy to decrease secretion is directed toward inhibition of cholinergic pathways and/or decreasing CCK-stimulated pancreatic exocrine secretion. Owyang et al. performed perfusion studies in humans to evaluate neural and hormonal control of the intestinal phase of human pancreatic enzyme secretion.[27,28] They stimulated pancreatic exocrine secretion with intraduodenal phenylalanine and found that when phenylalanine and trypsin were perfused together, pancreatic enzyme secretion was decreased to 63% of the response to phenylalanine alone. Intravenous atropine caused phenylalanine-stimulated pancreatic enzyme secretion to decrease to 38% of the response to phenylalanine alone, and when intravenous atropine and intraduodenal perfusion of trypsin were combined, the pancreatic enzyme response to phenylalanine stimulation was completely blocked. Although the relative contribution of hormonal and neural stimulation to the postprandial pancreatic exocrine response remains controversial, these studies demonstrate that nutrients such as phenylalanine stimulate pancreatic secretion primarily through release of CCK, and the osmolality and volume of a meal evoke a pancreatic response through cholinergic mechanisms. Therefore, both mechanisms must be considered when medical therapy designed to decrease pancreatic secretion is being planned.

Animal studies have been performed to evaluate cholinergic influences on the enteropancreatic reflex.[36] Although human studies have been initiated, no clinical studies have been completed that evaluate the effect of anticholinergics and intraduodenal proteases on pain relief in patients with CP. However, two studies have reported partial relief of pain in a significant number of patients with CP who were treated with high-dose oral pancreatic enzyme supplements.[14,34] Those two studies (Table 19-4) suggest that the patients who are most likely to demonstrate a decrease in pain scores while being treated with oral pancreatic enzyme supplements are those with non-alcohol-induced CP, especially female patients. In fact, it appears that up to 80% of female patients with idiopathic CP may experience a significant decrease in their painful symptoms when treated with oral enzyme supplements. Conversely, male patients with alcohol-associated CP are much less likely to respond to such treatment. Regardless of the etiology of CP or the gender of the patient, we suggest that oral administration of pancreatic extracts should always be the first line of therapy.

Oral pancreatic enzymes appear to inhibit pancreatic exocrine secretion, and thus decrease pain, through a negative-feedback mechanism involving intraduodenal proteases and the pancreas. Owyang et al. performed elegant studies in humans that demonstrated that intraduodenal trypsin modulates pancreatic exocrine secretion by regulating CCK release.[27] Simply stated, the presence of trypsin in the proximal duodenum appears to suppress CCK release and thus inhibit pancreatic enzyme secretion. Lu et al. clarified the mechanisms involved.[22] They demonstrated the existence of a trypsin-sensitive intestinal peptide that, if intact, can stimulate CCK release. Therefore, since patients with CP have decreased intraduodenal protease activity secondary to a damaged gland, they may not be capable of inactivating the intraduodenal peptide that stimulates CCK release. In patients with painful symptoms associated with CP, oral pancreatic enzyme supplements may provide relief of pain by supplementing endogenous protease inacti-

TABLE 19-4. EFFECT OF ORAL PANCREATIC ENZYMES ON PAIN SCORES IN PATIENTS WITH CP

	Pain Score Decrease of ≥70%	
	Isaksson and Ihse[14] (%)	Slaff et al.[34] (%)
All patients	53	55
Females	75	82
Female non-EtOH CP	75	78
Males	36	22
Male EtOH CP	33–36	13
Male and female mild to moderate CP	—	75
Male and female severe CP	—	25

vation of CCK-stimulating peptide. Inactivation of this peptide would result in decreased CCK release, which in turn decreases pancreatic stimulation and may thereby decrease pain. Support for this mechanism is provided by several studies[7,10,16,32,35] that have demonstrated increased CCK levels in patients with CP. Slaff et al. also demonstrated that fasting CCK levels decreased in patients who were treated with oral pancreatic enzyme supplements.[35] These studies clarify the mechanisms involved in the intraluminal feedback regulation of pancreatic exocrine secretion and the rationale for using oral pancreatic enzymes to relieve painful symptoms.

Specific Considerations in Medical Therapy

Medical therapy for patients with pain characteristic of CP, compatible clinical and historical findings, and an abnormal drainage test (e.g., secretin test) should not be delayed while waiting for other diagnostic studies. Initial therapy should be a conventional oral pancreatic enzyme supplement with meals and at bedtime (Fig. 19-1). Since intraluminal feedback regulation of the exocrine pancreas occurs in the proximal duodenum, the newer enteric-coated microspheres should not be used to treat pain as they may not dissolve until they pass beyond the proximal duodenum. In addition, enteric-coated microspheres should not be used in combination with H_2 antagonists, antacids, sodium bicarbonate, and so forth, as the microspheres may dissolve in the stomach and the enzymes be irreversibly inactivated by gastric acid.

Although little orally ingested enzyme actually reaches the proximal duodenum, it is frequently adequate to relieve pain. If painful symptoms do not improve within 1 month of initiating therapy with oral pancreatic enzymes, another agent should be added in an attempt to "protect" the enzyme from being inactivated by gastric acid. Traditionally, sodium bicarbonate (1300 mg q.i.d.), H_2 antagonists, or antacids were used. Studies by Graham demonstrated that sodium bicarbonate and aluminum hydroxide are much more effective than magnesium hydroxide, calcium carbonate, or cimetidine in improving clinical efficacy of a small amount of replacement enzyme.[9] In practice, however, second-line therapy generally includes pancreatic enzymes with either sodium bicarbonate or an H_2 antagonist. The reasons for selecting these agents over others include convenience, compliance, and studies by Regan et al. supporting the use of H_2 antagonists.[31] Lamers and Jansen reported two patients with severe steatorrhea secondary to CP who experienced more than 50% less steatorrhea when treated with pancreatic enzymes and omeprazole compared with treatment with pancreatic enzymes and H_2 antagonists.[18] In summary, second-line therapy for the pain associated with CP should include a non-enteric-coated oral pancreatic extract combined with an agent to protect the enzymes from inactivation by gastric acid. Currently, sodium bicarbonate and H_2 antagonists are the most frequently used adjuncts, but in the future, potent inhibitors of gastric acid secretion (e.g., inhibitors of parietal cell H^+-K^+ adenosine triphosphatase) may become the adjunct of choice.

Future directions in the medical management of the pain associated with CP will probably involve simultaneous inhibition of both cholinergic and CCK stimu-

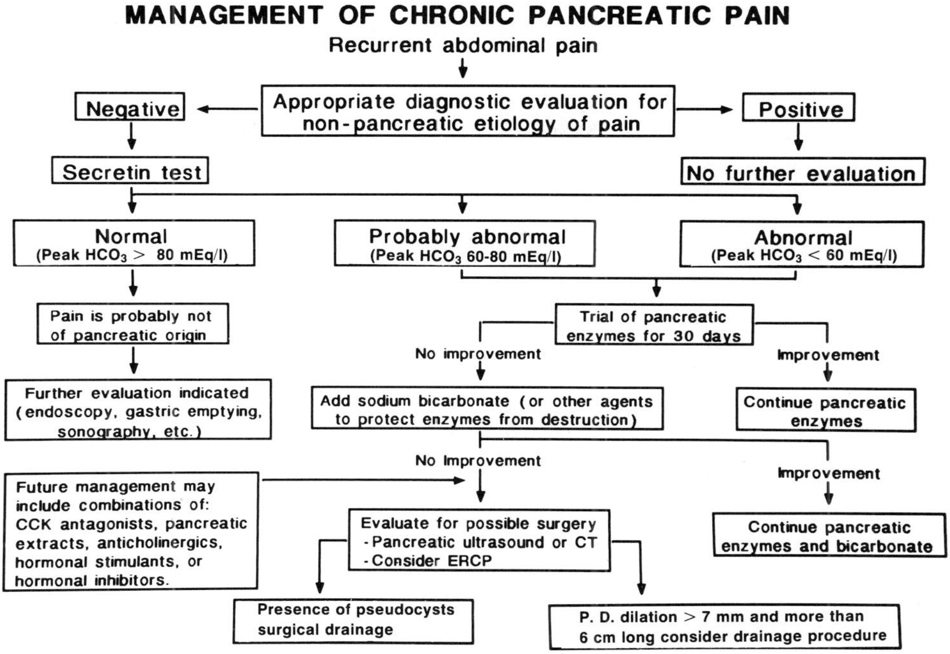

Figure 19-1. Algorithm for managing pain associated with CP in patients who do not experience pain relief with standard therapy (Table 19-3). (Reproduced with permission: Greenberger NJ. Chronic pancreatitis and exocrine insufficiency. Hosp Pract 20:44, 1985, and Slaff JI. Management of pain in chronic pancreatitis. Hosp Pract 20:61, 1985.)

lation of the pancreas. Although intraduodenal perfusion of trypsin is very effective in inhibiting amino acid[34]- and phenylalanine[28]-stimulated pancreatic exocrine secretion, orally administered pancreatic extracts may not be as effective due to dilution, inactivation, and other factors. Also, pancreatic extracts do not inhibit the cholinergic stimulation of exocrine secretion associated with a meal. Therefore, clinical studies designed to evaluate the efficacy of anticholinergics and oral pancreatic enzymes in patients with chronic pancreatitis and pain have been initiated. In addition, extremely potent CCK antagonists should become available, and these agents are capable of directly inhibiting CCK-stimulated acinar cell secretion. In addition, Lluis et al. reported that peptide YY can inhibit nutrient-, hormonally, and vagally stimulated pancreatic exocrine secretion in the dog,[21] and its mechanism of action appears to be independent of cholinergic innervation. Therefore, maximal medical therapy for patients with pain and CP should exploit several of the mechanisms that regulate pancreatic exocrine secretion. If the mechanism for reducing the pain of CP is inhibition of pancreatic exocrine secretion, some combination of oral pancreatic extract or CCK antagonist or anticholinergic or hormonal suppression should significantly improve the results of medical management in the future.

If medical therapy does not provide significant pain relief in 6 to 8 weeks, the patient will require further diagnostic studies to determine whether surgery is indicated. If ultrasonography or computed tomography of the pancreas was not performed to exclude a pseudocyst, such a procedure should be performed. To evaluate pancreatic ductal anatomy and to determine appropriateness of surgery, an ERCP should be considered. If a pancreatic pseudocyst is found, both Jensen et al.[15] and Ammann et al.[1] indicate a significant chance for pain relief if the pseudocyst is decompressed. If pancreatic ductal dilation of ≥8 mm and more than 6 cm in length is found, the patient is more likely to experience satisfactory pain relief from surgical drainage procedures.[4] If none of these abnormalities are found, resection rather than decompression can be considered, but long-term results are poor.

Percutaneous Celiac Plexus Block (PCPB)

This procedure is performed under fluoroscopic guidance and involves bilateral injection of short- and/or long-acting topical anesthetics in the paravertebral area caudal to the 12th rib. The most frequent complications include hypotension and misdirected injections (e.g., intravascular, subarachnoid, intraperitoneal, and intrathoracic injections). In fact, Leung et al.[19] found that 13% of patients with CP who underwent PCPB for pain control experienced significant neurologic complications, and one of these patients has persistent loss of anal and bladder sphincter control. However, PCPB can be an effective method for controlling the pain of CP. Unfortunately, the duration of its effect is very short (Table 19-5). Unlike patients with pancreatic cancer, who have a short life expectancy, patients with CP regularly outlive the effect of PCPB. If celiac plexus blocks are performed in patients with CP for pain relief, they will need to be repeated frequently, realizing the attendant risk of complications. Madsen and Hansen performed a controlled

TABLE 19-5. PAIN RELIEF FROM PERCUTANEOUS CELIAC PLEXUS BLOCK IN PANCREATIC DISORDERS

	Bell et al.[2]	Leung et al.[19]	Madsen and Hansen[23]	Hegedus[12]
		Chronic Pancreatitis		
Patients	16	23	8	9
Short-term improvement	81%	78%	75%	—
Short-term relief	—	52%	—	—
Long-term relief	63%	Avg. duration 2 months	0%	33%
		Pancreatic Cancer		
Patients	—	13	—	36
Short-term improvement	—	100%	—	64%
Short-term relief	—	85%	—	—
Pain-free at death	—	64%	—	—

randomized trial of celiac plexus block and pancreaticogastrostomy for control of pain in patients with CP. They found that pancreaticogastrostomy was superior to PCPB in providing lasting pain relief. PCPB is rarely recommended in the management of pain associated with CP since it provides only short-term pain relief, must be repeated frequently, and can be associated with significant complications. However, in the occasional patient in whom medical therapy fails and who is a high-risk surgical candidate, this is a viable option.

Medical Viewpoints on the Surgical Management of the Pain of CP

The role of surgery in the treatment of pancreatic pain is controversial, and interpretation of studies is difficult since the patients are rarely randomized to surgical or medical therapy and followed long-term. However, if a surgical procedure is required for control of painful symptoms associated with CP, most physicians agree that preservation of pancreatic tissue by selecting a drainage procedure rather than resection is most appropriate. This is associated with lower morbidity from endocrine and exocrine insufficiency and a higher incidence of pain relief. It is also generally agreed that patients with CP, a pancreatic pseudocyst, and painful symptoms that are unresponsive to medical therapy should undergo decompression of the pseudocyst. In addition, abstinent patients with a pancreatic duct that is dilated to more than 8 mm for at least 6 cm of length and persistent painful symptoms that have not responded to medical therapy should be considered for surgery. However, it is important to remember that painful symptoms resolve in 75% to 85% of patients with CP over time. Therefore, surgical procedures should be carefully considered. Delays do not appear to significantly influence outcome. In fact, Warshaw et al.[38] has demonstrated that decompression of the dilated pancreatic duct does not prevent continuing destruction of pancreatic glandular tissue.

Overall, impressive short-term pain relief has been obtained in most surgical series of appropriately selected patients. However, Bradley[4] and others suggest that, depending on the type of surgical procedure performed, good long-term (5 years or more following surgery) relief of pain occurs in only 34% to 66% of patients. These results would probably be better if more patients were able to remain abstinent. Additionally, only approximately one half the patients have ductal anatomy suitable for a lateral pancreaticojejunostomy. These patients bring up two important questions: first, is the mechanism of pain relief associated with surgical procedures due to decompression of the pancreatic duct or interruption of neural pathways? If the latter is the mechanism, more procedures directed at interrupting neural pathways should be performed. Second, if 75% to 85% of patients experience spontaneous pain relief after 3.3 to 4.5 years, do surgical procedures actually decrease the chance of experiencing spontaneous pain relief? Since the results of surgical treatment are not entirely satisfactory, new approaches to the surgical management of the pain associated with CP are proposed from year to year. It will be interesting to see what new surgical approaches to this old disease will be developed.

SUMMARY

1. The natural history of painful, alcohol-induced CP is one of progression to a pain-free state within 3 to 5 years.

2. Painful, idiopathic CP may resolve spontaneously or may progress.

3. Ductal morphology (presence of strictures, dilation, etc.) in patients with CP does not appear to correlate with severity of pain (unless a pseudocyst is present).

4. First-line therapy in patients with CP and painful symptoms should be a trial of oral pancreatic enzymes. If significant pain relief does not occur, an adjunct should be added to protect the enzyme from inactivation by gastric acid.

5. Patients with pancreatic pseudocysts and pain should have the cysts decompressed.

6. PCPB provides adequate short-term pain relief in patients with CP and in patients with pancreatic cancer. Due to the brief duration and potential complications, PCPB is unacceptable for pain management in most patients with CP.

7. The patients who are most likely to respond to medical therapy are females with non-alcohol-induced CP.

8. The patients who are most likely to respond to surgical therapy are those with alcohol-induced CP who are abstinent and undergo a lateral pancreaticojejunostomy.

9. Newer medical therapies directed at regulating neural and hormonal stimulation of the pancreas will become available in the near future.

REFERENCES

1. Ammann RW, Akovbiantz A, Largiader F, Schueler G. Course and outcome of chronic pancreatitis: Longitudinal study of a mixed medical-surgical series of 245 patients. Gastroenterology 86:820–828, 1984.
2. Bell SN, Cole R, Roberts-Thomson IC. Coeliac plexus block for control of pain in chronic pancreatitis. Br Med J 281(Dec 13):1604, 1980.
3. Bornman PC, Marks IN, Girdwood AH, et al. Is pancreatic duct obstruction or stricture a major cause of pain in calcific pancreatitis? Br J Surg 67:425–428, 1980.
4. Bradley EL. Long-term results of pancreatojejunostomy in patients with chronic pancreatitis. Am J Surg 153:207–213, 1987.
5. Bradley EL. Pancreatic duct pressure in chronic pancreatitis. Am J Surg 144:313–316, 1982.
6. Ebbehoj N, Barly L, Madsen P, Svendsen LB. Pancreatic tissue pressure and pain in chronic pancreatitis. Pancreas 1(6):556–558, 1986.
7. Ederle A, Vantini I, Harvey RF, et al. Fasting serum cholecystokinin immunoreactivity in chronic relapsing pancreatitis. Ric Clin Lab 8(3):199–206, 1978.
8. Girdwood AH, Marks IN, Bornman PC, Kottler RE, Cohen M. Does progressive pancreatic insufficiency limit pain in calcific pancreatitis with duct stricture or continued alcohol insult. J Clin Gastroenterol 3:241–245, 1981.
9. Graham DY. Pancreatic enzyme replacement the effects of antacids or cimetidine. Dig Dis Sci 27(6):485–490, 1982.
10. Harvey RF, Hartog M, Dowsett L, Read AE. A radioimmunoassay for cholecystokinin-pancreozymin. Lancet 2:826–828, 1973.
11. Hayakawa T, Kondo T. Surgical indication for chronic pancreatitis evaluated from the natural history of the disease. Jpn J Gastroenterol Surg 12:647–654, 1979.

12. Hegedus V. Relief of pancreatic pain by radiography-guided block. AJR 133:1101–1103, 1979.
13. Ink O, Labayle D, Buffet C, Chaput JC, Etienne JP. Pancreatite chronique alcoolique: Relations de la douleur avec le sevrage et la chirurgie pancreatique. Gastroenterol Clin Biol 8:419–425, 1984.
14. Isaksson G, Ihse I. Pain reduction by an oral pancreatic enzyme preparation in chronic pancreatitis. Dig Dis Sci 28:97–102, 1983.
15. Jensen AR, Matzen P, Malchow-Moller A, Christoffersen I. Pattern of pain, duct morphology, and pancreatic function in chronic pancreatitis. Scand J Gastroenterol 19:334–338, 1984.
16. Johnson AG, Marshall CE, Dowsett L, Harvey RF. The correlation of bioassay and radioimmunoassay of serum cholecystokinin. Gut 16(5):398–399, 1975.
17. Kugelberg CH, Wehlin L, Arnesjo B, Tylen U. Endoscopic pancreatography in evaluating results of pancreaticojejunostomy. Gut 17:267–272, 1976.
18. Lamers CBHW, Jansen JBMJ. Omeprazole as adjunct to enzyme replacement treatment in severe pancreatic insufficiency. Br Med J 293(Oct 18):994, 1986.
19. Leung JWC, Bowen-Wright M, Aveling W, Shorvon PJ, Cotton PB. Coeliac plexus block for pain in pancreatic cancer and chronic pancreatitis. Br J Surg 70:730–732, 1983.
20. Levrat M, Descos L, Moulinier B, Pasquier J. Evolution au long cours des pancreatites chroniques. Arch Fr Mal Appar Dig 59:5–18, 1970.
21. Lluis F, Gomez G, Fujimura M, Greeley GH, Thompson JC. Peptide YY inhibits nutrient-, hormonal-, and vagally-stimulated pancreatic exocrine secretion. Pancreas 2:454–462, 1987.
22. Lu L, Louie DS, May D, Owyang C. Regulation of pancreatic enzyme secretion by a trypsin-sensitive, intestinal peptide that stimulates cholecystokinin release. Dig Dis Sci 32:1175, 1987. Abstract.
23. Madsen P, Hansen E. Coeliac plexus block versus pancreaticogastrostomy for pain in chronic pancreatitis. Scand J Gastroenterol 20:1217–1220, 1985.
24. Marks IN, Girdwood AH, Bank S, Louw SB. The prognosis of alcohol induced calcific pancreatitis. S Afr Med J 57:640–643, 1980.
25. Miyake H, Harada H, Kunichika K, Ochi K, Ikuro K. Clinical course and prognosis of chronic pancreatitis. Pancreas 2:378–385, 1987.
26. Novis BH, Bornman PC, Girdwood AW, Marks IN. Endoscopic manometry of the pancreatic duct and sphincter zone in patients with chronic pancreatitis. Dig Dis Sci 30:225–228, 1985.
27. Owyang C, Louie DS, Tatum D. Feedback regulation of pancreatic enzyme secretion-suppression of cholecystokinin release by trypsin. J Clin Invest 77:2042–2047, 1986.
28. Owyang C, May D, Louie DS. Trypsin suppression of pancreatic enzyme secretion—Differential effect on cholecystokinin release and the enteropancreatic reflex. Gastroenterology 91:637–643, 1986.
29. Pap A, Berger Z, Varro V. Complementary effect of cholecystokinin-octapeptide and soy flour treatment in chronic pancreatitis. Mt Sinai J Med 51:254–257, 1984.
30. Phillip J, Koch H, Rosch W, et al. Significance of endoscopic retrograde pancreatography for therapy of chronic pancreatitis: Results of a follow up study. Gastroenterology 72:1113, 1977. Abstract.
31. Regan PT, Malagelada JR, DiMagno EP, Glanzman SL, Go VLM. Comparative effects of antacids, cimetidine and enteric coating on the therapeutic response to oral enzymes in severe pancreatic insufficiency. N Engl J Med 297:854–858, 1977.
32. Schafmayer A, Becker HD, Werner M, Folsch UR, Crutzfeldt W. Increased plasma CCK concentrations in patients with chronic pancreatitis. Digestion 32:136–139, 1985.
33. Scuro LA, Vantini I, Piubello W, et al. Evolution of pain in chronic relapsing pancreatitis: A study of operated and nonoperated patients. Am J Gasteroenterol 78:495–501, 1983.
34. Slaff J, Jacobson D, Tillman CR, Curington C, Toskes P. Protease-specific suppression of pancreatic exocrine secretion. Gasteroenterology 87:44–52, 1984.
35. Slaff JI, Wolfe MM, Toskes PP: Elevated fasting cholecystokinin levels in pancreatic

exocrine impairment: Evidence to support feedback regulation. J Lab Clin Med 105:282–285, 1985.
36. Solomon TE, Grossman MI. Effect of atropine and vagotomy on response of transplanted pancreas. Am J Physiol 236:E186–E190, 1979.
37. Tympner F, Rosch W. The treatment of chronic recurrent pancreatitis with depot secretin. Hepatogastroenterology 33:159–162, 1986.
38. Warshaw AL, Popp JW, Schapiro RH. Long-term patency, pancreatic function, and pain relief after lateral pancreaticojejunostomy for chronic pancreatitis. Gastroenterology 79:289–293, 1980.

CHAPTER

20

PANCREATIC PAIN: SURGICAL ASPECTS

Thomas Taylor White

Acute and chronic pancreatitis and cancer of the pancreas are the most common causes of pancreatic pain. I will discuss the three together because the pain in pancreatitis is virtually indistinguishable from that of cancer.

Inflammatory invasion of the surrounding structures occurs in all three diseases with pain localized either to the upper abdomen or to the left or right costovertebral angles. The pain may be due to involvement of the nerves posterior to and within the pancreas by inflammatory reaction, scarring, or tumor. Pain can also be due to distension of a pancreatic duct behind an obstruction due to scarring secondary to pancreatitis, calculi in the pancreatic duct, obstruction of the distal duct by a stricture of the ampulla of Vater, or a tumor at the right end of the duct.

Distended pancreatic cysts are another cause of extreme pain. Patients with pancreatic fistulas and/or sinuses may develop severe wound pain secondary to erosion of the surrounding skin by activated enzyme secretions. A few patients with acute pancreatitis may develop an acute abdomen due to release of fluid and kinins into the lesser and/or greater sac of the abdominal cavity with secondary peritoneal irritation.

Both patients with carcinoma of the pancreas and those with acute and chronic pancreatitis are now admitted to the hospital at about the same rate, 1 per 500 to 700 admissions. The relative incidence of cancer of the pancreas has tripled in the United States since 1940, while pancreatitis has remained at a relatively constant rate. For that reason, the number of patients seen with cancer of the pancreas that can be confused with pancreatitis is much greater than it was 30 or

40 years ago. Postoperative pancreatitis, pancreatic fistulas, sinuses, and cysts occur at a rate proportional to the amount of stomach, biliary, and pancreatic surgery and pancreaticobiliary endoscopy done and the excellence with which it is performed.

PATHOPHYSIOLOGY

About 60% of human pancreatitis is secondary to the passage of gallstones. It has been shown that virtually all patients with known gallstones who develop pancreatitis pass into the intestinal tract gallstones that can be collected from the stool. It appears that reflux of duodenal contents into and obstruction of the pancreatic duct during migration of a gallstone into the duodenum is responsible for the autoactivation or premature activation of pancreatic proteases within the pancreas.[19] About 15% of the total number of patients with pancreatitis are alcoholic, 10% have duodenal ulcer, and another 10% have operative or external trauma as the basis for the problem, with the remaining 5% divided between metabolic diseases such as hyperparathyroidism and hyperlipidemia, congenital strictures of the bile and pancreatic ducts, and various other congenital enzymatic abnormalities.[4] Just why activation occurs only rarely in the intrapancreatic ducts and why it causes acute pancreatitis, chronic pancreatitis (CP), or pancreatitis behind a carcinoma at the head of the pancreas is unknown at the present time. Some light may have been shed on the problem by the three-dimensional reconstructions of resected pancreases by Nakamura et al.,[15] which showed that patients with CP have different lesions from patients with obstruction of the main duct or normal individuals. The characteristics found in calcifying pancreatitis were as follows:

1. The lesions were distributed irregularly and were related to the ducts.
2. Protein plugs were frequently found in the ducts, occasionally containing mucoproteins, which may evolve into calculi by the deposition of calcium upon the surfaces.
3. Significant lesions were present in all sizes of ducts.

This protein material coagulates and eventually becomes deposited within the pancreatic ducts as calculi that can locally obstruct individual ducts; generally obstruct the entire ductal system, producing numerous areas of local inflammation; or produce one large dilated duct. Patients with acute pancreatitis average about 53 years of age as opposed to patients with CP, who average about 38. For this reason, it seems unlikely that CP is secondary to repeated attacks of acute pancreatitis. Furthermore, very few patients with CP have gallstones. The 20% of patients having pancreatitis secondary to duodenal ulcer or trauma probably develop autoactivation of the duct system secondary to those diseases that account for their acute pancreatitis. Pancreatitis can also be secondary to congenital strictures of the bile and pancreatic ducts with dilatation of one or the other system.[5,17] Patients with pancreas divisum are now being related to this obstruction of the system.[3]

The pain related to acute or chronic pancreatitis is due to

1. Diffusion of activated enzymes into the peritoneal cavity.
2. Inflammatory invasion of the structures surrounding the pancreas as well as the intrapancreatic nerve ganglia and surrounding sympathetic and parasympathetic network.
3. Distension of the pancreatic duct or a peripancreatic pseudocyst.

NERVE SUPPLY

There are both sympathetic and parasympathetic nerves to the pancreas. The sympathetic innervation passes to the pancreas through the splanchnic nerves. The greater splanchnic nerves derive from the 5th to the 10th thoracic ganglia. These branches join at the level of D10 or D11 to become the greater splanchnic nerve. They pass through the diaphragm and join the semilunar ganglia. The lesser splanchnic nerves arise variably from the 9th and 10th dorsal ganglia and then drop posterolaterally through the diaphragm to join the semilunar ganglia. There is a relay for all the sympathetic nerves at the celiac plexus (Fig. 20-1).

There is an exchange between the right and the left splanchnic nerves at the level of the celiac ganglia with the result that the tail of the pancreas receives a few fibers from the right, and the head of the pancreas receives some fibers from the left, splanchnic nerve. The postganglionic fibers travel with those of the parasympathetic nervous system after coming together in the celiac plexus. They pass along the gastroduodenal artery toward the head of the pancreas, the inferior portion of the common bile duct, and the sphincter of Oddi. They also pass along the hepatic artery toward the anterior and posterior hepatic plexuses, the gallbladder, and the hepatic bile ducts, along the splenic artery toward the body and tail of the pancreas. The sympathetic fibers appear to contain the principal afferent pain fibers.

The parasympathetic innervation is represented by the prepanglionic vagus nerves, which are not interrupted at the level of the celiac plexus. The posterior vagus nerve, after having given several branches to the lesser curvature of the stomach, gives off a celiac division that, after sending fibers around the lesser curvature of the stomach to the liver, advances directly to the celiac plexus. The biliary tree, including the sphincter of Oddi, is almost entirely innervated by the right vagus nerve, but the innervation is apparently only sensory. The vagus nerves pass through the celiac plexus without any ganglionic station. The sympathetic and parasympathetic fibers pass together from this level toward the pancreas and bile ducts. The very short postganglionic parasympathetic fibers connect with the adjacent viscera. The vagus nerves play an important part in the control of pancreatic secretions, while the pain fibers are primarily sympathetic. The sympathetic fibers also appear to play some part in the control of the vascular supply and to a lesser extent in the secretion of the pancreas.

Alcohol plays an important part in the precipitating attacks of pancreatitis in many patients, but there are a few who drink in order to relieve their pain. One particularly notable case in my experience was that of a man whose pancreatitis

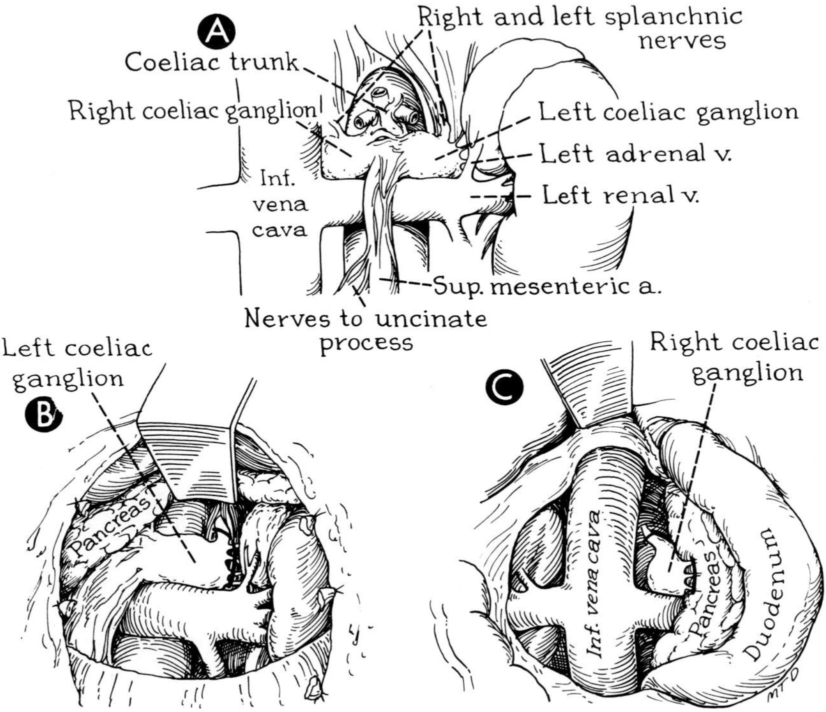

Figure 20-1. (A) The right and left celiac ganglia in relation to the superior mesenteric artery, inferior vena cava, adrenal vein, and celiac axis. (B) The exposure of the left celiac ganglion after the mesentery on the inferior surface of the pancreas has been divided and the pancreas dissected free from the posterior abdominal wall. (C) The right celiac ganglion after the duodenum and common duct have been freed together with the pancreas from the right to the left side. The solid lines represent the points at which the resection should begin. (From White TT. Pancreatitis. Baltimore, Williams & Wilkins, 1966, with permission.)

had been attributed for a number of years to an excessive alcohol intake. At operation, he was found to have a localized area of scarring in the region of the ampulla of Vater that was completely obstructing the principal pancreatic duct so that it had been dilated immediately to the left of this point to about 1 cm in diameter. In reviewing this patient's history at a later date, I became aware that this area of sclerosis was secondary to an abdominal injury that occurred some 30 years before in a fall from a horse; the fall had been followed by persistent abdominal pain that had followed him all the way through high school and college. Thus, it is possible that a localized area of obstruction secondary to posttraumatic scarring or due to congenital narrowing of the duct or even pancreatic cancer can cause left-sided obstructive pancreatitis.

The localization of the pain is greatly influenced by the position of the principal lesions. Localized obstruction of the pancreatic duct in the head of the pan-

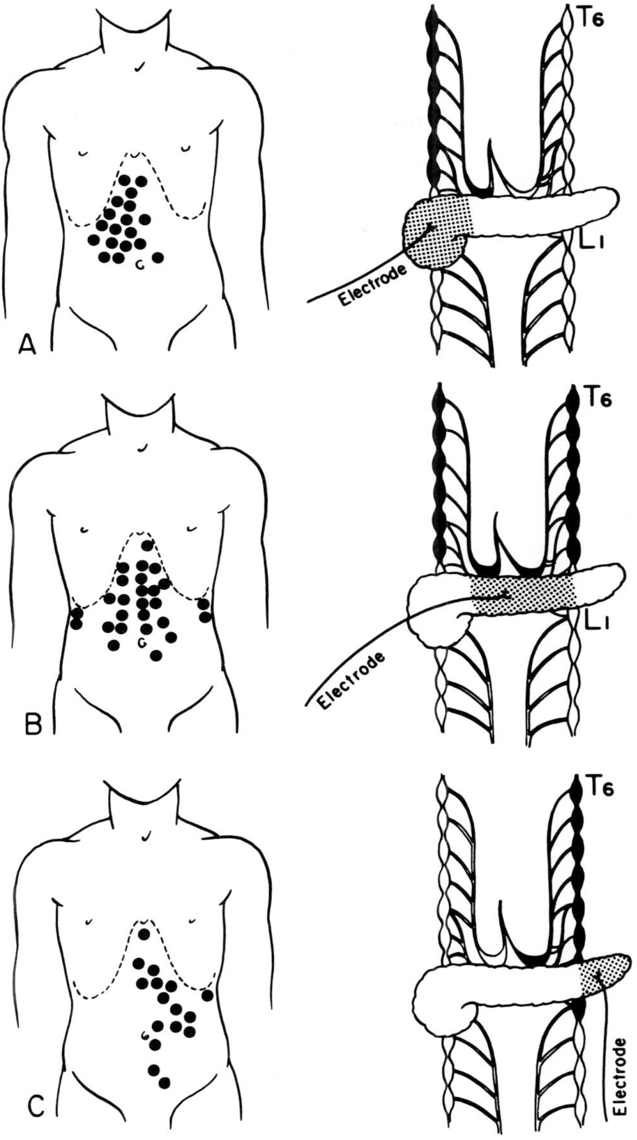

Figure 20-2. (A) Stimulation of the head of the pancreas with an electrode produces a predominantly right-sided pain, as indicated by the dots. (B) Stimulation of the central portion of the pancreas produces pain on both sides of the abdominal wall. (C) Stimulation of the tail of the pancreas produces predominantly left-sided pain. it is clear that there is some crossover in each instance. The blackened area of sympathetic chain illustrates the theoretical pathways involved. (From White TT. Pancreatitis. Baltimore, Williams & Wilkins, 1966, with permission.)

creas can often cause abdominal pain because of secondary dilatation of the pancreatic duct behind this obstruction. On the other hand, if the right-sided lesion is a large cyst, the principal pain is usually in this area. Some light was thrown on the pain pathways by the studies of Ray and Neil[17] and Bliss et al.[5] These authors studied patients by electric stimulation of the pancreas during abdominal operations performed under local anesthesia. Stimulation of the left side of the gland produced predominantly left-sided pain, and that on the right side produced right-sided pain. Stimulation of the central portion of the pancreas produced pain on both sides of the abdominal wall. There was some crossover in each instance (Fig. 20-2).

The pain from cancer of the pancreas seems to be due either to distension of the pancreatic duct behind the tumor or to the left of it and to invasion of the surrounding structures and nerve ganglia. As in other types of pancreatic pain, intraductal activation of pancreatic zymogens seems to be a major cause of pancreatic inflammation since the size of the palpable mass usually is much larger than that of the tumor, the peripheral portions of the mass consisting chiefly of inflammatory tissue that often shows only CP on biopsy.

Our studies of secretions collected from a patient with carcinoma of the head of the pancreas with a T tube left in the pancreatic duct to relieve pain from ductal distension behind the tumor showed no traces of proteolytic activity in the pancreatic juice for several days.[2,19] The patient's secretions became bloody and decreased in volume and protein output, and active chymotrypsin was present in all of the bloody specimens. At the same time, the patient developed an attack of acute abdominal pain. When the pain subsided, the flow rate and protein output of pancreatic juice returned to normal, and no free proteolytic activity was found again. This left us with the speculation whether the pancreatitis and pancreatic pain seen in connection with cancer, and the acute pancreatitis and pain seen in connection with gallstone disease, and CP seen in alcoholics, all develop by the same mechanism. It is well known that some tumor cells produce a proteolytic enzyme that will break down plasminogen. A substance of this type may activate the zymogens in cancer patients. We feel that the pancreatitis and pain seen in cancer patients may sometimes be due to obstruction of the duct and in other instances to the above mechanism of developing pancreatitis.

CLINICAL PICTURE OF PAIN

Pain is nearly always the primary complaint in acute pancreatitis, striking because of its severity and the speed with which it reaches maximum intensity. The pain sometimes becomes slightly less severe an hour or two after an acute onset and then worsens again. The pain may shift from the epigastric region to the right or left lower quadrants of the abdomen over a period of several hours. The pain and tenderness may be in the right or left lower quadrants without significant upper abdominal symptoms or signs if the physician does not see the patient immediately after the onset of the attack. Such pain is usually secondary to a localized area of fat necrosis in the right or left iliac fossa.

The characteristic pain of acute pancreatitis is so severe that the patient may faint. It is little affected by small doses of narcotics. It is knifelike, twisting, or bandlike, but rarely burning. It is often accompanied by flushing and shortness of breath. Most patients have upper abdominal pain, particularly in the right upper quadrant, at the beginning. Later, the pain may be present in the right or left scapular region. Sometimes the patient may have left chest pain mimicking pleurisy or there may be pain in both lower chest regions suggesting a pulmonary or cardiac lesion. The pain most commonly radiates to the back at the level of the lower thoracic vertebrae, as opposed to the pain of a gallbladder attack, which tends to localize at the level of the tips of the scapulae. The pain is typically excruciating, and, if epigastric, is located more frequently on the right side than on the left. Persistence of the pain and resistance to analgesics are very characteristic features of an acute attack of pancreatitis. The patient is obviously overcome by an abdominal catastrophe, searches for a position of comfort, and leans forward in a sitting position or lies on his or her side in a knee–chest position.

MANAGEMENT OF PAIN IN ACUTE PANCREATITIS

The treatment of acute pancreatitis varies depending on whether the disease is edematous, hemorrhagic, necrotic, related to cysts, or manifests itself in some other way. The initial treatment of patients with acute pancreatitis is always nonoperative unless there is a question as to the diagnosis—in other words, a question whether the patient has a perforated ulcer or a gangrenous section of intestine.

The management of shock, the control of vomiting, and reduction of pancreatic secretion are the main early problems related to the treatment of pain. Secondary infections of necrotic material tend to occur late in the course of a severe attack and are not an immediate cause of pain. I normally use continuous morphine in very large doses (10–15 mg/h) to control the pain. Hydromorphone hydrochloride (Dilaudid) (1–3 mg/h) is another suitable drug. Epidural anesthesia with bupivacaine hydrochloride (Marcaine) may be helpful if these drugs are ineffective. We no longer use celiac ganglion blocks during the acute phase of this disease.

The first priority aside from that of managing pain is always the treatment of hypovolemia and shock with sufficient and appropriate colloids so that the patient does not develop further complications such as renal failure secondary to shock. It is also important to differentiate the acute shock due to hypovolemia from that secondary to circulating vasoactive substances. The administration of a large volume of colloids, albumin, or dextran is usually quite effective as a volume expander, but blood transfusions must be given whenever there is a sharp drop in hematocrit. Trasylol is ineffective for the treatment of either the pain or the shock related to hemorrhagic pancreatitis.[3] The pain as well as some of the other complications are said to be be relieved by peritoneal dialysis as well as by the usual supportive measures of transfusions, nasogastric suction, and so forth.

About 90% of those with a clinical diagnosis of acute pancreatitis have the edematous type, which improves rapidly without surgical intervention. These patients can be evaluated later for the presence of gallstones, cholesterol crystals, duodenal ulcer, or alcoholism and treated electively. A careful history should be taken from all patients. Patients found to be alcoholic should be warned to stop drinking and told that continued drinking will cause recurrent attacks and eventually cause a crippling painful type of pancreatic disease. The other major group of nonalcoholic patients should be investigated for evidence of biliary disease and/or duodenal ulcer. Ultrasonography may be diagnositic for gallbladder calculi once the acute ileus has abated, even when gallstones have not been seen in prior examinations. Cholecystograms taken 2 to 3 weeks following an acute attack are largely ineffective because of poor liver function at that time.

Cholecystectomy with removal of common bile duct stones is the treatment of choice for patients with known gallstones. The surgery should be carried out as soon as the acute episode of pancreatitis has subsided in order to prevent the recurrence of acute pancreatitis or cholecystitis with attendant pain.[1] Patients with symptoms and signs of biliary disease in addition to pancreatitis without demonstrable stones or sludge can be evaluated for microcalculi by duodenal drainage, with cholesterol crystals and/or calcium bilirubinate sought in the duodenal aspirate. The decision for cholecystectomy depends on clinical evidence for the presence of biliary calculi or crystals. Cholangiography should accompany primary cholecystectomy to ensure that no further stones will pass and cause further attacks of pancreatitis. Patients in whom x-ray films show no passage of dye into the duodenum should be considered to have persistent stones or sphincter spasm and have a transduodenal sphincteroplasty performed as well.

Patients with a prior history of cholecystectomy for gallstones who now have recurrent acute pancreatitis should be reinvestigated for possible recurrent or residual stones. Endoscopic retrograde cannulation of the bile and pancreatic ducts is the best method for searching for recurrent gallstones, as well as being useful in the detection of pancreatic strictures or cysts. Most recurrent gallstones can be released by endoscopic sphincterotomy during a quiescent period after the acute attack of pancreatitis. I delay the use of this type of endoscopic surgery 2 or more weeks after an acute attack because of a fear of provoking pancreatitis immediately after the attack.

SPHINCTEROPLASTY

Sphincteroplasty at least 25 mm in length is used when endoscopic sphincterotomy is not practical (Fig. 20-3). A longitudinal incision in the duodenum allows complete exploration of the interior for neoplasms or granulomatous lesions that are occasionally the basis for pancreatitis rather than gallstone-related disease. I push the posterior duodenal wall and sphincter mechanism into the open duodenum with a large Bakes dilator. A smaller probe tends to pass through the sphincter so that it is is hard to see on the posterior duodenal wall. Once the papilla is found, a suture is placed on either side of the probe to hold the mucosa and muscular layer taut. Iris or sharp-pointed dura or vascular scissors should cut a 30-degree wedge from the sphincter about 15 degrees to the right and left of the common bile duct for a pathologic specimen. Allis clamps on the sides of the opening will control bleeding until the mucosal edges are oversewn. A children's feeding tube is passed into the pancreatic duct as an identifying marker until the sutures are in place. Pancreatic secretion can be induced with repeated small

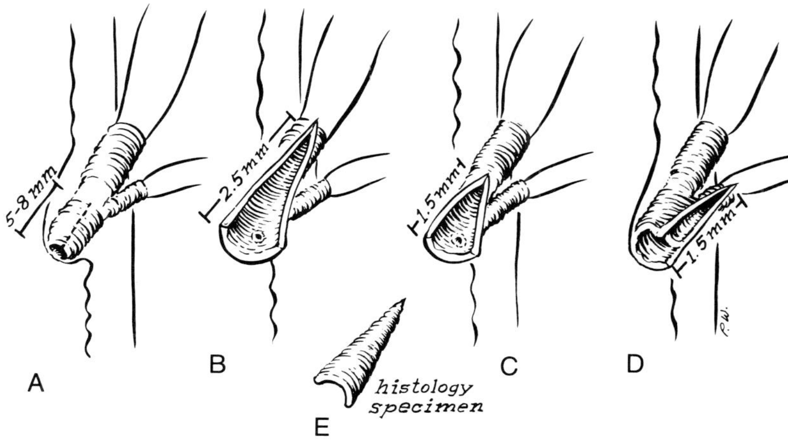

Figure 20-3. (A) The usual papillotomy for removal of a gallstone. (B, C) Sphincteroplasties from 15 to 25 mm in length extending into the distal bile duct. The longer cut (B) will divide all the sphincters. The shorter cut (B) will not. (D) The cut required to divide all the pancreatic duct sphincters. Long incisions will extend into and damage the pancreas. A wedge biopsy (E) can be taken in conjunction with this operation.

doses (10 units at a time) of secretin to demonstrate hard-to-find pancreatic ducts. The duct usually enters the side of the papilla at about a 30-degree angle from the entry of the bile duct. A No. 5 French pediatric feeding tube can then be inserted into the duct when identified and show rapid flow of clear juice.

The strictured orifice of the pancreatic duct that is causing pain and repeated attacks of acute pancreatitis must be identified to prevent continued symptoms.[13] The pancreatic duct must be identified and opened up from within the sphinctero-plasty. The three most common locations of the pancreatic duct opening relative to the common bile duct opening into the duodenum are as follows:

1. The usual position of the opening is within the distal end of the ampulla and just to the patient's left.
2. Next often the position is slightly distal to the papilla and also to the left.
3. The least frequent position is proximal to the papilla and to the left.

Identification also prevents oversewing of the pancreatic duct during a primary sphincteroplasty, which will in turn cause further attacks of acute abdominal pain on the basis of pancreatitis following a primary sphincteroplasty.

CP

This diagnosis is usually made after a pancreatic mass is found on ultrasound or CT scan, calcification of the pancreas, distortion of the pancreatic duct on endoscopic retrograde cholangiopancreatography (ERCP), together with the elimination of all other causes of upper and abdominal and back pain. The diagnosis of pancreatic cysts can be made using ultrasonography alone, or by a CT scan. Specific upper gastrointestinal x-ray techniques such as hypotonic duodenography and percutaneous cholangiography are not useful, as a rule, unless inflammatory mass or cystic structure secondary to CP or cancer compresses the digestive tube. The diagnosis of pancreatic cancer can be made by fine needle biopsy but is often reached at laparotomy after all prior test results have been negative.

PAIN IN CP

Pain is the most important clinical sign in chronic as well as acute pancreatitis although never of the terrible intensity found in the latter. The pain fluctuates greatly but tends to be continuous. The pain is usually least intense before a meal and reaches its peak after eating. Many patients cease eating because of this severe postprandial pain and, as a result, lose a lot of weight.

Patients complain of a variety of types of pain, but it is often the same as in acute pancreatitis, usually located in the upper midabdomen. The pain may appear in both subcostal regions as well, or in the lower anterior thorax. Inhibition of respiration and chest pain are rare unless a pancreatic cyst has ruptured through the diaphragm into the chest.

The principal treatments for CP are

1. Celiac ganglionectomy or alcohol block of the celiac ganglia for unremitting pain in the presence of an unobstructed duct.
2. Resection of part or all of the pancreas.
3. Roux en Y drainage of the opened dilated pancreatic duct for patients with dilatation of the ductal system.

NERVE BLOCKS AND OPERATIONS

The majority of sensory nerves to the pancreas pass through the celiac ganglia and splanchnic nerves, a fact that can be demonstrated by direct injection of anesthetic agents, such as procaine or lidocaine, into the area of these ganglia anterior to the aorta and adjacent to the celiac axis. Mallet-Guy[12] and others observed this phenomenon years ago and have used left or bilateral splanchnicectomy with or without partial ganglionectomy as the treatment of pain of pancreatitis. I believe that operations of this nature do not alter the long-term course of the disease and merely relieve pain for varying periods of time. I do not believe that this operation controls reflex irritation of the pancreas and agree that perineural infiltrate secondary to pancreatitis is a more likely cause of pain.[10]

Dramatic complete relief of pain of pancreatitis or pancreatic cancer can be first obtained with bilateral celiac ganglion test block with an anesthetic agent such as bupivacaine. The technique of blocking the ganglia is simple (Fig. 20-4), accomplished with the patient on his or her right side on a hard surface like an

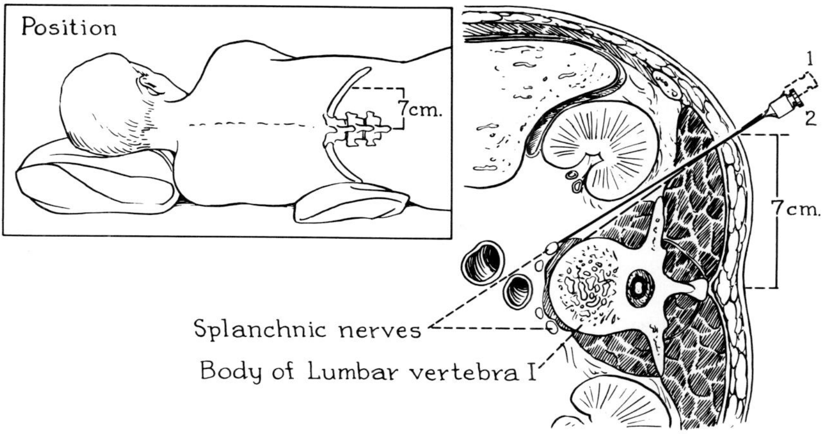

Figure 20-4. The technique for celiac ganglion block with the patient in the lateral position. The first lumbar process is identified. The needle is introduced as in position 1 until it impinges on the spinal column. It is then withdrawn and reinserted as in position 2 for injection of the retroperitoneal tissues, celiac ganglia, and splanchnic nerves. (From White TT. Pancreatitis. Baltimore, Williams & Wilkins, 1966, with permission.)

operating room or x-ray table so that the position of the needles can be checked with an image intensifier. Most of these blocks are performed in the operating room using a C-arm x-ray unit. When a patient with pancreatic cancer is relieved of pain after such a block, a further injection of 50 mL of 50% ethanol at that time or a day later will produce a long-lasting effect. We do not use alcohol blocks in the treatment of pain due to CP, only diagnostic blocks prior to a celiac ganglionectomy. The patient can sit up and talk 15 to 20 minutes after the procedure. The main complications of this procedure are those of temporary postural hypotension and diarrhea. Patients with recurrent pain secondary to cancer can be reblocked at 4- to 6-month intervals.

Continuous epidural anesthesia blocks not only the visceral but also the somatic nerve fibers. With this technique, a catheter placed in the epidural space can be used for injection of small quantities of anesthetic agents or morphine at intervals to produce continuous anesthesia over a long period of time.[6]

Celiac ganglionectomy is used occasionally to relieve pain in young patients with CP of unknown origin with a small, hard pancreas and unobstructed ducts in preference to resection. It is ineffective for the relief of pain in patients with ampullary or common bile duct stones, pancreatic duct calculi, dilated pancreatic ducts, or pancreatic cysts.[11] I have used the procedure in patients with inadequate drainage of the pancreas by pancreaticojejunostomy or in whom resection has been unsuccessful in relieving the pain. Injections of anesthetic agents have been shown to relieve pain but injections of alcohol have not. I do not feel that this alters the course of the disease other than by allowing patients to regain their appetite through reduction of pain.

Technic of Celiac Ganglionectomy

Celiac ganglionectomy can be performed through either a 12th rib or an abdominal approach.

The 12th-rib-bed approach (Fig. 20-5) is essentially the same as one often used for left adrenalectomy. Most of these operations are carried out on the left side because it is easier to perform on this side. The peritoneum is reflected forward until the left crus of the diaphragm is identified. The left kidney and adrenal lie immediately on top of the ganglion. The splanchnic nerves can be seen emerging from behind the crura. The two semilunar ganglia and splanchnic nerves lie medial to the adrenal on the superior surface of the renal vessels and adjacent to the celiac artery between the crura of the diaphragm. The nerves can be dissected out with a nerve hook and divided between clips that will control bleeding. Partial removal of the ganglia and a segment of splanchnic nerves on each side will be sufficient to relieve pain. A drop in blood pressure will indicate that the nerves have indeed been ablated. It is important to be sure that a ganglion and not scar or lymph glands has been removed before concluding the operation. On the right side, the operation is a little more difficult because one must retract the inferior vena cava for exposure.

Retropancreatic resection is the simpler of the two transabdominal operations available when a laparotomy is needed for diagnostic purposes. The pancreas is dissected off the posterior abdominal wall by an extended Kocher maneu-

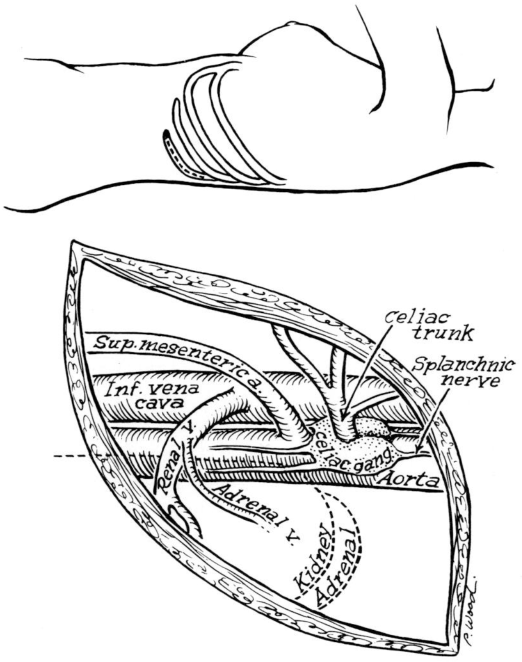

Figure 20-5. The celiac ganglion and splanchnic nerves are approached on the left side through a 12th-rib approach medial to the adrenal and adjacent to the superior mesenteric and celiac arteries and below the crura of the diaphragm. (From White TT, Harrison RC. Reoperative Gastrointestinal Surgery. Boston, Little Brown, 1979, with permission.)

ver, which mobilizes the duodenum, pancreas, and portal triad forward from the inferior vena cava and aorta (Fig. 1C).[20] The renal vessels, the superior mesenteric artery, and the celiac axis can then be identified. The right celiac ganglion is located in the 2- to 3-cm space between the two vessels and dissected as above. The dissection can be carried out to the left of the aorta if desired, but this is usually not necessary.

The celiac axis can be reached only with some difficulty through the gastrohepatic ligament because the ganglia are located just above and behind the pancreas. Here the gastrohepatic ligament is divided first, the stomach is retracted caudad, and the celiac axis is located at the upper border of the pancreas and then followed down posteriorly to the aorta. This approach is difficult because of the inflammatory adhesions usually present under these circumstances.

PANCREATICOJEJUNOSTOMY

This operation is useful only for patients with chronically dilated ducts 8 mm in diameter or greater throughout their length with or without cyst formation. It is not useful for patients with smaller ducts or when all cysts cannot be drained. The remaining cysts will continue to be painful. The five main techniques for anastomosis of the pancreas to the jejunum in the past 40 years have been[8,9,11,16]

1. Lateral–lateral anastomosis over a T-tube
2. Terminal–lateral anastomosis without a T-tube
3. Terminal–terminal anastomosis
4. Invagination of pancreas into the jejunum
5. Long lateral–lateral anastomosis

The first three operations have been largely ineffective in the management of pain from CP (Fig. 20-6). The latter two have relieved pain in about 75% of instances. Invagination of the widely opened pancreas after splenectomy into a Roux en Y loop has largely been abandoned in favor of side-to-side anastomosis without splenectomy because of the relative simplicity of the latter operation (Fig. 20-7). This approach is also a useful method of the treating failures from all the operations with a small anastomosis because the entire ductal system can be opened away from the original opening so that free drainage is attained.

The primary side-to-side anastomosis without splenectomy is constructed after opening the pancreatic duct longitudinally from just to the right of the tip of the tail to 2 cm from the duodenum either using a guarded Dura scissors or by means of electrocautery over a grooved director. This simple cut will cause the upper and lower edges of a small hard pancreas to spring open, leaving a wide aperture on the surface of the pancreas. On the other hand, where a large duct lies within an enormously proliferative pancreas, a strip of anterior pancreas as wide as 15 mm must be removed to form a wide enough opening for drainage into the jejunum.

A Roux en Y loop 40 to 50 cm long is then fashioned by division of the jejunum approximately 5 cm below the ligament of Treitz if it has not already been

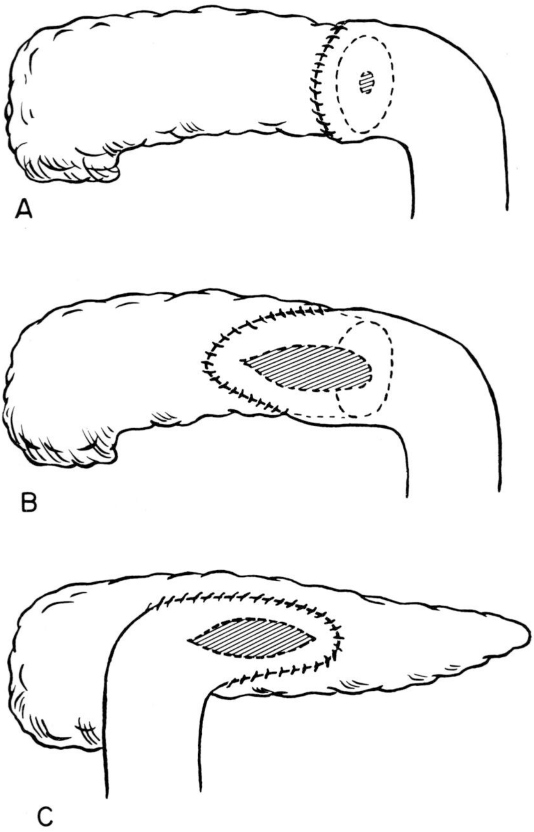

Figure 20-6. The three unsatisfactory methods of pancreaticojejunostomy: (A) end-to-end, (B) end-to-end with fish-mouth extension, (C) small end-to-side anastomosis. (From White TT, Harrison RC. Reoperative Gastrointestinal Surgery. Boston, Little Brown, 1979, with permission.)

created. We feel that unusually short loops created at the first operation should be lengthened. We use the gastrointestinal anastomosis (GIA) stapling clamp (manufactured by the Auto-Suture Co., a division of the United States Surgical Corp., 205 W. Main St., Stamford, CN 06902) for this purpose. The end of the loop is then inverted over the staples, and the other end is dropped back into the abdo-

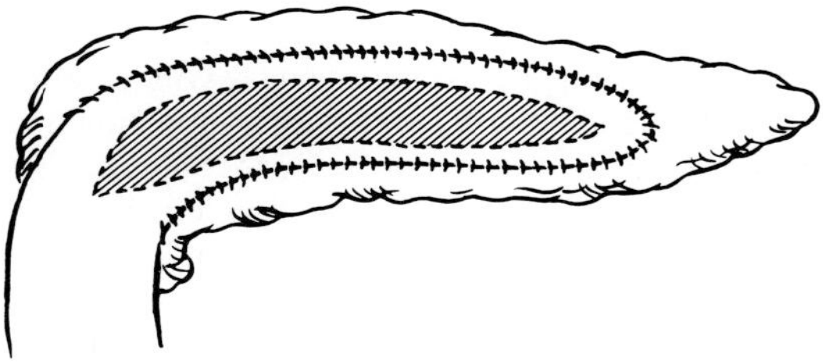

Figure 20-7. The type of anastomosis most commonly in use today. (From White TT, Harrison RC: Reoperative Gastrointestinal Surgery. Boston, Little Brown, 1979, with permission.)

men until it is time to construct the jejunojejunostomy. The loop is then passed through the mesocolon to the pancreas. The lower antimesenteric surface of the loop is sewn to the lower portion of the pancreas with interrupted No. 0 silk sutures on a heavy Mayo or even a cutting needle. After this line of tacking of sutures is complete, the jejunum is opened for about 8 cm adjacent to the suture line. A longer incision results in too large a jejunal opening because the jejunum tends to relax after the initial spasm that is related to the making of the incision has passed. The lower lip of the opened jejunum is then sewn to the lower edge of the opened pancreas with a continuous No. 0 chromic catgut or PDS locking sutures. A heavy needle is again used. The upper row of the anastomosis is placed in much the same fashion as the lower one was placed.

Left pancreatectomy to the aorta is mainly used for removal of a cyst in a localized area of painful CP. It may also be used as a first step in making a pancreaticojejunostomy when there is a large cyst of the tail and residual chronic disease to the right. Here, the spleen is mobilized from the posterior abdominal wall by division of the lienorenal ligaments and the attachments between the spleen, diaphragm, and posterior abdominal wall. The gastrosplenic ligament is divided between ligatures. The peritoneum above and below the pancreas is cut so that the pancreas can be gradually mobilized. The spleen and tail of the pancreas are dissected free from the stomach and diaphragm and then pulled forward away from the posterior abdominal wall. An attempt is then made to identify the splenic artery and vein, which are ligated with 2-0 silk, the artery first, then the vein. The pancreas is then sharply divided front to back, and bleeders are cauterized or oversewn with 3-0 silk. After hemorrhage is controlled, a descending pancreatogram may be taken to ensure that all obstructions to the pancreatic duct have been removed. I do not attempt to suture the capsule together in these circumstances because the pancreas is usually too hard. This operation has been effective in relieving pain in both alcoholic and nonalcoholic patients. Failure to relieve pain following this type of operation has been chiefly due to the presence of multiple strictures to the right of the point of resection, continuing chronic alcoholism, unsuspected cancer of the pancreas, and cysts in the head of the pancreas. Operative trauma has been a less important factor.

The extension of left-to-right pancreatectomy to the right of the portal vein and almost to the duodenum, and total pancreatectomy, have been used extensively in the past in an effort to relieve the painful symptoms of CP.[7] These operations are little used today both because of severe secondary problems with diabetes and malabsorption and because the pain was not eradicated.

Pancreaticoduodenectomy for the relief of pain from CP when the bulk of the lesion was localized to the right of the great vessels has been second only in success to that of pancreaticojejunostomy, but, again, much more successful in the treatment of nonalcoholic than alcoholic patients.[14] The complications of diabetes are much less severe after this operation than after the major 80% to 95% resections used in the recent past.

I am impressed at how often my patients with CP later turn out to have cancer of the pancreas. This failure to diagnose a tumor is a major cause for continued pain after operations for pancreatitis. Patients with stage 3 or 4 carcinoma of the pancreas are best treated by decompression of the biliary tree and/or stomach without resection. We have found that intraoperative injection of celiac ganglia with 50 to 60 mL of 50% alcohol has been a very effective means of relieving pain in these patients. The ganglia can be injected percutaneously with alcohol as described above if operative injection fails.[18]

REFERENCES

1. Acosta JM, Rossi R, Galli OR, et al. Early surgery for acute gallstone pancreatitis. Evaluation of a systematic approach. Surgery 83:367–370, 1978.
2. Allan BJ, Tournut R, White TT. Intraductal activation of pancreatic zymogens behind a carcinoma of the pancreas. Gastroenterology 65:412–418, 1973.
3. Banks PA. Acute pancreatitis. Gastroenterology 681:382–397, 1971.
4. Banks PA. Pancreatitis. New York, Plenum Publishing, 1979.
5. Bliss WR, Burch B, Martin MM, Zollinger RM. Localization of reflex pancreatic pain induced by electrical stimulation. Gastroenterology 16:317–323, 1950.
6. Dupen SL, Peterson DG, Bogosian AC, et al. A new permanent exteriorized epidural catheter for narcotic self-administration to control cancer pain. Cancer 59:986–993, 1987.
7. Frey CF, Child GC, Fry WJ. Pancreatectomy for chronic pancreatitis. Ann Surg 184:403–413, 1977.
8. Hart MJ, Miyashita H, Morita N, White TT. Pancreaticojejunostomy. Report of a 25 year experience. Am J Surg 145:567–570, 1983.
9. Jordan GL, Sirug BS, Crowder WE. Current status of pancreaticojejunostomy in the treatment of chronic pancreatitis. Am J Surg 122:46, 1971.
10. Keith RG, Keshavjee SH, Kerenyi NR. Neuropathology of chronic pancreatitis in humans. Can J Surg 28:207–211, 1985.
11. Leger L, Lenriot JP. Five to twenty year follow-up after surgery for chronic pancreatitis in 148 patients. Ann Surg 180:185–191, 1974.
12. Mallet-Guy PA. Late and very late results of resections of the nervous system in the treatment of chronic relapsing pancreatitis. Am J Surg 145:234–238, 1983.
13. Moody, FG, et al. Transampullary septectomy for postcholecystectomy pain. Ann Surg 186:415–423, 1977.
14. Moreaux J, Warshaw AL, Ranson JHC. Long-term follow-up studies of 50 patients with pancreaticoduodenectomy for chronic pancreatitis. World J Surg 8:346–353, 1984.
15. Nakamura K, Sarles H, Payan. Three dimensional reconstruction of the pancreatic ducts in chronic pancreatitis. Gastroenterology 62:942–949, 1972.
16. Potts JR, Moody FG. Surgical treatment for chronic pancreatitis: Selecting the appropriate approach. Am J Surg 142:654–659, 1981.
17. Ray BS, Neill CL. Abdominal visceral sensation in man. Ann Surg 126:709–724, 1947.
18. Sarr MG, Cameron JL. Surgical palliation of unresectable carcinoma of the pancreas. World J Surg 8:906–918, 1984.
19. White TT, Allan BJ. Intrapancreatic activation of proteases in the etiology of pancreatitis or cancer of the pancreas. Med Clin North Am 58:305–310, 1974.
20. White TT, Lawinski M, Stacher G, et al. Treatment of pancreatitis by left splanchnicectomy and celiac ganglionectomy. Am J Surg 112:195–199, 1966.

CHAPTER

21

BIOPSY OF PANCREATIC MASSES

A. R. Moossa

EDITORIAL COMMENT

Percutaneous fine needle aspiration has been a significant advance in diagnosing pancreatic malignancy, with an accuracy of close to 90%. It requires the presence of a skilled and experienced cytopathologist. In the operating room, fine needle aspiration of masses in the head of the pancreas is much safer than open biopsy or Tru-cut needles. Open biopsy, either wedge or shave, is not technically difficult when the mass is in the body, in the tail, or extrapancreatic.

Dr. Moossa is opposed to percutaneous aspiration biopsy for small potentially resectable lesions because of sampling errors and the theoretical possibility of seeding along the needle tract. We do not hesitate to perform fine needle biopsy in such patients, believing that a positive cytologic examination preoperatively is of considerable value, a negative result means nothing, and the risk of seeding is minute. We also use preoperative needle aspiration in jaundiced patients even when surgery is contemplated for palliation, to confirm the diagnosis and to reduce the operative time. As pointed out by Dr. Moossa, a small group of patients remain with a resectable lesion in the head of the pancreas; in such patients all attempts at biopsy do not show malignant cells. Here the experienced surgeon will have to make a deliberate decision to proceed with a major resection on clinical evidence alone, and in a few patients a major resection will be done for "benign" disease. This possibility should be discussed with the patient before operation.

CONTROVERSY

For years surgeons were apprehensive about cutting into a suspicious pancreatic mass, especially in the head of the pancreas, for a tissue diagnosis. Fear of fistula, infection, and bleeding led to patients being treated for carcinoma without an initial positive histologic diagnosis. The interpretation of biopsy material by the pathologist often results in equivocal reporting because of sampling errors and the presence of association pancreatitis. The introduction of fine needle biopsy or aspiration cytology has helped to avoid some of the problems of open biopsy but raises other questions regarding timing, interpretation, and possible tumor seeding. These issues are addressed in the present chapter.

The late Lord Cohen of Birkenhead once remarked that the feasibility of an operation is not an indication for its performance. We can safely borrow from this aphorism and state that the availability of a technique or procedure is not an indication for ordering it. The plethora of published papers on pancreatic biopsy is often a source of confusion and misinterpretation to many physicians. As a result, perceived errors in patient management, often with ensuing medicolegal problems, have been a poor advertisement for our understanding of the place of pancreatic biopsy in our diagnostic armamentarium. The aim of this chapter is to rationalize the continued use of various techniques of pancreatic biopsy in a *sensible* and *selective* way so as to provide maximum benefit with minimum risks to each individual patient.

Any review is bound to show some strong bias unless assessments are rendered as objective as possible. Thus, previous reports on pancreatic biopsy have emphasized sensitivity, specificity, predictive values, and so forth, without paying attention to the extent or stage of disease and to the prevalence of the disease in the population biopsied. Sensitivity and specificity are what the individual investigators like to report. The term *sensitivity* indicates the percentage of positive results obtained when a test is applied to patients known to have the disease under investigation. Thus, if the population studied consists of patients who have far advanced disease, the sensitivity is likely to be close to 100%. Specificity indicates the percentage of negative results obtained when the test is applied to subjects who are free of the disease. Predictive values are what the clinician needs to know for decision making and indicates the degree of reliance that can be placed on a positive or a negative result. Thus, the predictive value of a positive test answers the following question: If a positive result is reported, how often is the test correct? The predictive value of a negative test answers the opposite question: If the result of the test is negative, how often does this exclude the disease under investigation?

The rationale of pancreatic biopsy is based on the following assumptions.

1. An accurate tissue diagnosis is essential for the rational treatment of malignant disease in the gland.

2. The sensitivity, specificity, and predictive values of the biopsy are very high while the complication rate is very low.

The term *biopsy* has a finite meaning. According to Dorland's medical dictionary, it is defined as the removal and examination, usually microscopic, of tissue from the living body, performed to establish a precise diagnosis.[8] The term is often used to include cytologic biopsy, which is a procedure in which cells are obtained by various methods (usually needle aspiration) for cytologic (as opposed to histologic) examination.[19] Biopsy techniques are to two types, described in the following sections.

CLOSED OR NEEDLE BIOPSY OF THE PANCREAS

This may be performed percutaneously under ultrasonography or CT scan guidance or under direct vision intraoperatively. If a fine needle is used, the material obtained is suitable for cytologic examination. If a large needle (i.e., Tru-cut) is employed to cut out a cylindrical core of tissue, enough material can be obtained for histologic examination. There are four potential problems with needle biopsy of the pancreas: (1) Only a limited number of needle passes can be made into any lesion without causing excessive trauma or hemorrhage. (2) Sampling error is clearly the greatest disadvantage. Cancer and associated pancreatitis invariably coexist. Thus, a negative report for malignant disease does not exclude cancer. (3) There is a danger of implanting cancer cells along the needle tract. This often goes unnoticed or unreported. Hence estimates of incidence are unusually low. (4) Traumatic pancreatitis and its attending sequelae such as pseudocyst, abscess, or fistula formation. Again, for reasons mentioned later, there is probably gross underestimation of such complications in the literature.

OPEN BIOPSY OF THE PANCREAS

This can only be done through a formal laparotomy. The open biopsy can be of an *incisional* or of an *excisional* type.

Incisional Biopsy:

An open biopsy is of an incisional nature when a portion of the lesion is directly removed for pathologic examination. It is ideally performed in situations in which if the tumor cells are spilled at the time of the biopsy, the incisional wound can be encompassed and totally excised at the time of the curative surgical procedure. Thus, incisional biopsy should, in general, have much less sampling error than needle biopsy. However, the risk that the surgeon may seed cancer cells into the operative wound or that adjacent lymphatics can be opened to transport cancer cells to distant sites is more real. The type of incisional biopsy that is performed in pancreatic masses is usually termed a *wedge* biopsy. It implies removal of a triangular segment of pancreas by incising into the gland with a scalpel. This specimen is usually taken from areas believed to contain a malignant tumor, but it often includes adjacent normal or inflamed pancreas. Transection of pancreatic ducts is a major hazard, and risks of serious complications such as hemorrhage, fistula, pancreatitis, and abscess are more likely. Thus, the term *wedge* biopsy is a dangerous one, since it implies that the surgeon has to cut deep into relatively normal pancreatic tissue. McIlrath has rightly recommended that the term *shave* biopsy be used instead.[16] Clearly if a neoplastic lump is sticking out of the pancreatic surface, a piece of the tissue can be "shaved off" for histologic examination. The scalpel can be safely used for this specific situation. It is usually applicable to patients with masses in the body and tail of the pancreas where part of the neoplastic mass often protrudes through the anterior surface of the gland and a thin slice of the tumor can be easily and safely taken. *This incision must be limited to abnormal tissue so that injury to adjacent normal pancreas is avoided.* Such a shave incisional biopsy is rarely, if ever, indicated for lesion around the head of the pancreas because periampullary tumors are usually deeply located in the gland and are only truly accessible by needle punctures.

Excisional Biopsy:

Excisional biopsy implies total removal of the local lesion, usually with a margin of surrounding normal tissue. It may be used as definitive treatment for a malignant lesion, that is, segmental mastectomy in selected cases of breast cancer. Unfortunately, an excisional biopsy for a lesion in the head of the pancreas usually implies at least a pancreaticoduodenectomy. Similarly, an excisional biopsy of a lesion in the body and tail of the pancreas entails at least a distal pancreatectomy and splenectomy. The mortality and morbidity from such an excision can be prohibitive, and it should not be entertained lightly.

OPERATIVE BIOPSY OF THE PANCREAS

Surgeons have been biopsying the pancreas at laparotomy for over 4 decades and, in the past, have made major strategic and interpretative errors when handling pancreatic mass lesions. As a result, they have a responsibility to educate the interventional radiologists and the internist-endoscopists who are new to the field in order to avoid repetition of previous errors and pitfalls. Surgical options in the treatment of a lesion in the head of the pancreas is totally different from that of a lesion in the body and tail of the gland. Until 1950 serious complications followed attempts at wedge biopsies of mass lesions in the head of the pancreas. This led Kirtland in 1951 to recommend the use of the Vim-Silverman needle as a safe method of pancreatic biopsy.[13] This procedure was modified by other surgeons into one using the Tru-cut disposable needle as a method of removing a cylindrical core of tissue from a suspicious area in the head or uncinate process of the pancreas for microscopic examination. The technique of performing such a biopsy is important, and an adequate Kocher maneuver should be performed and the surgeon's left hand be placed behind the mass with the palm upward and with the thumb anterior. Palpation with the thumb and index finger permits accurate assessment of the mass in question and provides appreciation of the tumor margin. The needle is inserted through the wall of the duodenum and into the mass held by the left hand. It is essential to limit the depth to which the needle is inserted in the appropriate area of the head of pancreas, care being taken not to penetrate the major vessels. Two or three cores of tissue can be removed to ensure that specimens representative of the mass lesion are sent to the pathologist. The specimens should be examined immediately after preparation by frozen section techniques. Hemorrhage, when encountered, is best controlled by finger pressure. If direct pancreatic puncture, as opposed to transduodenal puncture, is deemed necessary, figure-eight silk sutures are occasionally needed for hemostasis and are preferable to clamping and tying at the puncture site. Absorbable sutures should never be used in this location since they will be rapidly digested in the presence of trypsin spilled from the gland. The surgeon must never biopsy any part of the pancreas "behind" an obstructed duct since this guarantees the formation of a pancreatic leak with potential for pseudocyst, abscess, and fistula formation.

What Are The Results?

Cote et al., reporting the experience with pancreatic biopsy in 83 patients at the Mayo Clinic between 1949 and 1954, and a 60% accuracy rate with a low incidence of complications.[6] Their conclusion was that they would hesitate to subject a patient who has a mass in the head of the pancreas to the risk of a Whipple type of operation unless a positive diagnosis of malignancy was obtained. In 1957, another series of 68 consecutive patients with "peri-ampullary masses" was analyzed; the analysis revealed that the frozen-section diagnosis was correct in greater than 90% of patients and there were only three complications.[23] Shultz and Sanders reported in 1963 a group of 159 patients treated by a number of different surgeons. They found a much higher complication rate of 9.5%; six of these complications were considered fatal. The accuracy rate was only 65%.[22] The University of California, San Francisco UCSF group evaluated a series of 171 patients who underwent intraoperative pancreatic biopsy between 1952 and 1970 using the needle or wedge biopsy techniques.[14] They reported an 86% accuracy rate with no false positives for cancer. They felt that in general a wedge biopsy was safer and more accurate than a needle biopsy, but it is clear that the most advanced tumors were the ones that were most amenable to a wedge biopsy. They reported a morbidity of 3% with wedge biopsy, 14% with direct needle biopsy, and 10% with transduodenal needle biopsy. There was a 9% mortality associated with direct needle biopsy and 5% with transduodenal biopsy.

A larger experience from the Mayo Clinic was published in 1974; the authors analyzed the results of operative pancreatic biopsy in 527 patients.[12] They reported complications in 14 patients, and 3 of these were deemed fatal. Malignant neoplasm was strongly suspected in 16 patients based on gross operative findings but could not be confirmed microscopically by biopsy. Later follow-up studies showed that 8 of these 16 patients did in fact have malignant disease of the pancreas. Pancreatic biopsy was the sole procedure in 112 of these 527 patients. Seven complications occurred in these 112 patients and included 4 wound infections, 2 cases of pancreatitis, and 1 subphrenic abscess due to pancreatitis. No mortality was attributable to pancreatic biopsy alone. The overall morbidity for both needle and wedge biopsies was 6.2%, and if wound infection was deemed incidental to the laparotomy itself, the morbidity can be considered to be lower.

Weiss et al. reviewed the experience at Thomas Jefferson University Hospital in 1982 and attempted to separate those complications directly attributable to biopsy from complications emanating from other causes.[25] They attributed intraabdominal hemorrhage, pancreatitis, pancreatic fistulas, pseudocysts, and pancreatic abscesses to be specifically induced by the pancreatic biopsy. They published their data on patients with cancer separately from those or patients without cancer. They concluded that when the pancreatic masses were inflammatory in origin, there was a much higher incidence of postoperative pancreatitis, fistula, or peripancreatic fluid collection. Of 22 patients without histologic evidence of cancer after operative biopsy, followed for a minimum of 1 year, two developed evidence of cancer after the negative laparotomy with biopsy. Thus, there was a false-negative biopsy rate of at least 10% in this small series. Three years later the same authors[26] reviewing 32 patients with pancreatic cancer who underwent laparotomy and biopsy followed by a second laparotomy demonstrated that patients who underwent two or more operative biopsy procedures were at markedly increased risk of developing intraabdominal tumor seeding that was not detectable by preoperative computed, tomography (CT) or ultrasonography. They concluded that multiple biopsy procedures should be avoided and that surgeons not prepared to provide definitive care for pancreatic patients should refrain from exploring these patients to avoid extensive tumor manipulation and biopsies.

Reuben and Cotton surveyed in 1978 the practice of British surgeons with respect to operative pancreatic biopsy and noted that the majority of surgeons who find a lesion judged to be nonresectable at laparotomy proceeded to bypass or closure without biopsy.[21] Only half of them took material for later histologic examination and then from lymph nodes or metastasis when possible rather than by direct pancreatic biopsy. Factors that were considered to influence the biopsy policy of the surgeons included personal experience of complications, histologic errors, and traditional teaching.

It should be emphasized that all these reports of pancreatic biopsy date to the time when the quoted mortality and morbidity from pancreaticoduodenal resections was still very high. Many senior surgeons still regard pancreatic biopsy as inaccurate and dangerous. However, it is often difficult to decide whether the complications of pancreatic biopsies are directly attributable to the biopsy itself or to the concomitant surgical maneuvers and manipulations. In the United States, there is a general impression of an increasing trend toward more frequent pancreatic biopsies. With the more widespread availability of, and increasing corporation with, skilled cytopathologists, fine needle aspiration cytodiagnosis is quite rightly gaining in popularity both preoperatively and intraoperatively.

PREOPERATIVE PANCREATIC BIOPSY

Noninvasive imaging modalities, namely, CT and ultrasonography, are major advances that may delineate structural abnormalities in the gland. Changes in size, contour, and echo pattern of the gland or the presence of a pancreatic mass may be indicative of malignant disease in the gland. Invasive techniques such as endoscopic retrograde cholangiopancreatography (ERCP) and angiography will delineate ductal stenosis, occlusion, or dilatation, and encasement or occlusion of intrapancreatic and peripancreatic vessels. In addition, angiography may provide information about unresectability of a pancreatic mass when there is encasement or occlusion of major arterial or venous structures. Unfortunately, chronic pancreatitis (CP) often produces many of these structural abnormalities mentioned. Hence, the dilemma of diagnosis of pancreatic cancer versus CP remains unresolved. The problem is further complicated by the fact that virtually all pancreatic cancers are associated with varying degrees of histologic pancreatitis that is probably induced by ductal obstruction and glandular destruction. Thus, the definitive preoperative diagnosis of pancreatic cancer depends on cytologic studies of pancreatic or duodenal juice or fine needle aspiration of the pancreas obtained endoscopically or percutaneously. The success of all cytologic diagnoses rests on two factors:

1. The ability to collect representative material from the appropriate part of the pancreas
2. The expertise and experience of the involved cytopathologist

The sensitivity for pancreatic cancer by pancreatic or duodenal juice analysis is, at best, about 66%.[18] However, if the cancer is located in the head of the gland, the detection rate increases to around 79%. While a false-positive cytologic report is rare, a negative cytologic report does not exclude pancreatic cancer.

Fine needle aspiration of a pancreatic mass can be performed through the endoscope either transduodenally or transgastrically. In one retrospective analysis of 51 patients with pancreatic and periampullary lesions, fine needle aspiration of the pancreas was performed using a specially designed hydraulic needle biopsy system.[24] In this series 25 patients had periampullary or pancreatic carcinoma and 26 had CP or other benign conditions. Transduodenal biopsy alone was performed in 30 cases and together with transgastric biopsy was perfumed in an additional 4 cases; transgastric biopsy alone was performed in 17 cases. The yield for transduodenal biopsy was 70% of the patients with malignancy, while transgastric biopsy was positive in 21%, for an overall sensitivity of 84% (21 of 25). There was no false-positive result. No mention was made of the size and type of tumor or of resectability. One can only assume that most, if not all, of these patients had extensive pancreatic cancer.

The major complications of ERCP with or without pancreatic biopsy should not be underestimated and may occasionally be fatal. Injection pancreatitis, pancreatic sepsis, and cholangitic sepsis should be dreaded. Such complications can be largely avoided by meticulous disinfection of the endoscope and cannula, using prophylactic antibiotics starting before the endoscopic procedure, and continuing for 48 hours afterward. Other rarer complications such as instrumental injury, hemorrhage, aspiration pneumonia, paralytic ileus, cardiac arrythmias, drug reactions, and oversedation should also be remembered.

PERCUTANEOUS FINE NEEDLE ASPIRATION OF PANCREATIC MASSES

The landmark contribution to fine needle aspiration of the pancreas for cytologic examination was only published in 1970 when Christofferson and Poll reported their experience with the technique applied during 91 autopsies and 28 abdominal operations.[5] They were able to diagnose 66 out of 68 documented cancers. Two years later Holm et al. introduced ultrasonic-guided fine needle aspiration of abdominal masses.[10] Over the ensuing decade the rapid development of diagnostic imaging modalities, especially ultrasonography and CT, added a new dimension to fine needle aspiration cytology. Using either of these modalities for localization of pancreatic masses, a fine (21–23 gauge) thin wall needle (1/14 the diameter of the Vim-Silverman needle) is passed into the mass using the appropriate imaging technique for guidance, and suction is applied with a syringe. Frequently, the specimen obtained is so minute as to be invisible in the hub of the needle. However, by removing the needle, filling the syringe with air, and replacing the needle, the specimen can be expressed on a microscopic slide, smeared, fixed in 95% alcohol, and stained by the Papanicolaou or other method. If an experienced cytopathologist is available, a diagnosis can generally be rendered within 20 minutes of obtaining the biopsy.[1]

Since adenocarcinoma of the exocrine pancreas (commonly referred to as pancreatic cancer) is by far the commonest type of malignant disease of the gland, the diagnosis is not difficult when obvious signs of malignancy are present—single or irregularly arranged clusters of cells exhibiting cellular pleomorphism, large vesicular nuclei, and prominent nucleoli. However, such cytologic examination may sometimes fail to differentiate between an adenocarcinoma of the gland, a lymphoma, or even an islet cell cancer. In addition, a negative cytologic examination does not exclude cancer because of sampling error.

Proponents of routine percutaneous biopsy of all pancreatic masses emphasize the possibility of making a diagnosis preoperatively to help the surgeon in the planning of an operative strategy and to obviate the need for time-consuming diagnostic maneuvers on the operative table. In selected patients it can also eliminate the need to perform a purely diagnostic laparotomy. A positive diagnosis can be obtained in some 87% to 100% of cases, with few false-positive results reported. The sampling problem, however, persists, and false-negative results occur with relatively small tumors but are rarely, if ever, reported. It is clear that the number of complications increases with the number of needle passes, and complications include pancreatitis, pseudocysts, and pancreatic fistula. This author has seen three deaths directly resulting from complications of percutaneous needle biopsy, and in two instances the pancreatic tumors were missed by the needle, giving an associated false-negative cytologic result. While the absence of recorded cases in which puncture of the stomach or colon has resulted in an adverse outcome is often quoted, this author has seen several abscesses and fistulas resulting from colon perforation and pleads guilty for never having bothered to report such complications. Seeding of the needle tract is also a definite possibility. It has only rarely been reported, but it is clearly related also to the number of needle passes and to the stage of the cancer.

In this author's opinion, percutaneous aspiration biopsy of the pancreas is useful for masses in the body and tail of the gland since cancers in this location are usually unresectable, especially if there is angiographic or CT scan evidence of unresectability. It is especially valuable in the frail, elderly patient in whom one wishes to avoid a purely diagnostic laparotomy when surgical palliation is not indicated or warranted. The technique, however, should not be applied to small potentially resectable cancers because of sampling error and the theoretical possibility of seeding along the needle tract. It should not be applied to patients with jaundice and/or duodenal obstruction when surgical palliation is contemplated. Finally, it should not be performed on the relatively fit young patient in whom a histologic (as opposed to cytologic) diagnosis is essential prior to the administration of aggressive radiation therapy or chemotherapy. It is not totally unusual for a surgeon to explore a patient with a suspected cancer of the body and tail of the pancreas to find that the patient has an islet cell tumor or a lymphoma, both of which carry a much better prognosis than adenocarcinoma of the exocrine pancreas.

PERSPECTIVE ON THE VALUE OF PANCREATIC BIOPSY

The sampling and intrepretative errors of pancreatic biopsy as well as its potentially lethal complications continue to be offered as a strong argument against the procedure. Historically, as early as 1953, Cattell and Warren regarded pancreatic biopsy as being both dangerous and inaccurate.[4] Bowden in 1954 regarded pancreatic biopsy as noninformative and frankly erroneous.[2] As late as 1980 Maingot emphasized the potential hazards.[15] The presence of a neoplasm often induces acinar rupture with periacinar inflammation and fibrosis as well as distortion of ductal distribution. Such inflammatory changes are present to a variable degree with any malignant lesion, leading to a coexistence of histologic pancreatitis and pancreatic cancer. Atypical epithelial hyperplasia occurring in CP can sometimes be mistaken for cancer on frozen-section histologic analysis. False-negative results have been reported to range from 12% to as high as 54%. Moossa and Dawson reviewed the University of Chicago experience over a 5-year period and showed an overall accuracy of frozen section of 92.5% with 4 false negatives (all due to sampling error) and 1 false positive (due to misinterpretation of the frozen-section findings).[20] The University of California, Davis, group recently reported a sampling error of 15% and a interpretative error of 15% leading to failure to diagnose a pancreatic caner in as many as 30% of patients.[3] Hyland et al. developed criteria to prevent interpretative errors and classified the histologic findings into three major and five minor morphologic criteria based on the frequency of occurrence and reproducibility.[11] Major criteria are nuclear size variation of 4 to 1 or greater between ductal epithelial cells; incomplete ductal lumens; and disorganized duct distribution. Minor criteria include those features that are more difficult to assess and occur with variable frequency in carcinomas: huge, irregular epithelial nucleoli; necrotic glandular debris; glandular mitoses; glands unaccompanied by connective tissue stroma within smooth muscle fascicles (periampullary biopsies); and perineural invasion. Combined application of both major and minor criteria in frozen-section diagnosis is recommended for maximum accuracy, especially in cases complicated by CP.

There are three further instances in which pancreatic biopsies may be unreliable. The histologic differentiation between the benign cystic tumor (cystadenoma) and the malignant one (cystadenocarcinoma), or between a benign and malignant islet cell tumor, may be difficult unless the presence of distant metastases (in the liver or lymph nodes) is documented. Nesidioblastosis, the commonest lesion responsible for hyperinsulinism in infants below the age of 1 year, requires special histochemical techniques for its documentation. Hence, frozen-section biopsies are noncontributory in these instances.

RECOMMENDATIONS

Pancreatic biopsy should not be performed in a ‘‘knee jerk’’ fashion without any planning whenever a pancreatic abnormality is encountered during an imaging technique or at laparotomy. Before proceeding with a pancreatic biopsy the physician must plan how to proceed if the biopsy shows cancer and how to proceed if the biopsy does not. A reasonable general policy is as follows:

1. In patients with a potentially resectable lesion in the head of the pancreas, it is reasonable to attempt to obtain a positive cytologic diagnosis by ERCP or duodenal drainage studies. Routine endoscopic or percutaneous fine needle biopsy is to be deplored in this setting. Obtaining a preoperative tissue diagnosis is desirable but should not be an obsession in itself. Under favorable circumstances, such lesions should be resected irrespective of the biopsy result provided that an informed consent has been obtained.

2. Unresectable lesions in the body and the tail of the pancreas can be biopsied using either the percutaneous or the endoscopic needle technique, especially if the patient is frail and elderly, to spare the patient a purely diagnostic laparotomy. Such patients do not usually need surgical palliation. However, one must never hesitate to operate on the relatively fit, young patient to obtain proper histologic diagnosis and staging since occasionally both the surgeon and the patient will have the pleasant surprise to find a more favorable lesion.

3. If a nonresectable or metastatic tumor is found at laparotomy it must be biopsied until a definite diagnosis is made on frozen-section histologic examination, no matter how tedious and time-consuming the job may be. Biopsy of liver deposits or peritoneal seedings must always be done for metastatic lesions. The exact cellular origin of a tumor must always be identified. This not only obviates the need for a purely diagnostic second look laparotomy if the patient survives longer than expected but also may occasionally reveal that the tumor is of a more benign nature.

4. Operative pancreatic biopsy is not an absolutely benign procedure and must be performed with reasonable safety considering the total magnitude of the problem. Obsession with multiple biopsies of a potentially resectable lesion is often traumatic and overtly dangerous. Indeed, a positive diagnosis can sometimes only be achieved when the entire resected specimen is at the disposal of the pathologist.

5. Since the mortality and morbidity of pancreaticoduodenal resection has decreased drastically in the past decade, every surgeon should be prepared to accept an occasionally benign pathology report.[7,9] The earlier the tumor, the more difficult it is to achieve a positive diagnosis by any needle biopsy technique, and the only hope of averting the tragedy of not resecting a potentially curable lesion is by performing an ‘‘excisional biopsy’’ provided that it can be done safely.

The problem of pancreatic biopsy and pancreatic resection often involves the unspoken sensitive issue of surgical "macho." It is widely recognized that there are differences in professional competence in any field. An experienced surgeon who frequently performs many pancreatic operations clearly has much better results than the occasional surgeon who tackles one or two cases a year. Thus, the important factors are the following:

1. The surgeon and the surgeon's experience, expertise, and knowledge of his or her operative mortality and morbidity.

2. The patient and his or her disease as well as understanding of the "informed consent" that the patient has given to the surgeon.

3. The pathologist and the pathologist's interest and experience.

Biopsy of the pancreas to "diagnose pancreatitis" should be strongly condemned. The "occasional" pancreatic surgeon should not meddle in the area and manipulate the gland unless he or she is prepared to proceed with definitive treatment. The question of how to proceed if a surgeon incidentally finds a mass in the pancreas during the course of a laparotomy for some other procedure, for example a cholecystectomy, is often asked. Unless the surgeon is prepared (and the surgeon rarely is) to proceed with an immediate pancreatic resection if the biopsy is positive for cancer, he or she should not perform any biopsy at that time. A negative biopsy does not help. In addition, the surgeon should refrain from mobilizing and assessing resectability at that operation. Such manipulations and dissections will undoubtedly make evaluation by subsequent investigations exceedingly difficult to interpret and render the second laparotomy technically more difficult and even more dangerous. This author feels very strongly that all pancreatic operations should be planned well in advance and proper informed consent obtained from the patient and the relatives. Only in this way can the many current medicolegal problems be averted.[17]

REFERENCES

1. Beazley RM. Needle biopsy of pancreatic cancer. Cancer 47:1685–1687, 1981.
2. Bowden L. The fallibility of pancreatic biopsy. Ann Surg 139:403–405, 1954.
3. Campanale R, Frey CF, Farias LR, et al. Reliability and sensitivity of frozen section pancreatic biopsy. Arch. Surg 120:283–288, 1985.
4. Cattell RB, Warren KW. Surgery of the Pancreas. Philadelphia, WB Saunders, 1953.
5. Christofferson P, Poll P. Preoperative pancreas aspiration biopsy. Acta Pathol Microbiol Scand 212(suppl):28–32, 1970.
6. Cote J, Dockerty MB, Priestly JT. An evaluation of pancreatic biopsy with the Vim Silverman needle. Arch Surg 79:588–592, 1959.
7. Crist DW, Sitzmann JW, Cameron JL. Improved hospital morbidity and mortality and survival following the Whipple procedure. Ann Surg 206:358–365, 1987.
8. Dorland's Illustrated Medical Dictionary, 25th ed. Philadelphia, WB Saunders, 1974, 202.
9. Grace PA, Pitt HA, Tompkins RK, et al. Decreased morbidity and mortality after pancreatoduodenectomy. Am J Surg 151:141–149, 1986.

10. Holm HA, Kristensen JK, Rasmussen SN, et al. Ultrasound as a guide in percutaneous puncture technique. Ultrasonic 10:83–84, 1972.
11. Hyland C, Kheir SM, Kashlan MB. Frozen section diagnosis of pancreatic carcinoma—A prospective study of 64 biopsies. Am J Surg Pathol 5:179–182, 1981.
12. Isaacson R, Weiland LH, McIlrath DC. Biopsy of the pancreas. Arch Surg 109:227–230, 1974.
13. Kirtland HB Jr. A safe method of pancreatic biopsy—A preliminary report. Am J Surg 82:451–453, 1951.
14. Lightwood R, Reber HA, Way LW. The risk and accuracy of pancreatic biopsy. Am J Surg 132:189, 1976.
15. Maingot R. Pancreatic tumors and periampullary carcinoma. In: Maingot R, ed. Abdominal Operations. New York, Appleton-Century-Crofts, 1980.
16. McIlrath DC. Biopsy of the pancreas. In: Brooks JR, ed. Surgery of the Pancreas. Philadelphia, WB Saunders, 1983, pp 130–133.
17. Moossa AR. Re-operation for pancreatic cancer. Arch Surg 114:502–505, 1979.
18. Moossa AR. A shortened version of the secretin test for the diagnosis of pancreatic cancer. In: Moossa AR, ed. Tumors of the Pancreas. Baltimore. Williams and Wilkins, 1980, pp 391–396.
19. Moossa AR, Altorki N. Pancreatic biopsy. Surg Clin North Am 63:1205–1214, 1983.
20. Moossa AR, Dawson PJ. The diagnosis of pancreatic cancer. In: Ioachim HL, ed. Pathobiology Annual. New York. Raven Press, 1981, vol 2, pp 229–235.
21. Reuben A, Cotton T. Operative pancreatic biopsy—A survey of current practice. Ann R Coll Surg Engl 6:53–56, 1978.
22. Schultz NJ, Sanders RJ. Evaluation of pancreatic biopsy. Ann Surg 158:1053–1055, 1963.
23. Spjut HJ, Ramos AJ. An evaluation of biopsy—Frozen section of the ampullary region and pancreas—A report of 68 consecutive patients. Ann Surg 146:922–926, 1957.
24. Tsuchiya R, Henmi I, Kondo N, et al. Endoscopic aspiration biopsy of the pancreas. Gastroenterology 73:1050–1052, 1977.
25. Weiss SM, Skibber JM, Dobelbower RR, et al. Operative pancreatic biopsy: 10 year review of accuracy and complication. Am Surg 48:214–216, 1982.
26. Weiss SM, Skibber JM, Mohiuddin, et al. Rapid intraabdominal spread of pancreatic cancer—Influence of multiple operatic biopsy procedures. Arch Surg 120:415–416, 1985.

CHAPTER

22

LESIONS OF THE PANCREAS AND PERIAMPULLARY AREA CAUSING BILIARY OBSTRUCTION: PALLIATIVE SURGERY

Philippe Gertsch and Les H. Blumgart

EDITORIAL COMMENT (Chapters 22 and 23)

It is generally accepted that biliary stent placement is the procedure of choice in patients with jaundice due to pancreatic cancer who are aged, in poor nutritional state, have other severe disease, or show metastases on the usual scanning techniques. The authors provide evidence showing that dissemination is poorly diagnosed by our current techniques and that 95% of patients have unresectable disease. They do make the important point of detailed preoperative investigation in these patients, if resective surgery is contemplated, for better staging of the disease. In most patients, the prognosis appears to be determined by unknown biological determinants. The authors address important aspects such as the importance of diagnosing ampullary lesions, high mortality of jaundice that does not remit with therapy, potential risks of skinny needle biopsy if surgery is contemplated, and newer techniques of endoscopic stent placement in the face of total bile duct or duodenal obstruction. However, the authors do not discuss the complications of stenting and the fairly high incidence of stents requiring removal and replacement. This has influenced some surgeons to advocate a return to biliary and/or gastroduodenal bypass as the primary procedure in younger patients in good physical condition to obviate the necessity for repeating stent placement. No doubt there will continue to be advocates of both techniques, and perhaps there is a place for individualization of patient treatment according to physical status at first diagnosis.

Surgical exploration for bypass of biliary obstruction allows for possible resection of the tumor, if the conditions and staging are favorable, and should be preceded by percutaneous fine needle biopsy. The possibility of tumor seeding exists, but this is extremely rare, and the slight risk is outweighed by the advantage of having a preoperative diagnosis of malignancy that permits a frank discussion of the options with the patient and family.

Resection of small tumors by pancreaticoduodenectomy in the hope of cure may turn out to be a form of palliation in the long run if the tumor later metastasizes, as pointed out by Drs. Gertsch and Blumgart. For advanced tumors, biliary bypass can be combined with gastrojejunostomy for the treatment or prophylaxis of duodenal obstruction, thus avoiding a second hospital admission later in the course of what would be a rather short illness. In the elderly or high-risk patient or in those with ascites or liver involvement, endoscopic stenting is preferred to operation.

Two recent randomized trials of surgical versus endoscopic biliary decompression have been reported from England. One trial showed more readmissions to hospital in the stent group but shorter overall hospital stay. The other trial showed that the stent group had fewer early complications and a smaller 30-day mortality but more readmissions later for jaundice and duodenal obstruction. Clearly the final word is not yet in on this controversial topic.

CONTROVERSY

The high success rate of endoscopic stent placement in relieving jaundice in patients with pancreatic disease, taken in conjunction with the poor prognosis for pancreatic carcinoma, has resulted in an almost universal use of biliary stenting in such patients. However, advocates of surgical bypass have stressed that stenting has resulted in patients who might benefit from resection being overlooked, and that stents frequently result in cholangitis and need to be replaced, so that ultimate survival and cost may be similar in the two groups with less morbidity in the surgical group. The endoscopic and surgical aspects are discussed in the next two chapters.

The aim of palliative treatment, by definition, is to attenuate the manifestations of a disease. This definition should take into account the fact that the treatment will not cure the disease definitively, but will give temporary relief of symptoms. It also assumes that prediction of the evolution of the disease as well as the effect of the treatment is possible. This is of course not always the case. Palliative treatment might in some instances give what is to all intents and purposes definitive relief. Similarly, treatments intended to be curative might fail but nevertheless give good palliation. For example, intended curative surgery for periampullary cancer may only reveal its palliative nature when tumor recurs at a later date. The life expectancy of a patient, independent of the disease process, might also influence the judgment of a treatment regarding its curative or palliative nature. Thus clear-cut definition of a treatment as palliative or curative is often not possible. Palliation must therefore constantly be judged in relation to curative therapy or therapeutic abstention. The record of success of a particular treatment, its mortality, and its complications should be carefully considered before making therapeutic decisions.

Lesions of the pancreas and periampullary area commonly present some degree of obstruction of the biliary tract, and treatment should be directed not only at relief of biliary tract obstruction but also at removal or cure of the disease process. In some instances both aims can be realized, but in others only the relief of biliary obstruction is possible. It is particularly in the latter group that therapeutic decisions are difficult, and choices must be made between surgical relief of biliary obstruction and endoscopic or transhepatic intubational methods.

A wide variety of lesions of the pancreas and periampullary areas can cause biliary obstruction since the terminal part of the bile duct traverses the head of the pancreas. Small lesions in this part of the gland can cause obstruction, and expanding lesions in more distant parts of the gland might extend to the region of the biliary–pancreatic junction or compress the biliary duct proximally. Tumors localized in the periampullary area may arise from pancreatic, biliary, duodenal, or papillary epithelium, and the origin of the tumor may be difficult to define.

In this chapter we discuss the diseases of the pancreas and periampullary region that may cause biliary tract obstruction and the relationship of the characteristics of these diseases to the definition of palliative treatment.

PANCREATITIS

Acute Pancreatitis

Acute pancreatitis may be associated with biliary obstruction in a proportion of cases. Ever since the 1901 publication of Opie,[78] choledocholithiasis has been identified as a frequent association with acute pancreatitis, and many studies have confirmed this. However, the presence of jaundice in acute pancreatitis may not be due to gallstones but may be a direct consequence of the inflammation. Biliary obstruction in such circumstances might be incomplete and transient and in this instance is usually caused by severe edema of the head of the pancreas and compression of the intrapancreatic bile duct (Fig. 22-1).

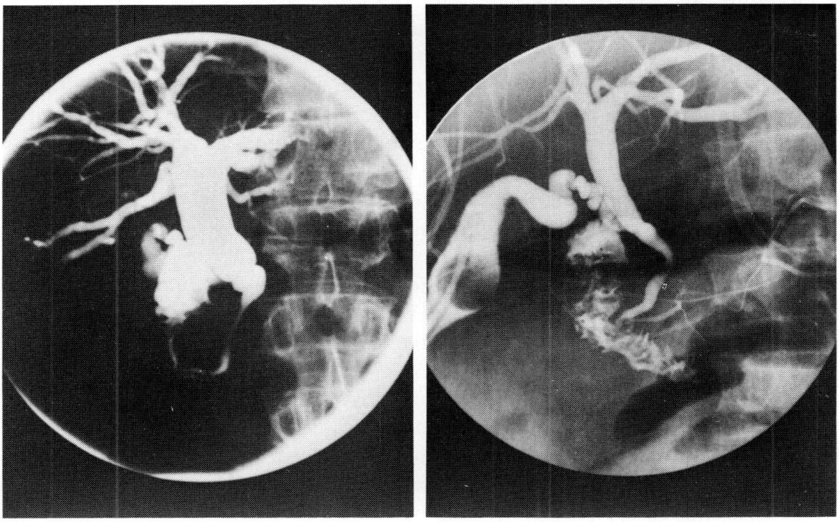

A B

Figure 22-1. Acute necrotizing pancreatitis with multiple pseudocysts. (A) Percutaneous cholangiography showing a stenosis of the distal choledochus. (B) Tube cholecystocholangiography 3 weeks after cholecystostomy and drainage of pancreatic pseudocysts. The figure shows a regression of the stenosis of the distal choledochus.

Pseudocysts in association with acute pancreatitis might also compress the distal bile duct, and this may appear as early as the first week.[97] It is, however, more usual to observe cyst formation some 2 to 3 weeks after the initial attack of pancreatitis, and although pseudocysts are estimated to occur in 13% of cases during the first attack of acute pancreatitis,[97] biliary obstruction as a result of compression is relatively rare. Spontaneous regression of pseudocysts in acute pancreatitis has been observed in 11% to 25% of cases.[20,67,97] The exact cause of jaundice in acute nonbiliary pancreatitis can be determined by imaging of the biliary tree. Percutaneous transhepatic puncture is probably the best method in the presence of pseudocyst. Endoscopic retrograde cholangiography requires a good visualisation of the papilla and this is usually difficult in such circumstances since compression of the duodenum by the pseudocyst is frequent.

Treatment

The place of surgical therapy in acute pancreatitis is still a matter of controversy. In particular the indications for surgery or endoscopic papillotomy in the acute phase of biliary-associated pancreatitis are hotly debated. We shall not consider this from the point of view of the attenuation or arrest of the process of pancreatic inflammation. However, the presence of progressive obstructive jaundice, with or without cholangitis, in a patient in the early phases of acute pancreatitis is probably a valid reason to consider either endoscopic papillotomy or exploration of the common bile duct. The choice of surgery for removal of gallstones in such circumstances will depend on a number of factors including particularly the presence of associated gallbladder inflammation that might require coincident therapy. Indeed, severe cases of acute biliary pancreatitis often occur in elderly women in whom judgment of whether there is coincident cholecystitis or threatened perforation of the gallbladder is extremely difficult.

In general terms the value of endoscopic papillotomy as a means of treating pancreatic inflammation is still debatable, and there are no good studies to demonstrate its value. Relief of biliary obstruction caused by stone remains the only firm indication for some form of interventional therapy.

In acute pancreatitis not associated with gallstones, there is seldom a need to treat biliary obstruction, which, as mentioned above, may be due to edema of the head of the pancreas or cyst formation. In such cases biliary obstruction can be isolated or be associated with other problems related to severe pancreatitis such as intraabdominal sepsis or bleeding. As far as possible, treatment should be conservative. If jaundice is, however, progressive, a precise diagnosis of its cause should be the first objective. Biliary pancreatitis and associated choledocholithiasis should of course be excluded and the presense or absence of a pseudocyst confirmed. Where it is judged that a pseudocyst is causing compression of the bile duct, ultrasound- or CT-guided percutaneous needle puncture of the cyst followed by insertion of a drain may relieve obstruction. If not, the bile duct may be drained by percutaneous transhepatic puncture. As far as possible no surgical therapy should be used, since edema and necrosis make surgical access to the choledochus hazardous. Usually when inflammation and edema subside, bile duct obstruction is also relieved.

Surgical drainage of a pseudocyst is indicated in a jaundiced patient when there is infection that is not relieved by percutaneous drainage, and particularly if there is clear slough present within the cyst and demonstrated by ultrasonography or CT.[104] Operation in such circumstances is always difficult. It should be remembered that an enlarged gallbladder with a demonstrated communication with the distended bile ducts can be drained by simple cholecystostomy and provide indirect bile duct decompression with minimal surgical risk. This is an appropriate approach in many cases and can be combined with cyst drainage and removal of slough.

Chronic Pancreatitis

The incidence of common bile duct stricture in chronic pancreatitis (CP) is estimated to be about 10%.[5,64,103,120] The degree of obstruction may vary with relapses of acute inflammation and consequent compression of the bile duct. Progressive fibrosis may be more insidious and remain asymptomatic for long periods. However serum alkaline phosphatase levels greater than twice the upper limit of normal, persisting for more than a few weeks, should alert the physician to such a complication.[64] Of the factors involved in cholestasis complicating CP, extrinsic compression of the common bile duct by pseudocyst or by concentric narrowing of the intrapancreatic duct are the most common.

Chronic pancreatitis presents with a pattern of histologic changes that may be associated with intense sclerosis,[114] thus explaining the well-known alterations of the bile ducts seen on cholangiography. The sclerosis traps the intrapancreatic bile duct leading to different degrees of stenosis or multiple areas with stenosis.[91,120] The diagnosis should be expected in alcoholic patients with chronic abdominal pain and with persistent symptoms of extrahepatic biliary tract obstruction. These can vary from persisting elevated levels of alkaline phosphatase to clinically apparent jaundice. A transient elevation of alkaline phosphatase levels has, however, been reported in 30% of patients during exacerbations of CP but may not be related to biliary obstruction,[64,90,122] radiologic examination failing to demonstrate any stricture in 90% of cases.[64] By contrast investigations performed in patients with persistent evidence of cholestasis reveals stricture in most instances.

A persistent elevation of the serum alkaline phosphatase level is the best index that biliary tract stenosis is present. The occurrence of frank jaundice is inconstant in this situation and is reported in only 3% to 27% of cases,[31,64,91] but the consequences of chronic and incomplete biliary stasis in CP is important in defining treatment since the potential secondary effects on the liver must be taken into account (see below).[117]

Pseudocysts of the pancreas may be a complication of chronic as well as of acute pancreatitis.[19] As they enlarge, pseudocysts cause compression and pain and might occasionally become infected. Perforation into an adjacent viscus, bleeding, or chronic leak causing pancreatic ascites have all been well documented. Common bile duct obstruction due to pancreatic pseudocyst has probably been overestimated in the past.[114] The criteria required to prove that obstruction is caused by direct compression of the biliary duct by the pancreatic cyst are that the common duct is demonstrably compressed by the pseudocyst and that relief of biliary obstruction by drainage of the pseudocyst is achieved.[98] The latter requirement is rarely defined in published cases and demonstrates the need for precise understanding of the condition for successful treatment (Fig. 22-2).

The preoperative diagnosis of the exact cause of obstruction in such cases is difficult, and no reliable technique has been described. Imaging of the biliary duct is probably insufficient, and a narrowed area of the bile duct apparently conforming to the pseudocyst in the head of the pancreas does not necessarily prove compression.[114] Disappearance of biliary obstruction after percutaneous evacuation of the cyst may provide confirmation.

Treatment

Since CP involves irreversible loss of glandular function, surgery should always be considered palliative. Surgical relief of biliary obstruction is necessary for persistent jaundice, cholangitis, or secondary biliary fibrosis.

However, the management of incomplete obstruction in asymptomatic patients is more difficult. Should asymptomatic bile duct stenosis be treated to prevent cholangitis or secondary biliary cirrhosis? Some believe that there is an absolute indication for surgery in these cases,[2,103,116] while others expect spontaneous resolution of the stenosis.[20] A study of the histopathologic changes in liver biopsies of patients with CP and cholestasis reveals that the liver shows very little irreversible damage consequent on clinical cholestasis in this situation.[35] There is

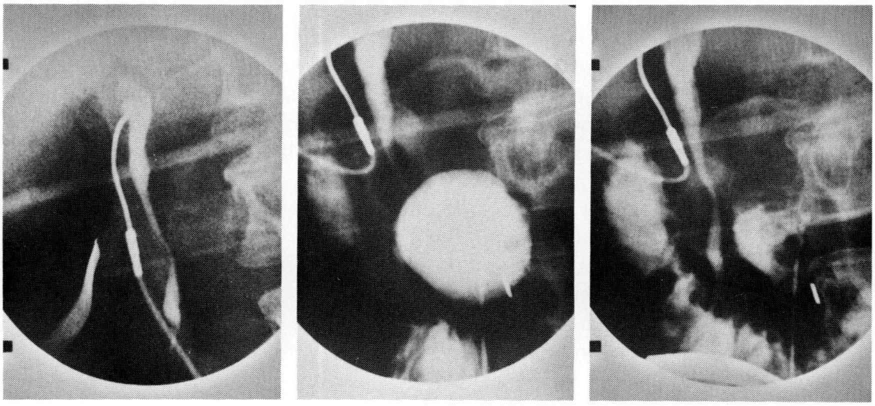

A B C

Figure 22-2. Chronic pancreatitis with a 5-cm pseudocyst in the head of the pancreas presenting with icterus. (A) The intraoperative cholangiography demonstrates a stenosis in the distal choledochus. (B) The intraoperative opacification of the pseudocyst demonstrates its relation with the distal bile duct. (C) The intraoperative cholangiography after evacuation of the pseudocyst demonstrates that the stenotic segment of the distal choledochus has remained unchanged.

also evidence that prolonged biliary obstruction usually results in a biliary fibrotic histologic change that only rarely proceeds to true cirrhosis.[15,117]

Stricture at the papilla with dilatation of both the common bile duct and the pancreatic duct is rare. In such circumstances, sphincteroplasty has been proposed and good long-term results claimed.[9,10,37,38] Other believe that this procedure is insufficient because the usual length of the biliary stricture involves 2 to 3 cm of the intrapancreatic bile duct.[103] Drainage is best achieved by choledochoduodenostomy or by choledochojejunostomy, preferably using an end-to-side technique.[5,73,103] Cholecystectomy is advised because of the risk of stone formation consequent on gall bladder stasis, and indeed biliary sludge or stones are often present within the gallbladder in such patients. The gallbladder may also be used for bypass, but this alternative is seldom mentioned in the literature dealing with biliary obstruction due to CP. Utilization of the gallbladder for bypass should not be entertained if it is judged that complete relief of biliary obstruction will not be achieved. It should not be employed if there is no clear cholangiographic evidence of a widely patent cystic duct joining the common bile duct above the level of the disease process.

It is important to note that an associated surgical procedure for other complications of CP may be required.[16] Thus in a series of 28 patients operated on for complications of CP, biliary obstruction was present in 16 cases. In only 37% was biliary obstruction an isolated complication, but it was associated with pancreatic obstruction in 44% and with duodenal obstruction in 19%. Duodenal obstruction can be relieved by gastrojejunostomy combined with truncal vagotomy.[107] If pain associated with pancreatic duct stenosis requires a drainage procedure of the duct of Wirsung, a Roux en Y loop may allow decompression of both the choledochus and the pancreatic duct.[40] Combined procedures on the bile duct and pancreatic duct have been necessary in up to 89% of cases submitted to operation.[40] The mortality of these operations varies between 0% and 3.5%.[40,65,107] Occasionally, pancreatic resectional procedures are necessary to treat severe pain in CP that is unassociated with dilatation of the duct of Wirsung, and such operations may also be combined with biliary enteric anastomosis for coincident biliary obstruction.[16,28]

Pseudocysts may be associated with biliary duct stenosis in CP (see above). Only rarely does simple drainage of the cyst relieve jaundice. In such cases intraoperative cholangiography should be obtained after decompression of the cyst (Fig. 22-2). If relief of biliary obstruction is not clearly demonstrated, complementary biliary–enteric bypass should be performed.[114]

PERIAMPULLARY TUMORS

A variety of benign and malignant tumors of the pancreas and of the periampullary region may be associated with biliary obstruction. Neoplasms arising at or within 1 cm of the papilla of Vater can take origin from cells at the distal common bile duct, duodenum, papilla of Vater, or pancreas. These tumors have often been described as a group because of their similarities, common clinical features, and sometimes indistinguishable histologic features. However, the prognosis, management, and results of therapy of these various tumors differ considerably. Although all usually present with jaundice of some degree, treatment is best selected on the basis of precise diagnosis whenever possible.

Benign Tumors of the Periampullary Region

Benign tumors, whether of biliary, papillary, or duodenal origin, all have malignant potential.[22,23,24] Malignant change results in an occult periampullary malignant tumor that may be undetected by simple inspection of the papilla and revealed only by ERCP as a filling defect at the lower end of the common duct.

Adenomatous polyps of the papilla of Vater are rare. Delpy et al., in a review of the literature, analyzed 77 cases.[34] Adenomata are diagnosed more rarely than ampullary carcinomata, probably because they cause symptoms late in their evolution at a time when malignant change has already supervened.[46,62] Jaundice occurred in 77%, pain in 64%, and gastrointestinal bleeding in 64% of cases.

Treatment

Treatment of benign tumors should be curative whenever possible since complete excision brings definitive cure.[35] Palliation therefore relates to cases with incomplete excision that might recur or when subsequent malignant change may supervene.

Vaterian and duodenal adenomas present a therapeutic dilemma. On one hand a small benign tumor does not seem to warrant wide excision, but on the other hand incomplete excision may result in early recurrence with possible malignant change, and indeed in such tumors malignant change may already have taken place and remain undiagnosed. Since these tumors develop malignant changes in 47% of cases,[34] and since systematic histologic examination in patients with carcinoma of the papilla of Vater reveals areas of adenomatous polyps in up to 81% of cases,[46,62] even apparently benign adenomatous polyps may conceal focal malignant change. Radical excision is recommended whenever possible, and indeed only systematic histologic examination of the entire specimen allows exclusion of malignancy, especially in large polyps.[46,62]

Polyps of the papilla of Vater may be excised locally. The resection, which is carried out transduodenally, should involve a portion of the duodenal wall and include all the sphincteric area with reimplantation of the distal bile duct and pancreatic duct. Such an operation allows complete histologic examination of the tumor and will cure most polyps.

Since obstruction of the distal common bile duct in its intrapancreatic course, even by a benign tumor, occurs in an anatomically complex location, excision may not always be possible, and a palliative bypass procedure may be electively chosen when operative risk seems to outweigh the threat represented by the tumor.

Endoscopic snare excision of an adenomatous polyp of the papilla of Vater should be used with caution in cases not suitable for surgical approaches.

In some patients polypoid lesions of the papilla of Vater causing biliary obstruction may be associated with multiple adenomas of the duodenum.[87] This is particularly so in patients presenting with Gardner's syndrome.[108] The tendency for malignant change of these adenomatous polyps has been well documented.[87,94,108] In such circumstances ampullectomy leaving in place other potentially malignant tumors should be regarded as palliative only. Duodenopancreatectomy is the curative surgical approach.[87]

Malignant Tumors of the Periampullary Region

Malignant tumors arising in the periampullary region are usually adenocarcinomata with varying degrees of differentiation.[4,112] Primary adenocarcinoma of the head of the pancreas is usually less well differentiated than primary adenocarcinoma of the bile duct, of the papilla, or of the duodenum, but, as already stated, the origin of this tumor cannot always be recognized preoperatively. In less than 5% of cases other tumors such as carcinoid lymphoma, adenoacanthoma, leiomyosarcoma, cystadenocarcinoma, islet cell tumors, haemangiopericytoma, or melanoma might arise in the periampullary area.[63,112]

Because of their location, periampullary tumors usually cause symptoms at an early and potentially curable stage. Signs of extrahepatic biliary obstruction may vary from persisting pruritus to frank icterus. Jaundice may fluctuate as these tumors undergo necrosis, and sloughing and bleeding may be an initial sign revealed by the presence of either anemia or melena.[84]

Treatment

There is no doubt that surgical excision allows a significantly better prognosis for periampullary malignant tumors than for tumors arising in the head of the pancreas. Five-year survival rates vary between 10% and 40%.[11,59,60,61,86,111]

The outcome after surgical therapy is influenced by the characteristics of the tumor and by its extent as well as by the surgical procedure chosen for treatment.[17,59,86]

Resection of periampullary malignant tumors by means of duodenopancreatectomy has been performed since the first report of Whipple (1935).[118] Mortality rates have steadily decreased over the years and now stand at less than 10% in most series and less than 5% in specialist centers.[59,86] Local ampullary excision first performed by Halsted[49] has recently been advocated as a curative treatment and as an alternative to pancreaticoduodenectomy.[77] Recent publications report a similar 5-year survival rate for radical surgery or for local excision.[61,86] Comparisons between the two surgical approaches should be careful and take into account patient selection in different series as well as operative mortality and long-term results.

A collective review of 514 pancreaticoduodenectomies for periampullary cancer and 138 cases of ampullary excision show mortality rates of 18.3 and 27.7%, respectively.[76] The higher mortality rate for local excision in comparison to radical resection has been noted in other series[68,73] and is almost certainly related to the poorer condition of patients selected for local excision. However, local excision remains a reasonable alternative in selected cases although the currently low operative mortality for radical removal makes it the procedure of choice in fit patients. Local excision is reserved for older or high-risk patients in whom the mortality for ampullectomy is almost certainly less than for radical excision.

Biliary enteric bypass without excision of tumor is clearly palliative but allows a mean survival of no more than 10 months[61,86] and still carries a significant operative mortality in older high-risk patients.

Endoscopic sphincterotomy or intubation for relief of jaundice may be used for the palliation of periampullary carcinoma and has also been proposed for biliary decompression before definitive surgery.[3,18] However, the benefits of preoperative biliary decompression in jaundiced patients has not been confirmed in controlled clinical studies,[53,68,69,80] and there are no controlled clinical studies examining specifically the benefits or disadvantages of endoscopic approaches for periampullary or pancreatic carcinoma.

Endoscopic sphincterotomy with or without introduction of endoprothesis is an alternative to surgery in some elderly and high-risk patients but should not be chosen as a primary approach when excision with potential cure is possible. Infection of the biliary tree after sphincterotomy may not be clinically evident but only become so when excisional or bypass surgery is performed at a later date in the presence of infected bile.

Palliative endoscopic procedures allow an approximate 5-month symptom-free interval with survival of 8 to 13 months.[55,88] This is an acceptable alternative for lesions that cannot be approached for surgical excision but should not be chosen for potentially curable candidates.

Bile Duct Cancer

Bile duct cancer in the periampullary region presents in an indistinguishable manner from pancreas cancer, but direct cholangiography may allow differentiation from other periampullary tumors. Despite thorough investigation there may be an incorrect diagnosis. Differentiation from carcinoma of the pancreas may be impossible, and in addition, low bile duct cancer can be confused with benign obstruction due to either stones or benign tumors in the distal bile duct.

Surgical resection remains the procedure of choice and is potentially curative. Recent reports emphasize that the mortality for pancreaticoduodenectomy is acceptable (see above). The 5-year survival rate is probably 15% to 20% and is significantly better than for carcinoma of the head of the pancreas. Thus, in 1984 Alexander et al. found 100% of 14 patients with distal bile duct tumors resectable with a median survival of 16 months (range 5 to 84 months) and 2 patients surviving 5 years.[4]

It should perhaps be emphasized that the results for excision or surgical palliative bypass for mid and low bile duct cancer appear to offer distinct advantages over intubational techniques. While the success rate for intubation of low and mid bile duct tumors is considerably higher than that for tumors at the confluence, this technique has still to demonstrate an improved 30-day mortality over current surgical figures and cannot offer any hope of cure. Surgical bypass gives excellent palliation from jaundice, and no further procedures are required. The period of palliation offered by intubational techniques is not longer than that for surgical approaches. Nevertheless, in selected patients endoscopic intubation may prove of value.[89]

TUMORS OF THE PANCREAS

Cystadenoma and Cystadenocarcinoma

Benign tumors of the pancreas are rare. *Cystadenoma* was described at the end of the last century, and fewer than 400 cases have been recorded. The true incidence is unknown, although cystadenoma probably represents 10% of pancreatic cysts.[13,72] In young patients the disease is relatively more common than adenocarcinoma.

Cystadenoma may be microcystic or present with mucinous cysts. Microcystic adenomas are well-circumscribed, multiloculated lesions that range from 1 to 25 cm. Mucinous cysts may reach similar size, and in these lesions the wall is usually thick and forms a single cavity containing dense, brown or red cloudy material. Mucinous cystadenomas occur more frequently in the head of the pancreas than the microcystic variety. The malignant potential of these lesions is well known.[8,83,95,115,123]

Pain is the most frequent presenting symptom and is often associated with loss of weight. Localization in the head of the pancreas is rare, but associated jaundice is reported in 8% of cases.[52,84,101] Bleeding occurs in 10% of cases. Association of cystadenoma with benign and malignant pancreatic and nonpancreatic neoplasms has also been described.[7,27,52,70,101] Differentiation from pseudocysts of the pancreas is not reliable by morphologic studies alone.

Cystadenocarcinoma of the pancreas represents 1% of all pancreatic malignancies. Predilection for women has been reported to be from 3 : 1 to 9 : 1,[27,30,33] but this is not confirmed in all series.[51] Symptoms are similar to those observed with cystadenoma. Pain is present in more than 80% of cases, but jaundice is more frequent than in cystadenoma and occurs in 29%.[51] The common bile duct may be compressed when invaded by the tumor[51] or obstructed by mucinous material leaking from the cyst.[57] Positive diagnosis by means of percutaneous aspiration cytology may be difficult as cystadenocarcinoma often has benign areas within the main lesion. For this reason diagnosis of a cystic neoplasm of the pancreas should always be accompanied by suspicion of malignancy.[8,83,95]

Cystadenoma or cystadenocarcinoma of the pancreas should be suspected when cystic lesions are discovered in patients without a history of alcoholism, pancreatitis, or trauma. Other tumors such as leiomyosarcoma, paraganglionoma, and islet cell tumors occasionally have a cystic appearance.

Malignant characteristics in cystic lesions[79] should be suspected on ultrasonography or CT scanning when infiltration of the surrounding structures or irregularity of the capsule is demonstrated. Similarly irregularity of the lining of the cyst may suggest malignancy. These changes are, however, not always present, and the simple presence of multiple cysts or internal septa raise the suspicion of benign or malignant tumor.[115] Transcutaneous aspiration of the cyst fluid for cytologic examination might give precise information. The amylase content is high in pseudocysts and normal in neoplastic cysts.[115]

Treatment

Benign tumors of the pancreas are usually amenable to curative treatment.[105] *Cystadenoma* should be completely excised by enucleation when the cyst has a well-defined capsule but otherwise by means of partial or total pancreatectomy. Recurrence after total removal is rare,[27,52] and the mortality for excision or the Whipple procedure is about 7%.[105] However, when the lesion is not resectable, either for general or local reasons, palliative operation may be performed. Partial excision of the cyst might relieve compression of the bile duct but carries the risk of spreading undetected malignant cells in cases of mucinous cyst adenoma.[31] There are insufficient data in the literature to assess the results of this procedure. Intraoperative cholangiography before and after decompression should allow precise assessment of its effect. Obstruction to the bile ducts caused by mucinous material issuing from the cyst may not be relieved by simple excision and may require bile duct exploration. Internal or external drainage of the cyst has also been performed in rare instances.[58,96,105] Biliary enteric bypass may be necessary if bile duct obstruction is not relieved by partial or total excision of the tumor. The mortality for palliation of cystadenoma of the pancreas is low, and when total excision or pancreaticoduodenectomy has been performed, a mortality rate of 7% or less is reported.[105]

Biliary obstruction caused by *cystadenocarcinoma* of the pancreas is a very rare condition. It may be caused by compression or invasion of the bile duct or by passage of mucus into the bile duct.[57] All efforts should be made to resect these tumors; curative resective surgery is possible even in presence of nodal metastasis. Palliation should be offered to patients with liver metastasis, or to those who are unfit for major surgery, although internal drainage of the cyst is usually condemned,[30,105,115] since the stiff neoplastic wall fails to collapse. Nevertheless, earlier publications have reported survival of 1 year with this procedure.[58,96] A biliodigestive anastomosis above the cyst is the best palliative procedure. As in pancreatic carcinoma, a gastroenterostomy might be added to the biliodigestive anastomosis.

Carcinoma of the Pancreas

Adenocarcinoma is the most common malignant tumor of the pancreas, and the bleak prognosis has not changed over the last 20 years despite the advent of new diagnostic imaging techniques. Its incidence has increased worldwide, and it is now the fourth cause of cancer death in the United States. The annual incidence approaches 10 cases per 100,000 inhabitants. Its incidence increases with age and is around 100 cases per 100,000 in patients over 70 years old.[48] Because of its retroperitoneal location, adenocarcinoma of the pancreas often remains asymptomatic until an advanced stage. Tumor infiltration causing loss of weight or pain or symptoms of compression of adjacent structures may often be the first signs of disease. Occlusion of the distal choledochus may be the earliest manifestation when a tumor is localized to the head of the pancreas, and this occurs in 60% to 80% of cases.[36] However, cancer localized in the uncinate process tends to present late, obstruction of the pancreatic duct occurring before the obstruction of the choledochus.

No tumor marker has sufficient specificity to be reliable as a screening test. The disease is therefore nearly always diagnosed when it becomes symptomatic. In icteric patients, Courvoisier's sign is often sufficient to raise a high suspicion of malignancy. Ultrasonography or CT scanning will then define the local extent of the tumor and sometimes demonstrate the presence of metastases. These imaging modalities, however, do not always give enough information, particularly in cases in which a diagnosis of CP is possible. Ultrasound- or CT-scan-guided fine needle puncture provides specimens for cytologic examination for which specificity is 100%[41,44,56] and is reported to yield a positive diagnosis in 60% to 100% of cases.[12,41,44] Complications are rare.[12]

Islet cell tumors of the pancreas are often small, solid, and benign but may be cystic, reach a large size, and be malignant. On occasion they may cause biliary obstruction by direct invasion or compression of the common bile duct.[109,110] It is important in discussing palliation of pancreatic malignancies to recognize these tumors since their prognosis differs significantly from adenocarcinoma even when liver metastases are present.

Treatment

When dealing with malignant tumors, palliation is often the only therapeutic possibility, curative resection being much less frequently feasible. In addition, many patients have technically resectable tumors but are either elderly or have coincident disease that renders the risk of radical resection too high. Malignant tumors of the pancreas are resectable only in some 10% of patients, and palliation is the main surgical option. The place of resection for palliation is discussed elsewhere in this book and will not be further discussed here.

In the vast majority of cases, obstructive jaundice is present,[50,76,102] and a relief of this obstruction is the main goal in patients with unresectable tumor. This not only influences obstructive jaundice and pruritus but also prevents hepatic dysfunction, coagulopathy, and nutritional disorders related to malabsorption.[21,42,81,85] Unfortunately, the median survival remains short, usually not exceeding 1 year even in the best series.[71,121]

Although different forms of biliary enteric bypass may be used for palliation in cancer of the head of the pancreas, no review has demonstrated any clear advantage of any particular technique. When the gallbladder is distended and clearly communicates with the biliary tree well above the obstruction, cholecystoenterostomy is the simplest procedure. However, using the gallbladder has several drawbacks. In 10% of patients, the cystic duct enters the common bile duct low down, near the upper border, or even within the pancreas and is prone to obstruction by the growth of the tumor. It is therefore to be expected that this form of anastomosis allows palliation and possibly survival for a shorter time than choledochoenteric bypass. A review of 19 reports comprising 1850 cases reveals that biliary bypass using the gallbladder is followed by an average survival of 5.3 months compared with 6.5 months when the common bile duct is used. In the same review the morbidity after cholecystoenteric bypass is greater than that after choledochoenteric bypass, cholangitis or recurrent jaundice occurring in 10% of cases in the former but being absent in the latter category. The mortality is similar for both techniques: 16% for cholecystoenterostomy and 20% for choledochoenterostomy.[92]

The use of side-to-side choledochoduodenostomy is advocated by some,[66,106] and although the technique has the advantage of simplicity, it is not generally used because of two theoretical drawbacks. First, the bypass lies in close proximity to the tumor, and second, duodenal obstruction by the tumor may supervene. However despite these supposed disadvantages, survival after such bypass does not seem to be shorter than anastomosis to the jejunum.[92]

A variety of biliary–jejunal bypass procedures can be performed. A Roux en Y limb has proved its superiority over loop jejunostomy. Thus in the treatment of benign biliary obstruction, intestinal biliary reflux and consequent cholangitis are far less common.[74,75] For that reason the use of the Roux en Y loop has been advocated for the palliation of pancreatic carcinoma.[7,47,51] However, many still favor the use of a jejunal loop since it is simple and allows a faster operation. A diverting enterostomy is advocated by some to prevent reflux,[39,50,82,119] but this adds time and complexity to the operation without preventing reflux.[74]

The survival of 1132 patients with pancreatic cancer treated by various means of surgical bypass showed no clear advantage for any particular approach.[92]

Obstruction of the duodenum by the tumor may destroy the palliation afforded by biliary digestive anastomosis and indeed necessitates reoperation in 15% to 34% of patients.[85,92,93] This complication usually occurs later than biliary obstruction, less than 5% presenting duodenal obstruction as the first manifestation of disease.[29,45] Nevertheless 30% of patients have signs suggesting abnormality of the duodenum at the time they become jaundiced.[14,26,29,45,54] There are therefore strong arguments to perform palliative gastroenterostomy as a routine at the same time as biliary enteric bypass even in the absence of duodenal obstruction. Several studies have demonstrated the advantage of this approach, which does not increase the operative risk associated with biliary enteric bypass, which remains at about 15%.[70,92] Stomal peptic ulceration occurs in less than 5% of cases,[92] and should this occur an H_2 antagonist is usually effective. In patients with known duodenal ulcer, vagotomy may be added to the procedure.

In some cases patients with cancer of the head of the pancreas initially complain of back pain, particularly on the left side. In such patients the disease has usually commenced in the uncinate process, obstructing the pancreatic duct prior to the bile duct; a dilated pancreatic duct can often be demonstrated at preoperative CT scanning or ultrasonography and can be palpated and punctured at operation. Decompression is then easily performed by Roux en Y pancreaticojejunostomy,[112,113] giving significant relief of pain according to some[24] or disappointing results according to others.[6] We use a simpler procedure, performing a pancreaticogastrostomy by means of a T tube introduced across the stomach and into the pancreatic duct. The anterior wall of the pancreas about the drain is attached to the posterior wall of the stomach. The anterior wall of the stomach is similarly fixed at the abdominal wall, where the drain is exteriorized. Ten days later the drain is removed, leaving an open pancreaticogastrostomy.

In cases in which pain is not associated with pancreatic ductal enlargement, the palliation of pain is more difficult. Rarely, biliary and duodenal bypass give some relief.[36,43,45,47,92] However, in the majority, extension of the tumor into the retroperitoneal tissues about the celiac axis is responsible for the pain. Chemical splanchnicectomy may be obtained by the injection of 50% alcohol or 5% phenol about the celiac axis, and pain is relieved in about 80% of cases without adding to the morbidity of the operation.[43]

Palliation of biliary ductal obstruction can also be obtained by endoscopic or percutaneous insertion of a prosthesis through the narrowed or obstructed bile duct.[100] What is the place of this technique compared with surgery? Comparisons are difficult, and no randomized study has compared surgery with endoscopic drainage. While surgery for palliation of biliary obstruction is an established treatment widely available for many years, endoscopic insertion of an endobiliary prosthesis is still a new technique available only in some institutions. Nevertheless, large series of more than 250 cases have recently been published.[99]

The success rate of endoscopic drainage is around 90%, hospital mortality varying from 12% to 18%,[99,32] this being similar to that for surgery.[92] The survival of 2 to 6 months[32,99] also does not differ significantly from that following surgical approaches. However, the mean period of hospitalization after endoscopic intubation is less than 4 days[99] and obviously shorter than after surgical operation. Obstruction of the prosthesis has, however, been a problem, occurring in 30% of cases within 3 months and in 70% within 6 months.[99] This can be managed by changing the prosthesis, but the procedure requires a further short hospitalization.

The advantages of the endoscopic approach—simplicity for the patient and short hospitalization—should not hide the fact that the procedure cannot be performed in all patients (large tumors of the head of the pancreas cause duodenal distortion), and cholangitis occurs in some 8% of patients with endoscopically placed tubes. Duodenal obstruction is rarely reported by endoscopists, probably because the majority of patients in whom endoscopic treatment is feasible do not have duodenal tumor involvement.

In general, it would seem that surgery is preferable for fit patients, since it offers a definitive palliation of biliary ductal obstruction without the need for repeated hospitalization and usually without cholangitis. In addition it allows prophylaxis of duodenal obstruction, which is known to occur in 20% to 30% of cases. Endoscopic intubation is preferred for frail patients without duodenal involvement or when a survival is assumed to be short because of liver metastasis or local extension of the tumor. The percutaneous insertion of an endobiliary endoprosthesis gives a palliation similar to that achieved by endoscopic means.[32] In general, the endoscopic approach is preferable, but local conditions and expertise may dictate therapy.

Biliary obstruction associated with islet cell tumors is uncommon. In general these lesions are best treated by resection even in the presence of liver metastasis, since adjuvant chemotherapy administered systemically or intraarterially may be effective. Palliation of biliary ductal obstruction can be performed by techniques similar to those used for adenocarcinoma, but in general intubational approaches are not to be encouraged since the patients usually survive for long periods and surgical debulking has a clear palliative role even if this is extended to duodeno-pancreatectomy.[109]

In conclusion, palliative therapy in malignant lesions of the pancreas and periampullary area causing obstructive jaundice may be by means of surgical bypass or by means of endoscopic or interventional radiologic intubation. In general, surgical approaches offer excellent relief of symptoms without the need for repeated procedures and are preferable except in patients with carcinoma of the head of the pancreas who are frail and unfit for operation or in whom there are coincident metastases suggesting a short term of survival.

REFERENCES

1. Acosta JM, Ledsesma CL. Gallstone migration as a cause of acute pancreatitis. N Engl J Med 290:484–487, 1974.
2. Afroudakis A, Kaplowitz N. Liver histopathology in chronic common bile duct stenosis due to chronic alcoholic pancreatitis. Hepatology 1:65–72, 1981.
3. Alderson D, Lavelle M, Venables CW. Endoscopic sphincterotomy before pancreatico-duodenectomy for ampullary carcinoma. Br Med J 282:1109–1111, 1981.
4. Alexander F, Rossi RL, O'Brian M, et al. Biliary carcinoma: A review of 109 cases. Am J Surg 147:503–509, 1984.
5. Anderson MC, Stroud WH. Complications of chronic pancreatitis. In: Dent TL, ed. Pancreatic Disease. Diagnosis and Therapy. New York, Grune & Stratton, 1981.
6. Apalakis A, Dussault J, Knight M, Smith R. Relief of pain from pancreatic cancer. Ann R Coll Surg Engl 59:401–403, 1977.
7. Aspestrand F. Angiographic demonstration of simultaneous appearance of cystadenoma and non-functioning insulinoma of the pancreas. Roefo 132:587–588, 1980.
8. Ayella A, Howard J, Grotzinger P. Cystadenoma and cystadenocarcinoma of the pancreas. Am J Surg 103:242–246, 1962.
9. Bagley FH, Braash JW, Taylor RH, Warren KW. Sphincterotomy or sphincteroplasty in the treatment of pathologically mild chronic pancreatitis. Am J Surg 141:418–421, 1981.
10. Barlett MK, Nardi GL. Treatment of recurrent pancreatitis by transduodenal sphincterotomy and exploration of the pancreatic duct. N Engl J Med 262:643–648, 1960.
11. Barton RM, Copeland EM. Carcinoma of the ampulla of Vater. Surg Gynecol Obstet 156:297–301, 1983.
12. Beazley, TM. Needle biopsy of pancreatic cancer. Cancer 47:1685–1687, 1981.
13. Benson R, Gordon W. Cystadenoma of the pancreas. Presentation of one case and review of twenty-eight cases collected from the medical literature. Surgery 21:353–361, 1947.
14. Bernard LJ, Royal JC, Taylor BJ. The surgical management of carcinoma of the pancreas. J Natl Med Assoc 63:37–39, 1971.
15. Blumgart LH. Benign biliary stricture. In: Blumgart LH, ed. Surgery of the Liver and Biliary Tract. Edinburgh, Churchill Livingstone, 1988. Chapter 58.

16. Blumgart LH, Imrie CW, McKay AJ. Surgical management of chronic pancreatitis. J Clin Surg 1:229–235, 1982.
17. Blumgart LH, Kennedy A. Carcinoma of the ampulla of Vater and duodenum. Br J Surg 60:33–40, 1973.
18. Borsch G, Schmidt G, Schafer K, et al. Advanced periampullary carcinoma: Endoscopic palliation by sphincterotomy. South Med J 78:1251–1253, 1985.
19. Bradley EL, Clements JL, Gonzales AC. The natural history of pancreatic pseudocysts: A unified concept of management. Am J Surg 137:135–141, 1979.
20. Bradley EL, Gonzales AC, Clements JL. Acute pancreatic pseudocysts: Incidence and complications. Ann Surg 184:734–737, 1976.
21. Bufkin WJ, Smith PE, Krementz FT. Evaluation of palliative operations for carcinoma of the pancreas. Arch Surg 94:240–242, 1967.
22. Burhans R, Myers RT. Benign neoplasms of the extrahepatic biliary ducts. Am Surg 37:161–168, 1971.
23. Caroli J. Diseases of the intrahepatic biliary tree. Clinc Gastroenterol 2:147–153, 1973.
24. Cattell RB, Pytrek LJ. Premalignant lesions of the ampulla of Vater. Surg Gynecol Obstet 90:21–25, 1950.
25. Cattell RB. Anastomosis of the duct of Wirsung. Surg Clin North Am 27:636–643, 1947.
26. Collure DWD, Burns GP, Schenk WG Jr. Clinical, pathological and therapeutic aspects of carcinoma of the pancreas. Am J Surg 128:683–689, 1974.
27. Compagno J, Oertel J. Microcystic adenomas of the pancreas (glycogen-rich cystadenomas). A clinicopathologic study of 34 cases. Am J Clin Pathol 69:289–298, 1978.
28. Cooper MJ, Williamson RCN, Benjamin IS, et al. Total pancreatectomy for chronic pancreatitis. Br J Surg 74:912–915, 1987.
29. Copping J, Willix R, Kraft R. Palliative chemical splanchniectomy. Arch Surg 98:418–420, 1969.
30. Cornes JJ, Azzopardi JG. Papillary cystadenoma of the pancreas (with report of two cases). Br J Surg 47:139–142, 1959.
31. Cornet A, Debesse B, Barbier J-P, El Hadad A, Carnot F. Les cystadenomes du pancreas. À propos de deux observations. Sem Hop Paris 49:2985–2993, 1975.
32. Cotton PB. Endoscopic methods for relief of malignant obstructive jaundice. World J Surg 8:854–861, 1984.
33. Cullen P, Kemine WH, Dahlin DC. A clinicopathological study of cystadenocarcinoma of the pancreas. Surg Gynecol Obstet 117:189–192, 1963.
34. Delpy JC, Bruneton JN, Aubanel D, Lecomte P. Vaterian duodenal adenomas. Fortschr Rontgenstr 138:623–625, 1983.
35. Di Bisceglie AM, Paterson AC, Segal I. The liver in biliary obstruction due to chronic pancreatitis. Liver 5:189–195, 1985.
36. Diamond D, Fisher B. Pancreatic cancer. Surg Clin North Am 55:363–376, 1975.
37. Doubilet H, and Mulholland JH. Eight-year study of pancreatitis and sphincterotomy. JAMA 160:521–528, 1956.
38. Dreiling DA, Greenstein RJ. State of the art: The sphincter of Oddi, sphincterotomy and biliopancreatic disease. Am J Gastroenterol 72:665–670, 1979.
39. Du Plessis DJ. The palliative operation for obstructive jaundice due to carcinoma of the pancreas. S Afr J Surg 8:11–14, 1970.
40. Eckhauser FE, Knoll JA, Strodel WE, Achem S, Nostrant T. Common bile duct strictures associated with chronic pancreatitis. Am Surg 49:350–358, 1983.
41. Evander A, Ihse I, Lunderquist A, et al. Percutaneous diagnosis of carcinoma of the pancreas and bile duct. Ann Surg 188:90–92, 1978.
42. Feduska MJ, Dent TL, Lindenauer SM. Results of palliative surgery for carcinoma of the pancreas. Arch Surg 103:330–334, 1971.
43. Flanigan DP, Kraft RO. Continuing experience with palliative chemical splanchniectomy. Arch Surg 113:509–511, 1978.
44. Forsgren L, Orell S. Aspiration cytology in carcinoma of the pancreas. Surgery 73:38–42, 1973.

45. Gallitano A, Fransem H, Martin RG. Carcinoma of the pancreas. Cancer 22:939–944, 1968.
46. Gertsch P, Preitner J, Fontolliet C. Carcinome de l'ampoule de Vater et états précurseurs. Schweiz Med Wochenschr 117:1098–1100, 1987.
47. Glenn F, Thorbjanarson B. Carcinoma of the pancreas. Ann Surg 159:945–958, 1964.
48. Gordis L, Gold EB. Epidemiology of pancreatic cancer. World J Surg 8:808–882, 1984.
49. Halsted WS. Contributions to the surgery of the bile passages, especially of the common bile duct. Boston Med Surg J 141:645–654, 1899.
50. Hertzberg J. Pancreatico-duodenal resection and bypass operation in patients with carcinoma of the head of the pancreas, ampulla, and distal end of the common duct. Acta Chir Scand 140:523–527, 1974.
51. Hodgkinson DJ, ReMine WH, Weiland LH. A clinicopathologic study of 21 cases of pancreatic cystadenocarcinoma. Ann Surg 188:679–684, 1978.
52. Hodgkinson D, ReMine W, Weiland L. Pancreatic cystadenoma. A clinicopathologic study of 45 cases. Arch Surg 113:512–519, 1978.
53. Hotfield ARW, Terblanche J, Fataar S, Marks IN. Preoperative external biliary drainage in obstructive jaundice. Lancet 2:896–899, 1982.
54. Howard JM, Jordan GL Jr. Cancer of the pancreas. Curr Probl Cancer, 2:5–52, 1977.
55. Huibregtse K, Katon RM, Tytgat GN. Endoscopic management of biliary and periampullary cancer. In: Blumgart LH, ed. Surgery of the Liver and Biliary Tract. Edinburgh, Churchill Livingstone, 1988,
56. Ihre T, Pyk E, Raaschou-Nielsen T, Seligson U. Percutaneous fine needle aspiration biopsy during endoscopic retrograde cholangiopancreatography. Scand J Gastroenterol 13:657–662, 1978.
57. Ito Y, Blackstone MO, Frank PH, Skinner DB. Mucinous biliary obstruction associated with a cystic adenocarcinoma of the pancreas. Gastroenterology 73:1410–1412, 1977.
58. Johnson RR. Cystadenocarcinoma of the pancreas with staged pancreatoduodenectomy. NY State J Med 74:865–868, 1974.
59. Jones BA, Langer B, Taylor BR, Girotti M. Periampullary tumors: Which ones should be resected? Am J Surg 149:46–52, 1985.
60. Kellum JM, Clark J, Miller HH. Pancreatoduodenectomy for resectable malignant periampullary tumors. Surg Gynecol Obstet 157:363–366, 1983.
61. Knox RA, Kingston RD. Carcinoma of the ampulla of Vater. Br J Surg 73:72–73, 1986.
62. Kozuka S, Tsubone M, Yamagushi A, Hachisuka K. Adenomatous residue in cancerous papilla of Vater. Gut 22:1031–1034, 1981.
63. Legg MA. Brooks JR, eds. Surgery of the Pancreas. Philadelphia, WB Saunders, 1985.
64. Littenberg G, Afroudakis A, Kaplowitz N. Common bile duct stenosis from chronic pancreatitis: A clinical and pathological spectrum. Medicine 58:385–412, 1979.
65. Lygidakis NJ. Biliary stricture as a complication of chronic relapsing pancreatitis. Am J Surg 145:804–806, 1983.
66. Madden JL, Chun JY, Kandalaft S, Parekh M. Choledochoduodenostomy: An unjustly maligned surgical procedure. Am J Surg 119:45–54, 1970.
67. McConnel DB, Gregory JR, Sasaki TM. Pancreatic pseudocyst. Am J Surg 143:599–601, 1982.
68. McPherson GAD, Benjamin IS, Habib NA. Percutaneous trans-hepatic drainage in obstructive jaundice: Advantages and problems. Br J Surg 69:261–264, 1982.
69. McPherson GAD, Benjamin IS, Hodgson HJF, et al. Pre-operative percutaneous transhepatic biliary drainage. The results of a controlled trial. Br J Surg 71:371–375, 1984.
70. Meinke WB, Twomey PL, Guernsey JM, et al. Gastric outlet obstruction after palliative surgery for cancer of the head of the pancreas. Arch Surg 118:550–553, 1983.
71. Monge JJ. Survival of patients with small carcinomas of the head of the pancreas: Biliary intestinal bypass vs pancreaticoduodenectomy. Ann Surg 166:908–912, 1967.

72. Monzan A. Cystadenoma of the pancreas. Am J Surg 81:204–214, 1951.
73. Moossa AR. Surgical treatment of chronic pancreatitis: An overview. Br J Surg 74:661–667, 1987.
74. Morgenstern L, Shore JM. Selection of an optimal procedure for decompression of the obstructed common bile duct. Am J Surg 119:38–43, 1970.
75. Musgrove JE, Grindlay JH, Karlson AG. Intestinal-biliary reflux after anastomosis of common duct to duodenum or jejunum. Arch Surg 91:579–589, 1952.
76. Nakase A, Matsumoto Y, Uchida K, Honjo I. Surgical treatment of cancer of the pancreas and the peri-ampullary region. Cummulative results in 57 institutions in Japan. Ann Surg 185:52–57, 1977.
77. Newmann RJ, Pittam MR. Local excision in the treatment of carcinoma of the ampulla of Vater. J R Coll Surg Edinb 27:154–157, 1982.
78. Opie EL. The etiology of acute hemorrhagic pancreatitis. Johns Hopkins Med J 12:182–186, 1901.
79. Persaund V. Carcinoid tumor and cystadenoma of the pancreas. Arch Pathol 92:28–30, 1971.
80. Pitt HA, Gomes AS, Lois JF, et al. Does preoperative percutaneous biliary drainage reduce operative risk or increase hospital cost? Ann Surg 201:9–16, 1985.
81. Pope NA, Fisch JC. Palliative surgery for carcinoma of the pancreas. Am J Surg 121:271–272, 1971.
82. Porter EA. Carcinoma of the pancreas. NZ Med J 71:288–292, 1970.
83. Probstein J, Blumenthal H. Progressive malignant degeneration of cystadenoma of the pancreas. Arch Surg 81:683–689, 1960.
84. Remigio P. Pancreatic cystadenoma and biliary tract disease. Am J Gastroenterol 54:603–608, 1970.
85. Richards AB, Sosin H. Cancer of the pancreas: The value of radical and palliative surgery. Ann Surg 177:325–331, 1973.
86. Robertson JFR, Imrie CW, Hole DJ, Carter DC, Blumgart LH. Management of periampullary carcinoma. Br J Surg 74:816–819, 1987.
87. Ryan DP, Shapiro RH, Warshaw AL. Villous tumors of the duodenum. Ann Surg 203:301–306, 1986.
88. Safrany L. Palliative endoscopic therapy of ampullary cancer. Gastrointest Endosc 26:77, 1980.
89. Salmon PR. Interventional endoscopy surgery of the liver and biliary tract. In: Blumgart LH, ed. Surgery of the Liver and Biliary Tract. Edinburgh, Churchill Livingstone, 1988, pp 467–472.
90. Sarles H, Sahel J. Cholestasis and lesions of the biliary tract in chronic pancreatitis. Gut 19:851–857, 1978.
91. Sarles H, Sarles JC, Camatte R, et al. Observations on 205 confirmed cases of acute pancreatitis, recurring pancreatitis, and chronic pancreatitis. Gut 6:545–549, 1965.
92. Sarr MG, Cameron JL. Surgical palliation of unresectable carcinoma of the pancreas. World J Surg 8:906–918, 1984.
93. Sarr MG, Gladen HF, Beat RW, Van Heerden JA. Role of gastroenterostomy in patients with unresectable pancreatic carcinoma. Surg Gynecol Obstet 152:597–600, 1981.
94. Sarre RG, Frost AG, Jagelman DG, et al. Gastric and duodenal polyps in familial adenomatous polyposis: A prospective study of the nature and prevalence of upper gastrointestinal polyps. Gut 28:306–314, 1987.
95. Sawyer K, Spencer R, Lubchenco A. Proliferative cysts of the pancreas. Ann Surg 135:548–554, 1952.
96. Schulman AG, Lippman RW, Miller W. Internal drainage of malignant pancreatic cysts as an effective palliative procedure. Am J Surg 102:470–472, 1961.
97. Schulze S, Baden P, Brandenhoff P, et al. Pancreatic pseudocysts during first attack of acute pancreatitis. Scand J Gastroenterol 21:1221–1223, 1986.
98. Sidel VW, Wilson RE, Shipp JC. Pseudocyst formation in chronic pancreatitis: A cause of obstructive jaundice. Arch Surg 77:933–939.

99. Siegel JH, Snady H. The significance of endoscopically placed prostheses in the management of biliary obstruction due to carcinoma of the pancreas: Results of nonoperative decompression in 277 patients. Am J Gastroenterol 81:634–641, 1986.
100. Soehendra N, Reynders-Frederix V. Palliative Gallengangsdrainage. Eine neue Methode zur endoskopischen Einführung eines inneren Drains. Dtsch Med Wochenschr 104:206–207, 1979.
101. Solway H. Constitutional abnormalities associated with pancreatic cystadenomas. Cancer 18:1297–1300, 1965.
102. Spohn K, Fux HD, Tewew G, Hahn K. Das Pankreas-Carcinom, palliative Operationen. Langenbecks Arch Chir 339:267–273, 1975.
103. Stabile BE, Wilson SE, Passaro E. Stricture of the common bile duct from chronic pancreatitis. Surg Gynecol Obstet 165:121–126, 1987.
104. Stone HH, Strom PR, Mullins RJ. Pancreatic abscess management by subtotal resection and packing. World J Surg 8:340–345, 1984.
105. Strodel WE, Eckhauser FE. Cystic neoplasms of the pancreas. In: Dent TL, ed. Pancreatic Disease. Diagnosis and Therapy. New York, Grune & Stratton, 1981, pp 363–377.
106. Stuart M, Keo T, Hermann RE, Hoerr SO. Palliation of malignant obstruction of the common bile duct by side to side choledochoduodenostomy. Am J Surg 121:505–509, 1971.
107. Sugerman HJ, Barnhart GR, Newsome HH. Selective drainage for pancreatic, biliary, and duodenal obstruction secondary to chronic fibrosing pancreatitis. Ann Surg 203:558–567, 1986.
108. Sugihara K, Muto T, Kamiya J, et al. Gardner's syndrome associated with periampullary carcinoma, duodenal and gastric adenomatosis. Dis Colon Rectum 25:766–771, 1982.
109. Thompson NW, Eckhauser FE. Malignant islet-cell tumors of the pancreas. World J Surg 8:940–951, 1984.
110. Thompson NW, Eckhauser FE, Vinik AI, et al. Cystic neuroendocrine neoplasms of the pancreas and liver. Ann Surg 199:158–164, 1984.
111. Warren KW, Choe DS, Plaza J, Relihan M. Results of radical resection for periampullary cancer. Ann Surg 181:534–540, 1975.
112. Warren KW, Braasch JW, Thum CW. Carcinoma of the pancreas. Surg Clin North Am 48:601–618, 1968.
113. Warren KW, Braasch JW, Thum CW. Diagnosis and surgical treatment of carcinoma of the pancreas. Curr Probl Surg 6:3–70, 1968.
114. Warshaw AL, Rattner DW. Facts and fallacies of common bile duct obstruction by pancreatic pseudocysts. Ann Surg 192:33–37, 1980.
115. Warshaw AL, Rutledge PL. Cystic tumors mistaken for pancreatic pseudocysts. Ann Surg 205:393–398, 1987.
116. Warshaw AL, Schapiro RH, Ferrucci JT, Galbadini J. Persistent obstructive jaundice, cholangitis, and biliary cirrhosis due to common bile duct stenosis in chronic pancreatitis. Gastroenterology 70:562–565, 1976.
117. Weinbren HK, Hadjis NS, Blumgart LH. Structural aspects of the liver in patients with biliary diseases and portal hypertension. J Clin Pathol 38:1013–1020, 1985.
118. Whipple AD, Parsons WB, Mullins CR. Treatment of carcinoma of the ampulla of Vater. Ann Surg 102:763–779, 1935.
119. White TT, Murat J, Morgan A. The immediate surgical management of a mass in the head of the pancreas. Northwest Med 67:731–734, 1968.
120. Wisloff F, Jakobsen J, Osnes M. Stenosis of the common bile duct in chronic pancreatitis. Gut 19:851–857, 1978.
121. Wong J, Kim STK, Lam KH, Ong GB. Unresectable malignant obstruction of the bile ducts. Aust NZ J Surg 48:503–509, 1978.
122. Yadegar J, Williams RA, Passaro E, et al. Common duct stricture from chronic pancreatitis. Arch Surg 115:582–586, 1980.
123. Yamaguchi K, Enjoji M. Cystic neoplasms of the pancreas. Gastroenterology 92:1934–1943, 1987.

CHAPTER

23

PALLIATIVE MANAGEMENT OF LESIONS OF THE PANCREAS CAUSING BILIARY OBSTRUCTION

David S. Zimmon

ENDOSCOPIC OVERVIEW

Endoscopic retrograde cholangiopancreatography (ERCP) allows the precise delineation of pancreatic and biliary anatomy at a level of accuracy not yet possible with other imaging techniques. Since the papilla of Vater is approached through the mouth and gastrointestinal tract lumen, the morbidity is relatively low. The painless procedure is often performed on an ambulatory basis. Radiographic visualization of the pancreatic duct differentiates pancreatic adenocarcinoma from pancreatitis and other periampullary cancers when imaging by ultrasonography, computed tomography (CT), magnetic resonance imaging, and angiography are negative or not decisive.[35]

Both pathologic and anatomic differentiation of periampullary and more proximal bile duct cancer from extension of pancreatic cancer is essential to plan appropriate therapy. Patients with cancer of the terminal bile duct or papilla of Vater with appropriate histopathologic lesions and the absence of visible dissemination in the duodenum may be submitted to local excision or radical resection.[15] Endoscopic local excision with combined intraluminal and external radiation therapy is an important low-risk alternative to surgery in selected patients.[20] Carcinoma of the duodenum is unlikely to be resected successfully.[4] Local endoscopic laser therapy is palliative.

Overall, 95% of patients with adenocarcinoma of the pancreatic head presenting as bile duct obstruction are not resectible for cure at the time of diagnosis.[9] Even when all imaging methods fail to reveal metastasis, at least 50% of patients show intraabdominal dissemination at laparoscopy.[5] Furthermore, some of these intraabdominal metastases would have been missed for resection at laparotomy because of their location under the liver, on the under surface of the diaphragm, or deep in the pelvis.[33] Therefore, more than 95% of patients with adenocarcinoma of the pancreas and bile duct obstruction are candidates for palliative endoscopic management of bile duct obstruction, since "cure" by resection is impossible.

THE PROBLEM

The cause of this dismal prognosis in adenocarcinoma of ductal origin is the intrinsic aggressive nature of the majority of these cancers and the small duct system where they originate. Since the pancreas has no serosa, extension through the duct wall into the pancreatic parenchyma is tantamount to dissemination.[29] Therefore, only pancreatitis or pain arising from duct obstruction, in the absence of extension beyond the duct, might be considered early (i.e., predissemination) symptoms. In view of the rapid growth of these cancers,[27] identifying a patient at this early stage when other imaging modalities yield a presumptive diagnosis of pancreatitis by failing to document a mass would require prompt ERCP.[24,32] Even this vigorous early diagnostic approach is unlikely to change the results of surgical therapy, as implantation of tumor by aspiration biopsy[7,14] or percutaneous stents that penetrate biliary mucosa is well documented. On the other hand, a few fortunate individuals survive with a localized tumor[22] after palliative surgical resection or without therapy.[8] Unknown biological determinants appear to dominate prognosis for adenocarcinoma of the pancreas.

PATIENT SELECTION

Jaundice accompanying carcinoma of the pancreas is a multifactoral sign. Approximately 75% of patients who have technically successful biliary decompression do not have complete resolution of jaundice.[2] Imaging methods do not identify the most unfavorable 50% of patients who fail to respond to biliary decompression and have an 88% 30-day operative mortality.[25] Some 25% of patients have partial resolution of jaundice and gain from reduced pruritus and improved digestion. Thus, of patients who have successful biliary decompression, only 25% could be considered for surgical resection if resolution of jaundice were a prerequisite. Identifying this relatively favorable 25% of patients is the burden of nonsurgical therapy of bile duct obstruction arising from cancer of the pancreatic head. On examination, this group contains patients with mid and proximal bile duct obstruction as well as metastases that preclude surgical resection. The remainder would be reduced by at least 50% if laparoscopic examination were used to demonstrate intraabdominal dissemination.[33] If all of these criteria for operability were met, less than 5% of patients with adenocarcinoma of the pancreas would be candidates for surgery. Consequently, 95% are candidates for nonoperative palliation of bile duct obstruction.

CLINICAL STAGING

Bile duct obstruction from carcinoma of the pancreas is a complex clinical entity. The sign of jaundice may result from a minute (less than 1 cm) tumor with adjacent pancreatitis that is invisible by CT scan or demonstrates only a vague enlargement of the head of the pancreas or a huge tumor mass invading the porta hepatis with gross hepatic metastasis and obstruction of the duodenum. This diversity of presentation and the often rapid progression are responsible for the dismal results of therapy. Clinical staging by endoscopy, direct cholangiography (ERCP or percutaneous transhepatic cholangiography [PTC]), a trial of nonsurgical biliary decompression, and laparoscopy is essential prior to laparotomy or attempted resection. External biliary drainage is not satisfactory since malabsorption, immunologic competence, and reticuloendothelial function are regained only after restoration of bile flow to the gut.[28,30] Brief trials of external biliary drainage are of little value except to demonstrate that jaundice will respond, in part, to decompression and is not the result of advanced disease. Undoubtedly, in adenocarcinoma of the pancreas, a delay prior to resection might allow substantial tumor growth and perhaps dissemination. This is the conundrum of pancreatic adenocarcinoma. Attempted resection without staging must carry a high risk since 95% of patients are unresectable and occult dissemination is present in 50% of patients after a complete imaging evaluation proves negative.[33]

THE PATIENT'S VIEWPOINT

One to 3 months of vague premonitory abdominal or constitutional symptoms precede the first visit to a physician. Irritable bowel syndrome or ulcer is usually presumed and often treated empirically. Hepatitis that will resolve is a common initial diagnosis followed by a period of delay. Identification of a dilated biliary tree or fever raises the issue of stones or tumor.[27] Pity the 30% of female or 10% of male patients over age 60 who have cholelithiasis and are submitted to a simple biliary operation only to find their life expectancy is 6 months or less. If the correct diagnosis is suspected, by the time the patient recovers from the palliative diagnostic laparotomy, pancreatic cancer has tightened its grip and there are few good days remaining. A substantial number never leave the hospital, as laparotomy for exploration and bypass carries a 20% to 30% 30-day mortality.[6]

Patients are rarely referred to a surgeon with sufficient experience in the 10% mortality, high-morbidity pancreatic resection.[17] Furthermore, the operation has probably been delayed too long to be of value because of the patient's reluctance to consult a physician and the initial methodical evaluation. Additional impediment to prompt resectional surgery for the 5% in whom it might be appropriate is the necessity of obtaining informed consent for high-risk surgery without a substantiated diagnosis. In my opinion, percutaneous aspiration biopsy should not be performed if curative surgery is contemplated, since dissemination by the needle track is well documented. ERCP with pancreatography and cholangiography to exclude pancreatitis and other periampullary neoplasms and provide complete definition of preoperative gastric, duodenal, biliary, and pancreatic anatomy is essential.[32]

In the occasional patient it is impossible to differentiate localized pancreatitis with bile duct compression from pancreatic cancer. I suggest treatment to relieve obstruction and pain with biliary and pancreatic stents as indicated, then laparoscopy to show intraabdominal dissemination and seek a positive biopsy. If laparoscopy is negative, the ERCP should be repeated in 4 to 6 weeks to reevaluate progression. In the absence of progression, reevaluation should be done in 6 months. If progression suggests pancreatic cancer, the physician should consider resection but remember that the operative mortality is 10%, the morbidity substantial, and the long-term salvage similar to that for no therapy (1% 5-year survival).[26] Is the initial cost of surgery in terms of mortality and lost good time worth a rare good result? Only the patient can decide.

TECHNICAL CONSIDERATIONS

The palliation of bile duct obstruction resulting from malignant or benign pancreatic disease is mechanically straightforward.[34] A biliary stent or stents is passed through the obstructed segment.[11] The endoscopic retrograde approach is preferred since it is painless[12,19,23] and of low risk.[3,31] It also provides the diagnostic yield of ERCP in differentiating benign disease from periampullary neoplasia[15,16] and visualizing the pancreatic duct as well as an opportunity to place the pancreatic stents for pain relief in benign pancreatic disease.[36]

If the bile duct obstruction cannot be passed by the retrograde endoscopic route or cannot be serviced because of actual or incipient duodenal disease (edema, ulceration, compression), the percutaneous route is utilized.[1] Endoscopic evaluation of the duodenum showing a large ulcerating neoplastic mass in a good-risk patient is a strong indication for laparotomy with combined duodenal and biliary bypass. Where the patient's condition does not allow laparotomy, a percutaneous gastrostomy with a tube passed through the duodenum into the jejunum maintains a lumen at least for liquids. Alternatively, when duodenal obstruction is complete and cannot be traversed, a percutaneous gastrostomy for gastric decompression may be combined with a percutaneous transhepatic bile-duct-to-jejunal feeding tube. This is placed beside the biliary stent and allows enteral nutritional support and administration of pain medication. In fact, a major indication for biliary stents is to counter the malabsorption of total biliary tract obstruction.

Benign inflammatory stenosis of the bile duct resulting from pancreatitis is readily managed by stent insertion for a period of 6 months to 1 year. The stent is then removed, and the lumen generally remains patent.[10] The confounding problems of hemobilia, intractable infection, and proximal progression of adenocarcinoma are absent. Long-term follow-up (10 years) is lacking, but the simplicity, low risk, effectiveness, and repeatability of biliary endoprosthesis insertion in these patients renders surgical alternatives obsolete.

Technical success for placement of endoscopic biliary prosthesis in experienced hands is approximately 85% in cancer patients.[18] The remainder are managed by placing a percutaneous transhepatic 480-cm wire guide into the duodenum when appropriate for endoscopic therapy. The wire is grasped endoscopically and brought out of the patient's mouth. The endoscope is then repassed into the duodenum with the guide wire within the instrument channel. With the endoscope used as an overtube, the stenosis can be dilated with teflon dilators and a stent(s) used. This combined technique limits the hepatic trauma, risk, and pain of manipulating large transhepatic dilators and stents.[21] With the endoscopic route, in most cases, the patient is ambulatory throughout and may be dismissed immediately after stent insertion. In complex cases with proximal bile duct obstruction by cancer, use of combined percutaneous and endoscopic methods allows placement of stents in the three major hepatic ducts when necessary. Technical success of endoscopic stents for benign bile duct obstruction is greater than 90%.

CONCLUSIONS

The rapid evolution of endoscopic and percutaneous nonoperative methods for the management of bile duct obstruction associated with pancreatic disease has made laparotomy unnecessary unless an additional goal of benefit to the patient is apparent. The staging of these complex diseases by laparotomy rarely allows informed consent on the part of the patient or performance of the preferred operation by the surgeon. Since dissemination and unresectability is present in 95% of patients with adenocarcinoma of the pancreas at the time of diagnosis and median life expectancy is only 6 months, surgical palliation with its pain, cost, and obligatory convalescence should be reserved for the special case in which gastroenterostomy for duodenal obstruction is required or recurrent bleeding and cholangitis with stent obstruction force hepatojejunostomy. Careful evaluation of each patient requires cholangiopancreatography, inspection of the duodenum, and laparoscopy to establish a precise anatomic and histopathologic diagnosis if resection is considered seriously. With this information in hand, the appropriate individualized care required for this terrible disease may be provided.

REFERENCES

1. Brambs HJ, Billman P, Pausch J, Hostege A, Salm R. Non-surgical biliary drainage: Endoscopic conversion of percutaneous transhepatic into endoprosthetic drainage. Endoscopy 18:52–54, 1986.
2. Burcharth F. Nonsurgical drainage of the biliary tract. Semin Liver Dis 2:275–286, 1982.
3. Carasco CH, Zamoza J, Bechtel WJ. Malignant biliary obstruction: Complications of percutaneous drainage. Radiology 152:343–346, 1984.
4. Cooperman A. Periampullary cancer, 1983. Seminars in liver disease 3:181–192, 1983.
5. Cuschiera A, Hall AW, Clark J. Value of laparoscopy in the diagnosis and management of pancreatic carcinoma. Gut 19:672–677, 1987.
6. Feduska NJ, Dent TL, Lindenauer SM. Results of palliative operations for carcinoma of the pancreas. Arch Surg 103:330–334, 1971.
7. Ferrucci JT Jr, Wittenbert J, Margolies MN, Carey RW. Malignant seeding of the tract after thin-needle aspiration biopsy. Radiology 130:345–346, 1979.
8. Gudjonsson B, Livstone E, Spiro HM. Cancer of the pancreas. Cancer 42:2494–2506, 1978.

9. Herman RE, Cooperman AM. Cancer of the pancreas. N Engl J Med 301:482–485, 1979.
10. Huibregtse K, Katon RM, Tytgat GN. Endoscopic treatment of postoperative biliary strictures. Endoscopy 4:133–137, 1986.
11. Huibregtse K, Katon RM, Coene PP, et al. Endoscopic palliative treatment of pancreatic cancer. Gastrointest Endosc 32:334–338, 1986.
12. Jaques PF, Mandel VS, Delany DJ, Nath PH. Percutaneous transhepatic biliary drainage: Advantages of the left-lobe subxiphoid approach. Radiology 145:534–536, 1982.
13. Kerlan RK, Ring EJ, Pogony AC, Jeffrey RB. Biliary endoprosthesis insertion using a combined peroral-transhepatic method. Radiology 150:828–830, 1984.
14. Kim WS, Barth KH, Zinner M. Seeding of pancreatic carcinoma along the transhepatic catheter tract. Radiology 143:427–428, 1982.
15. Knox RA, Kingston RD. Carcinoma of the ampulla of Vater. Br J Surg 73:72–73, 1986.
16. Leese R. Pseudotumor of the papilla of Vater. Gut 27:1186–1192, 1986.
17. LaFerla G, Murray WR. Carcinoma of the head of the pancreas: Bypass surgery in unresectable disease. Br J Surg 74:212–213, 1987.
18. Marks WM, Freeny PC, Kosarek RA, Ball TJ. Endoscopic retrograde biliary drainage: An alternate method of drainage. Semin Intervent Radiol 2:74–80, 1985.
19. Mendez G Jr, Russell E, LePage JR, et al. Abandonment of endoprosthetic drainage technic in malignant biliary obstruction. AJR 143:617–622, 1984.
20. Molt P, Hopfan S, Watson RC, Botet JF, Brennan MF. Intraluminal radiation therapy in the management of malignant biliary obstruction. Cancer 57:536–544, 1986.
21. Mueller PR, Ferrucci JT, Teplick SK, et al. Biliary stent endoprosthesis: Analysis of complications in 113 patients. Radiology 156:637–639, 1985.
22. Nagai H, Kuroda A, Morioka Y. Lymphatic and local spread of T1 and T2 pancreatic cancer. Ann Surg 65–71, 1986.
23. Neff CC, Mueller PR, Ferruci JT, et al. Serious complications following transgression of the pleural space in drainage procedures. Radiology 152:335–341, 1984.
24. Neff CC, Sineone JF, Wittenberg J, Mueller PR, Ferrucci JT Jr. Inflammatory pancreatic masses. Radiology 150:35–38, 1984.
25. Neff RA, Frankuchen EJ, Cooperman AM, et al. The radiological management of malignant bile obstruction. Clin Radiol 34:143–146, 1983.
26. Nix GAJJ, Schmitz PI, Wilson OH, et al. Carcinoma of the head of the pancreas. Gastroenterology 87:37–43, 1984.
27. Okuda C, Tsuchiya Y, Ohto M. Percutaneous transhepatic cholangiography and its relevant techniques. In: Kawai K, ed. Early diagnosis of Pancreatic Cancer. Tokyo, New York, Igaku-Shoin, 1980, pp 164–174.
28. Pitt H, Cameron JL, Postier RG, Gadacz TR. Factors affecting mortality in biliary tract surgery. Am J Surg 141:66–72, 1981.
29. Shirakabe H. Foreward in Early Diagnosis of Pancreatic Cancer ed K. Kawai Igaku-Shoin, Tokyo-New York 1980.
30. Smith RC, Pooley M, George CR, et al. Preoperative percutaneous transhepatic internal drainage in obstructive jaundice: A randomized controlled trial examining renal function. Surgery 97:641–647, 1985.
31. Speer AG, Cotton PB, Russell RCG, et al. Randomized trial of endoscopic vs. percutaneous stent insertion in malignant obstructive jaundice. Lancet 2:57–62, 1987.
32. Stadelmann O, Safrany L, Loffler A, et al. Endoscopic retrograde cholangiography in the diagnosis of pancreatic cancer. Endoscopy 6:84–93, 1974.
33. Warshaw A. Laparoscopy in carcinoma of the pancreas. Am J Surg 151:76–80, 1986.
34. Zimmon DS. New uses of endoscopic retrograde cholangiopancreatography in the management of biliary tract and pancreatic disease. In: Jerzy Glass GB, Sherlock P, eds. Progress in Gastroenterology. Grune & Stratton, 1983, pp 477–504.
35. Zimmon, DS. Gastrointestinal endoscopy in the diagnosis and management of hepatobiliary disease. In: Schiff L, Schiff ER, eds. Diseases of the Liver. Philadelphia, JB Lippincott, 1987, pp 311–340.
36. Zimmon DS, Clemmett AR. Endoscopic stents and drains in the management of pancreatic and bile duct obstruction. Surg Clin North Am 62:837–844, 1982.

CHAPTER

24

THE ROLE OF RESECTION IN THE MANAGEMENT OF PANCREATIC CANCER

Henry A. Pitt and Pierce A. Grace

EDITORIAL COMMENT

We agree with the authors' statement that for patients with cancer of the head of the pancreas, resection remains the only modality of treatment offering the possibility of cure. Tumors of the body and tail are rarely resectable and almost never curable. Indeed, for lesions in the head over 90% are unresectable because of local or distant spread, and the mainstay of treatment is palliation of biliary and gastric obstruction and pain.

The mortality of the Whipple procedure in experienced hands is now around 2% to 3%, and in a small number of recent series the 5-year survivorship lies between 15% and 18%. These results should promote cautious optimism. It is not clear whether the improvement lies in the lesser surgical mortality, better pre- and postoperative care, the use of postoperative radiotherapy, or perhaps the inclusion of some periampullary tumors. The more extensive resections such as Fortner's regional pancreatectomy and total pancreatectomy have not been justified by the results and are unlikely to receive routine acceptance.

CONTROVERSY

The controversial role of radical resection in pancreatic cancer stems from the almost universally dismal results even in carefully selected patients. Some physicians maintain that resection should not be considered a therapeutic option and that similar or better results can be obtained by palliative bypass procedures. This chapter looks at the role of resection and the place of more extensive procedures and adjuvant therapy.

The incidence of carcinoma of the pancreas has increased[13,67] and now represents 10% of all gastrointestinal neoplasms.[54] Adenocarcinoma of the pancreas remains a disease that is difficult to diagnose and unsatisfactory to treat.[42] While only 10% to 20% of patients with carcinoma of the head of the pancreas are found to be resectable at the time of laparotomy,[27,60,80,85] resection remains the only modality of treatment offering the possibility of cure. Older reports documented high mortality and morbidity rates following pancreaticoduodenectomy.[65,82] More recent advances in diagnostic techniques and improvements in operative and perioperative management have lessened the risk of pancreatic resection.[9,15,40,60,119] Controversy, still exists, however, regarding the philosophy of management of patients with pancreatic cancer.

Three different approaches to the management of patients with pancreatic carcinoma have been advocated. Trede has characterized these philosophies as "nihilism, activism, and realism."[120] The nihilistic view is that high operative mortality and morbidity and poor long-term survival rates preclude radical resection for pancreatic cancer. Therefore, the nihilists advocate palliation even for potentially curable lesions.[19] The activists, adhering to the Halstedian philosophy of achieving a cancer cure by more radical resections, recommend extensive regional pancreatectomy whenever possible.[29] The realists argue that pancreatic resection can now be undertaken with an acceptably low mortality and morbidity[39,40,119] and that an occasional patient with carcinoma of the head of the pancreas is cured by resection. Moreover, the duration and quality of palliation are improved and the chance of resecting a more favorable periampullary malignancy is not overlooked.[70] Therefore, the realists advocate exploration for selected patients with tumors that appear resectable.[40,71] The purpose of this review is to discuss the role of resection in the management of patients with pancreatic cancer with particular reference to newer diagnostic and operative techniques as well as adjuvant therapies.

HISTORICAL ASPECTS

At the Congress de Paris in 1900, Mayo-Robson credited Billroth with having removed the entire pancreas from a patient in 1884 because of its involvement in a growth. The patient was said to have survived, although no operative details were available.[106] Sauve in 1908 collected the reports of 11 patients who had undergone various operations on the pancreas.[106] Included in this report was a procedure attributed to Codvilla, which was performed in 1898. Finding a cancer in the head of the pancreas and involving the duodenum, Codvilla resected en bloc the head of the pancreas, a major portion of the duodenum, and the pyloric end of the stomach. He reestablished alimentary continuity with a Roux en Y gastroenterostomy, and a cholecystoenterostomy was performed with a Murphy button. The patient survived for 24 days but died with progressive cachexia and glycosuria.

In 1912 Kausch[62] in Germany performed a successful two-stage partial pancreatectomy, while in 1922 Tenani[113] in Italy also undertook a successful two-stage resection of the proximal portion of the head of the pancreas with a segment of the duodenum. The modern era of pancreatic surgery, however, was initiated by Whipple and his colleagues[132] in 1935 with their report of a successful, two-stage radical en block resection of the head of the pancreas and duodenum.

Whipple's Original Operation

Whipple in his original report described a radical en block excision of an ampullary tumor by a two-stage procedure.[132] In the first stage, the patient underwent a gastrojejunostomy, ligation of the distal common bile duct, and cholecystogastrostomy (Fig. 24-1). In the second stage, an en block excision of the second part of the duodenum including the ampulla of Vater, the lower common bile duct, and surrounding portion of the head of the pancreas was performed. The cut end of the pancreatic duct was ligated, and the pancreatic stump was sutured with interrupted fine silk sutures (Fig. 24-1).

This procedure, while initially successful, was associated with a number of complications that rapidly led to further modifications. Ascending cholangitis due to narrowing of the cholecystogastrostomy stoma and the passage of infected material into the gallbladder was soon recognized.[131] Thus, in 1937, Brunschwig replaced the cholecystogastrostomy with a cholecystojejunostomy.[11] Brunschwig was also the first to report a successful pancreaticoduodenectomy for carcinoma of the head of the pancreas.

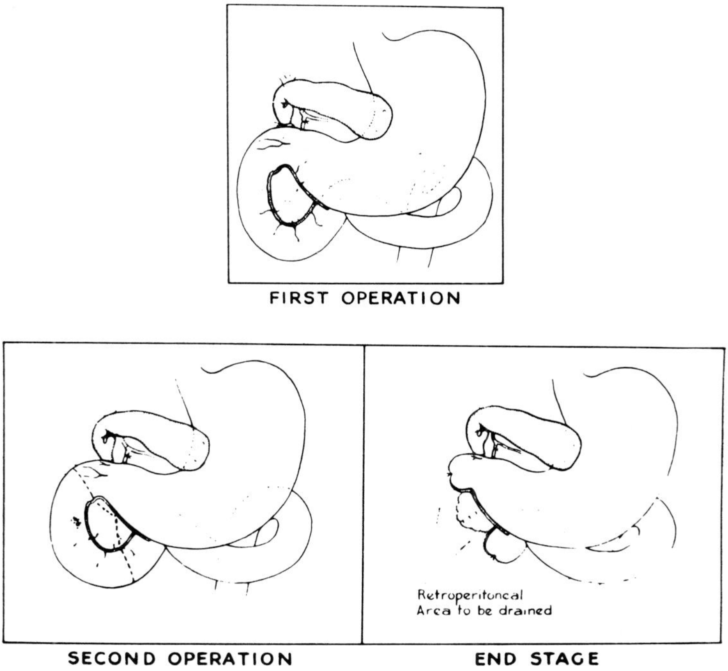

Figure 24-1. Whipple's original operation was performed in two stages. The first operation included a cholecystogastrostomy and a gastrojejunostomy. The second operation consisted of local resection of the pancreatic head with oversewing of the pylorus, pancreas, and duodenum (end stage).

Biliary fistula was also a frequent occurrence following the original Whipple procedure.[121,131] This problem was due to the breakdown of the closure used to tie off the distal common bile duct. Recognition of this problem led both Trimble et al.[121] and Whipple[131] to simultaneously advocate choledochojejunostomy. Trimble also proposed resection of the distal stomach and the creation of a gastrojejunostomy. This modification eliminated the suture line in the proximal duodenum, a potential source of leakage. Both Trimble et al. and Whipple felt that this modified procedure could be performed safely as a one-stage operation, and in 1941 they independently reported successful one-stage radical pancreaticoduodenectomies.[121,131]

Trimble's Operation

In Trimble's operation, the first and second portions of the duodenum together with the pyloric end of the stomach, the distal end of the common bile duct, and the head of the pancreas were resected en masse (Fig. 24-2).[121] Alimentary continuity was achieved by a Polya antecolic gastrojejunostomy. The stump of the common duct was inserted into the jejunum 20 cm distal to the gastrojejunostomy, and the cut surface of the pancreas was transfixed with catgut sutures.

In light of subsequent experience, it is interesting to note that on the 16th postoperative day, Trimble's first patient developed a severe upper gastrointestinal hemorrhage that responded to conservative management. Warren in 1957 noted the development of three jejunal ulcers in 23 patients,[126] and in 1967 Warren et al. reported the occurrence of jejunal ulcers in 7.5% of patients following pancreaticoduodenectomy.[128] This experience led him to advocate high gastric resection or vagotomy when undertaking pancreaticoduodenectomy.

In the early pancreaticoduodenectomies the pancreatic stump was universally ligated and oversewn.[11,121,131,132] In 1941 Hunt introduced pancreaticojejunostomy, arguing that this procedure was safer and physiologically more acceptable than pancreatic stump ligation.[56] In 1948 Cattell reported a two-layer anastomosis of the pancreatic stump to the jejunum using the pancreatic duct as an inner layer surrounded by an outer serosal muscularis capsular suture.[14] He suggested that this type of anastomosis was suitable for a firm pancreas with a dilated duct. However, for soft glands with small ducts, he believed that the end of the pancreas should be inserted into the open end of the jejunum, the so-called dunking procedure. Such an anastomosis was originally described by Desjardins in 1907.[21] Recently, pancreaticogastrostomy has also been advocated as a method for dealing with the pancreatic stump.[26,76]

Current Whipple Operation

The acceptance of the various modifications described above has resulted in the evolution of the current standard ''Whipple'' operation. In this procedure, the head and uncinate process of the pancreas are resected together with the sur-

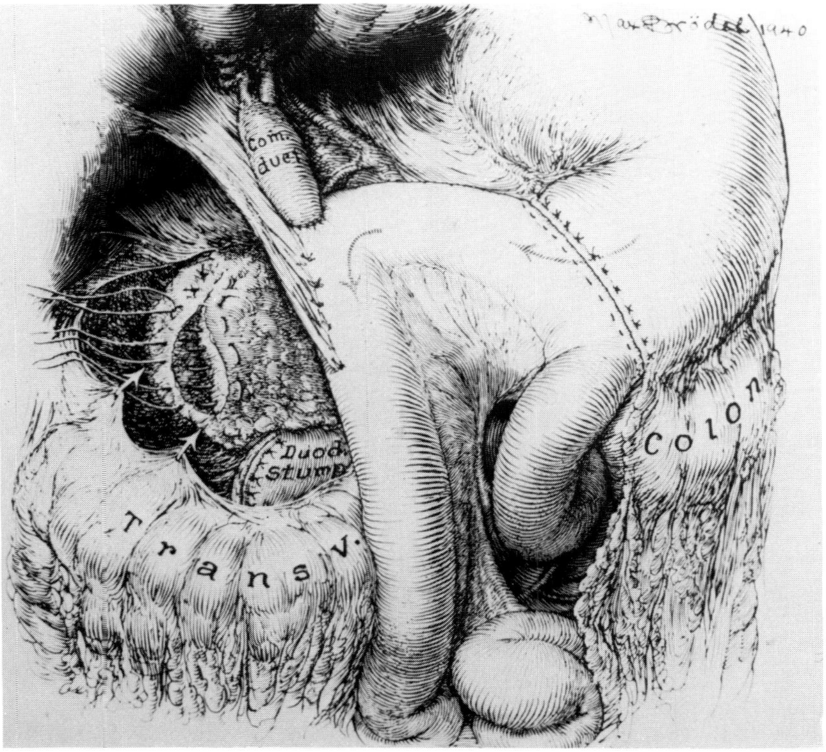

Figure 24-2. Trimble's operation was a one-stage procedure. The antrum of the stomach, pancreatic head, duodenum, and gallbladder were removed. Reconstruction consisted of a gastrojejunostomy, a choledochojejunostomy, and oversewing of the pancreatic stump. (From Trimble et al.[121] with permission.)

rounding duodenum, lower end of the common bile duct, gallbladder, and distal stomach with or without the addition of a truncal vagotomy. Reconstruction is achieved by (1) mucosa-to-mucosa or dunking pancreatojejunostomy with or without stenting, (2) end-to-side choledochojejunostomy, and (3) antecolic gastrojejunostomy (Fig. 24-3).

While a 50% to 70% gastrectomy is now customarily performed during pancreatoduodenectomy, Watson, as early as 1944, argued that preservation of the intact stomach and pylorus would facilitate digestion, improve the patient's nutrition status, and prevent the formation of jejunal ulceration.[130] Similarly, Traverso and Longmire in 1978 argued that removal of the pylorus might predispose the patient to postgastrectomy symptoms of dumping, diarrhea, or dyspepsia, and the risks of jejunal ulceration.[117] Their report of the pylorus-preserving pancreaticoduodenectomy in 1978 heralded a new era in pancreatic surgery.

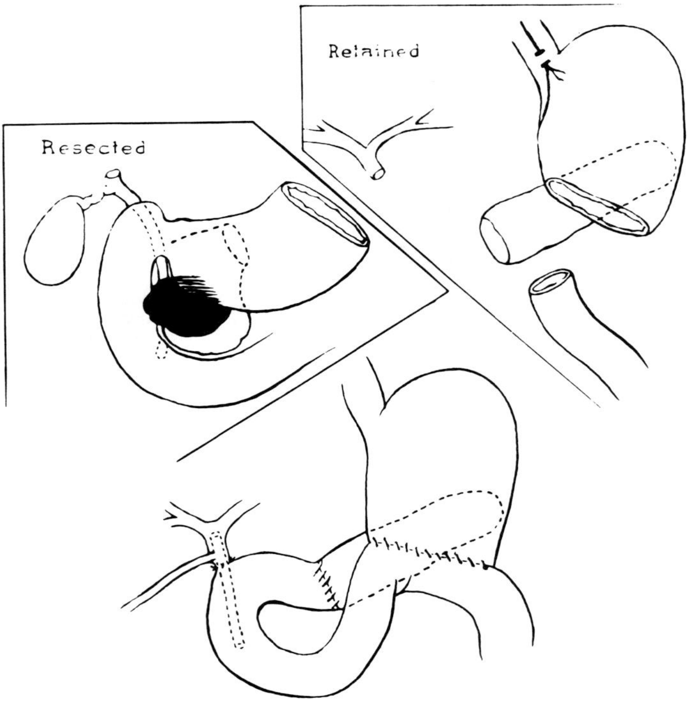

Figure 24-3. The current Whipple operation includes en block resection of the antrum, duodenum, pancreatic head, distal bile duct, and gallbladder. A relatively normal pancreatic remnant is invaginated into the end of the proximal jejunum. Choledochojejunostomy and gastrojejunostomy are also performed.

Pylorus Preservation Pancreaticoduodenectomy

In 1978 Traverso and Longmire introduced the pylorus-preserving pancreaticoduodenectomy for benign disease of the pancreas.[117] In such patients, extensive margins of resection are unnecessary. By preserving the pylorus, gastric emptying is controlled physiologically, thus preventing the exposure of the jejunum to excessive amounts of acid. Although the operation was originally introduced for benign disease, a number of recent reports include details of patients who have undergone the pylorus preservation procedure for various malignant tumors.[39,59,87]

In the pylorus preservation operation, the duodenum is divided approximately 2 cm distal to the pylorus. The head of the pancreas, surrounding duodenum, and lower end of the common bile duct are resected en block (Fig. 24-4). Pancreatic and choledochal anastomoses are fashioned as in the standard Whipple operation, and alimentary continuity is restored by a two-layer duodenojejunostomy.

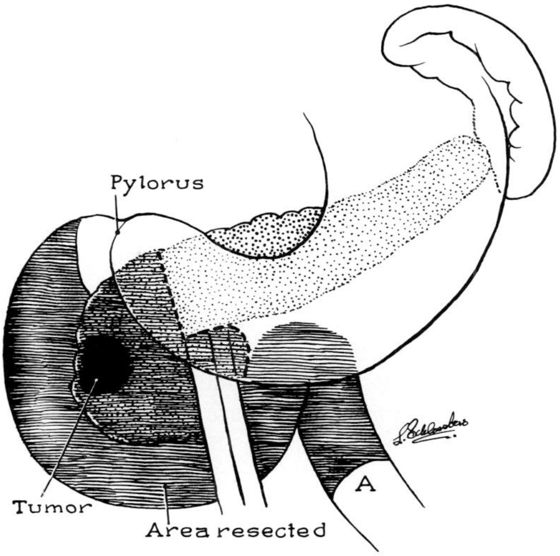

Figure 24-4. The pylorus-preserving pancreaticoduodenectomy of Traverso and Longmire[117] includes the same resected area as the current "Whipple" operation except that the pylorus and first few centimeters of pylorus are preserved. (From Grace et al.[39] with permission.)

Resection of the head of the pancreas and duodenum with preservation of the pylorus has a number of theoretical advantages over the current Whipple operation. Duodenojejunostomy is technically simpler than gastrojejunostomy; and by avoiding gastric resection and vagotomy, operating time is reduced. Furthermore, preservation of the pylorus may ameliorate some of the malabsorption problems that are in part caused by the gastric resection. A concern expressed about pylorus preservation has been its adequacy as a cancer operation. Two groups of investigators have observed that survival of patients with periampullary carcinoma[87] and ductal pancreatic cancer[39] treated by pylorus preservation was similar to that for the current Whipple resection. Thus, the pylorus preservation procedure can be considered in the operative management of carcinoma of the head of the pancreas.

Total Pancreatectomy

The quest for improved survival following pancreatic resection for carcinoma of the head of the pancreas has led some surgeons to advocate total pancreatectomy for this condition.[10,100] the first total pancreatectomy was performed by Rockey in 1942, but his patient died postoperatively as a result of a bile leak.[102] Two years later, however, Priestly et al. reported the first successful total pancreatectomy in a patient with an insulinoma.[99] Recently, some investigators have reported mortality rates for total pancreatectomy comparable to those currently being achieved for partial pancreatectomy.[38] Others, however, have failed to observe any improvement in mortality with this procedure in recent years.[15,40,122,123]

The theoretical advantages of total pancreatectomy are (1) the elimination of potential pancreatic fistulas by avoiding pancreaticojejunostomy, (2) eradication of multicentric disease within the pancreas, and (3) more complete regional lymphatic dissection. Disadvantages include an increased incidence of anastomotic jejunal ulceration, pancreatic exocrine insufficiency, and definite diabetes millitus, which may be difficult to control and may lead to death in some instances.[2,40,123]

Improved survival following total pancreatectomy has been reported by some authors,[10,27] but others[40,122] have not observed any improvement in long-term survival after this procedure. Thus, the routine use of total pancreatectomy for adenocarcinoma of the head of the pancreas cannot be recommended. However, total pancreatectomy may be indicated in patients whose tumor involves the line of pancreatic resection and those whose pancreatic remnant is so friable that anastomotic complications are inevitable.[70,119]

Regional Pancreatectomy

Fortner, adhering to the principle of en bloc resection of a primary cancer with both a wide tissue margin and regional lymphatic drainage, has advocated an extensive regional pancreatectomy for adenocarcinoma of the head of the pancreas.[28,29] Fortner's operation includes a total pancreatectomy with removal en bloc of a generous margin of soft tissue around the pancreas. The regional lymph nodes, including those around the porta hepatis, celiac axis, and superior mesenteric artery, are also removed. Resection of the portal vein, celiac axis, and superior mesenteric artery followed by reconstruction of these vessels is undertaken when they are involved in the tumor. A subtotal gastrectomy is also included in this procedure. Major disadvantages of regional pancreatectomy are that it takes 12 to 14 hours to perform and that the incidence of enterocutaneous fistulas is high.

While Fortner's aggressive approach may increase the resectability rate of patients with pancreatic cancer, no evidence demonstrates that it has resulted in improved survival. Fortner has reported his experience with 61 patients who underwent regional pancreatectomy, of whom 35 had carcinoma of the head of the pancreas.[29] The operative mortality was 26%. Ten patients (28%) died of recurrent cancer and nine patients (26%) of other causes, leaving seven patients (20%) alive who had survived for between 3 and 18 months.

PREOPERATIVE ASSESSMENT

The aims of preoperative assessment of a patient suspected of having carcinoma of the head of the pancreas are to establish the diagnosis, determine the extent of disease, evaluate resectability, and determine whether the patient will survive the operation. A wide range of diagnostic techniques are now available for preoperative assessment. Evaluation of the patient is usually initiated by noninvasive studies, proceeding to more invasive techniques if further information is required.

An assessment of various patient risk factors is also undertaken before embarking on radical surgical procedures.

Radiologic Assessment

Ultrasonography and CT Scanning

In 1967 Holmes reported the first pancreatic masses detected by ultrasound.[51] Ultrasonography is a very safe and easy examination for the patient and is relatively inexpensive. Ultrasound examination of the pancreas is not always successful, however, failing in 12% to 15% of patients.[58,72,73] The commonest cause of failure is the presence of overlying bowel gas.[72] A further disadvantage is failure to evaluate the retropancreatic area for perivascular invasion and lymphadenopathy.

The sensitivity of ultrasonography in detecting pancreatic cancer is variously reported as 76% to 94%.[98,124] Makie and his colleagues were able to correctly identify pancreatic cancer in 81% of patients.[72] Their overall results for ultrasonography were a sensitivity of 87% and a specificity of 74%. In one series, 94% of tumors located in the head of the pancreas could be diagnosed on ultrasonography, and lesions as small as 1.5 cm could be detected.[8]

In this same study, CT was highly successful in demonstrating the pancreas in from 93% to 100% of the patients.[8] The typical appearance of a pancreatic carcinoma on CT is the presence of a localized mass in the pancreas (Fig. 24-5). Edema or atrophy of the tail of the pancreas, dilatation of the biliary tree and/or the pancreatic duct, obliteration of the peripancreatic fat planes, and the presence

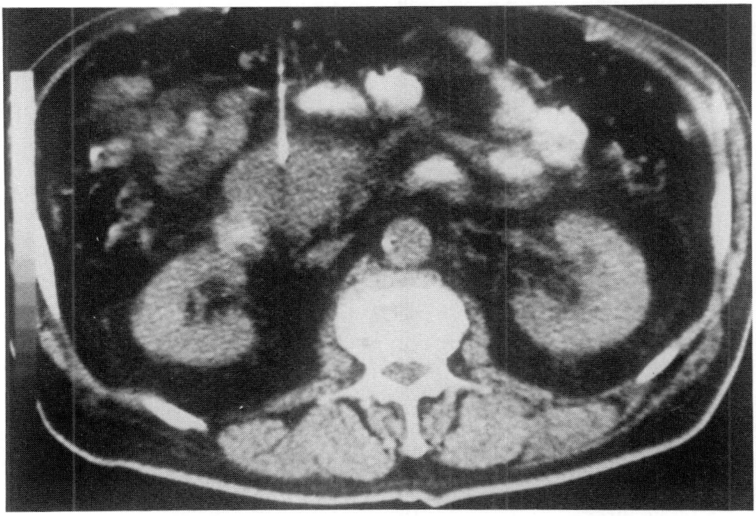

Figure 24-5. CT scan demonstrating a mass in the head of the pancreas. Note that a CT-guided fine needle aspiration is being performed.

of hepatic metastases are additional signs indicative of carcinoma.[8] CT scanning may also provide information on extrapancreatic spread of tumor. Perivascular extension to the celiac or superior mesenteric arteries is also reported in 30% and 60% of patients, respectively.[125]

Ultrasonography and CT are the two most frequently used noninvasive imaging techniques for evaluation of patients with suspected pancreatic disease.[1,137] An earlier study comparing ultrasonography and CT scanning demonstrated no superiority with either examination.[5] More recently, however, a number of reports indicate that CT scanning is more accurate than ultrasonography in evaluating the pancreas.[50,68] Hessell and his colleagues, in a prospective study, reported that CT scanning has a sensitivity of 87% and a specificity of 90% in the evaluation of patients with pancreatic disease compared with a sensitivity and specificity of 69% and 82%, respectively, for ultrasonography.[50] Furthermore, these authors reported that 16% of the ultrasound examinations were technically unsatisfactory, whereas all CT examinations were satisfactory. CT scanning is also reported to be three times more accurate in providing etiologic information.[137]

Cholangiography

Endoscopic retrograde cholangiopancreatography (ERCP) is one of the most important techniques for diagnosing pancreatic cancer. Technical success with ERCP usually parallels endoscopic experience. However, practiced endoscopists report a technical failure rate of only 10% in achieving a complete study.[81] The radiologic findings most suggestive of pancreatic carcinoma on ERCP include pancreatic duct stricture or obstruction. Freeny and associates, in a study of 40 ERCPs, felt that the most useful signs in identifying cancers were (1) obstruction of the pancreatic duct showing an irregular, eccentric or ''rat tail'' termination, (2) stenosis of the pancreatic duct with a nodular appearance suggesting tumor encasement, and (3) the double duct sign, in which there is an abnormality of the bile duct contiguous to that seen in the pancreatic duct (Fig. 24-6).[33]

The accuracy of ERCP in diagnosing carcinoma of the pancreas is very high. Reported sensitivities range from between 80% and 95% and specificities from 88% to 90%.[32,34,101] A further advantage of ERCP is that the examination can be combined with brushings or duct aspiration for cytologic examination.[57,91] More recently, an extension of the ERCP technique has been the development of endoscopic biliary drainage as a therapeutic maneuver in the management of malignant obstructive jaundice.[38]

Percutaneous transhepatic cholangiography (PTC) is also a very accurate diagnostic method in the investigation of the pancreatoduodenal region, especially in jaundiced patients.[32] The usual radiographic finding of pancreatic carcinoma is partial or complete obstruction of the distal common bile duct. The distance from the hepatic ducts to the level of obstruction may give some indication of resectability, which is more likely with greater distance.[105] Like ERCP, PTC can also be used to obtain samples for cytologic examination and therapeutically to achieve either external or internal biliary drainage.[31]

Although ERCP may be a less traumatic procedure than PTC, ERCP is probably more difficult to perform. The choice between these two techniques will

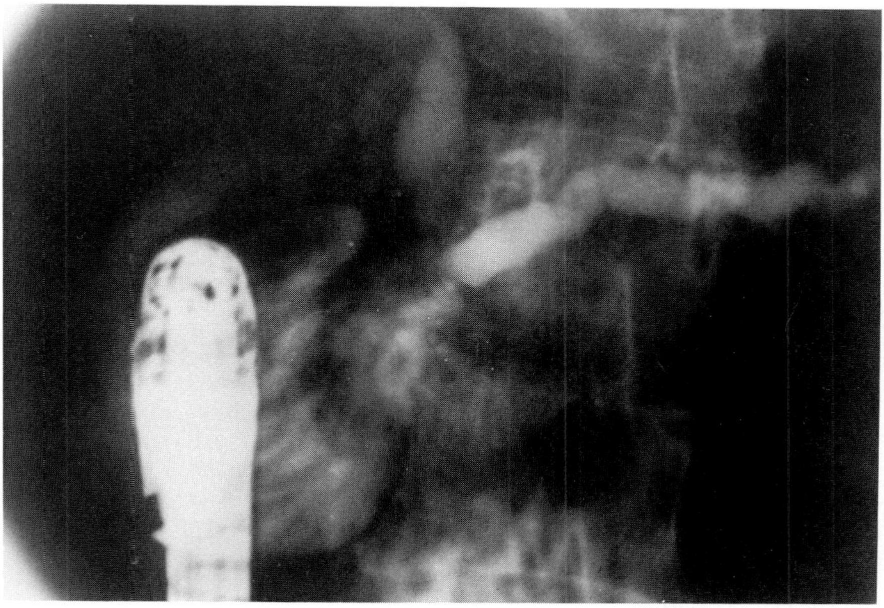

Figure 24-6. ERCP demonstrating strictures of the bile duct and pancreatic duct in the pancreatic head, the double duct sign. Note the dilatation of the proximal biliary and distal pancreatic ducts.

depend on the availability of the necessary endoscopic or radiologic expertise. In patients with a severe coagulopathy, ERCP may be safer. Moreover, with lesions in the region of the pancreatic head, ERCP has the advantages of visualization and biopsy of the ampulla and of providing a pancreatogram.

Arteriography

During the 1960s and 1970s, arteriography appeared to be unrivaled as an imaging test for pancreatic cancer. However, arteriography has now been superceded by less invasive pancreatic imaging tests.[75] In contradistinction to most organ tumors, which exhibit "neovascularity" on arteriography, carcinomas of the pancreas are usually relatively avascular. Other arteriographic findings in tumors of the pancreas are arterial encasement, abrupt occlusion of large or small arteries, and venous involvement.[75]

A prospective study[74] from the University of Chicago reported a sensitivity and specificity of 72% and 71%, respectively, for arteriography in pancreatic carcinoma. Angiography may be a useful preoperative study in those patients who are being considered candidates for exploration. Major arterial or venous encasement is virtually pathognomonic of nonresectability. In patients with large tumors of the pancreatic body or tail, angiography in combination with fine needle aspiration cytologic examination may prevent an unnecessary exploration. Angiography also provides important information on foregut vascular variations, which may be present in 25% of patients.[75]

FINE NEEDLE ASPIRATION CYTOLOGY

In 1951 Kirtland proposed "a safe method of pancreatic biopsy" that employed the intraoperative use of the Vim Silverman needle.[63] The Tru cut disposable needle subsequently replaced the Vim Silverman needle. In 1970 Christoffersen and Poll first reported the preoperative use of fine needle aspiration for cytologic examination.[16] The desire to obtain preoperative histologic confirmation of a mass in the head of the pancreas and, thus, avoid laparotomy in selected patients led to the development of percutaneous fine needle aspiration cytology.

In 1972, Oscarson and his colleagues reported their experience of 20 patients with angiographically guided fine needle aspiration cytologic examination of pancreatic and gastric masses.[90] In seven patients who had documented pancreatic malignancy, aspiration cytology successfully diagnosed all seven cases. In 1975 Hancke and colleagues reported the use of ultrasound localization as a method of directing percutaneous aspiration.[45] A year later, Haaga et al. used CT-guided percutaneous fine needle aspiration (Fig. 24-7).[44] Guidance has also been provided by fluoroscopy during ERCP and PTC.[24]

The diagnostic accuracy of fine needle aspiration is very high. The technique has an overall sensitivity of 90% and a specificity of essentially 100%.[37,78] Percutaneous fine needle aspiration is also extremely safe.[6] Theoretical concerns with fine needle aspiration seeding the needle tract, however, are with tumor cells or peritoneum.[25] Percutaneous aspiration cytology may help to avoid an operation when a large mass is present in the body or tail of the pancreas or when a patient may be a poor risk for anesthesia. With lesions in the region of the pancreatic head, the value of percutaneous cytologic examination is less obvious. These periampullary tumors may originate from the distal duct, the duodenum, or the ampulla of Vater. Each of these adenocarcinomas has a much better prognosis than those that originate in the pancreas. Thus, a positive cytologic examination would not deter the authors from exploring a patient with a tumor in the region of the pancreatic head.

Operative Risk

When contemplating surgery for carcinoma of the pancreas, a number of patient factors have to be considered. Epidemiologic studies have shown that approximately 80% of pancreatic cancers occur between the ages of 60 and 80 years.[18] Some authors have cautioned against performing radical pancreatic surgery in patients over 70 years.[27,89] Obertop and colleagues reported a significantly higher operative mortality in patients over 70 years of age (27% vs. 3%).[89] However, recent studies by Grace et al.[40] and Kairaluoma and coworkers[61] found no difference in operative mortality or survival in patients over 70 years of age

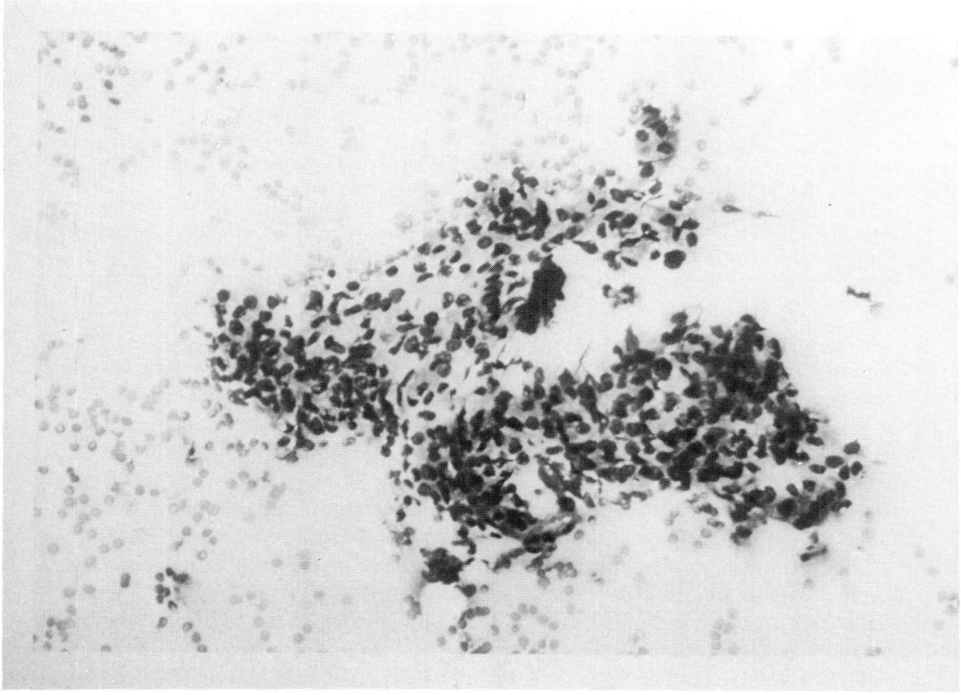

Figure 24-7. Malignant cells aspirated from the pancreas with the aid of a CT-guided fine needle (Fig. 24-5).

compared with patients under 70 years of age. These authors argue that the decision to operate should not be based on an arbitrary age limit but rather on physiologic age.

The observation that biliary tract surgery in the presence of jaundice is associated with a high mortality and morbidity has led a number of investigators to seek potential predictive risk factors.[7,22,55,69,96] Pitt and colleagues, in an analysis of 155 consecutive patients undergoing a variety of biliary tract operations excluding cholecystectomy, identified 10 parameters that correlated significantly with hospital mortality.[96] These risk factors were the presence of malignant disease, age >60 years, fever >38°C, hematocrit <30%, white blood count >10,000/mm^3, and levels of blood urea nitrogen >20 mg/dL, creatinine >1.3 mg/dL, albumin <3.0 g/dL, bilirubin >10 mg/dL, and alkaline phosphatase >100 IU. Furthermore, they observed that patients with five or more risk factors had an increased risk of developing major complications or dying after the operation.

Blamey and his coworkers used linear discrimination analysis of risk factors in a study of 186 biliary operations.[7] These investigators showed that the only independent predictors of mortality were levels of serum creatinine, serum albumin, and serum bilirubin, in that order. However, these authors also observed

TABLE 24-1. LITTLE'S MORTALITY INDEX*

$$\text{Mortality index} = 0.0016 \times [\text{creatinine}] - 0.0227 \times [\text{albumin}] + 0.0641 \times \text{cholangitis score} + 0.6935$$

An index of 0.4 or higher is associated with a higher risk of death. Creatinine is expressed in micromoles per liter, and albumin in grams per liter. Cholangitis is scored 0 if the patient is afebrile, 1 if the temperature is <37.5°C, 2 if >37.5°C without sepsis or right upper quadrant pain, 3 if >37.5°C with rigors and/or right upper quadrant pain, and 4 if fever with shock and/or mental obtundation is present.

* From Little.[69]

that the presence of six or more positive predictive factors, similar to those described by Pitt et al.[96] was associated with a postoperative mortality of 77.4% compared with 7.6% if fewer than six factors were positive, a relative risk of 10.2 : 1. A similar relationship between increasing risk factors and mortality has been recognized by Dixon et al.[22] These authors showed that elevated bilirubin levels, a decreased hematocrit, and malignancy were associated with a 60% mortality. When these three factors were absent, the mortality was only 5%.

Hunt and his colleagues have identified the presence of fibrin degradation products and circulating endotoxin as significant risk factors for patients undergoing biliary tract surgery.[55] A recent study by Sandler et al. has also identified diabetes as a risk factor in biliary surgery.[104] In this series of 126 patients, the mortality was sevenfold higher in the diabetic group compared with the nondiabetic group. Foshi et al. have also demonstrated that the majority of patients with pancreatic tumors have some degree of malnutrition.[30] Their data suggest that nutritional parameters such as weight loss and serum albumin levels may predict outcome. Most recently, Little has defined a mortality index (Table 24-1) that relies on serum albumin levels, serum creatinine levels, and a cholangitis score.[69] In a prospective study of 40 patients, Little's mortality index was 100% accurate in predicting outcome.

Thus, application of predictive models, such as Little's mortality index or Pitt's biliary risk factors,[96] should allow better patient selection before pancreatic surgery. With these models a small percentage of patients can be identified in whom the risks of major pancreatic resection are very high. In these patients preoperative maneuvers, such as parenteral or enteral nutrition and internal biliary drainage to decrease operative risk may be indicated before embarking on surgery.

PREOPERATIVE PREPARATION

Percutaneous Transhepatic Biliary Drainage

A number of authors have postulated that percutaneous decompression of the obstructed biliary tree by lowering bilirubin concentrations would reduce postoperative mortality and morbidity.[20,36,80,86,112] A number of earlier studies with either historical controls or concurrent but unrandomized controls supported this attractive proposition.[20,43,88] However, three more recent prospective, randomized analyses have found no advantage for routine percutaneous biliary drainage prior to surgery.[47,77,97] Moreover, one analysis demonstrated that the excess hospitalization associated with preoperative percutaneous biliary drainage costs over $6000 per patient.[97]

In each of these randomized studies, however, preoperative drainage was relatively short (10–18 days), many patients were drained externally and not internally, and preoperative nutritional status was not assessed.[47,77,97] The work of Koyama and associates on the recovery of hepatic function after relief of obstructive jaundice suggests that adequate recovery depends not only on the duration of biliary decompression but also on the duration of jaundice prior to decompression.[64] These authors suggest a minimum period of 4 to 6 weeks of biliary drainage before definitive surgery. Hepatic reticuloendothelial and mitochondrial function as well as lymphocyte and polymorphonucleocyte function also take at least 6 weeks to return to normal after relief of obstruction. Recent animal studies also suggest that internal biliary drainage reduces risk in comparison to external biliary drainage.[103] These facts may, in part, explain why trials of short-term preoperative, usually external, biliary drainage have not demonstrated any benefit in postoperative mortality or morbidity.

Preoperative Bile Salts

As early as 1941, Whipple, advocating his one-stage operation, observed that jaundiced patients could be prepared preoperatively with vitamin K and bile salts, thus decreasing operative risk.[131] Recently, a number of authors have studied the influence of preoperative oral bile salts on prevention of endotoxemia in jaundiced patients.[12,115] Postoperative renal failure occurs in 9% of jaundiced patients[93] and is a contributing factor in up to 50% of postoperative deaths.[135] Gut-derived endotoxins have been shown to be associated with renal failure in jaundiced patients.[93] After surgery, endotoxins can be demonstrated in the peripheral blood of at least 50% of jaundiced patients.[4,12] Moreover, whereas renal impairment is common in patients with endotoxemia, renal insufficiency is rare in the absence of endotoxemia.[4,134]

A recent study in both animals and humans has demonstrated that preoperative treatment with oral bile salts—sodium deoxycholate and sodium taurocholate—prevents endotoxemia and protects renal function.[12] Oral lactulose was similarly shown in a prospective study of 24 patients to lower systemic endotoxemia and to protect renal function in jaundiced patients.[92] Thus, in the preoperative preparation of high-risk, jaundiced patients, administration of oral bile salts or lactulose may be a consideration when internal biliary drainage is not possible.

Total Parenteral Nutrition (TPN)

Malnutrition and cachexia are common in cancer patients, and the presence of a decreased serum albumin level in patients undergoing biliary tract surgery is

TABLE 24-2. PERCUTANEOUS TRANSHEPATIC DRAINAGE PLUS HYPERALIMENTATION*

	PTD	PTD + Hyperalimentation
Patients (No.)	32	34
Internal drainage (%)	10	12
PTD time (days)	15	20
Postop morbidity (%)	49	13†
Postop mortality (%)	18	4†

* Adapted from Foshi et al.[30]
† $p < .05$

associated with higher postoperative mortality and morbidity.[7,30,69,96] Several studies have attempted to establish whether preoperative nutritional replacement reduces postoperative morbidity.[48,79,84,136] These analyses have been criticized because of small numbers; but when considered in aggregate, the patients given TPN had a statistically significant advantage in terms of improved morbidity.[108]

A study examining the role of preoperative nutrition in jaundiced patients has recently been published by Foshi et al.[30] These authors found that the combination of 20 days of preoperative hyperalimentation and percutaneous transhepatic drainage (PTD) resulted in a significantly lower morbidity and mortality when compared with preoperative percutaneous biliary drainage alone (Table 24-2). Thus, high-risk patients may become candidates for pancreatic resection after a period of preoperative internal biliary drainage and hyperalimentation.

OPERATIVE TECHNIQUE

Patients with a large mass in the body or tail of the pancreas have such a low probability of cure that exploration may not be warranted if a tissue diagnosis of adenocarcinoma can be established with percutaneous aspiration cytology. On the other hand, we believe that patients who have a reasonable operative risk and a localized mass in the region of the pancreatic head should be explored for possible resection. Moreover, in these latter patients the lesion may originate in the distal bile duct, duodenum, or ampulla and, as a result, may have a much better prognosis than pancreatic cancer.

Determining Resectability

Adequate exposure is essential for assessment of resectability of the pancreas and subsequent pancreaticoduodenectomy. The head of the pancreas can be approached through either a midline or a right subcostal incision. If a resection is to be undertaken, this incision can easily be converted to a bilateral subcostal (Chevron) incision. In a thin patient with a narrow costal angle, a midline upper abdominal incision may be preferable. A full and comprehensive laparotomy is performed initially to detect metastases in the liver, lymph nodes, peritoneum, or omentum. A Kocher maneuver is performed, and the head of the pancreas evaluated for size and location of the primary lesion. Invasion of contiguous structures such as the portal vein, superior mesenteric artery, and common hepatic artery are also assessed.

If a preoperative histologic diagnosis has not been made, biopsy of the primary lesion and any lymph nodes may be considered. Biopsy material can be obtained by open scalpel biopsy of any superficial lesion, transduodenal Tru-cut needle biopsy of a pancreatic mass, or fine needle aspiration cytology of the lesion. The common duct may also be opened and biopsy material obtained from the distal common bile duct.

If adenocarcinoma is found in a lymph node and the primary is almost certainly in the pancreas, an argument can be made not to resect because of the extremely poor prognosis. However, if the primary is in the bile duct or ampulla and the positive node is in the field of resection, survival may not be adversely influenced, and, therefore, resection should still be considered.[9,39] Even with a pancreatic primary and a positive lymph node, resection may be undertaken as a palliative measure.

Controversy exists whether histologic proof of carcinoma of the head of the pancreas is necessary before embarking on pancreaticoduodenectomy. We agree with Longmire and Traverso, who have suggested that if the possibility of a resection for benign disease has been discussed with the patient, it is acceptable to perform pancreatectomy without a tissue diagnosis.[71] Thus, a potentially curable occult lesion is not overlooked. Others have argued that if pancreatitis is severe enough to be confused with malignancy, pancreatectomy is probably indicated in any case.[52,53]

If a diagnosis of pancreatic malignancy has been established or if the suspicion remains high, an assessment of resectability is undertaken. Dissection is continued along the third part of the duodenum to expose the superior mesenteric vein at the point where it crosses the duodenum and passes under the neck of the pancreas. A critical determination of resectability is the ability to separate the portal vein from the adjacent pancreas. Division of the bile duct with dissection from above also facilitates this decision. No major tributaries enter the portal vein on its ventral surface behind the pancreatic neck so that it should be possible to develop a plane between these two structures. If this can be achieved, the tumor is usually resectable. Further assessment of extension into the uncinate dorsal to the portal vein is facilitated by an extensive Kocher maneuver and bimanual palpation.

Technical Aspects

Either classic Whipple or pylorus-preserving pancreatectomy can be performed. In either case, the gastroduodenal artery should be isolated and divided at the junction with the hepatic artery. The common hepatic duct should be divided just proximal to the cystic duct and a cholecystectomy performed. The stomach is now transected in the region of the incisura or, if a pylorus-preserving procedure is to be performed, the duodenum is divided approximately 2 cm distal to the pylorus (Fig. 24-4). In the latter procedure, an intact neurovascular supply to the pylorus and the first part of the duodenum is essential. The right gastric artery is preserved (Fig. 24-8). The gastroepiploic vessels along the entire length of the greater curve of the stomach are carefully preserved as is the vagal innervation of the pylorus and antrum. The right gastroepiploic artery is divided at its origin from the anterior pancreatoduodenal artery on the head of the pancreas.

The pancreas should be transected across the surgical neck. Transfixion sutures placed along the upper and lower margins of the pancreas on either side of the line of transection will reduce bleeding from the cut surface of the pancreas. The uncinate process should now be carefully dissected from the lateral wall of the superior mesenteric and portal veins. Division of the jejunum distal to the ligament of Treitz and passage of this short segment to the patient's right beneath the mesenteric vessels facilitates the final uncinate dissection.

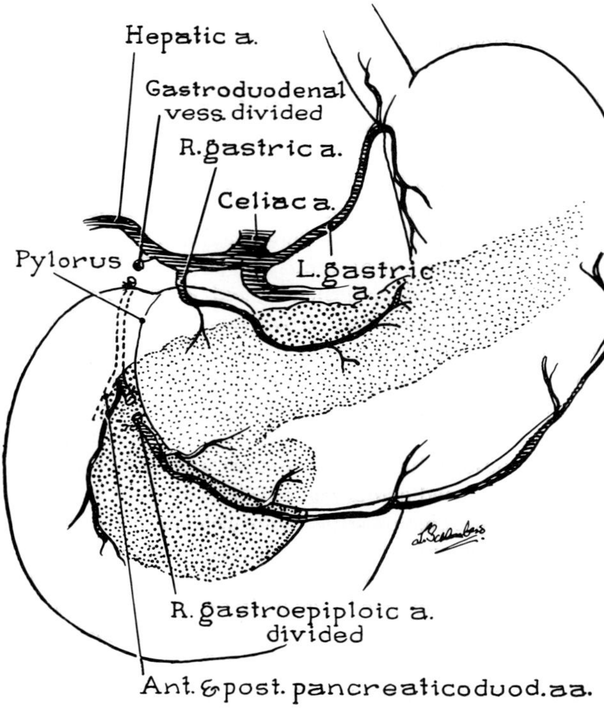

Figure 24-8. Vascular consideration during the pylorus-preserving pancreaticoduodenectomy. The right gastric artery, when present, is preserved. The gastroduodenal and right gastroepiploic vessels are divided adjacent to the pancreatic head. (From Grace et al.[39] with permission.)

Reconstruction Methods

Reconstruction of the alimentary tract is now undertaken. A number of methods of pancreaticojejunostomy are available. If the pancreas is soft with a small pancreatic duct, the safest method of handling the transected pancreatic stump may be to invaginate it into the proximal jejunum. However, if the duct is dilated and the pancreas is firm, a mucosa-to-mucosa anastomosis between the pancreatic duct and the jejunum can usually be performed. Our practice has been to create a very small opening in the jejunum that corresponds to the size of the pancreatic duct. The anastomosis is performed with a single layer of interrupted fine polypropylene sutures. We have also stented this anastomosis with a pediatric feeding tube, which is brought through the jejunum as an external stent (Fig. 24-9). The anastomosis is protected by an anterior and a posterior row of silk sutures from the pancreatic capsule to the jejunal serosa. An end-to-side choledochojejunostomy is then created and stented with a T tube. The duodenojejunostomy is now created 20 to 30 cm distal to the choledochojejunostomy (Fig. 24-9). Closed sump drains are placed adjacent to the pancreatic and choledochal anastomoses and brought out through separate stab incisions.

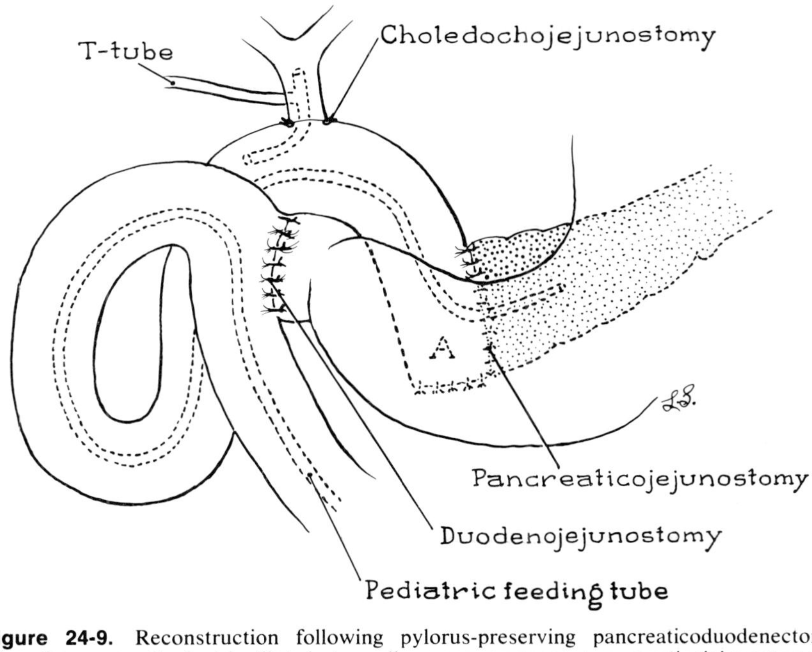

Figure 24-9. Reconstruction following pylorus-preserving pancreaticoduodenectomy when the pancreatic duct is dilated. A small, mucosa-to-mucosa pancreaticojejunostomy is performed and stented with a pediatric feeding tube. The choledochojejunostomy is stented with a T tube. The duodenojejunostomy is performed 2 to 3 cm from the pylorus. (From Grace et al.[39] with permission.)

POSTOPERATIVE MORTALITY

During the last 20 years, considerable improvement has occurred in postoperative mortality following pancreaticoduodenectomy. In 1968, Howard reported 41 consecutive Whipple procedures without a single death.[52] However, most of his contemporaries recorded operative mortalities of between 20% and 40% following the Whipple procedure (Table 24-3).[65,82] During the 1970s, operative mortality rates decreased to the 10% to 12% range.[3,27,127]

Five recent reports suggest, however, that pancreaticoduodenectomy can be performed with an operative mortality of 2% to 3% (Table 24-3).[9,15,40,60,119] In a recent study of 96 pancreaticoduodenectomies from UCLA, we reported an operative mortality of 10% between 1975 and 1979, and 2% between 1980 and 1985.[40] Similarly, Crist et al. have recently reported only one hospital death among 47 consecutive patients undergoing pancreaticoduodenectomy at Johns Hopkins since 1980.[15] Thus, at tertiary referral centers, pancreaticoduodenectomy now carries an acceptable operative risk. With these very acceptable mortality figures, we believe that pancreaticoduodenectomy, which is the only modality of treatment offering the possibility of cure, should be offered to patients with potentially resectable pancreatic cancer.

POSTOPERATIVE MORBIDITY

Pancreatic Fistula

Pancreatic fistula is the most common complication after pancreaticoduodenectomy. The reported incidence of this complication varies from 2.6% to 18.5%, but in most series pancreatic fistula occurs in about 12% of patients.[3,40,49,52,60,66] Moreover, pancreatic fistula has been associated with increased mortality rates. However, in five recent series, mortality among 565 collected cases has only been 2.3% despite a pancreatic fistula rate of 8.7%.[9,15,40,60,119] We believe that attention to detail in the placement of drains, monitoring of drain fluid for amylase levels, and postoperative TPN if a fistula develops have helped to reduce the lethality of this complication.

TABLE 24-3. CHANGING MORTALITY OF PANCREATICODUODENECTOMY

Author	Year	Patients	Mortality, %
Morris and Nardi[82]	1966	38	42
Aston and Longmire[3]	1973	65	10
Warren et al.[127]	1975	348	10
Forrest and Longmire[27]	1979	51	12
Lerut et al.[66]	1984	103	11
Jones et al.[60]	1985	87	3
Trede[119]	1985	199	3
Grace and Pitt[40]	1986	45	2
Braasch et al.[9]	1986	87	2
Crist et al.[15]	1987	47	2

The operative management of the pancreatic duct is a major factor in the development of pancreatic fistula following pancreaticoduodenectomy. Papachristou and colleagues reported a 70% rate of fistula occurrence in 37 patients in whom the duct was oversewn.[94] Lerut and his colleagues observed a 100% pancreatic fistula rate in two patients managed by duct ligation and four patients in whom rapidly hardening amino acids were used to occlude the pancreatic duct.[66]

In a previous analysis of 96 pancreaticoduodenectomies from UCLA, we also reported a 100% pancreatic fistula rate among four patients in whom the pancreatic duct was oversewn, compared with a rate of 14% in those who had a pancreatojejunostomy.[40] However, the type of pancreatic–jejunal anastomosis was not important, as the incidence of pancreatic fistulas was similar in patients who had a mucosa-to-mucosa anastomosis (14.5%) and in those in whom the cut end of the pancreas was invaginated into the jejunum (13.3%). We also observed a fistula rate of only 11% in 55 patients in whom stenting of the pancreaticojejunostomy was employed, compared with a 30% fistula rate in 10 patients without stents. This trend and the observation of high outputs of pancreatic fluid in the early postoperative period have led to a policy of routine stenting of this anastomosis.

Hemorrhage

Intraabdominal and upper gastrointestinal hemorrhage are also major complications following pancreaticoduodenectomy. Intraabdominal hemorrhage may occur in up to 6% of patients despite meticulous hemostasis before closing the abdomen.[40] The usual sources of bleeding in postoperative gastrointestinal hemorrhage are erosive gastritis and anastomotic ulceration. These complications carry a 20% to 70% mortality.[60,66] The reported incidence of postoperative gastrointestinal hemorrhage varies from 5% to 14%,[40,60,127] whereas that of anastomotic ulceration ranges between 2% and 17%.[3,41,66,107]

In an attempt to reduce the incidence of postoperative anastomotic ulceration, Scott and his colleagues have recommended that truncal vagotomy be performed concomitantly with pancreaticoduodenectomy.[107] In an analysis of 41 pancreatoduodenal resections, he observed anastomotic ulceration in 36% of patients without vagotomy compared with no anastomotic ulceration in patients who had undergone vagotomy. The pylorus-preserving pancreaticoduodenectomy is also associated with a very low incidence of anastomotic ulceration. In a recent review of the literature, Itani and coauthors found only six jejunal anastomotic ulcers in a collected series of 252 pylorus-preserving pancreaticoduodenectomies, an incidence of 2%.[59] Only two of these six patients required vagotomy and antrectomy. The remaining four patients were treated successfully with H_2-receptor blocking agents.

Gastric Emptying

A concern expressed about the pylorus-preserving pancreaticoduodenectomy has been whether the stomach would empty satisfactorily following the procedure. Itani and coauthors[59] reported delayed gastric emptying in the early postoperative period as the most common complication following pylorus-preserving pancreaticoduodenectomy.[59] In their review this problem occurred in 30% of patients. Newman et al., in an analysis of 35 patients, reported that nasogastric intubation was required for a longer period after pylorus preservation.[87] Warshaw and Torchiana also reported a significant delay in achieving full diet in patients following the pylorus-preserving procedure compared with the standard Whipple resection (16 vs. 9.8 days).[129]

In comparison, Grace et al. found that those patients in whom a pylorus preservation procedure had been performed required postoperative nasogastric intubation for a slightly shorter period than those in whom an antrectomy was carried out (7 vs. 9.3 days).[40] Similarly, Mosca et al., in an analysis of 30 patients, found that the resumption of oral feeding was satisfactory in all but two patients.[83] Traverso and Longmire, in a detailed study of gastric function in eight patients 2 to 12 months after pylorus preservation, found normal gastric emptying in all patients.[118]

In our experience, problems with gastric emptying in the postoperative period have usually been associated with postoperative pancreatitis or a leak at the pancreatic anastomosis that lies just dorsal to the duodenojejunostomy. When the pancreatitis resolves or the pancreatic fistula has healed, gastric emptying returns to normal. Moreover, recent data suggest that in the long term, gastric emptying is normal after pylorus preservation.[59] Thus, although temporary gastric outlet dysfunction has been reported after the pylorus-preserving pancreaticoduodenectomy, this problem is usually easily managed and does not have any long-term sequelae.

Other Complications

Infective complications may be seen in 8% to 14% of patients following pancreaticoduodenectomy.[40,49] Septic complications include intraabdominal abscess, wound infection, cholangitis, and septicemia. Intraabdominal sepsis is associated with considerable mortality and is often the result of an underlying biliary or pancreatic leak.[49] In the UCLA experience, we observed that 35% of septic complications were associated with an underlying pancreatic fistula.[40]

Renal failure associated with the hepatorenal syndrome may also occur following pancreaticoduodenectomy. However, prophylaxis with oral bile salts or lactulose and the maintenance of a good diuresis pre- and postoperatively should reduce the incidence of this complication. Enterocutaneous and biliary fistulae are infrequent complications that are largely preventable by meticulous surgical technique.

SURVIVAL

While the operative mortality has decreased steadily following pancreaticoduodenectomy, the long-term survival for patients with adenocarcinoma of the head of the pancreas has also recently shown some improvement. Earlier reports documented 5-year survival rates following pancreaticoduodenectomy of less than 5%.[27,85,109] However, isolated reports of 12% to 18% 5-year survival have appeared in the past.[65,127] More recently, we documented an estimated survival of 13% at 4½ years,[40] and Trede, in an analysis of 37 pancreatic resections, has observed that nine patients survived for more than 5 years.[120]

Three recent reports from Johns Hopkins,[15] The Lahey Clinic,[9] and the Gastrointestinal Tumor Study Group (GITSG)[35] document 5-year survivals of 15% to 18% following pancreatoduodenectomy for adenocarcinoma of the pancreas (Table 24-4). These improved survival statistics may be, in part, the result of lower operative mortality and postoperative adjuvant radiotherapy. Despite early promise, total pancreatectomy has not resulted in improved survival.[15,40] Moreover, pylorus preservation has proved to provide long-term survival comparable with that recently observed with the more traditional Whipple procedure.[39] Thus, resection has been the only treatment that has resulted in a cure and has often provided excellent palliation. More importantly, resection has permitted the removal of other malignant tumors in the periampullary area arising from the distal bile duct, ampulla, or duodenum.

In the UCLA experience,[40] the 5-year survival rate for periampullary nonpancreatic adenocarcinomas was 58% (Table 24-4). These figures are similar to those reported by Lerut and colleagues, who were able to document a 50% 5-year survival rate in 24 patients with ampullary carcinoma and a 60% rate at 5 years in patients without lymph node involvement.[66] Braasch et al. have also reported a 5-year survival of 65% among 30 patients with nonpancreatic periampullary adenocarcinoma undergoing pylorus-preserving pancreaticoduodenectomy.[9] Thus, the prognosis for nonpancreatic periampullary carcinomas may also be improving. Moreover, differentiation of pancreatic from other periampullary adenocarcinomas may not be possible without careful histologic examination of the entire specimen. Thus, a policy of nonresection of pancreatic masses would leave these more favorable tumors untreated and deny these patients the possibility of cure. Therefore, we believe that "therapeutic nihilism" is no longer defensible.

TABLE 24-4. RECENT SURVIVAL STATISTICS

Author	Year	Patients	5-year Survival, %
	Periampullary Adenocarcinoma		
Lerut et al.[66]	1984	24	50
Grace et al.[40]	1986	38	58
Braasch et al.[9]	1986	30	65
	Pancreatic Adenocarcinoma		
GITSG[35]	1985	43	15
Braasch et al.[9]	1986	14	17
Crist et al.[15]	1987	50	18

ADJUVANT THERAPY

The poor survival statistics associated with carcinoma of the pancreas, even following "curative" resections, have led a number of investigators to explore the impact of adjuvant radiotherapy and chemotherapy on this disease.

Radiotherapy

Until recently, radiotherapy was not considered as a treatment for pancreatic carcinoma. Prior to the development of high-energy radiotherapy machines, pancreatic carcinomas were generally regarded as radio-resistant. Only with the development of high-energy machines was it possible to deliver sufficient external beam radiation dosages to deep-seated tumors. With low-energy x-ray machines, the maximum dose was deposited at the skin surface, and the dose diminished rapidly as the beam traversed the tissue.[23]

Postoperative Radiation

Radiation in adequate doses can be an effective palliative modality for treating pain in selected patients with unresectable pancreatic cancer.[23] Until recently, the role of radiation as an adjunct to resection has not been clearly elucidated. The GITSG evaluated the impact of combined postoperative radiotherapy and 5-fluorouracil (5-FU) as an adjunct to curative surgery.[35] Forty-three patients received either surgery alone ($n = 22$) or surgery combined with irradiation (4000 cGy) and 5-FU (500 mg/m^2 IV) postoperatively ($n = 21$). The median disease-free survival of the combined treatment group was 11 months compared with 9 months for surgery alone. Recurrent disease developed in 71% of study patients and in 86% of controls. Moreover, the 5-year survival of 15% in the patients who received radiation was greater than that in the nonradiated controls.

Pilepich and Muller studied 17 patients with cancer of the pancreas who received preoperative radiation (4000–5000 cGy) to either unresectable or marginally resectable tumors.[95] Six patients subsequently underwent a Whipple procedure, and two of the six survived 5 years. Ongoing studies should determine the safety of preoperative radiotherapy. In the meantime, however, the GITSG's results have encouraged us to recommend postoperative radiation in resected patients.

Intraoperative Radiation Therapy

The delivery of adequate radiation dose to the tumor and not to the surrounding tissue is a basic principle of radiotherapy. To achieve this ideal, surgical implantation of radioactive sources (usually an intersititial ^{125}I implant) into the tumor or intraoperative radiation therapy (IORT) by electron beam can be utilized.[110] IORT by ^{125}I has a practical advantage over IORT by electron beam in that ^{125}I implantation can be administered in a conventional operating room, whereas IORT by electron beam requires substantial adaptation of the operation room or moving the patient preoperatively to a radiation treatment unit.

Shipley and colleagues have treated 10 patients with either an interstitial ^{125}I implant of the residual pancreas (n = 6) or IORT with electron beams to the tumor bed (n = 4).[110] The results in this small group were disappointing. The median survival was only 7 months, and 50% of patients have developed recurrent disease. Similarly, recent data from the National Institutes of Health have not demonstrated any distinct advantage for IORT in patients with pancreatic cancer.[111]

Chemotherapy

The therapy of pancreatic carcinoma with cytotoxic agents has not been associated with much success. The use of several single agents has been assessed in pancreatic cancer. However, only three agents, 5-FU, mitomycin C, and streptozotocin, appear to have response rates greater than 20%.[46] Efforts to combine chemotherapeutic agents have used these marginally active single agents. In unresectable tumors, response to combination chemotherapy with streptozotocin, 5-FU, and mitomycin C may occur in up to 43% of patients. Moreover, in one report, response appeared to be associated with increased survival.[133]

The isolation of high concentrations of estrogen receptors in the cytoplasm and nucleus of pancreatic adenocarcinoma suggests that pancreatic cancer might be a hormone-responsive neoplasm, similar to carcinoma of the breast and prostate.[42] Two Scandinavian reports using tamoxifen in small numbers of patients with unresectable pancreatic carcinoma have suggested an increase in median survival and an increased number of patients with long survival.[114,116] Randomized trials with larger numbers of patients will be necessary, however, to determine whether antiestrogen therapy will play a role in pancreatic cancer.

CONCLUSIONS

We believe that surgery, when possible, remains the most effective therapeutic modality in the management of adenocarcinoma of the pancreas. Resection of the tumor provides the only possibility of cure and improves the duration and quality of palliation. Moreover, with this policy the chance of resecting a more favorable nonpancreatic periampullary tumor is not overlooked. In 1979, Lord Smith of Marlow wrote, "Although the average long-term results of pancreaticoduodenectomy for cancer are poor, no man is an average and resection does provide the only chance of cure. Individually, many patients might well opt for a considerable operative hazard with a small chance of cure rather than an inconsiderable hazard and no chance of cure." Pancreatic resection today can be performed with an acceptably low operative risk. Thus, the proposition that patients should not be subjected to pancreaticoduodenectomy because of its attendant high operative mortality and morbidity is no longer tenable.

Controversy still exists as to the extent of surgical resection. More extensive resections have not been shown to result in longer survival and may be associated with greater morbidity. Pancreaticoduodenectomy with pancreaticojejunostomy and choledochoduodenostomy still remains the operation of choice for resectable adenocarcinoma of the head of the pancreas. Serious consideration, however, should be given to the use of the pylorus preservation operation, as it has a number of advantages over the classic Whipple resection and does not compromise survival in patients with malignant disease.

REFERENCES

1. Anacker H, Lamarque JL, Pistolesi GF. Efficiency of different radiodiagnostic techniques in pancreatic disorders. Eur J Radiol 1:79–84, 1981.
2. Andren-Sandberg A, Ihse I. Factors influencing survival after total pancreatectomy in patients with pancreatic cancer. Ann Surg 198:605–610, 1983.
3. Aston SJ, Longmire WP. Pancreatoduodenal resection: Twenty years experience. Arch Surg 106:813–817, 1973.
4. Bailey ME. Endotoxin, bile salts and renal function in obstructive jaundice. Br J Surg 63:774–778, 1976.
5. Barkin J, Vining D, Nuale A Jr., et al. Computerized tomography, diagnostic ultrasound and radionuclide scanning: Comparison of efficacy in diagnosis of pancreatic carcinoma. JAMA 238:2040–2042, 1977.
6. Beazley RM. Needle biopsy diagnosis of pancreatic cancer. Cancer 47:1685–1687, 1981.
7. Blamey L, Fearon KCH, Gilmour H, Osborne DH, Carter DC. Prediction of risk in biliary surgery. Br J Surg 70:535–538, 1983.
8. Bowie JD, Moossa AR. Ultrasonography and computed tomography in the diagnosis of pancreatic tumors. In: Moosa AR, ed. Tumors of the Pancreas. Baltimore, Williams & Wilkins, 1980.
9. Braasch, JW, Deziel DJ, Rossi RL, Watkins E, Winter PF. Pyloric and gastric preserving pancreatic resection—Experience with 87 patients. Ann Surg 204:411–418, 1986.
10. Brooks JR, Calebras JM. Cancer of the pancreas: Palliative operation, Whipple procedure or total pancreatectomy. Am J Surg 131:516–520, 1976.
11. Brunschwig A. Resection of head of pancreas and duodenum for carcinoma—Pancreatoduodenectomy. Surg Gynecol Obstet 65:681–684, 1937.
12. Cahill CJ. Prevention of postoperative renal failure in patients with obstructive jaundice—The role of bile salts. Br J Surg 70:590–595, 1983.
13. Carter DC. Surgery for pancreatic cancer. Br Med J 1:744–746, 1980.
14. Cattell RB. A technique for pancreatoduodenal resection. Surg Clin North Am 28:761–775, 1948.
15. Crist DW, Sitzmann JV, Cameron JL. Improved hospital morbidity, mortality, and survival after the Whipple procedure. Ann Surg 206:358–365, 1987.
16. Christoffersen P, Poll P. Preoperative pancreas aspiration biopsies. Acta Pathol Microbiol Scand 212(suppl):28–32, 1970.
17. Cohen I, Colp R. Cancer of the perampullary region of the duodenum. Surg Gynecol Obstet 45:322–346, 1927.
18. Cordis L, Cold EB. Epidemiology of pancreatic cancer. World J Surg 8:808–821, 1984.
19. Crile G Jr. The advantages of bypass operations over radical pancreatoduodenectomy in the treatment of pancreatic cancer. Surg Gynecol Obstet 130:1049–1053, 1970.
20. Denning DA, Molnar W, Carey LC. Preoperative percutaneous transhepatic biliary decompression lowers operative mortality in patients with obstructive jaundice. Am J Surg 141:61–65, 1981.
21. Desjardins A. Technique de la pancreatectomie. Rev Chir 35:945–973, 1907.
22. Dixon JM, Armstrong CP, Duffy SW, Davies GC. Factors affecting morbidity and

mortality after surgery for obstructive jaundice: A review of 373 patients. Gut 24:845–852, 1984.

23. Dobelbower RR, Milligan AJ. Treatment of pancreatic cancer by radiation therapy. World J Surg 8:919–928, 1984.
24. Evander A, Ihse I, Lunderquist A, Tylen U, Akerman M. Percutaneous cytodiagnosis of carcinoma of the pancreas and bile duct. Ann Surg 188:90–92, 1978.
25. Ferrucci JT, Wittenberg J, Margolies MN, Carey RW. Malignant seeding of the tract after thin needle aspiration biopsy. Radiology 130:345–346, 1979.
26. Flautner L, Tihanyi T, Szecseny A. Pancreatogastrostomy: An ideal complement to pancreatic head resection with preservation of the pylorus in the treatment of chronic pancreatitis. Am J Surg 150:608–611, 1985.
27. Forrest J, Longmire WP Jr. Carcinoma of the pancreas and periampullary region: A study of 279 patients. Ann Surg 189:129–138, 1979.
28. Fortner JG. Regional resection of cancer of the pancreas: A new surgical approach. Surgery 73:307–320, 1973.
29. Fortner JG. Regional pancreatectomy for cancer of the pancreas, ampulla and other related sites. Ann Surg 199:418–425, 1984.
30. Foshi D, Cavagna G, Callioni F, Morandi E, Rovati V. Hyperalimentation of jaundiced patients on percutaneous transhepatic biliary drainage. Br J Surg 73:716–719, 1986.
31. Frank PH, Moossa AR. The value of standard radiological investigations in the diagnosis of pancreatic neoplasms. In: Moossa AR, ed. Tumors of the Pancreas. Baltimore, Williams & Wilkins, 1980,
32. Freeny PC, Ball TJ. Endoscopic retrograde cholangiopancreatography (ERCP) and percutaneous transhepatic cholangiography (PTC) in the evaluation of suspected pancreatic carcinoma. Diagnostic limitations and contemporary roles. Cancer 47:1667–1678, 1981.
33. Freeny PC, Bilbao MK, Katon RM. "Blind" evaluation of endoscopic retrograde cholangiopancreatography (ERCP) in the diagnosis of pancreatic carcinoma: The "double duct" and other signs. Radiology 119:271–274, 1976.
34. Frick MP, Feinberg SB, Goodale RL. The role of endoscopic retrograde cholangiopancreatography in patients with suspected carcinoma of the pancreas and indeterminant computed tomography results. Surg Gynecol Obstet 155:177–182, 1982.
35. Gastrointestinal Tumor Study Group. Pancreatic cancer: Adjuvant combined radiation and chemotherapy following curative resection. Arch Surg 120:899–903, 1985.
36. Gobien RP, Stanley JH, Soucek CD, et al. Routine preoperative biliary drainage: Effect on management of obstructive jaundice. Radiology 152:353–356, 1984.
37. Goldstein HM, Zoronoza J, Wallace S, et al. Percutaneous fine needle aspiration biopsy of pancreatic and other abdominal masses. Radiology 123:319–322, 1977.
38. Grace PA, Pitt HA. Biliary tract surgery: The role of percutaneous and endoscopic biliary drainage. In: ReMine WH, ed. Problems in General Surgery. Philadelphia, JB Lippincott Company, 1986, pp 157–169.
39. Grace PA, Pitt HA, Longire WP Jr. Pancreatoduodenectomy with pylorus preservation for adenocarcinoma of the head of the pancreas. Br J Surg 73:647–650, 1986.
40. Grace PA, Pitt HA, Tompkins RK, DenBesten L, Longmire WP Jr. Decreased morbidity and mortality after pancreatoduodenectomy. Am J Surg 151:141–149, 1986.
41. Grant CS, van Heerden JA. Anastomotic ulceration following subtotal pancreatectomy. Ann Surg 190:1–5, 1979.
42. Greenway BA. Carcinoma of the exocrine pancreas: A sex hormone responsive tumor. Br J Surg 74:441–442, 1987.
43. Grundy SR, Strodel WE, Knol JA, Eckhauser FE. Efficacy of preoperative percutaneous biliary decompression in patients with obstructive jaundice. Arch Surg 119:703–708, 1984.
44. Haaga JR, Alfidi RJ. Precise biopsy localization by computed tomography. Radiology 118:603–607, 1976.
45. Hancke S, Holm HH, Koch F. Ultrasonically guided percutaneous fine needle biopsy of the pancreas. Surg Gynecol Obstet 140:361–364, 1975.

46. Harvey JH, Schein PS. Chemotherapy of pancreatic carcinoma. World J Surg 8:935–939, 1984.
47. Hatfield ARW, Terblanche J, Fataar S, et al. Preoperative external biliary drainage in obstructive jaundice. Lancet 2:896–899, 1982.
48. Heatley RV, Williams RHP, Lewis MH. Preoperative intravenous feeding: A controlled trial. Postgrad Med J 55:541–545, 1979.
49. Hertner FP, Cooperman AM, Ahlborn TN, Antinori C. Surgical experience with pancreatic and periampullary cancer. Ann Surg 195:274–281, 1982.
50. Hessel SJ, Siegelman SS, McNeill BJ, et al. A prospective evaluation of computed tomography and ultrasound of the pancreas. Radiology 143:129–133, 1982.
51. Holmes JH. Diagnosis of tumor by ultrasound. Prog Clin Cancer 3:135–150, 1967.
52. Howard JM. Pancreaticoduodenectomy: Forty-one consecutive Whipple resections without an operative mortality. Ann Surg 168:629–640, 1968.
53. Howard JM, Jordan GL. Cancer of the pancreas. Curr Probl Cancer 2:5–52, 1977.
54. Hsu YH, Guzman LG. Carcinoma of the pancreas: Diagnosis and treatment. South Med J 75:972–984, 1982.
55. Hunt DR, Allison MEM, Prentice CRM, Blumgart LH. Endotoxemia, disturbance of coagulation, and obstructive jaundice. Am J Surg 144:325–329, 1982.
56. Hunt VC. Surgical management of carcinoma of the ampulla of Vater and of the periampullary portion of the duodenum. Ann Surg 114:570–602, 1941.
57. Ihre TL, Pyk E, Raaschou-Nielsen T, Seligson U. Percutaneous fine needle aspiration biopsy during endoscopic retrograde cholangiopancreatography. Scand J Gastroenterol 13:657–662, 1978.
58. Ihse I, Isaksson G. Preoperative and operative diagnosis of pancreatic cancer. World J Surg 8:846–853, 1984.
59. Itani KMF, Coleman RE, Akwari OE, Meyers WC. Pylorus preserving pancreatoduodenectomy: A clinical and physiological appraisal. Ann Surg 204:655–664, 1986.
60. Jones BA, Langer B, Taylor BR, Girotti M. Periampullary tumors: Which ones should be resected? Am J Surg 149:46–52, 1985.
61. Kairaluoma MI, Kiviniemi H, Stahlberg M. Pancreatic resection for carcinoma of the pancreas and the periampullary region in patients over 70 years of age. Br J Surg 74:116–118, 1987.
62. Kausch W. Das Carcinoma der Papilla duodeni und seine radikale Entfernung. Beitr Z Klin Chir 78:439–486, 1912.
63. Kirtland HB Jr. A safe method of pancreatic biopsy: A preliminary report. Am J Surg 82:451–457, 1951.
64. Koyama K, Takagi Y, Ito K, et al. Experimental and clinical studies on the effect of biliary drainage in obstructive jaundice. Am J Surg 142:293–299, 1981.
65. Lansing PB, Blalock JB, Oschner JC. Pancreaticoduodenectomy: Retrospective review, 1949–1969. Am J Surg 38:79–86, 1972.
66. Lerut JP, Gianello PR, Othe JB, Kestens PJ. Pancreaticoduodenal resection. Ann Surg 199:432–437, 1984.
67. Levin DL, Conelly RR, Devesa SS. Demographic characteristics of cancer of the pancreas: Mortality, incidence and survival. Cancer 47:1456–1468, 1981.
68. Levitt RG, Stanley RJ, Sagel SS, Lee JKT, Weyman PJ. Computed tomography of the pancreas. Three second scanning versus 18-second scanning. J Comput Assist Tomogr 6:259–267, 1982.
69. Little JM. A prospective evaluation of computerized estimates of risk in the management of obstructive jaundice. Surgery 102:473–476, 1987.
70. Longmire WP Jr. The vicissitudes of pancreatic surgery. Am J Surg 147:17–24, 1984.
71. Longmire WP Jr, Traverso WL. The Whipple procedure and other standard operative approaches to pancreatic cancer. Cancer 47:1706–1711, 1981.
72. Mackie CR, Bowie JD, Cooper MJ, Kunzmann A, Moossa AR. Prospective evaluation of gray scale ultrasonography in the diagnosis of pancreatic cancer. Am J Surg 135:575–581, 1978.
73. Mackie CR, Cooper MJ, Lewis MH, Moossa AR. Non-operative differentiation between pancreatic cancer and chronic pancreatitis. Ann Surg 189:480–487, 1979.

74. Mackie CR, Lu CT, Noble HG, et al. Prospective evaluation of angiography in the diagnosis and management of patients suspected of having pancreatic cancer. Ann Surg 189:11–17, 1979.
75. Mackie CR, Moossa AR, Frank PH. The place of angiography in the diagnosis and management of pancreatic tumors. In: Moossa AR, ed. Tumors of the Pancreas. Baltimore, Williams & Wilkins, 1980,
76. Mackie JA, Rhoads JE, Park CD. Pancreaticogastrostomy: A further evaluation. Ann Surg 181:541–545, 1975.
77. McPherson GAD, Benjamin IS, Jodgson JHF, et al. Preoperative percutaneous transhepatic biliary drainage: The results of a controlled trial. Br J Surg 71:371–375, 1984.
78. Mitty HA, Efremidis SC, Yeh HC. Impact of fine needle biopsy on management of patients with carcinoma of the pancreas. Am J Roentgenol 137:1119–1121, 1981.
79. Moghiss K, Hornshaw J, Teasdale PR, Davies EA. Parenteral nutrition in carcinoma of the esophagus treated by surgery: Nitrogen balance and clinical studies. Br J Surg 64:125–128, 1977.
80. Moossa AR. Pancreatic cancer: Approach to diagnosis, selection for surgery and choice of treatment. Cancer 50:2689–2698, 1982.
81. Moossa AR, Levin B. Collaborative studies in the diagnosis of pancreatic cancer. Semin Oncol 6:298–308, 1979.
82. Morris PJ, Nardi GL. Pancreaticoduodenal cancer. Arch Surg 92:934–837, 1966.
83. Mosca F, Giulianotti PC, Arganini M, Brandi LS, Selli M. Pancreaticoduodenectomy with pylorus preservation. Ital J Surg Sci 14:313–320, 1984.
84. Muller JM, Dienst C, Brenner U, Pichlmaier H. Preoperative feeding in patients with gastrointestinal carcinoma. Lancet 7:68–71, 1984.
85. Nakase A, Matsumoto Y, Uchida K, Honjo I. Surgical treatment of cancer of the pancreas and periampullary region: Cumulative results in 57 institutions in Japan. Ann Surg 185:52–57, 1977.
86. Nakayama T, Ikeda A, Okuda K. Percutaneous transhepatic drainage of the biliary tree: Technique and results in 104 patients. Gastroenterology 74:554–559, 1978.
87. Newman KD, Braasch JW, Rossi RL, O'Campo-Gonzales S. Pyloric and gastric preservation with pancreatoduodenectomy. Am J Surg 145:152–156, 1983.
88. Norlander A, Kalin B, Sundblad R. Effect of percutaneous drainage upon liver function and postoperative mortality. Surg Gynecol Obstet 155:161–166, 1982.
89. Obertop H, Bruining HA, Elftinck-Schattenkerk M, Eggink WF, Jeekel J, VanHouten H. Operative approach to cancer of the head of the pancreas and periampullary region. Br J Surg 69:573–576, 1982.
90. Oscarson J, Stormley N, Sundgren R. Selective angiography in fine needle aspiration cytodiagnosis of gastric and pancreatic tumors. Acta Radiol Diagn (Stockh) 12:737–748, 1972.
91. Osnes M, Sereck-Hanssen A, Kristensen D, et al. Endoscopic retrograde brush cytology in patients with primary and secondary malignancies of the pancreas. Gut 20:279–283, 1979.
92. Pain JA, Bailey ME. Experimental and clinical study of lactulose in obstructive jaundice. Br J Surg 73:775–778, 1986.
93. Pain JA, Cahill CJ, Bailey ME. Perioperative complications in obstructive jaundice: Therapeutic considerations. Br J Surg 72:942–945, 1985.
94. Papachristou DN, D'Agostino H, Fortner JG. Ligation of the pancreatic duct in pancreatectomy. Br J Surg 67:260–262, 1980.
95. Pilepich MV, Miller HH. Preoperative irradiation in carcinoma of the pancreas. Cancer 46:1945–1949, 1980.
96. Pitt HA, Cameron JC, Postier RG, Gadacz TR. Factors affecting mortalty in biliary tract surgery. Am J Surg 141:66–72, 1981.
97. Pitt HA, Gomes AS, Lois JF, et al. Does preoperative percutaneous biliary drainage reduce operative risk or increase hospital cost? Ann Surg 201:545–553, 1985.
98. Pollock D, Taylor JW. Ultrasound scanning in patients with clinical suspicion of pancreatic cancer: A retrospective study. Cancer 47:1662–1665, 1981.
99. Priestly JT, Comfort MW, Radcliffe J Jr. Total pancreatectomy for hyperinsulinism

due to an islet cell adenoma: Survival and cure at sixteen months after operation. Presentation of metabolic studies. Ann Surg 119:211–221, 1944.
100. ReMine WH, Priestly JT, Judd ES, King JN. Total pancreatectomy. Ann Surg 172:595–604, 1970.
101. Reuben A, Cotton PB. Endoscopic retrograde cholangiopancreatography in carcinoma of the pancreas. Surg Gynecol Obstet 148:179–184, 1979.
102. Rockey EW. Total pancreatectomy for carcinoma: Case report. Ann Surg 118:603–611, 1943.
103. Roughneed PT, Gouma DJ, Kulkarni AD, Fanslow WF, Rowlands BJ. Impaired specific cell-mediated immunity in experimental biliary obstruction and its reversibility by internal biliary drainage. J Surg Res 41:113–125, 1986.
104. Sandler RS, Maule WF, Balthus ME. Factors associated with postoperative complications in diabetes after biliary tract surgery. Gastroenterology 91:157–162, 1986.
105. Sato J, Saitoh Y, Koyama K, Wantanabe K. Preoperative determination of operability in carcinomas of the pancreas and periampullary region. Ann Surg 168:876–881, 1968.
106. Sauve L. Des pancreatectomies et specialement de la pancreatectomie cephalique. Rev Cir 37:355–385, 1908.
107. Scott WH, Dean RH, Parker T, Avant G. The role of vagotomy in pancreaticoduodenectomy. Ann Surg 191:688–696, 1980.
108. Shanbhogue LKR, Chwals WJ, Weintraub M, Blackburn GL, Bistrian BR. Parenteral nutrition in the surgical patient. Br J Surg 74:172–180, 1987.
109. Shapiro TM. Adenocarcinoma of the pancreas: A statistical analysis of biliary bypass vs Whipple resection in good risk patients. Ann Surg 182:715–721, 1975.
110. Shipley WU, Tepper JE, Warshaw AL, Orlow BA. Intraoperative radiation therapy for patients with pancreatic cancer. World J Surg 8:929–934, 1984.
111. Sindeler WF, Hoekstia HJ, Kinsella TJ. Surgical approaches and techniques in intraoperative radiotherapy for intraabdominal, retroperitoneal, and pelvic neoplasms. Surgery 103:247–256, 1988.
112. Takada T, Hanyu F, Kobayashi S, Uchida Y. Percutaneous transhepatic cholangial drainage: Direct approach under fluoroscopic control. J Surg Oncol 8:83–97, 1976.
113. Tenani O. Contribution to the surgery of the papilla of Vater. Policlinico 29:291–300, 1922.
114. Theve NO, Pousette A, Carlstrom K. Adenocarcinoma of the pancreas—A hormone sensitive tumor? A preliminary report on Nolvadex treatment. Clin Oncol 9:193–197, 1983.
115. Thompson JN, Cohen J, Blenkharn JI, et al. A randomized clinical trial of oral urodeoxycholic acid in obstructive jaundice. Br J Surg 73:634–636, 1986.
116. Tonnesen K, Kamp-Jensen M. Antioestrogen therapy in pancreatic carcinoma: A preliminary report. Eur J Surg Oncol 12:69–70, 1986.
117. Traverso LW, Longmire WP Jr. Preservation of the pylorus in pancreaticoduodenectomy. Surg Gynecol Obstet 146:959–962, 1978.
118. Traverso LW, Longmire WP Jr. Preservation of the pylorus in pancreaticoduodenectomy. Ann Surg 192:306–310, 1980.
119. Trede M. The surgical treatment of pancreatic carcinoma. Surgery 97:28–35, 1985.
120. Trede M. Treatment of pancreatic carcinoma: The surgeon's dilemma. Br J Surg 74:79–80, 1987.
121. Trimble, IR, Parsons JW, Sherman CP. A one stage operation for the cure of carcinoma of the ampulla of Vater and the head of the pancreas. Surg Gynecol Obstet 73:711–722, 1941.
122. vanHeerden JA. Pancreatic resection for carcinoma of the pancreas: Whipple versus total pancreatectomy. An institution perspective. World J Surg 8:880–888, 1984.
123. vanHeerden JA, ReMine WH, Weiland LH, McIlrath LH, Ilstrup DM. Total pancreatectomy for ductal adenocarcinoma of the pancreas. Am J Surg 142:308–311, 1981.
124. Walls WJ, Gonzalez G, Martin NC et al. B-scan ultrasound evaluation of the pancreas: Advantages and accuracy compared to other diagnostic techniques. Radiology 114:127–134, 1975.

125. Ward EM, Stephens DH, Sheedy PR. Computed tomographic characteristics of pancreatic carcinoma: An analysis of 100 cases. Radiographics 3:547–550, 1983.
126. Warren KW. Complication of pancreatic surgery. Surg Clin North Am 36:683–693, 1957.
127. Warren KW, Choe DS, Plaza J, Relihan M. Results of radical resection for periampullary cancer. Ann Surg 181:534–540, 1975.
128. Warren K, Veidenheimer MD, Pratt HS. Pancreaticoduodenectomy for periampullary cancer. Surg Clin North Am 47:639–645, 1967.
129. Warshaw AL, Torchiana DL. Delayed gastric emptying after pylorus preserving pancreaticoduodenectomy. Surg Gynecol Obstet 160:1–4, 1985.
130. Watson K. Carcinoma of the ampulla of Vater: Successful radical resection. Br J Surg 31:368–373, 1944.
131. Whipple AO. The rationale of radical surgery for cancer of the pancreas and ampullary region. Ann Surg 114:612–615, 1941.
132. Whipple AO, Parsons WB, Mullens CR. Treatment of carcinoma of the ampulla of Vater. Ann Surg 102:736–776, 1935.
133. Wiggans RG, Woolley PV, Macdonal JS, Ueno W, Schein PS. Phase II trial of streptozotocin, mitomycin C and 5-fluorouracil (SMF) in the treatment of advanced pancreatic cancer. Cancer 41:387–391, 1978.
134. Wilkinson SP, Moodie H, Stamatakis JD, Kakkar VV, Williams R. Endotoxemia and renal failure in cirrhosis and obstructive jaundice. Br Med J 2:1415–1418, 1976.
135. Williams RD, Elliot DW, Zollinger RW. The effect of hypotension in obstructive jaundice. Arch Surg 81:335–340, 1960.
136. Williams RHP, Heatley RV, Lewis MH. A randomized controlled trial of preoperative intravenous nutrition in patients with stomach cancer. Br J Surg 63:667–670, 1976.
137. Wittenberg J, Ferrucci JT, Warshaw AL. Contribution of computed tomography to patients with pancreatic adenocarcinoma. World J Surg 8:831–838, 1984.

CHAPTER

25

PANCREATIC ENDOCRINE TUMORS: MEDICAL MANAGEMENT

Aaron I. Vinik, Ali Reza Moattari, Ivana Pavlic-Renar, and Norman W. Thompson

EDITORIAL COMMENT (Chapters 25 and 26)

The early reports of suspected gastrointestinal hormone–producing tumors and the discovery, sequencing, and synthesizing of the multiple polypeptides have provided one of the remarkable physiologic medical stories of the last few decades. The story began when Zollinger and Ellison enumerated the clinical characteristics of their syndrome and Bank and others showed almost simultaneously that the serum of these patients contained a circulating gastric secretagogue. Then Gregory and Tracy demonstrated the presence of gastrin in the tumor and metastases, and subsequently the gastric polypeptide was synthesized. This was followed closely by suggestions from Marks and Bank that the Verner Morrison syndrome (or WDHA syndrome as they named it) was due to an intestinal secretory gastric-inhibitory hormone that could be affected by steroids and finally the discovery of vasoactive intestinal polypeptide by Said. The advances have continued, largely due to the remarkable technical discoveries of radioimmunoassay, electronmicroscopy, fluorescent antibody techniques, and immunoperoxidase studies. Since then, vast strides have been made in the methods of diagnosis, polypeptide identification, and treatment of the apudomas. Further hormonal syndromes will undoubtedly be discovered, and current diagnostic and therapeutic methods will be improved, modified, or discarded.

Many questions still remain unanswered, including the best method of treatment of the hormonal effects of the tumors and the approach to the primary tumor with the alternatives of either surgery or chemotherapy. Dr. Vinik and his colleagues have outlined the hormonal changes, diagnostic technology, provocative tests, hormonal content of the various apudomas including insulinoma and carcinoid tumors, and classification of the chemical structures, that is, peptides, amines, and prostaglandins, and the clinical features such as flushing, diarrhea, diabetes, hypercalcemia, abdominal pain, and so forth. Even these comprehensive state-of-the-art diagnostic methods (1) do not diagnose all the tumors, (2) fail to completely categorize the exact incriminating hormone in many apudomas, (3) do not explain why the tumors occur in the pancreas, where the cells of origin do not seem to exist, (4) do not always explain why some tumors have multiple polypeptides, amino acids, and prostaglandins with only one or more expressing themselves, (5) do not explain why non-functioning tumors may contain pancreatic polypeptide yet no functional effects are apparent, and lastly, (6) do not explain why so many of the apudomas exhibit hormonal syndromes only after they have already metastasized. It is this last manifestation that still defies a rational approach to treatment. With modern medical therapy for example, H_2-receptor antagonists, omeprazole, somatostatin, steroids, and indomethacin, to affect the end organ function of the tumors, what is the place for surgery today, and does it in fact prolong life? There is a prevailing attitude that these malignant apudomas have a good prognosis after surgical eradication and are often associated with a long life span. This is true when compared with pancreatic carcinoma with its dismal outlook, but most patients have a bad prognosis once metastases have occurred, and it is unusual for such patients to survive more than 3 to 5 years after diagnosis.

The surgical aspects of endocrine tumors of the pancreas are addressed by Drs. Seymour and Andersen. We agree with their concept that, if feasible, surgical removal of the tumor should occur at any early point in every patient's management. This ideal can be achieved in many patients with insulinomas and cure obtained by simple enucleation of the tumor. However, for the less common glucagonomas and somatostatinomas, the diagnosis is often late, the tumor already metastatic, and the results of exploration poor. For gastrinomas the surgical removal of the tumor for sporadic cases has resulted in apparent cures in 20%. Unfortunately MEN-1 patients have a poor prognosis, either due to the multiplicity of the lesions or to more aggressive tumors. For all patients with small lesions, the use of endoscopic and intraoperative ultrasonography is an important advance and has facilitated the localization of the tumor.

CONTROVERSY

One of the most rapidly progressive fields of medicine has been the discovery, recovery, and synthesis of gastrointestinal hormones and elucidation of their role in the syndromes associated with apudomas. Equally rapid has been the progression in the methods of diagnosing the tumors and constantly evolving changes in the best treatment. Because of these rapid advances, the authors have been given leeway to expand on the subject in detail. Further advances may be expected in the near future.

There are now over 200 hormonally active agents that have been identified in the gut. Very few have been shown to have biological functions, and even fewer are associated in a cause–effect relationship with a clinically recognizable syndrome. It is the purpose of this chapter to outline the syndromes whose characteristics have been clearly defined but, nonetheless, continue to present medical problems of management. Management, however, has prerequisites: correct diagnosis; localization of the tumor(s); determination of the peptide, amines, and so forth, secreted; and embarkation on a decision tree based upon a reasonable assumption when facts are of limited availability. In the sections that follow we will give a brief overview of the tumors of the gastroenteropancreatic (GEP) axis, their clinical manifestations, and means whereby they may be diagnosed and localized, and we will dwell at some length on the controversial issues pertinent to current views on management.

OVERVIEW

Tumors of the GEP axis occur predominantly in the pancreas and rarely in the duodenum and stomach. Occasionally, tumors secreting GEP hormones may even be found in ectopic sites in the kidney, ovary, thyroid (C cell), lung (bronchial carcinoid), or adrenal medulla, or even be apparently confined to a solitary lymph node.

The various hormone-secreting cells are not evenly distributed but are found in defined areas of the gastrointestinal tract and in the pancreas.[60,152,187] Within the pancreatic islet, the central portion of the islet is composed almost entirely of islet cells that synthesize and secrete insulin, whereas the mantle of the islet contains cells that secrete glucagon, somatostatin, and pancreatic polypeptide. While the pancreas remains the major site of presentation of GEP tumors and is the prime site for gastrinomas and vipomas, it is of interest that the adult human pancreas does not contain gastrin or vasoactive intestinal polypeptide (VIP) cells. It thus appears that these tumors must derive from a pluripotential cell or at least one that is capable of differentiating into a cell capable of secreting a hormone capable of producing the syndrome. This nonhomogeneity of hormone content is, in part, reflected in portal venous concentrations, and a thorough knowledge of the anatomy, especially of the variability of the venous drainage of the pancreas and proximal gut, is required to allow interpretation of measurements made in the portal venous system (PVS) in humans.

It is now established that GEP tumors are of neuroendocrine origin and derive from a primitive stem cell that may differentiate into any one of a variety of adult endocrine-secreting cells: B cell and insulinoma: A cell and glucagonoma; D cell and somatostatinoma; the pancreatic polypeptide (PP) cell and PPoma; cells capable of producing corticotropin, growth hormone–releasing hormone (GHRH), VIP, substance P, gastrin-releasing factor (GRF), and calcitonin; and the enterochromaffin (EC) cell with its ability to cosecrete amines such as serotonin and the peptide motilin. At any one point in time, these cells may secrete one hormone, whereas at other times the peptide or amine secreted may differ and yield an entirely different clinical syndrome. Indeed, metastases are known to secrete hormones that differ from the parent tumor, and different metastases may secrete different hormones.

Of all GEP tumors, carcinoids account for 55%, insulinomas 17%, tumors of unknown types (probably PPomas) 15%, gastrinomas 9%, vipomas 2%, and the remainder secreting a variety of peptides, including somatostatin, glucagon, neurotensin, and sundry others, 2%. The incidence of these tumors is around 1.5 cases per 100,000 of the general population. Although the tumors are relatively rare, the interesting clinical syndromes, the testing of diagnostic acumen, the controversies in management, and the application of knowledge of physiopathology are a challenge to physicians, and this perpetuates an intense interest in the area. To further complicate the issue, these tumors tend to grow very slowly and often do not manifest symptoms until the tumors are fairly advanced and often not before they have metastasized. They are very difficult to locate and often blend with the surrounding tissue by having characteristics that make them isodense with the surrounding pancreas. Even with the most sophisticated means of scrutiny, they go undetected. The tumors are often small (<2 cm), below the resolving capacity of current means of detection. What is often needed is a keen awareness of the symptom complexes and the means for diagnostic evaluation, to avoid much unnecessary suffering and needless attribution of the symptoms to a variety of syndromes, mostly of the neurotic or anxiety-state variety.

While insulinomas constitute the greatest proportion of islet tumors, tumors secreting gastrin,[262] glucagon,[97] somatostatin (SRIF),[50,79,80,124,127,136] human PP (hPP),[137] VIP,[18,207] and thyrocalcitonin;[185] multiple endocrine neoplasia (MEN);[135] and diffuse islet cell adenomatosis,[34] hyperplasia, and nesidioblastosis[82] have all been described as producing clinical syndromes. Although well over 100 different peptides have now been described in the gastrointestinal tract, the clinical syndromes that have been ascribed to a known peptide are indeed limited.

The accurate preoperative localization of islet cell tumors may be essential to the appropriate operative approach in some cases. Most islet cell tumors are small, ranging from 0.5 to 3.0 cm,[78] and may not be readily palpable at operation owing to a texture similar to that of the normal pancreatic tissue.[3,149,172,232] Blind pancreatic resection and unnecessary dissection of the pancreas increase operative morbidity and may result in incomplete cure or even require repeat exploration with an increased risk of morbidity and mortality.[3,233] The advent of computerized tomography (CT), magnetic resonance imaging (MRI), and ultrasonography, all noninvasive techniques, has considerably enhanced our diagnostic skills, but angiography remains the gold standard.

Percutaneous transhepatic portal venous sampling (THVS) for localization of hormone production has proved a valuable tool for localizing many endocrine tumors. This technique has been applied to localization of gut or pancreatic tumors, but several important problems have arisen and require detailed discussion.[270,271]

We will review our experiences with the clinical syndromes, their secretory products, diagnostic tests CT, MRI, ultrasonography, angiography, and transhepatic venous sampling with hormone assay in the localization of GEP tumors. We will also present the most current forms of medical management of these tumors and where surgery is the only option defer to chapter 26.

TABLE 25-1. SECRETORY PRODUCTS OF NEUROENDOCRINE TUMORS*

Peptides	Amines	Miscellaneous
Corticotropin, neurokinins, calcitonin, growth hormone, motilin, substance P, VIP, MSH, PTH, ADH, neurotensin, glucagon, enteroglucagon, insulin, gastrin, HCG subunits, releasing peptides (TRH, GRP, GHRH), CGRP, NSE, chromogranin	Serotonin, 5HTP, 5HIAA, histamine, dopamine, norepinephrine	Prostaglandins

* VIP = vasoactive intestinal polypeptide; MSH = melanocyte stimulating hormone; PTH = parathyroid hormone; ADH = antidiuretic hormone; HCG = human chorionic gonadotrophin; TRH = thyrotropin releasing hormone; GRP = gastrin releasing polypeptide; GHRH = growth hormone releasing hormone; CGRP = calcitonin gene-related peptide; NSE = neuronspecific enolase; 5HTP = 5 hydroxytryptophan; 5HIAA = 5 hydroxy indole acetic acid.

THE CLINICAL SYNDROMES

Gastrinoma

The Zollinger-Ellison syndrome is characterized by persistent basal gastric acid hypersecretion due to hypergastrinemia. The syndrome has been the subject of several extensive recent reviews[165] and will not be reviewed here. What may not be appreciated is that up to 25% of patients do not have ulcer disease, that 33% have diarrhea as the major presenting symptom, and that in 15% of cases diarrhea is the sole manifestation of the disease. Indeed, diarrhea that is responsive to treatment with an H_2-receptor blocking drug demands that the presence of a gastrin-secreting tumor be sought and excluded as the cause. No other diarrhea improves with H_2-receptor blocking drugs. It has been increasingly recognized that the Zollinger-Ellison syndrome can exist in multiple forms: benign sporadic, malignant metastatic, as part of the MEN-I syndrome, and as a G cell hyperplasia syndrome apart from those rare cases in which acid hypersecretion cannot be ascribed to gastrin.[270,271] From various series, it appears that about 66% of gastrinomas are sporadic.[165] Most sporadic tumors are solitary and have been malignant in about 60% to 85% of cases. These are usually found in older subjects but may be seen in children or adolescents. Sporadic tumors generally occur in the pancreas, although primary tumors may also occur in the body of the stomach, duodenum, or jejunum and account for up to 23% of tumors found at operation.[165] The incidence of malignancy is around 60% for tumors arising from the pancreas, whereas it is less than 40% in those arising outside the pancreas. Ectopic tumors have also been identified in peripancreatic lymph nodes;[72,75,165,222] in the splenic hilum; in the root of the mesentery, omentum, liver, and gallbladder, and in the ovary.[14,165] Solitary tumors in these sites are less likely to be malignant, and the overall "cure" is higher than that reported for pancreatic tumors.[10] The likelihood of the surgeon finding a tumor in these sites, however, has been less than 50% in the past. There are still difficulties finding tumors in these locations, leading to operative failures,[226,246,281] dictating a need for improved techniques for localization.

About 33% of gastrinomas are associated with the MEN-I syndrome.[51,74,132,153,170,244] The problems attending gastrinoma in the MEN-I syndrome are quite different from those associated with the sporadic variety. These are not usually associated with a family history but may also occur sporadically, whereas 50% to 60% of MEN-I patients develop gastrinoma, >90% have hyperparathyroidism. Refined testing may be needed to uncover the presence of gastrinoma in ulcer patients with hyperparathyroidism.[13] Tumors in the MEN-I syndrome are usually multiple, often small or undetectable, and less frequently (5%–7%)[51,74,132,153,170] malignant. However, most cases are discovered at a younger age than in the sporadic cases, and the incidence of malignancy may indeed be considerably higher. The multiplicity of the tumors and their small size may make it difficult to find the specific tumors secreting gastrin, and the likelihood of recurrence or persistence after excision militates against laparotomy without identifying a specific site or sites of origin for the hypergastrinemia.

The G cell hyperplasia syndrome has been considered by some to be a part of the gastrinoma syndrome, but in general the distinction from a tumor can be made on the basis of equivocal responses to secretin and an exaggerated response to food ingestion, directing attention to the appropriate site of gastrin overproduction, the antrum.[268] There is seldom a need to pursue localization procedures.

Metastases from gastrinoma are predominantly located in the liver. The presence of gastrinoma in peripancreatic lymph glands should not be taken to indicate incurable malignancy.[14,133,226,227,268,281] The presence of metastases in lymph nodes no longer precludes removal of the primary tumor for possible cure. Some have advocated resection or a debulking procedure[133,227,243,285] or even gastrectomy, which has been reported to cause regression of the primary tumor.[75,177] It nonetheless becomes of vital importance to identify metastases, as the tumor-related mortality can be as high as 79%.[226]

The gastrin gene is known to encode 101 amino acids.[183] Gastrin precursors are encoded with a nonapeptide COOH-terminal extension, a 17–amino acid NH_2 extension, a 55–amino acid precursor, and a preprogastrin. Perhaps the single most important observation is that posttranscriptional processing of the gastrin molecule occurs from the COOH-terminal end to yield gastrin 17. The COOH-terminal phenylalanine becomes amidated, so that antisera to gastrin 17 do not recognize precursors. This may lead to false-negative measurement of gastrin if a gastrin-17-specific antiserum is used. Therefore, knowledge of the specificity of the antiserum used to detect gastrin is a prerequisite for the diagnosis of gastrinoma to be excluded with any degree of certainty.[261] This is probably of utmost importance in those situations in which the clinical syndrome appears to be the gastrinoma syndrome with acid hypersecretion, yet the gastrin values appear at first sight to be within the normal range. High serum levels of gastrin 17 compared with gastrin 34 may be of value,[61,108] or, if available, measurement of the NH_2/COOH terminal gastrin ratio[122,193] to determine the presence of metastases and to monitor the course of treatment. Elevated levels of circulating HCG subunits strongly favor the presence of metastases.[166] In such cases, any curative surgical attempts are unlikely to succeed.

Insulinoma

The classification of causes of insulinoma and the symptom complexes that derive therefrom have recently been reviewed in detail[62] and will not be presented here. Organic hyperinsulinism may be due to a variety of causes of insulin oversecretion. A single benign adenoma occurs in the majority of cases, whereas microadenomatosis, islet cell carcinoma, and the syndrome of multiple endocrine neoplasia each account for about 10% of the remainder of the cases. Nesidioblastosis, a disease generally of childhood, nonetheless occurs in adulthood and needs to be distinguished from diffuse hyperplasia. The table indicates the clinical features, the nature of the abnormality, and the diagnostic tests used to determine the cause of organic hyperinsulinism.

TABLE 25-2. DIAGNOSTIC TESTS FOR ORGANIC HYPERINSULINISM

Clinical feature		Fasting hypoglycemia		
Pathologic findings		Single benign adenomas		68%
		Scattered microadenomatosis		10%
		Islet cell carcinoma		8%
		Nesidioblastosis		5%
		Hyperplasia		?
		MEN-I		10%
Diagnostic glucose tests	Level (mg/dL)	Insulin IRI/G (μU/mL)	Corrected IRI/G	
Overnight fast	<60 (50%)	>24 (50%) >0.3 (95%)	>50 (100%)	
72 h fast	<35 (not in females)	>24 >0.3 (100%)	>50 (100%)	
Proinsulin		>22% (85%)		
C-peptide suppression		Suppression of C peptide to <2 ng/mL with the infusion of insulin		
Calcium infusion test		Too many false negatives		
Secretin test	Administration of 2 U/kg fails to stimulate the release of insulin in a single adenoma and in nesidioblastosis, but with multiple tumors and hyperplasia there is excessive release of insulin			
Insulin and insulin-receptor antibodies	Differentiates insulin autoimmune receptor antibody and some cases of factitious hypoglycemia			
Insulin HPLC	Differentiates some cases of factitious hypoglycemia and autoimmune hypoglycemia when a mutant insulin is secreted			
Localization	See section on tumor localization			

Only 50% of individuals with insulinomas have an overnight fasting blood glucose level of <60 mg/dL. Prolonging the fast to 72 hours in men results in a further slight fall in the blood glucose concentration but not to <55 mg/dL. A value of <35 mg/dL is highly suggestive of organic hypoinsulinism. It is, however, not uncommon for the blood glucose level to fall below 35 mg/dL in women. Therefore, the blood glucose level alone cannot be taken as diagnostic of insulinoma.

The absolute insulin level is not elevated in all patients with organic hyperinsulinism; hence, a normal level does not rule out the diagnosis. A fasting insulin level of <24 μU/mL is 2 standard deviations above the mean for normal nonobese adults, and a value above this in the absence of obesity or other causes of hyperinsulinism is strongly suggestive of organic hyperinsulinism. However, this is found only about 50% of the time. With prolongation of the fast, both normal males and normal females have a fall in their plasma insulin concentration to 4–7 μU/mL, and values greater than this are strongly suggestive of organic hyperinsulinism.

The normal proinsulin/insulin ratio is <22%, and in the absence of uremia, thyrotoxicosis, and liver disease, a value of >24% is found in 85% to 100% of patients with insulinomas.[62]

The accuracy of the insulin and proinsulin measurements can be considerably improved by determining the insulin/glucose ratio. Values of >0.3 are found in

95% of cases with organic hyperinsulinism after an overnight fast and in 100% of cases after fasting for 72 hours. For improvement in the sensitivity of the test, Turner and colleagues have recommended that the insulin/glucose ratio be corrected for a value of glucose of 30 mg/dL, at which level insulin has normally disappeared ($<1\ \mu$U/mL) from the circulation in all healthy subjects. The ratio is

$$\frac{\text{Insulin } (\mu\text{U/mL})}{\text{Glucose}-30 \text{ (mg/dL)}} \times 100$$

and values have been >50 in all cases of proven insulinoma. When these tests are done in practice it may be found that a single value during a fast is normal, but the characteristic of the individual with an insulinoma is that with increasing duration of the fast the test tends to become more abnormal, in contrast to the improvement found in healthy nonhypoglycemic subjects. A number of miscellaneous tests of insulin secretion have been proposed by others and are in use elsewhere but have not proved to be any more successful in our hands than the tried and tested measures outlined above. Suppression of C peptide by the infusion of insulin testifies to the autonomy of insulin secretion but does not help to distinguish its cause. The administration of calcium has been popularized by some authors but yields inconsistent results. Glucagon and/or tolbutamide infusions and the administration of leucine have fallen by the wayside, since most of these tests yield falsely negative results and offer no advantage over prolongation of the fast. A glucose tolerance test, which is almost always requested for the patient with organic hyperinsulinism, has no diagnostic value whatsoever!

As a useful marker for malignancy, the measurement of the levels of the subunits of HCG may be helpful inasmuch as a normal value for the α subunit is always found in patients with benign disease and in 43% of patients with metastases. Thus an abnormal value always heralds the presence of malignancy though a normal value does not exclude it.

Perhaps one of the greatest diagnostic dilemmas is the distinction of organic hyperinsulinism from the subtle presentation of autoimmune hypoglycemia syndrome and from factitious hypoglycemia; the patient with the latter condition can try the ingenuity of even the most careful and astute physician. Surreptitious administration of insulin may cause not only high insulin values but, because of the cross-reaction of antibodies to insulin that are generated, also spuriously high proinsulin values. Measurement of the C-peptide values generally exclude this possibility. However, there are instances in which proinsulin and C-peptide values will not separate these conditions, and provided it is available, characterization of the insulin by high-performance liquid chromatography (HPLC) will identify the insulin as pork, bovine, or human, depending on the species that is present.[119] With the advent of human insulin preparations, even this sophisticated approach may be mitigated by the determined individual aware that human insulin cannot be differentiated in the human serum and generally does not generate antibodies. Autoimmune hypoglycemia can usually be identified in older people with recurrent severe episodes of hypoglycemia, artificially high insulin levels due to interference with the assay by the circulating insulin antibodies, and high C-peptide levels, presumably due to the pancreatic overcompensation for the inactivation of insulin by binding to the antibody.[217] A very rare subgroup of people have antibodies to the insulin receptor or idiotypic antibodies to insulin antibody that are capable of activating the receptor and increasing glucose transport, thus mimicking organic hyperinsulinism. In these difficult cases measurement of these antibody levels may be diagnostic.

Hypoglycemia that accompanies the presence of large mesothelial tumors such as retroperitoneal fibrosarcoma and hepatomas generally does not present a diagnostic problem. The recent demonstration of activation of the glucose transporter by oncogene products has provided a long-awaited explanation for the mechanism of production of hypoglycemia but as yet has not reached the diagnostic arena.

Somatostatinoma

Somatostatin is a tetradecapeptide that inhibits numerous endocrine and exocrine secretory functions. Almost all gut hormones studied are inhibited by SRIF, including insulin, PP, glucagon, gastrin, secretin, GIP, and motilin.[255] In addition to the inhibition of the endocrine secretions, SRIF has direct effects on a number of target organs.[44] For example, it is a potent inhibitor of basal and pentagastrin-stimulated gastric acid secretion. It also has marked effects on gastrointestinal transit time, intestinal motility, and the absorption of nutrients from the small intestine. The major effect in the small intestine appears to be a delay in the absorption of fat and reduced absorption of calcium. The salient features of the somatotstatinoma syndrome, therefore, are diabetes, diarrhea or steatorrhea, gallbladder disease, hypochlorhydria, and weight loss.[127,136]

The first cases of the somatostatinoma syndrome were reported in 1977 by Ganda et al., and recently Krejs et al. reported another case and reviewed the six other cases that had appeared in the literature prior to 1980.[80,127]

We have examined the literature between 1980 and 1986 and describe here the features now recognized to be a part of the syndrome. For convenience, we have divided the cases into pancreatic and extrapancreatic tumors.[269]

Twenty-seven cases of pancreatic and 18 cases of intestinal somatostatinomas have been reported. The mean age of the 27 patients was 53 years (range, 26–84 years). Most patients were between 40 and 60 years of age. Of the 27 patients, 18 were female and 9 were male, suggesting a female preponderance, in contrast to the equal sex incidence in other islet tumors.[43]

TABLE 25-3. DIFFERENTIATION OF PANCREATIC AND INTESTINAL SOMATOSTATINOMAS

Feature	Pancreatic	Intestinal
Age	26–84	26–77
Sex (M : F)	9 : 18	12 : 6
Diabetes	20/27	2/18
Gallbladder disease	16/27	5/18
Diarrhea	9/27	11/18
Hypochlorhydria	7/8	1/8
Weight loss	9/27	4/18
Associated disorders	None	Café au lait spots, neurofibromatossis, hypertension

The mean SLI concentration in patients with pancreatic somatostatinoma was 50 times higher than normal (range 1–250 times). The plasma of many patients with somatostatinoma contained 3 to 4 different molecular forms of SLI, specifically, of SLI fractions with apparent molecular weights of 1600, 3000 to 4000, 6000 to 15,000, and greater than 30,000. Some of these molecular fractions may be SRIF precursors. Release into the circulation of abnormally large amounts of high-molecular-weight forms of polypeptide hormones is a characteristic feature of endocrine tumors, including insulinomas and glucagonomas. Conceivably, differences in the patterns of SLI in the circulation could account for differences in the clinical presentation.

Of 27 patients with pancreatic tumors, 20 had diabetes mellitus. In contrast, diabetes occurred in only 2 of 18 patients with intestinal tumors. In all instances, the diabetes was relatively mild and could be controlled with diet and/or hypoglycemic agents or with small doses of insulin except in two cases,[103,254] in whom ketonemia was present. Somatostatin is known to inhibit insulin responses to all major physiologic stimuli. The high incidence of diabetes mellitus, 75% in patients with pancreatic tumors who had high SLI levels, and the low incidence in patients with intestinal tumors with low SLI levels strongly suggest a cause-and-effect relationship between somatostatinoma, chronically elevated plasma SRIF concentrations, and diabetes mellitus. It is not clear whether differential inhibition of insulin and diabetogenic hormones can explain the usually mild degree of diabetes and the rarity of ketoacidosis in patients with somatostatinoma.

Four patients with pancreatic tumors had recurrent attacks of hypoglycemia, the hypoglycemia of one patient alternating with diabetes. Possible differences in the short- and long-term inhibitory effects of hypersomatostatinemia include other factors that determine the development and the degree of glucose intolerance. Suppression of glucagon rather than insulin by high-molecular-weight SLI could account for hypoglycemia, rather than diabetes, but suitable studies have not been carried out. Replacement of functional islet cell tissue with tumor in pancreatic tumors may be another reason for the development of diabetes in the majority of patients with pancreatic somatostatinoma, contrasting with the low incidence in those with intestinal tumors. These tumors are usually large and, therefore, destroy substantial portions of the pancreas. From the available evidence, it appears, therefore, that tumor size and location as well as the level of circulating SLI, its molecular species, and the relative effects on insulin and glucagon are all important determinants for the development of diabetes mellitus and/or hypoglycemia.[155]

Sixteen of the 27 patients with pancreatic tumors and 5 of 18 with intestinal tumors had gallbladder disease. The ability of SRIF to inhibit gallbladder contraction and secretion of bile[43,44,80,103,127,136,141,155,254,269] is compatible with the high incidence of gallbladder disease in patients with somatostatinoma.

Diarrhea consisting of 3 to 10 frequently foul-smelling stools per day and/or steatorrhea (20–76 g of fat per 24 hours) was reported in 9 and 11 pancreatic tumor patients, respectively. In some cases, the severity of diarrhea and steatorrhea paralleled the course of the disease, worsening as the tumor advanced and the metastatic disease spread and improving after tumor resection. Diarrhea and/or steatorrhea occurred in only three patients with intestinal tumors. Somatostatin has been shown to inhibit pancreatic secretion of proteolytic enzymes, water, and bicarbonate,[23] and gallbladder motility.[45] In addition, it has been demonstrated to inhibit absorption of lipids.[212] High blood concentrations of SRIF such as occur in patients with pancreatic somatostatinoma can, therefore, be anticipated to result in maldigestion, diarrhea, and steatorrhea.

Gastric acid secretion was evaluated in 13 patients with pancreatic tumors and 6 with intestinal tumors. Basal and stimulated acid secretion were inhibited in 7 of 8 patients with pancreatic tumors tested and in only 1 of 8 patients with intestinal tumors, in keeping with the known gastric antisecretory activities of SRIF.[17]

Weight loss ranging from 9 to 21 kg over several months was mentioned in fourteen case reports, nine of 27 patients with pancreatic tumors and four of 20 with intestinal tumors. The weight loss may be related to malabsorption and diarrhea, but in small intestinal tumors, anorexia, abdominal pain, and yet-unexplained reasons may be relevant.

Of great interest was the presence of café au lait spots, neurofibromatosis, and paroxysmal hypertension and pheochromocytoma in some patients with intestinal tumors.

Of the 47 primary tumors, 27 were found in the pancreas and 20 in the duodenum or jejunum. Of the pancreatic tumors, 14 were located in the head and 5 in the tail, while 2 tumors infiltrated the whole pancreas and 2 were found in the body. Twenty tumors had extrapancreatic locations, 9 originating in the duodendum, 10 in the ampulla, and 1 in the jejunum. Thus, about 60% of somatostatinomas originated in the upper intestinal tract, probably a consequence of the relatively large number of D cells present in this region.

Somatostatinomas tend to be large, similar to glucagonomas[15] but unlike insulinomas and gastrinomas, which are small as a rule.[62,105] In more recent cases within the intestine, the tumors have tended to be smaller. The symptoms associated with somatostatinomas and glucagonomas are less pronounced and probably do not develop until very high blood levels of the respective hormones have been attained. As a result, somatostatinomas and glucagonomas are likely to be diagnosed later.

Twenty-one of 27 patients with pancreatic tumors and 10 of 20 with intestinal tumors had evidence of metastatic disease. Metastatic involvement of the liver was reported most frequently, and regional lymph node involvement and metastases to bone less frequently. Thus, in approximately 31 of 45 cases, metatastic disease was present at the time of diagnosis. This is similar to the high incidence of malignancy in glucagonoma[15] and in gastrinoma,[105] but it is distinctly different from the low incidence of malignant insulinoma.[62] The high prevalence of metastatic disease in somatostatinoma may also be a consequence of late diagnosis but is apparently not dependent upon the tissue of origin.

Diagnosis

In the reported series somatostatinomas were found more or less accidentally. In the majority of cases, the tumors were found either during exploratory laparotomy or during upper gastrointestinal x-ray studies, CT scans, or ultrasound or endoscopic studies performed because of various symptoms including unexplained abdominal pain, melena, hematemesis, or persistent diarrhea, or in search of insulinomas or corticotropin-secreting tumors. Once found, the tumors were identified as somatostatinomas by demonstration of elevated tissue concentrations of SLI[266] and/or prevalence of D cells by immunocytochemistry or by the demonstration of elevated plasma SLI concentrations. Thus, the events leading to the diagnosis of somatostatinoma have occurred in reverse order. In other islet cell tumors, the clinical symptoms and signs usually suggest the diagnosis, which is then established by the demonstration of diagnostically elevated blood hormone levels, following which efforts are undertaken to localize the tumors. It can be expected that the same sequence of diagnostic procedures will be followed in the future for the diagnosis of somatostatinoma, mainly for two reasons.[1] (1) There is increasing familiarity of physicians with the clinical somatostatinoma syndrome. This symptom complex, while not pathognomonic, is nevertheless sufficiently characteristic for somatostatinoma to suggest the correct diagnosis.[2] (2) The greater availability of reliable radioimmunoassays for the determination of SLI in blood has increased the yield.[266] Presently these assays are complicated by the need for cumbersome extraction procedures and are not readily available. However, it should be recognized that the syndrome is rare. Of 1199 cases screened for somatostatinoma at the University of Michigan between 1982 and 1986, 8 have had diagnostic levels of SLI.

The diagnosis of somatostatinoma at a time when blood SLI concentrations are normal or only marginally elevated, however, will require reliable provocative tests. Increases in plasma SLI concentrations have been reported after intravenous infusion of tolbutamide and arginine. Decreases in SLI concentrations have been observed after intravenous infusion of diazoxide. Arginine is a well-established stimulant for normal D cells and thus is unlikely to differentiate between normal and supranormal SRIF secretion. The same may be true for diazoxide, which has been shown to decrease SLI secretion from normal dog pancreas as well as in patients with somatostatinoma.[208] Tolbutamide stimulates SLI release from normal dog and rat pancreas,[23,45,208] but Pipeleers and colleagues[198] found no change in circulating SLI concentrations in three normal human subjects after intravenous injection of 1 g of tolbutamide. At present, therefore, tolbutamide appears to be a candidate for a provocative agent most useful in the diagnosis of somatostatinoma. Clearly, however, its reliability will have to be established in a greater number of patients and controls. Until then, it may be necessary to measure plasma SLI concentrations during routine workups for postprandial dyspepia and gallbladder disorders as suggested by Krejs,[67,127] diabetes without a family history, and unexplained steatorrhea, inasmuch as these symptoms appear to be very early signs of somatostatinomas. The distinctive clinical features of duodenal somatostatinomas and the good prognosis of those with amyloid and psammoma bodies make it important for clinicians to be aware of this newly described clinical entity.

PPoma

Pancreatic polypeptide was discovered by serendipity. In 1972, working in separate laboratories, Chance and Jones,[87] and Kimmel et al.[116] purified a single major protein from a crude insulin preparation; the protein was named pancreatic polypeptide.[37] In mammals 93% of the cells producing PP are located in the pancreas. These have been found both within the islets, scattered in the exocrine parenchyma, and lining the ducts. Within the islets, the PP cells are located mainly in the periphery, wedged between the A and B cells, and where nerves make their entry into the islets. This latter observation appears to be important in view of the extreme sensitivity of PP cells to autonomic perturbation. The PP cells are more abundant in the head than in the body and tail. Orci et al.[187] have recently isolated a lobe that is particularly rich in PP cells separate from the remainder of the head of the pancreas. They have suggested that this lobe represents persistence of the ventral primordia consistent with the embryologic development of the pancreas. This uneven distribution of PP within the pancreas has relevance when attempts are made to localize PPomas by portal venous sampling.

Several assays are available for the measurement of PP in the circulation. Although little is known about the physiologic functions of PP, the fasting levels increase with age, prolonged fasting, uncontrolled diabetes, and exercise.[71] Ingestion of nutrients is followed by an extremely rapid rise in the circulating concentration of PP, and the elevation persists for 4 to 8 hours. The descending order of potency of nutrients is protein, fat, and carbohydrate. Circulating nutrients have little or no effect, suggesting the importance of the gastrointestinal tract in mediating signals to the pancreas.[71] A unique and interesting dependence of these gastrointestinal signals on extravagal cholinergic mediation has been shown, since responses to meals can be abolished by the administration of the muscarinic cholinergic blocker atropine.[81] Apart from the nutrient effect, there is clearly a cerebral or neural phase and one mediated by gastrointestinal hormones. The PP levels increase markedly with administration of secretin, cholecystokinin, and bombesin, but less so with gastrin and pentagastrin.[71,81,83,87]

Despite these very dramatic effects of meal ingestion, cerebral stimulation, and hormone administration on circulating levels of PP, a biological role for PP has not been established. The only physiologic effects in humans are inhibition of

TABLE 25-4. COMPARISON OF VIPOMA AND GASTRINOMA

Symptom or Sign	Vipoma	Gastrinoma
Diarrhea	Secretory	Nonsecretory (0.5–6 L/day)
	Usually >2 L/day	
	No improvement with fasting	Improves with H_2 blockers
Ulcer	Nil	Severe
Abdominal pain	None	Marked
Acid secretion	Decreased	Increased
Gastric volume	Decreased	Increased
Steatorrhea	Rare	Frequent
Malabsorption	Rare	Frequent
Hypokalemia	Usual	Rare
Acidosis	Usual	Rare
Hypercalcemia	50%	Only MEN (15%)
Flushing	80%	None
Abnormal GTT	50%	None

gallbladder contraction and pancreatic enzyme secretion.[87] Thus, a tumor deriving from PP cells is predicted to be clinically *silent*. That this is not always the case is illustrated in Table 25-5.[26,27,57,76,91,134,137,150,154,180,199,225,237,247–249,275] Tomita et al. reported two patients, one of whom had persistent watery diarrhea and the other of whom had high levels of circulating PP and PP cell hyperplasia.[247] Bordi et al.[27] reported a PP tumor in a patient with chronic duodenal ulcer, and Ebeid et al. reported a patient with a tumor that invaded the bile ducts, producing biliary obstruction.[57] Larsson et al. suggested that the watery diarrhea syndrome may have its origin in PP overproduction.[137] The picture is further complicated by the fact that mixed tumors, PP cell hyperplasia in association with other functioning islet cell tumors, ductal hyperplasia of PP cells, nesidioblastosis, and multiple islet tumors producing PP have also been described either alone or as part of the MEN-I syndrome.[134,199] Basal concentrations of PP in plasma may be raised above 1000 pg/mL in 22% to 77% of cases of all endocrine-secreting tumors, and in 29% to 50% of patients with the carcinoid syndrome, even if the carcinoid is located outside the pancreas. Among 53 patients with adenocarcinomas of the pancreas, in no instance was an elevated basal concentration of PP found.[268,271] The diagnostic accuracy of elevated basal PP concentrations as a marker for endocrine-secreting tumors can be marginally increased to around 50% to 60% by determining the response of PP to secretin administration.[262,264] A response of greater than 5000 pg/min per milliliter is more than 2 standard deviations above that observed in healthy subjects. It appears, however, that many of the cases of so-called nonfunctional tumors are indeed PPomas, since it is our experience that 50% to 75% of these have raised basal PP levels, and in 67%, the response to secretin is exaggerated. Thus, in the absence of factors such as chronic renal failure that are known to cause marked elevation of PP levels, in an older healthy patient, a markedly elevated PP level may occasionally be indicative of a nonfunctioning pancreatic endocrine tumor. Differentiation of a high basal concentration in a healthy subject from that appearing in patients with tumor has been difficult. Schwartz suggested that administration of atropine would suppress concentrations in healthy subjects and would fail to do so in patients with tumors, but this has not been subject to extensive examination.[213]

Increased PP cells are found in 20% to 67% of functioning and nonfunctioning tumors of the pancreas.[186] There does not appear to be a relationship between the number of cells and their function, since islet tumors containing subnormal, normal, or supernormal concentrations of PP compared with the normal pancreas may be associated with normal or high levels of circulating PP. There are now at

TABLE 25-5. CAUSES OF SECRETORY DIARRHEA

Vipoma
PPoma, somatostatinoma, calcitoninoma, prostaglandinoma
Carcinoid
Medullary carcinoma of the thyroid
Villous adenoma of the rectum
Surreptitious laxative abuse
Hyperthyroidism (apparent)
Idiopathic

least 21 patients in the literature with PPomas. The age ranged from 20 to 74 years with a mean of 51. Twelve were males and 9 were females. Diabetes was found in only 2 cases. Diarrhea, which was formerly thought to be a part of the syndrome,[137] occurred in 6 out of 16 cases in which it was recorded, and steatorrhea was found in 5 out of 5 patients in whom it was sought. Decreased acid secretion was documented in only 2 of 6 people studied. Eleven presented with weight loss. We have come to recognize the PPoma syndrome as silent. These tumors are often found by serendipity in patients with hepatomegaly (8 out of 20) or abdominal pain (6 out of 20); due to metastases to the liver; jaundice due to obstruction of the common bile duct; or upper GI bleeding that may be due to invasion of the wall of the duodenum or thrombosis of the splenic or portal veins and the development of varices. Not infrequently, they are recognized by the radiologist as highly vascular tumors with metastases to the liver. Six of the reported cases had PPomas as part of the MEN-I syndrome.

Vipoma

The syndrome was first described by Verner and Morrison in 1958,[258] and in 1974 they reviewed 55 patients.[259] The clinical features of the syndrome are a secretory diarrhea of 0.5 to 6.0 L/day, hypokalemia, hypochlorhydria, flushing, hypercalcemia, an abnormal glucose tolerance test, tetany, and a dilated gallbladder. The major constant feature of the syndrome is the diarrhea, which is generally profuse and watery. Because of this predominant feature, the syndrome has been given various names that include pseudocholera syndrome; the Verner Morrison syndrome; and WDHHA, to represent, watery diarrhea, hypokalemia, hypochlorhydria, and alkalosis. However, in all instances that we have encountered, the bicarbonate wasting that accompanies the diarrhea is so severe that invariably the patients present with the paradox of hypokalemia and acidosis. In the series reported by Long and colleagues,[145] the commonest site for these tumors is in the pancreas, presumably derived from either the primitive stem cell or alternatively from nervous tissue within the pancreas. Ten children of the 62 patients with the disease reported by Long had ganglioneuroblastomas. Any diarrhea that persists with fasting should alert the physician to the possibility of a vipoma, but the condition can be difficult to distinguish from other causes of secretory diarrhea. The diarrhea can be confused with that of the Zollinger-Ellison syndrome, but there are certain distinguishing features that allow the separation to be made at the bedside.

The common findings in the vipoma syndrome can be rationalized on the basis of the known actions of the hormone. The increase in intestinal secretions is a direct function of VIP. The structural similarity with the pancreatic secretogogue secretin accounts for the increase in pancreatic bicarbonate secretion, and the similarities with glucagon and GIP for the hyperglycemia and reduction in gastric acid secretion, respectively. VIP also relaxes smooth muscle in the gallbladder, and a dilated gallbladder is highly suspicious. The high incidence of flushing attacks may be related to the vasodilatory properties of VIP but may also be due to cosecretion of other vasoactive agents. The mechanism for the hypercalcemia is ill-understood; it may be due to VIP's stimulating effect on the osteoclast.

By simple definition the diagnosis is made by detecting an elevated VIP level of >150 pg/mL, which distinguishes this disease from other causes of secretory diarrhea.

Thus, when a patient presents with the syndrome, it is usually prudent to estimate other agents in urine or blood known to be implicated in the diarrhea syndrome and to exclude conditions such as hyperthyroidism, although the diarrhea is usually one of hyperdefecation and not secretory. The diarrhea of medullary carcinoma of the thyroid is not often as profuse, but that of tumors of the pancreas that secrete calcitonin can be and is more refractory to management than that of vipomas. Even with a broad array of measurements, one is not infrequently left with a patient who has the syndrome but in whom no tumor can be identified; some of these patients have gone on to total pancreatectomy without success. Indeed we have identified tumors free in the mesentery, in the skin, and in the ovary, and in one patient with a hypernephroma, diarrhea preceded evidence of the tumor by almost 2 years!

Glucagonoma

The glucagonoma syndrome presents a constellation of features that now has become reasonably easy to identify. In 1966 McGavran[167] first described a syndrome with diabetes and glucagon-producing tumors, and Wilkinson in 1973 and Sweet in 1974 drew attention to the rash that almost alway accompanied the syndrome. There are now well over 200 cases that have been reported in the literature, and the syndrome has several important distinguishing features: necrotizing migratory erythema associated with angular stomatitis; onycholysis and a red beefy tongue due to glossitis; diabetes; a normochromic normocytic anemia; marked weight loss; oftentimes severe depression; and a tendency toward thromboembolic disease. The skin rash is essentially a bullous dermatosis that may be extremely polymorphic, but the waxing and waning and the natural progression of lesions are, if not classic, typical and should help to differentiate it from other dermatologic conditions. The lesions commence with an erythematous papule that enlarges to form a vesicle that spreads to become confluent with other vesicles. The vesicles then erode, ulcerate, and discharge a white flaky material that is the necrotic epidermis. The lesions then heal, leaving a brown depressed pigmented patch. The rash is widely distributed over the body but involves especially the fissures in the groin, perineum, and buttocks, under the breasts, and in other intertriginous areas. The differential diagnosis includes other deficiency states, acrodermatitis enteropathica, zinc deficiency, fatty acid deficiency, pellagra, psoriasis, pemphigus, and moniliasis. Indeed the association of *Monilia* with diabetes is not infrequently confused with the glucagonoma syndrome. The histologic features of the rash are typical, with necrolysis of the upper epidermis, liquefaction of the granular layer, and subcorneal blister formation. The diagnosis is difficult to make, and several biopsies may be necessary for confirmation. With the ready availability of glucagon assays it seems that in doubtful cases a single estimation of the plasma glucagon level is not an unreasonable test.

A number of patients have now been described in whom diabetes is the only manifestation of the disease. Diabetes in an older individual without a family history of diabetes should alert one to the possibility of a glucagon-producing tumor. The diabetes is mild and unaccompanied by ketoacidosis. This is somewhat surprising in view of the known ketogenic activity of glucagon. The high rate of thromboembolic phenomena and the depression are invariably sufficient to warrant further investigation provided that the physician is aware of the constellation of symptoms and signs that make up the disease.

Once the condition is suspected, the diagnosis need not be very complicated. All cases thus far reported have had inordinately elevated glucagon levels, and the only diagnostic dilemma is the familial hyperglucagonemia syndrome, in which there is no associated diabetes or skin rash.[22,189] Earlier diagnosis in individuals with normal glucagon levels may be disclosed by the finding of an exaggerated glucagon response to the hormone secretin, much as is the case in gastrinoma patients. Hypoaminoacidemia is also a characteristic feature, but amino acid analyses are not available as readily as the glucagon radioimmunoassay.

In spite of the ready availability of radioimmunoassays for glucagon, the incidence is still rare ($\pm 2\%$ of all gut endocrine tumors), and it seems that a number of these cases must have been and still are being missed. The constellation of features erroneously leads to diagnoses of vitamin, fatty acid, and zinc deficiency and the thrombophlebitis to a carcinoma lurking somewhere. A fruitful search for these cases may be done in the offices of psychiatrists, who may have treated the depression for years without recognition of the true underlying pathologic condition. The very fact that almost all these tumors are very large at the time of diagnosis testifies to the delay in diagnosis and is supported by the high incidence (50%–70%) of malignancy and metastases at the time of diagnosis. The possibility of metastases may be substantiated by the finding of elevated levels of the β subunit of hCG or carcinoembryonic antigen and recently by elevated levels of carbohydrate antigen (CA 19-9).[6]

Carcinoid

Although carcinoids are classically tumors of enterochromaffin and argentaffin cells of the digestive tract, the term *carcinoid tumor* can be expanded to cover "gut" tumors of paracrine- and endocrine-like cells of unknown function.[224,276]

The clinical and biochemical features of carcinoid tumors depend on their site of origin. The classic features of carcinoid syndrome are seen in midgut carcinoid. There are, however, certain distinguishing features of carcinoid tumors of the foregut. The syndrome is often atypical, wheezing is prominent, symptoms occur in the absence of metastases, the flush is often protracted and involves the upper trunk, and the major excretion product is the serotonin precursor 5HTP, rather than serotonin. Attempts to separate pancreatic carcinoids from those of the rest of the gut on the basis of the hormonal profile have, however, not proved uniformly successful.

TABLE 25-6. CLINICAL FEATURES OF CARCINOID TUMORS

	Foregut	Midgut	Hindgut
Localization	Pancreas, stomach, duodenum, ileum	Jejunum, rectum, bronchial tree	Transverse colon–ascending colon
Secretion products	5HTP, histamine, multiple peptides, somatostatin, calcitonin	5HT, bradykinins, prostaglandins, substance P	No known substances
Functional manifestations	Atypical carcinoid, ZE, acromegaly	Carcinoid syndrome, Cushing's, etc.	Silent
Staining	Argyrophil	Argentaffin	Nonreactive

The tumors are slow-growing and may be present for years without overt symptoms, thus escaping attention. In the early stages, vague abdominal pain goes undiagnosed and is invariably ascribed to "irritable bowel or spastic colon." With metastases to the liver, the correct diagnosis is generally arrived at with a latency, however, of many years. Even then, mistaken identity is not uncommon, and unless biopsy material is examined for the neuronal glycolytic enzyme neuron-specific enolase or the secretory peptide chromogranin,[221] tumors may be erroneously labeled as adenocarcinomas, with a negative impact upon survival and attitudes to management.

Carcinoid syndrome occurs in less than 10% of patients with carcinoid tumors. The principal features of carcinoid syndrome include flushing, sweating, wheezing, diarrhea, abdominal pain, cardiac fibrosis, and pellagra dermatosis. Diarrhea is found in 83% of cases, flushing in 49%, dyspnea in 20%, and bronchospasm in 6%.[238] The relationship between diarrhea and flushing is variable. One can occur without the other, and there may be no temporal relationship between the two. The specific etiologic agent(s) for each of the protean manifestations of the carcinoid tumors is not known. Serotonin,[67,169] prostaglandins,[209] 5-hydroxytryptophan,[5,184,196] substance P,[236,279] kallikrein,[147] histamine,[195] dopamine,[66] and neuropeptide K[242] are thought to be involved in the clinical manifestations of carcinoid tumors. In addition, symptoms may be related to overproduction of peptides of the proopiomelanocortin family, β endorphin, and enkephalin. Pancreatic polypeptide and motilin levels are often raised,[68,270] which may be impor-

TABLE 25-7. CLINICAL MANIFESTATIONS OF THE CARCINOID SYNDROME

Manifestation	Patients Affected (%)
Cutaneous flushing	49
GI hypermotility	83
Signs of heart disease	37
Bronchoconstriction	6
Pellagra pigmentation	5

tant markers of tumor activity and provide a means of monitoring tumor growth and response to therapy rather than contributing to specific symptomatology.

DIAGNOSIS OF THE CLINICAL SYNDROMES

With this brief overview of the major clinical syndromes, it is important to be able to recognize the constellation of features that combine to represent a gut hormone–producing tumor and to be aware of the hormones that may be implicated. Although tentative, Table 25-8 presents a reasonable fascimile of the symptom complexes and the hormones that may be implicated and that are deserving of measurement. Only in those instances in which assays are sufficiently reliable for clinical use have these been listed. Clearly there are other agents that may be involved in the generation of the symptom complex, but it is premature to list these until we have better means of measurement.

LOCALIZATION OF ISLET CELL TUMORS

Angiography, Ultrasonography and Radionuclide Imaging

For many years arteriographic studies have been the most sensitive means of localizing islet cell adenomas, with success rates ranging widely among reported series.[3,149,204] Most insulinomas are small,ranging from 0.5 to 3 cm[78] and may not

TABLE 25-8. CLINICAL SYNDROMES AND AGENTS TO MEASURE

Symptom or Disease	Agent(s) Implicated
Ulcer disease	Gastrin
Diabetes (no family history, late in life)	Glucagon, somatostatin, corticotropin, VIP, GHRH
Diarrhea	VIP, gastrin, somatostatin, PP, calcitonin, 5HT, 5HTP, glucagon, prostaglandins
Dermatosis (migratory, necrolytic erythema)	Glucagon
Flushing and hypotension	Substance P, VIP, 5HT, prostaglandins, calcitonin, neurokinins, histamine
Gallbladder disease	Somatostatin, VIP, glucagon
Hypercalcemia	PTH, VIP
Hypoglycemia	Insulin
Spastic colon (irritable bowel)	5HT, substance P, neurokinins, PP, motilin
Hepatomegaly (pain RUQ)	PP
Acromegaly (without pituitary tumor)	Growth hormone, GHRH
Cushing's (normal adrenal and pituitary)	Corticotropin, Corticotrophin Releasing Factor (CRF)
Suspect neuroendocrine tumor	Neuron-specific enolase, chromogranin, calcitonin gene-related peptide

be readily visible because they have a texture similar to that of normal pancreatic tissue.[3,78,172,222] Angiograms may falsely localize lesions and in unusual cases demonstrate only one of several when multiple adenomas are present.[78,121] We have previously reported false localization of tumors due to (1) an opaque shadow in the duodenal bulb and (2) an apparent tumor that was a splenunculus.[268] In other islet cell tumors, particularly small insulinomas and gastrinomas, we have been singularly unsuccessful but have had some measure of success with large tumors, as in the case of malignant glucagonomas. Our success rate differs from that reported by other authors (60%–85%),[3,149,204,232] reflecting upon the nature of our referral pattern. We are a tertiary-care institution, and only those tumors that are occult and have not been identified by angiography carried out elsewhere are referred for diagnosis and localization. With metastatic tumors such as PPomas, angiography can prove very helpful, and the demonstration of highly vascular metastases usually means a neuroendocrine tumor. The silent clinical nature of the PPoma often causes it to be confused with an adenocarcinoma and can be distinguished by the highly vascular nature of the metastases.

Ultrasonography is now receiving more attention as a potential tool in the localization of these tumors, especially when used by the endoscopic route.

Somatostatin receptors have been detected in a variety of neuroendocrine tumors.[201b] Autoradiography of endocrine pancreatic tumors and carcinoids revealed high density of binding sites[201a] and led to the use of iodine (^{123}I) labeled somatostatin analog as a new imaging technique for localization of tumor tissue.[127a,131a]

CT

Functioning pancreatic islet cell tumors are often small at presentation. Tumors less than 2 cm in diameter cause no significant deformation of the pancreatic contour. Such small tumors are usually invisible on noncontrast CT scans. These lesions generally, however, become hyperdense because of their hypervascularity compared with adjacent normal pancreatic parenchyma on scans obtained shortly after an intravenous bolus injection of contrast material; thus, they may be detected at CT when a contrast bolus and rapid, thin section scanning (contiguous 5-mm slices) are used. Rarely, these tumors are hypodense on contrast-enhanced scans.[70,88] CT detects most tumors larger than 3 cm because of pancreatic contour abnormalities as well as density differences on postcontrast scans. Tumor calcifications may be present. Multiple tumors are a frequent occurrence, particularly for gastrinomas. Extrapancreatic tumor foci can blend in with adjacent bowel loops and thus be difficult to detect.

Nonfunctional tumors, on the other hand, are usually large when the patient first seeks medical attention. These lesions range in size from 1 to 24 cm in diameter[58,113] and are generally detected on noncontrast CT scans due to alteration of the pancreatic contour.

Tumor size, rather than tumor histologic lesions, is the major determinant of CT detectability. Most intrapancreatic tumors that are missed at CT are less than 2 cm in diameter. Thus, most nonfunctional endocrine tumors and glucagonomas, which are also usually large, are detected by CT. Extrapancreatic tumor location also contributes to the difficulty in identifying small lesions at CT; this compounds the problem in assessing gastrinomas, which are often both small and extrapancreatic. Generalizations regarding CT assessment of other islet cell tumors, such as somatostatinomas, VIPomas, or PPomas, cannot be made since few of these tumors have been reported.

Islet cell tumors may calcify, and large lesions often have low-density areas of necrosis. In some series, calcifications at CT showed a positive correlation with malignant tumor histologic lesions.[29,58,98,251] The calcifications are typically coarse and clumped, in contrast to the fine, punctuate, diffuse calcifications seen in chronic pancreatitis at CT. Pancreatic ductal adenocarcinomas rarely calcify. Other differentiating features between islet cell tumors and ductal carcinomas include the vascular blush of the former following administration of an intravenous contrast bolus: ductal adenocarcinomas are usually hypodense on contrast-enhanced scans. In addition, although large islet cell tumors can invade adjacent vessels and retroperitoneal structures, encasement of the celiac or superior mesenteric arteries is much more commonly found in ductal adenocarcinoma; this feature is usually well demonstrated using CT.[168]

With carcinoid tumors there may be multiple small (0.5–1.0 cm) focal mesenteric densities, consistent with lymphadenopathy and fibrotic change, as well as a linear, radiating pattern of desmoplastic mesenteric retraction.[42] Localized small bowel wall thickening and occasionally malignant ascites are present. These changes are usually evident on CT scans.

Hepatic metastases from pancreatic and extrapancreatic endocrine tumors are generally hypodense compared with normal liver parenchyma on noncontrast CT scans; due to the hypervascularity of these lesions, many become isodense or hyperdense on postcontrast scans. In some patients, hepatic metastases are visible only on noncontrast images or only on postcontrast images, but not on both. Bressler et al. reviewed CT scans of 28 patients with hepatic metastases from hypervascular primary tumors: these included 13 carcinoid and 10 islet cell tumors.[30] Dynamic incremental scanning was performed after administration of a 100 to 150-mL intravenous bolus of 60% contrast material. In four patients with islet cell tumors and four with carcinoid tumors, metastases visible on noncontrast examinations became isodense or nearly isodense with normal liver on contrast-enhanced scans. Only 2 of 62 metastases were evident on contrast-enhanced scans and invisible on the precontrast studies; histologic type for these two lesions was not specified. The timing of intravenous contrast administration and scan acquisition are critical in order to maximize the difference in enhancement between normal hepatic tissue and hepatic metastases.[4,30,35,284]

MRI

Large primary pancreatic endocrine tumors can be detected at MRI by pancreatic contour abnormalities. The tumors are typically hypointense compared with normal pancreas on T1-weighted images and hyperintense on T2-weighted images. More work needs to be done to establish the detectability and characteristics of small, non-contour-deforming lesions.[88,229,230]

Hepatic metastases from endocrine tumors are typically hypointense compared with normal liver on T1-weighted and moderately to extremely hyperintense on T2-weighted sequences. Approximately two thirds of endocrine tumor metastases in our series (unpublished data) were so intense that they simulated cavernous hemangiomas (lesion/normal liver intensity ratio >1.4 on a T2-weighted sequence).[84] However, hemangiomas are typically homogeneous in appearance, whereas the hepatic metastases were often heterogeneous. In equivocal cases at MRI, comparison with bolus dynamic CT scanning may be necessary to distinguish between these two types of lesions.[250]

Percutaneous Transhepatic Venous Sampling

Ingemansson et al. first demonstrated the feasibility of THVS of blood in the venous effluent at the site of the tumor.[102] This technique has been employed by several groups in the successful localization of insulinomas.[102,148,173,185,253] Tumors secreting gastrin,[34,101] glucagon,[99] somatostatin,[82] and mixed endocrine tumors,[42,268,270] have been localized by hormone concentrations in the portal effluent. Aside from tumors, nesidioblastosis, hyperplasia, G cell hyperplasia, and multiple adenomatosis may be diagnosed by this technique.[82,100,262]

The appreciation of gradients across the liver may be important with regard to the possible diagnosis of metastatic disease since we have shown that the hepatic vein/portal gradient disappears.[268,270] In the case of gastrin and motilin, which are not extracted by the liver, higher levels in the hepatic vein than in the portal vein would suggest hepatic metastases.

An awareness of the effects of catheter placement is necessary in interpreting concentrations of hormones in the THVS. Insertion of the catheter tip into small tributaries and occlusion of the vessel lumen can give erroneously low values. It is for this reason that we contend that superselective sampling is unnecessary and may even be misleading. It is not unusual to find levels declining during the course of the procedure, possibly due to stress-related factors. The need to take simultaneous arterial samples to avoid differences due to rapid oscillations or changing hormone levels is stressed.

It is now our belief that *regionalization* of the tumor is more critical than exact localization, since the correct operative procedure can usually be determined depending on whether it is established that the tumor is located in the head, neck, or body of the pancreas.

The Insulinoma Syndrome

In patients with single adenomas even when pancreatic angiography and abdominal CT and ultrasonography failed to localize tumor, all tumors were localized by the maximum hormone level in the PVS.

The maximum insulin concentrations ranged from 64 to 2600 μU/mL. The mean $\pm$ SE of insulin concentrations in samples drawn simultaneously from the celiac artery was 62 $\pm$ 19 μU/mL, and that in veins draining the uninvolved pancreas was 58 $\pm$ 18 μU/mL. The gradients corresponding to the tumor site ranged from 39 to 2547 μU/mL. Tumors in the head of the pancreas had high insulin levels in the area of drainage of the superior pancreaticoduodenal vein. Tumors in the uncinate lobe gave high values in the superior mesenteric close to the anastomosis with the splenic vein. Tumors in the neck drained into the proximal portal vein or near the confluence of splenic and portal close to the junction of the superior mesenteric and splenic veins. Tumors in the tail of the pancreas drain directly into the distal splenic vein but may give erroneously high values in the gastrocolic trunk due to a venous connection between the tail of the pancreas and the superior mesenteric vein via the gastroepiploic vein.[185,268,270]

Both nesidioblastosis and hyperplasia or multiple adenomatosis give nonhomogeneous elevation and insulin levels; this cannot be used to distinguish these conditions.[82,100] They can, however, be clearly delineated from single adenomas, defining an entirely different surgical approach to that of the single adenoma.

The Gastrin Hypersecretion Syndrome

Although both CT and selective visceral angiography were found effective in identifying nearly all patients with metastatic disease to the liver and in some cases retroperitoneal lymph nodes, these studies failed to identify primary tumors in more than half the patients seen with biochemical proof of Zollinger-Ellison syndrome (ZES). Furthermore, up to 40% of patients explored without positive preoperative imaging studies had negative findings at operation.[226,285]

The use of percutaneous transhepatic portal, pancreatic, and hepatic venous gastrin sampling by Ingemansson et al. in 1977[101] and Burcharth et al. in 1979[34] and subsequently by Vinik and colleagues[85,265,268,270] and others[191] suggested that this technique was of value in those gastrinoma patients without liver metastases or a primary gastrinoma that was not detected by conventional imaging methods. Our initial studies were undertaken in 1978.[191,265,268,270] It has been possible to predict the presence or absence of liver metastases and, in two patients, solitary resectable primary liver gastrinomas. Our results in patients with gastrin hypersecretion indicated that the technique may be very valuable in sporadic or ectopic gastrinomas,[265,268,270] though false-negative results have been reported by others.[38,181] It is clear, however, that the surgeon would have found at least half the tumors without the aid of THVS. Our approach has been aggressive, and if there has been a gradient, corresponding to the triangle of the head of the pancreas, first portion of the duodenum, and pylorus of the stomach, the surgeon has pursued duodenotomy and Kocherization of the head of the pancreas, a procedure not agreed upon by all surgeons because of the relatively benign course of those patients in whom no tumor is found at laparotomy.[165,270]

The high incidence of false-positive localizations found by some authors[38,181] is likely due to the tumors' being in the head of the pancreas, peripancreatic lymph nodes, or wall of the duodenum.[51,170,191,205,244,257] Failure to find a tumor carries a good prognosis, and none have died in a 8.5-year follow-up[227] in contrast with the 37% reported perioperative morbidity and mortality resulting from explorations of the head of the pancreas reported by some[205] but the <2% in the hands of others.[75,226,246] We aggressively seek these tumors if the THVS results suggest regionalization to the head of the pancreas and have not thus far failed to identify tumor tissue.

Multiple Endocrine Neoplasia

The management of MEN-I patients, who constitute about a third of all patients with the ZES, remains controversial. There are an increasing number of groups that favor only medical management because of the conclusion that these patients cannot be cured of their diffuse pancreatic islet cell disease.[51,153,165,191,257] Early detection and excision may, however, prevent tumor-related deaths. During the past 5 years, all our MEN-I patients ($n = 14$) with ZES had THVS. Most of these patients have had multiple or diffuse sources of gastrin secretion from the pancreas or duodenum. Removal of the major tumor did not restore gastrin levels, gastric acid secretion, or the responses of gastrin to secretin stimulation to normal. However, in four patients, localized gastrin secretion was found and at operation, pancreatic tumors were enucleated. It cannot be claimed that these patients are cured, because they continue to demonstrate abnormal responses to secretin stimulation. Resection of only an imaged lesion in the pancreas of an MEN-1 patient on the basis that it represents a gastrinoma may be futile. They can, in fact, be secreting any of a number of hormones not contributing to the clinical picture.[268,270] In each of our patients who was successfully palliated, by selective venous sampling we detected a localized site of hypergastrinemia that corresponded to a palpable tumor that could be excised at operation. In patients with diffuse or multiple sites of hypergastrinemia detected by venous sampling,[191,268] operative intervention has been unsuccessful in alleviating the ZES syndrome and operation is justifiable only on the basis of excising gross tumors.

Carcinoid Syndrome

Carcinoid tumors that have not metastasized may be notoriously difficult to localize. It appears that serotonin concentrations may be misleading and that substance P levels more accurately localized the tumor.[158,236]

MANAGEMENT

Gastrinoma

The treatment of the ZES has undergone significant changes since the first case was described in 1955.[286] Until the development of drugs to control the excessive acid production,[52,162,171] the purpose of operative intervention was to excise the acid-secreting stomach, which was the major cause of morbidity and mortality from massive hemorrhage or perforation.

Subsequent to the introduction of H_2 blockers in 1974[52,162,171] and other major antisecretory drugs since that time,[272] management of the ZES patient has undergone a number of important changes. These drugs, which for the first time controlled the hypersecretory state, allowed elective operations, which, in turn, decreased the mortality from total gastrectomy and also allowed more efforts to find and excise the tumor when localized. It was found that in some patients, tumor excision without gastrectomy was possible, and this was proved successful by follow-up gastrin levels that remained normal. Nevertheless, some physicians became so impressed with the results of drug therapy that they considered only those patients who did not respond to drug therapy for exploration and possible gastrectomy. Because of the possibility of a curative procedure and concern about the malignant potential, others recommended routine exploration when no liver metastases were present but limited any gastric procedure to selective vagotomy because of its augmentation of the effects of H_2-blocking agents.[197,202]

Studies carried out in the past 10 years in several species, including humans, have shown that somatostatin and its analogs exert inhibitory actions on the basal and stimulated secretion of both gastrin and gastric acid.[59,120,140,146,215,283] With the availability of a long-acting somatostatin analog,[273] it is now feasible to treat patients with the ZES.

In eight of our patients with gastrinoma in whom we were able to evaluate acid secretion, a long-acting analog of somatostatin, octreotide (sandostatin), in doses of 50 to 100 μg every 6 to 12 hours suppressed basal gastric acid secretion and restored the BAO/MAO ratio to normal.[273] The rapid and complete inhibition of gastric acid secretion led to a striking clinical improvement and made it possible to carry out surgery without other forms of preoperative preparation. A single 50-μg injection of octreotide was sufficient to control acid secretion for the duration of operation.[251] Hypotension did not occur, and blood glucose levels remained stable throughout the surgical procedures.

Long-term therapy with octreotide reduces basal and pentagastrin-stimulation acid secretion with a return of responsiveness to pentagastrin and a normal BAO/MAO ratio. This occurs simultaneously with the reduction in basal and secretin-stimulated gastrin levels, suggesting that octreotide is not only capable of acutely reducing the gastric acid secretory response and serum gastrin but that it can over the longer term reduce the effective parietal cell mass, equivalent to a medical gastrectomy. This, however, remains to be proved.

Two of our patients were quite unresponsive to octreotide. The nonresponsive patients who had high levels of gastrin had high NH_2-/COOH-terminal ratios. We have shown this to predict metastases, and the ratio is of value in monitoring progress.[123] We have not, however, determined the impact of octreotide on different molecular species of gastrin. The only apparent correlate of tumor response was with the level of the initial gastrin. It could not be predicted by the presence or absence of metastases. The failure of octreotide to lower gastrin levels did, however, appear to parallel the lack of effect on tumor mass monitored by serial CT. Six of eight patients had excellent biochemical and clinical responses without evidence of tumor regression, but with an apparent cessation of tumor growth.

At least 60% of gastrinomas are malignant, and at operation more than 50% have already metastasized to the liver.[153,163,226] Various drugs and specific chemotherapeutic agents such as streptozotocin,[175,228] 5-fluorouracil,[175,245] doxorubicin,[105] tubercidin,[287] mitomycin, or irradiation[192] have been used for the management of unresectable or metastatic gastrinomas. These therapeutic modalities may provide palliative relief for some patients, as was demonstrated in one patient, but the overall results have been disappointing.[164] Both experimental[211] and clinical findings[41,125,283] suggest that it might be possible to use octreotide as hormonal therapy for some malignant GEP endocrine tumors. Gastrinomas appear to be resistant to octreotide, although it has been reported that symptomatic improvement occurred in six of nine patients with metastases treated with the analog.[129] In our patients in whom chemotherapy failed, octreotide did not control tumor growth or the serum gastrin levels.

We believe that octreotide is a useful addition to currently available therapeutic agents for the treatment of the heterogenous forms of gastrinoma syndrome. It acutely lowers gastric acid and serum gastrin levels, contrasting with the rise in gastrin levels with H_2 blockers. In the long term it may reduce tumor gastrin secretion and parietal cell mass. Tumors that elaborate large amounts of gastrin appear to be refractory, and there seems to be a relationship between cessation of tumor growth and the biochemical response. It appears worthwhile pursuing long-term therapy in patients refractory to other measures to control gastrin secretion and tumor growth in an endeavor to identify those factors that determine responsiveness. Currently omeprazole is the drug of choice in doses of 20–100 mg per day.

Insulinoma

The treatment of this condition is amelioration of hypoglycemia by either surgical or medical means.[112] If the tumor is easily localized and/or accessible, surgery is the treatment of choice and is curative.[62] Medical therapy is reserved for patients who are not able to undergo operation because of their poor medical condition or inoperable islet cell carcinoma or when surgical treatment is refused. Medical treatment is also valuable in controlling patients who are still symptomatic after partial or subtotal resection of the pancreas, or if surgery has to be delayed for any reason. Frequent meals to avoid hypoglycemia are useful but may be bothersome, especially if time intervals between feedings are short and the patient has to wake up at night to eat to avoid hypoglycemia. Some patients have unacceptable weight gain as a result of frequent eating.[112]

Diazoxide has been used for the treatment of organic hypoglycemia.[63,64,86,156,157] Addition of a thiazide diuretic to diazoxide not only has a synergistic hyperglycemic effect but may prevent or decrease water retention, which is a major side effect of diazoxide. Dilantin,[32,96] propranolol,[21,179,218] chlorpromazine,[65] calcium-channel blockers such as diltiazem,[240] and verapamil[49] have been used with variable success for treatment of organic hypoglycemia. However, none of the current medical therapies for organic hyperinsulinism is ideal. The naturally occurring form of the neuropeptide somatostatin-14 or one of its analogs has been used for control of neonatal hypoglycemia[20,28,49,95,117,206] and the hypoglycemia due to insulinoma.[1,40,46,145,214] The first reports of the use of somatostatin-14 in the control of blood glucose levels in insulinoma came simultaneously from Curnow et al.[46] and Christensen et al.,[40] who both used somatostatin-14 by infusion, to suppress insulin secretion in malignant and benign insulinomas. Although infusion of somatostatin-14 was useful in suppressing the elevated insulin levels and alleviating the symptoms in these cases, the main problem was the very short half-life of somatostatin-14,[219] which necessitated a constant intravenous infusion. Octreotide has been used successfully to control hypoglycemia in some cases of benign[142] and one case of malignant insulinoma.[188] Hypoglycemia on fasting improves in some patients and worsens in others after short-term administration of octreotide. The differences in the responses appear to be related to variable and unpredictable effects on glucose homostasis.

We have not achieved a normal 72-hour fasting profile in spite of apparently adequate suppression of insulin. Suppression of gluconeogenic hormones by octreotide and depletion of liver glycogen storage may contribute to failure to normalize the ability to fast. It is clearly related to the degree of suppression of hepatic glucose production or the decrease in circulating glucagon levels.[40]

Some patients demonstrate a postprandial drop in plasma glucose levels and a delay in the rise and time of the peak in plasma glucose levels with octreotide. This could be the result of an action of octreotide on the gastrointestinal tract with a delay in the gastric emptying time as occurs with somatostatin-14[19,39] and/or a decrease in digestion and absorption of glucose and other nutrients.[106,107] Although somatostatin delayed and increased the peak level of glucose in two of our patients, we could not use this action as a measure to prolong fasting. Suppression of plasma levels of glucagon would explain why one of our patients had a decrease in plasma glucose levels following treatment with the analog. During the meal studies, we examined the effects of octreotide on glucose, insulin, and glucagon levels. The combination of depressed glucagon levels and delayed absorption of nutrients may have shortened the hypoglycemia-free interval and increased its severity despite frequent feeding. Giving the analog 2 hours postprandially does not have any effects on improvement in the plasma glucose levels.

Patients unresponsive to octreotide may respond to diazoxide. By substitution with diazoxide, we were able to extend the feeding interval from every 4 hours to every 6 hours and achieve prolonged euglycemia in patients refractory to octreotide. This suggests that the mechanism of action of these two agents is different, although both diazoxide and somatostatin seem to act through calcium translocation in the B cells.[9]

For malignant insulinomas, streptozotocin appears to be the most effective tumor agent: about 50% of patients have an objective response in tumor mass and about 17% have complete remission. Streptozotocin has serious side effects on the kidney and hematopoietic system. Urinary protein levels should be monitored, and repeated doses should be administered only when the urine is free of protein. A weekly schedule of 1 to 2 g/m^2 may be useful in a 4- to 6-week regime; this, however, requires further trials. Other drugs such as L-asparaginase, 5-fluorouracil, tubericidin, doxorubicin, and mithramycin have been used in selected cases, but in general toxicity has precluded adequate therapy.

Somatostatinoma

Eight of 20 patients with somatostatinoma died at intervals ranging from 1 week to 14 months after diagnosis. Two patients died in hypoglycemic coma, the remaining one as a result of metastatic disease. Twelve patients were alive from 6 months to 5 years after diagnosis. Thus, the syndrome tends to be associated with a malignant potential. It is, therefore, important to be aggressive in the management and attempt to remove all tumor tissue in benign cases. In those in whom metastases have already occurred at the time of diagnosis, the optimal form of chemotherapy remains to be determined.

PPoma

It is our contention that not every patient with raised PP levels has a tumor, but if a tumor can be identified and localized, it should be removed.[186,262,264,268,271] Raised PP levels occur as part of the MEN-I syndrome and may reflect nesidioblastosis of PP cells or multiple adenomata not amenable to resection. The rate of malignancy of these tumors is not established, and resection should be reserved for those patients with clearly identified solitary lesions.

It has been suggested that every patient who has a markedly elevated level of PP should undergo exploratory laparotomy and careful inspection of the pancreas.[76] This has not been our experience. Malignant PPomas are best treated with streptozotocin. PPomas may occur outside the pancreas, and carcinoid tumors can present a real dilemma, since these may occur in the chest and elsewhere. Laparotomy is not advised. We content that THVS, and if necessary total body venous sampling, should be performed to localize the source of PP overproduction. If such a locus is found, then abdominal or other exploration should be performed. In patients who have metastatic tumors and those refractory to other forms of treatment, the use of the somatostatin analog octreotide proves to be useful and is worthy of trial.

Vipoma

The initial treatment of the diarrhea syndrome is a replacement of fluid, electrolyte, and potassium losses and the correction of hypokalemia and the acidosis. The magnitude and the route of fluid and electrolyte administration should be individualized and dictated by the severity of the deficits observed. Once the fluid deficit has been corrected, attempts to control the diarrhea should be made. The variety of agents that have been used in the treatment of the diarrhea are listed in Table 25-9. Prednisone or corticosteroids have been shown to control the diarrhea in a majority of patients.[8,139] Although the exact mechanism of action is obscure, it is not by lowering the VIP concentration. A number of agents including the α_2-adrenergic agonists and norepinephrine[69,161,201] have been shown to enhance absorption of fluid and electrolytes, and they improved the diarrhea. In contrast, agents that inhibit secretion, indomethacin,[2,104] lithium carbonate,[190] somatostatin,[36,53,54] phenothiazines,[55,223] propranolol, and other inhibitors of adenylate cyclase[151,274] have been used in attempts to control the secretory diarrhea. The mechanism of diarrhea in this syndrome is complex, and although VIP may be the dominant agent activating adenylate cyclase and cyclic AMP production, other agents may also be implicated, in which case mechanisms that embrace calcium translocation and increase in tissue prostaglandin levels may be important. Thus, the phenothiazines may decrease cytosolic calcium levels[118] and decrease the activation of calcium calmodulin. Indomethacin de-

TABLE 25-9. THERAPY OF VIPOMA SYNDROME

Supportive	Intravenous fluids Oral glucose and electrolytes Correction of hypokalemia and acidosis
Diarrhea	
Enhance absorption	Corticosteroids α_2-Adrenergic agonists Angiotensin II
Inhibit secretion	Indomethacin Lithium carbonate Phenothiazines Somatostatin Opiates β-Adrenergic blockers Calcium-channel blockers Adenylate cyclase inhibitors
Tumor	
Surgery	Pancreatectomy Excision or debulking
Chemotherapy	Streptozotocin 5-fluorouracil Chlorozotocin Somatostatin Interferon

creases intestinal prostaglandin production, and the calcium-channel blockers may add to the reduction in calcium translocation. The mechanism of action of somatostatin is not entirely known but may be by a calcium-channel-blocking action as well. The current notion is that lithium carbonate acts by decreasing phosphoinositide turnover. These differences in mode of action have proved useful in being able to use the addition effects of the two agents.

The primary treatment of a VIP-secreting tumor is resection once the diagnosis has been established and the site of the tumor localized. Single localized tumors occur in about 80% of patients, and about 50% of these are benign and, therefore, potentially resectable. However, there are about 20% in whom islet cell hyperplasia or microadenomatosis accounts for the clinical syndrome. Transhepatic venous sampling to localize VIP tumors has not proved successful in our hands but has occasionally been effective in those of others. Intraoperative ultrasonography, as well as angiography, may be of help. Our experiences indicate that some of these tumors may not be detectable at the onset of the clinical symptom complex, and longer-term follow-up is necessary. Tumors may appear in the skin[278] as hypernephromas[33] or as neuroblastomas, and CT scanning with contrast material may be the most helpful for identification of the tumor. In cases of inoperable lesions, a debulking operation may be carried out, and in those cases in which no tumor is found, some have responded to total pancreatectomy. In malignant metastatic tumors in which surgery has been of no avail, chemotherapy with streptozotocin and 5-fluorouracil[110,175] and more recently streptozotocin has been reported to yield a 60% to 70% response rate. Our own experience[272] as well as that of O'Dorisio is that these tumors even when metastatic may respond dramatically to the use of octreotide, which has proved to be helpful in the management of the diarrhea and flushing and has induced tumor regression and infarction in a limited series of cases.

Glucagonoma

Glucagon-producing tumors are, in general, malignant and very large when they are first detected. They are slow-growing, and it is not unusual to find patients with a 10-year or more history of the presence of tumor without treatment.[176] Management of the diabetes tends to be fairly simple; the diabetes responds to diet with the administration of small amounts of insulin.

The skin rash can prove to be intractable in its management, and various therapeutic topical agents, such as zinc, tar preparations, or steroid preparations, are often tried without success. The skin rash does tend to wax and wane, and the erroneous impression may be obtained of an improvement with one or other form of treatment. Since the exact pathogenesis of the skin rash is not clearly known and hypoaminoacidemia, zinc deficiency, and a direct toxic effect of glucagon have been implicated, it is not surprising that improvement has been observed with the administration of amino acids, intravenous alimentation with amino acid solutions, and even zinc therapy.[182,280]

The tendency to recurrent venous thrombosis appears to improve with successful removal of the tumor, as does the severe depression.

The primary goal of treatment is to remove the tumor in the 50% of cases in whom no metastases are present at the time of diagnosis. Successful removal of these tumors has been reported,[16,24,92,94,109,111,126,138,143,144,178,194,220,241,260,277] but recurrence is not unusual, even after complete removal of the primary tumor.[109,138,200,239,277] Operation even in those instances in which total removal is not successful (debulking or partial resection) may have beneficial effects with a long-term survival of 12 years or more.[12,94,256]

In patients in whom surgery is not feasible, encouraging results have been obtained with streptozotocin,[12,31,47,73] although disappointing results have been observed.[11,25,90,109,114,160,235] A combination of streptozotocin and 5-fluorouracil may give slightly better results,[115] but this has not been systematically studied. Others have claimed better results with dacarbazine (DTIC)[114] given intravenously in doses of 250 mg/m^2 daily for 5 days every 4 weeks.[160,200,235] Unfortunately, serious side effects such as thrombocytopenia may occur, and the drug may be ineffective.[56,90]

There are few studies in which new agents have been examined, and it appears that those cases resistant to the above forms of therapy may be responsive to octreotide. When this treatment fails, chemotherapy with a new agent, human leukocyte interferon, may be considered.

Carcinoid

The general prognosis in carcinoid is excellent. Based upon a world literature of some 2837 cases, the median survival for all cases is 82%.[174] If, however, the tumor is localized, then the 5-year survival is 94%, decreasing to 64% with regional lymph node involvement and 18% with distant metastases. Davis reported a mean survival of 38 months from the first episode of flushing in patients with the carcinoid syndrome, with 25% living for more than 6 years.[48] With regional lymph node involvement, the figure falls to about 14 months,[80] and with urinary 5HIAA levels in excess of 150 mg/24 hours or inoperable tumors, the median survival is only 11 months.[174]

Patients with carcinoid may suffer as a result of the endocrine syndrome and/or tumor growth. Surgical removal of the primary tumor is the treatment of choice for small and localized tumors or for alleviation of any obstructive symptoms, but surgical cure of carcinoid is almost impossible in the presence of intra-abdominal and hepatic metastases. Different chemotherapeutic agents and surgery or arterial embolization[159] have been used with variable success, but eventual relapse with increasing resistance to the drugs is encountered.[174] Since carcinoid is a slow-growing tumor, even patients with extensive metastatic disease can enjoy a normal quality of life so long as the endocrine syndrome is quiescent. Different chemical agents such as methylsergide, cyproheptadine, heparin, phenothiazines, α-adrenergic antagonists, corticosteroids, H_1 and H_2 antihistamine blockers, symptomatic treatment of diarrhea with opioids, and codeine have been tried with variable results.[174] Since somatostatin has very broad inhibitory effects, somatostatin-14 has been used successfully to suppress diarrhea and flushing in patients with carcinoid tumors,[89] but its clinical use is limited by its short half-life,[219] with the resulting need for continuous intravenous infusion. With the advent of octreotide,[10] it has been used in the treatment of different neuroendocrine tumors including carcinoid.

We have evaluated the effects of octreotide on clinical, biochemical, and tumor growth in 14 patients with carcinoid tumors. Our patients were a heterogenous group with advanced carcinoid tumors refractory to conventional chemotherapeutic agents, who were tried on the somatostatin analog with variable clinical and biochemical responses. We have previously shown a dramatic response of symptomatic flushing to treatment with somatostatin.[252] Frohlich and colleagues[77] have also reported on the value of native somatostatin given by continuous infusion as a means of reversing the pentagastrin-induced flushing in carcinoid patients. We, however, were unable to show that pentagastrin was a reliable means whereby flushing could be provoked in our patients. Kvols et al.[131] found that 19 of 24 patients with carcinoid tumors had a 50% reduction in flushing and 3 a minor response, and in 2 patients the drug failed. Richter et al. showed that 6 of 8 patients had improved symptoms.[203] Our more recent experience is that 64% of our patients presented with flushing as their major symptom. In all instances, the symptom complex improved with a clear decrease in the frequency of symptoms with doses of 1 to 2 μg/kg per day. In no instance was there resistance to the drug, tachyphylaxis did not occur, and withdrawal of the drug, or substitution with distilled water, was always followed by recurrence of the symptom complex. In contrast to another study,[203] relapse of flushing did not occur with continued treatment once it was under control. However, in contrast to the reduction in the number of episodes, in certain patients the severity decreased only slightly and the duration of each episode was essentially unchanged.

The extreme example of flushing is the carcinoid crisis with a profound fall in blood pressure. It is deemed unwise to submit a patient to anesthesia or operation without premedication with a combination of adrenergic blocker, steroids, thorazine, and aspirin. Kvols et al. have presented data on one such patient, who soon after induction of anesthesia had a fall in blood pressure unresponsive to intravenous fluid, calcium, neosynephrine, or epinephrine administration.[130] Within 1 minute of the intravenous administration of 100 μg of octreotide, blood pressure rose and the patient made an uneventful recovery.

Thus, while the mechanism of action of octreotide and the factors mediating flushing and vasodilatation are unclear, there can be no doubt that octreotide is a potent antidote to the vasoactive humors participating in the flush and hypotension. The drug may prove to be a useful adjunct in the preparation of patients for operative procedures and as a standby for the management of carcinoid crises. We have used octreotide intravenously during resection of metastases to successfully alleviate hypotension induced by tumor manipulation.

Diarrhea occurred in 86% of our patients and responded variably to octreotide. Acute administration of octreotide thus normalized the water and electrolyte transport across the proximal intestine, as has been shown in patients with WDHH syndrome.[210,272] Only 58% of our patients with diarrhea had complete remission, a finding that differs from the improvement in 19 of 25 patients reported by Kvols et al.[131] This could be because diarrhea in patients with carcinoid tumors has multiple causes, that is, secretory, increased motility, malabsorption, partial luminal lymphatic obstruction, bacterial overgrowth, and short bowel syndrome due to surgical resection. The diarrhea may even appear to worsen with the appearance of steatorrhea, and the physician is not infrequently faced with the confounding situation of not knowing to what to attribute the symptom. However, although somatostatin does inhibit exocrine pancreatic secretion,[7] addition of pancreatic enzyme supplementation has not uniformly decreased octreotide-induced steatorrhea.[234] We did not find any consistent changes in frequency or consistency of bowel movements in response to pancreatic supplement in those patients with steatorrhea before treatment or the bowel habits after therapy with octreotide, compatible with the notion that the steatorrhea has a complex pathogenesis and may be affected by alterations in bile flow and the direct effects of somatostatin on nutrient absorption and intestinal motility.[93]

There are conflicting reports regarding the biochemical responses of carcinoid patients to somatostatin. Richter et al. reported a significant drop in 5HT levels in 8 patients treated with 150 μg/day of octreotide, but no changes in urinary 5HIAA levels,[203] while others have found a drop in urinary 5HIAA levels.[282] When treatment of 4 of their patients was prolonged to 15–30 weeks, blood serotonin levels remained unchanged.[234] In our patients, urinary 5HIAA levels dropped in almost all patients and normalized in one third of the patients. There was no clinical correlation between clinical responses and the blood serotonin level. For contrast, in patients in whom the urinary 5HIAA levels fell, there was clinical improvement in one or more of the symptoms. This may reflect the fact that there are multiple etiologic factors involved in the symptomatology of carcinoid tumors. In our patients, those who responded clinically required no more than 500 μg/day to control their symptoms.

Due to the slow growth of carcinoid tumors, it is difficult to assess the effect of octreotide on the rate of tumor growth or regression. Shrinkage of liver metastases in patients with carcinoids[131,272] and other functioning pancreatic neurendocrine tumors[125] has been reported. We have had variable experiences but in general have found a cessation of further tumor growth in at least 40% of patients if therapy is continued for at least 1 year or more. The relationship between tumor size and growth and the biochemistry is not a simple one. Plasma serotonin levels appear to be unhelpful in monitoring progress, but the urinary 5HIAA level does decrease with a reduction in size of the tumor.

Miscellaneous

The management of MEN-I patients remains controversial. When the tumor is producing insulin and the syndrome is that of organic hyperinsulinism, then there can be no doubt that the management is excision of the tumor except in those rare instances when the tumor is malignant. If the presenting features are those of the ZES, there are an increasing number of groups that favor only medical management because of the conclusion that these patients cannot be cured of their diffuse pancreatic islet cell disease.[165] Total pancreatectomy is the only procedure that can be truly curative in the MEN-I patient without evidence of metastatic gastrinoma. This operation is contraindicated, however, because the benefits of the operation are outweighed by the operative mortality or long-term morbidity of insulin-dependent diabetes. Nevertheless, the malignant potential of small islet cell tumors in the MEN-I patients should not be ignored. Early detection and excision may prevent tumor-related deaths.

All lesions imaged in the pancreas of an MEN-I patient do not represent a secretory tumor and may not be accounting for the clinical syndrome. They can, in fact, be secreting any of a number of hormones not contributing to the clinical picture.[268,270] It is for this reason that in the MEN-I patients we routinely do THVS for a battery of gastrointestinal pancreatic hormones including glucagon, somatostatin, pancreatic polypeptide, insulin, and VIP, as well as gastrin. Only in those instances in which the tumor can be shown to be the source of hormone overproduction accounting for the symptom complex is it justifiable to resort to excision. In our total experience with the ZES in MEN-I patients, we have had only one patient who had no detectable tumor at operation. This patient had only diffuse islet cell hyperplasia as the source of hypergastrinemia. In each of our patients who were successfully palliated, we detected a localized site of hypergastrinemia by selective venous sampling that corresponded to a palpable tumor that could be excised at operation.

In patients with diffuse or multiple sites of gastrin overproduction detected by THVS, operative intervention has been unsuccessful in alleviating the ZES, and operation is justifiable only on the basis of excising gross tumors. Because of the ability to control hypersecretion of acid in most of these patients with the MEN-I syndrome and ZES, we believe that it is even more important now to treat the malignant potential of any detectable tumor in order to prevent a long-term cancer-related death.

The total experience at the Mayo Clinic, which was recently reviewed by van Heerden et al., included 25 patients who were treated between 1960 and 1984.[257] There were 14 patients diagnosed and treated prior to 1979, and 10 of these (71%) had pancreatic procedures that included 5 tumor enucleations and 1 total pancreatectomy. None of these patients was "cured" in reference to their hypergastrinemia. Subsequent to the use of H_2 antagonists in 1979, they have used antisecretory drugs as the primary treatment in 11 patients who have been followed for a mean interval of 26 months without significant problems from the drugs, although 1 did require a gastrectomy. Overall, 18 of their 25 patients required gastrectomy, including 13 total gastrectomies. They concluded that drug therapy may be the best means of managing their patients. Deveney et al. found that 29% of their 52 patients with ZES and gastrinoma had MEN-I; all had hyperparathyroidism.[40] They emphasized that multiple tumors were found in 6 of 7 patients in which partial pancreatectomies were done. One of their two postoperative deaths occurred in an MEN-I patient after a total gastrectomy. In two of their cases of ZES in MEN-I patients, they attempted curative operations on the pancreas (distal pancreatectomy including all gross neoplasm in 1 patient, and enucleation of 3 tumors in the pancreatic head in the other) as well as total gastrectomy. Neither patient was cured of hypergastrinemia. Their only "cure" was in a patient who was treated by total pancreatectomy for both gastrinomas and insulinomas. These authors did no systematic venous sampling for gastrin prior to their operations with the exception of one case. They, too, concluded that routine exploration and attempted cure of the MEN-I patient is futile because of the diffuse islet cell disease and they also favor H_2-antagonist therapy. Of 144 consecutive cases reported by Mignon et al.,[170] 35 patients had MEN-I disease. Seven of these had no operation at all. Mignon et al. found that therapy (attempted cure) failed in 16 of 26 patients in whom a surgical procedure was performed on the pancreas. Three of their patients developed malignancies during follow-up. Other endocrinopathies led to the death of 3 additional patients. Although these authors favor exploratory laparotomy in the sporadic cases of ZES without known metastases, they favor drug therapy for most patients with the MEN-I syndrome, providing they are easily controlled.

It would appear that the total number of patients with the MEN-I syndrome and ZES that have been carefully evaluated for possible palliative or curative pancreatic operations based on selective venous sampling has been so limited that a definitive statement about optimal management cannot be made at the present time. The low incidence of malignancy in the MEN-I patients dictates a less cavalier approach than in sporadic cases without evidence of MEN-I.

REFERENCES

1. Adrian TE, Barnes AJ, Long RG, et al. The effect of somatostatin analogs on secretion of growth, pancreatic and gastrointestinal hormones in man. J Clin Endocrinol Metab 53:675–681, 1981.
2. Albuquerque RH, Owens CWI, Bloom SR. A study of vasoactive intestinal polypeptide (VIP) stimulated intestinal fluid secretion in rat and its inhibition by indomethacin. Experientia 35:1496–1497, 1979.

3. Alfidi RJ, Bhyun DS, Crile G Jr, Hawk W. Arteriography and hypoglycemia. Surg Gynecol Obstet 133:447–452, 1971.
4. Alpern MB, Lawson TL, Foley WD, et al. Focal hepatic masses and fatty infiltration detected by enhanced dynamic CT. Radiology 158:45–49, 1986.
5. Alumets J, Hakanson R, Ingemannson S, Sundler F. Substance P and 5-HT in granules isolated from an intestinal argentaffin carcinoid. Histochemistry, 52:217–222, 1977.
6. Archembeaud Mouveroux, Cardinaud F, Verrot J, et al. Carbohydrate antigen (CA19-9) and malignant glucagonoma. N Engl J Med 315:1555, 1986.
7. Arnold R, Lankisch. Somatostatin and the gastrointestinal tract. Clin Gastroenterol 9:733–754, 1980.
8. Barraclough MA, Bloom SR. VIPoma of the pancreas. Observations on the diarrhea and circulatory disturbances. Arch Int Med 139:467, 1969.
9. Basabe J, Cresto J, Aparicio N. Studies on the mode of action of somatostatin on insulin secretion. Endocrinology 101:1436–1443, 1977.
10. Bauer W, Briner U, Doepfner W. SMS 201–995: A very potent and selective octapeptide analogue of somatostatin with prolonged action. Life Sci 31:1133–1140, 1982.
11. Belchetz PE, Brown CL, Makin HLJ, et al. ACTH, glucagon and gastrin production by a pancreatic islet cell carcinoma and its treatment. Clin Endocrinol 2:307–316, 1973.
12. Beltzer-Garelli E, Cesarini JP, Cywiner-Golenzer CH, et al. Lesions cutanees revelatrices d'un glucagonome. Sem Hop Paris 56:579–582, 1980.
13. Betts JB, O'Malley BP, Rosenthal FD. Hyperparathyroidism: A prerequisite for Zollinger-Ellison syndrome in MEA-I: Report of a further family and a review of the literature. Q J Med 193:69–76, 1980.
14. Bhagavan BS, Slavin RE, Goldberg J, Rao RN. Ectopic gastrinoma and Zollinger-Ellison syndrome. Hum Pathol 17:584–592, 1986.
15. Bhathena SJ, Higgins GA, Recant L. Glucagonoma and glucagonoma syndrome. In: Unger RH, Orci L, eds. Glucagon. New York, Elsevier North Holland, 1981, p 413.
16. Binnick AN, Spencer SK, Landon Dennison W, Horton ES. Glucagonoma syndrome. Report of two cases and literature review. Arch Dermatol 113:749–754, 1977.
17. Bloom SR, Mortimer CH, Thorner MO, et al. Inhibition of gastrin and gastric-acid secretion by growth-hormone-release-inhibiting hormone. Lancet 2:1106–1109, 1974.
18. Bloom SR, Polak JM, Pearse AGE. Vasoactive intestinal polypeptide and watery diarrhea syndrome. Lancet 2:14–16, 1973.
19. Bloom SR, Ralphs DN, Besser GM, et al. Effect of somatostatin on motilin levels and gastric emptying. Gut 16:834, 1975.
20. Bloomgarden ZT, Sundell H, Rogers LW, O'Neill JA, Liljenquist JE. Treatment of intractable neonatal hypoglycemia with somatostatin plus glucagon. J Pediatr 96:148–151, 1980.
21. Blum I, Doron M, Laron Z, Atsmon A. Prevention of hypoglycemic attacks by propranolol in a patient suffering from insulinoma. Diabetes 24:535–537, 1975.
22. Boden G, Owen OE. Familial hyperglucagonemia—An autosomal dominant disorder. N Engl J Med 296:534–538, 1977.
23. Boden G, Baile CA, McLaughlin CL, et al. Effects of starvation and obesity on somatostatin, insulin and glucagon release from an isolated perfused organ system. Am J Physiol 241:E215, 1981.
24. Boden G, Owen OE, Rezvani I, et al. An islet cell carcinoma containing glucagon and insulin. Diabetes 26:128, 1977.
25. Boden G, Wilson RM, Owen OE. Effects of chronic glucagon excess on hepatic metabolism. Diabetes 27:643–648, 1978.
26. Bordi C, Sivelli R, Lampugnani R, Zanella E, Fajans SS. Hormonal studies in a patient with PP-producing tumors. Horm Metabol Res 17:467–470, 1985.
27. Bordi C, Togni R, Baetens M. Human islet cell tumor storing pancreatic polypeptide. J Clin Endocrinol Metab 56:215–219, 1978.
28. Bougneres PF, Landier F, Garnier P, Job JC, Chaussain JL. Treatment of insulin excess by continuous subcutaneous infusion of somatostatin and glucagon in an infant. J Pediatr 106:792–794, 1985.

29. Breatnach ES, Han SY, Rahatzad MT, Stanley RJ. CT evaluation of glucagonomas. JCAT 9:25–29, 1985.
30. Bressler EL, Alpern MB, Glazer GM, Francis IR, Ensminger WD. Hypervascular hepatic metastases: CT evaluation. Radiology 162:49–51, 1987.
31. Broder LE, Carter SK. Pancreatic islet cell carcinoma, II: Results of streptozotocin treatment in 52 patients. Ann Intern Med 79:108, 1973.
32. Brodows RG, Campbell RG. Control of refractory fasting hypoglycemia in a patient with suspected insulinoma with diphenylhydentoin. J Clin Endocrinol Metab 38:159–161, 1974.
33. Brown-Aldrich L, Moattari AR, Vinik AI. Distinguishing features of idiopathic flushing and carcinoid syndrome. Arch Int Med 148:2614–2618, 1988.
34. Burcharth F, Stage JG, Stadil F, Jensen LI, Fischermann K. Localization of gastrinomas by transhepatic portal catheterization and gastrin assay. Gastroenterology 77:444–450, 1979.
35. Burgener FA, Hamlin DJ. Contrast enhancement of hepatic tumors in CT: Comparison between bolus and infusion techniques. AJR 140:291–295, 1987.
36. Carter RE, Bitar KN, Zfass AM, Makhlouf GM. Inhibition of VIP stimulated intestinal secretion and cyclic AMP production by somatostatin in the rat. Gastroenterology 74:726–730, 1978.
37. Chance RE, Jones WE. Polypeptides from bovine, ovine, human, and porcine pancreas. US Patent Office 842(3):063, 1974.
38. Cherner JA, Doppman JL, Norton JA, et al. Selective venous sampling for gastrin to localize gastrinomas: A prospective assessment. Ann Intern Med 105:841–847, 1986.
39. Chernish SM, Miller RE, Rosenak BD, Brunelle RL. Effect of D-Val D-Trp^{8}-somatostatin on the motility of the stomach, duodenum and jejunum. Am J Gastroenterol 75:36–40, 1981.
40. Christensen SE, Hansen AP, Lundbaek K, Orskow H, Seyer-Hansen K. Somatostatin and insulinoma. Lancet 1:1426, 1975.
41. Clements D, Elias E. Regression of metastatic VIPoma with somatostatin analogue SMS 201-995. Lancet 1:874–875, 1985.
42. Cockey BM, Fishman EK, Jones B, Siegelman SS. Computed tomography of abdominal carcinoid tumor. JCAT 9:38–42, 1985.
43. Crain EL Jr, Thorn GW. Functioning pancreatic islet cell adenomas. Medicine 28:427, 1949.
44. Creutzfeldt W, Arnold R. Somatostatin and the stomach: Exocrine and endocrine aspects. First International Somatostatin Symposium, Freiberg, Germany. Metabolism 27(suppl):1309–1315, 1978.
45. Creutzfeldt W, Lankisch PG, Folsch UR. Hemmung der Secretin und Cholezystokinin-Pankreozymin-induzierten Saft und Enzymsecretion des Pancreas und der Gallenblasen-Kontraktion beim Menschen durch Somatostatin. Dtsch Med Wochenschr 100:1135, 1975.
46. Curnow RT, Carey RM, Taylor A, Johanson A, Murad F. Somatostatin inhibition of insulin and gastrin hypersecretion in pancreatic islet-cell carcinoma. N Engl J Med 292:1385–1386, 1975.
47. Danforth DN, Triche T, Doppman JL, et al. Elevated plasma proglucagon-like component with a glucagon-secreting tumor. Effect of streptozotocin. N Engl J Med 295:242–245, 1976.
48. Davis Z, Moertel CG, Mc Iirath DC. The malignant carcinoid syndrome. Surg Gynecol Obstet 137:637–644, 1973.
49. De Marinis L, Barbarino A. Calcium antagonist and hormone release. Effects of verapamil on insulin release in normal subjects and patients with islet-cell tumor. Metabolism 29:599–604, 1980.
50. deNutte N, Somers G, Gepts W, Jacobs M, Pipeleers D. Pancreatic hormone release in tumor associated hypersomatostatinemia. Diabetologia 15:227, 1978.
51. Deveney CW, Deveney KE, Stark D, et al. Resection of gastrinomas. Ann Surg 198:546–553, 1983.
52. Deveney CW, Stein S, Way LW. Cimetidine in the treatment of Zollinger-Ellison syndrome. Am J Surg 146:116–123, 1983.

53. Dharmsathaphorn K, Binder JJ, Dobbins JW. Somatostatin stimulates sodium and chloride absorption in the rabbit ileum. Gastroenterology 78:1559–1565, 1980.
54. Dharmsathaphorn K, Sherwin RS, Dobbins JW. Somatostatin inhibits fluid secretion in the rat jejunum. Gastroenterology 78:1554–1558, 1980.
55. Donowitz M, Elta G, Bloom SR, Nathanson L. Trifluoroperazine reversal of secretory diarrhea in pancreatic cholera. Ann Intern Med 93:284–285, 1980.
56. Duncan LA, Marynick SP. Glucagonoma and dacarbazine. Ann Intern Med 97:930, 1982.
57. Murray PD, Fischer JE. Vasoactive intestinal peptide and the watery diarrhea syndrome. Ann Surg 187:411–416, 1978.
58. Eelkema EA, Stephens DH, Ward EM, Sheedy PF. CT features of nonfunctioning islet cell carcinoma. AJR 143:943–948, 1984.
59. Ellison EC, Woltering EA, Mekhjian TS, et al. Characterization of somatostatin inhibition of gastrin secretion in vivo and in vitro. Proceedings of the Symposium on Gut Endocrinology. Clinical and Therapeutic Impact. Am J Med 815:55–64, 1986.
60. Erlandsen SL, Hegre OD, Parsons JA, McEroy RC, Elde RP. Pancreatic islet cell hormones: Distribution of cell types in the islet and the evidence for the presence of somatostatin and gastrin within the D cell. J Histochem Cytochem 24:883–897, 1976.
61. Fabri PJ, Johnson JA, Ellison EC. Prediction of progressive disease in Zollinger-Ellison syndrome—Comparison of available preoperative tests. J Surg Res 31:93, 1981.
62. Fajans SS, Vinik AI. Diagnosis and treatment of insulinoma. In: Santen RJ and Manni A, eds. Diagnosis and Management of Endocrine Related Tumors. Boston, Martinus Nijhoff, 1984, pp 235–304.
63. Fajans SS, Floyd JC Jr, Knopf RF, et al. Benzothiadiazine suppression of insulin release from normal and abnormal islet tissue in man. J Clin Invest 45:481–492, 1966.
64. Fajans SS, Floyd JC Jr, Thiffault CA, et al. Further studies on diazoxide suppression of insulin release from abnormal and normal islet tissue in man. Ann NY Acad Sci 150:261–280, 1968.
65. Federspil G, Casara D, Stauffacher W. Chlorpromazine in the treatment of endogenous organic hyperinsulinism. Diabetologia 10:189–191, 1974.
66. Feldman JM. Increased dopamine production in patients with carcinoid tumors. Metabolism 34:255–260, 1985.
67. Feldman JM. Urinary serotonin in the diagnosis of carcinoid tumor. Clin Chem 32:840–844, 1986.
68. Feldman J, O'Dorisio TM. Role of neuropeptides and serotonin in the diagnosis of carcinoid tumors. Am J Med 81(suppl 6b):41–48, 1986.
69. Field M, McColl I. Ion transport in rabbit ileal mucosa, III: Effects of catecholamines. Am J Physiol 225:852, 1973.
70. Fink IJ, Krudy AG, Shawker TH, et al. Demonstration of an angiographically hypovascular insulinoma with intraarterial dynamic CT. AJR 144:555–556, 1985.
71. Floyd JC Jr, Vinik AI, Glaser B, et al. Pancreatic polypeptide. In: Waldhusl W, ed. Proceedings of the 10th Congress of the International Diabetes Federation. Amsterdam, Excerpta Medica, 1979, p. 490.
72. Fox PS, Hoffman JW, DeCosse JJ, Wilson SD. The influence of total gastrectomy on survival in malignant Zollinger-Ellison tumors. Ann Surg 180:558, 1974.
73. Freedberg IM, et al. Case record of the Mass General Hospital. N Engl J Med 292:1117, 1975.
74. Friesen SR. The development of endocrinopathies in the prospective screening of two families with MEA-I. World J Surg 3:753–764, 1979.
75. Friesen SR, Bolinger RE, Pearse AGE, McGuigan JE. Serum gastrin levels in malignant Zollinger-Ellison syndrome after total gastrectomy and hypophysectomy. Ann Surg 172:504, 1970.
76. Friesen SR, Kimmel JR, Tomita T. Pancreatic polypeptide as screening for pancreatic polypeptide apudomas in multiple endocrinopathies. Am J Surg 139:61–72, 1980.
77. Frohlich J, Bloomgarden Z, Oates J, et al. The carcinoid flush provocation by pentagastrin and inhibition by somatostatin. N Engl Med 299:1055-1057, 1978.
78. Fulton RE, Sheedy PF, McIllrath, DC, Ferris DO. Preoperative angiographic locali-

zation of insulin producing tumors of the pancreas. Am J Gastroenterol 123:367–377, 1975.
79. Gahmiche JP, Conlin R, Dubois PM, et al. Calcitonin secretion by a pancreatic somatostatinoma. N Engl J Med 299:1252, 1978.
80. Ganda PO, Weir GC, Soeldner JS, et al. Somatostatinoma: A somatostatin-containing tumor of the endocrine pancreas. N Engl J Med 296:963, 1977.
81. Glaser B, Floyd JC Jr, Vinik AI, et al. Evidence for extravagal cholinergic dependence of pancreatic polypeptide responses to beef ingestion in man. Clin Res 27:336, 1979.
82. Glaser B, Valtysson G, Fajans SS, et al. Gastrointestinal/pancreatic hormone concentration in the portal venous system of nine patients with organic hyperinsulinism. Metabolism 30(10):1001–1010, 1981.
83. Glaser B, Vinik AI, Sive AA, et al. Plasma human pancreatic polypeptide responses to administered secretion effects of surgical vagotomy, cholinergic blockage and chronic pancreatitis. J Clin Endocrinol Metab 50:1094–1099, 1980.
84. Glazer GM, Aisen AM, Francis IR, et al. Hepatic cavernous hemangioma: Magnetic resonance imaging. Radiology 155:417–420, 1985.
85. Glowniak J, Shapiro B, Vinik AI, et al. Percutaneous transhepatic venous sampling of gastrin. N Engl J Med 307:293–297, 1982.
86. Graber AL, Porte D Jr, Williams RH. Clinical use of diazoxide and mechanism for its hyperglycemic effects. Diabetes 15:143–148, 1966.
87. Greenberg GR, McCloy RF, Adrian TE, et al. Inhibition of pancreas and gallbladder by pancreatic polypeptide. Lancet 2:1280–1282, 1978.
88. Gunther RW, Klose KJ, Ruckert K, et al. Localization of small islet-cell tumors. Preoperative and intraoperative ultrasound, computed tomography, arteriography, digital subtraction angiography, and pancreatic venous sampling. Gastrointest Radiol 10:145–152, 1985.
89. Gyn NE, Kayasseh L, Keller IJ. In: Bloom SR, Polak JM, ed. Gut Hormones, 2nd ed. Edinburgh, Churchill Livingstone, 1981, pp 581–585.
90. Hallengren B, Dymling JF, Manhem P, et al. Unsuccessful DTIC-treatment of a patient with glucagonoma syndrome. Acta Med Scand 213:317–318, 1983.
91. Hayes MMM. Report of a pancreatic polypeptide-producing islet-cell tumor of the pancreas causing the watery diarrhea, hypokalemia, achlorhydria syndrome in a 55 year old Zimbabwean African male. Cent Afr J Med 26:195, 1980.
92. Helland S, Thorsen E, Holst JJ, Ingemansson S. Glukagonomsyndrometnekrolytisk migrerende erythem. Tidsskr Nor Laegeforen 99:638, 1979.
93. Hengl G, Prager J, Pointner H. The influence of somatostatin on the absorption of triglycerides in partially gastrectomized subjects. Acta Hepatogastroenterol 26:392–395, 1979.
94. Higgins GA, Recant L, Fischmann AB. The glucagonoma syndrome: Surgically curable diabetes. Am J Surg 137:142–148, 1979.
95. Hirsch HJ, Loo S, Evans N, et al. Hypoglycemia of infancy and nesidioblastosis: Studies with somatostatin. N Engl J Med 296:1323–1326, 1977.
96. Hofeldt FD, Dippe SE, Levin SR, et al. Effects of diphenylhydantoin upon glucose-induced insulin secretion in three patients with insulinoma. Diabetes 23:192–198, 1973.
97. Holst SS, Hellend S, Ingemannson S, Bang Pedersen N, von Schenck H. Functional studies in patients with glucagonoma syndrome. Diabetologia, 17:151–156, 1979.
98. Imhof H, Frank P. Pancreatic calcifications in malignant islet cell tumors. Radiology 122:333–337, 1977.
99. Ingemansson S, Holst J, Larson LE, Lunderquist A. Localization of glucagonomas by catheterization of the pancreatic veins and with glucagon assay. Surg Gynecol Obstet 145:509–516, 1977.
100. Ingemansson S, Holst J, Larsson LI, Lunderquist A, Nobin A. Islet cell hyperplasia localized by pancreatic vein catheterization and insulin radioimmunoassay. Am J Surg 133:643–645, 1977.
101. Ingemansson S, Larsson LI, Lunderquist A, Stadil F. Pancreatic vein catheterization

with gastrin assay in normal patients and in patients with Zollinger-Ellison syndrome. Am J Surg 134:558–563, 1977.
102. Ingemansson S, Lunderquist A, Lundquist I, Loudahl R, Tibbin S. Portal and pancreatic vein catheterization with radioimmunologic determination of insulin. Surg Gynecol Obstet 141:705–711, 1975.
103. Jackson J, Raju U, Fachnie JD, et al. Malignant somatostatinoma presenting with diabetic ketoacidosis. Clin Endocrinol 26:609–621, 1987.
104. Jaffe BM, Kopen DF, DeSchryver-KecsKemeti K, et al. Indomethacin-responsive pancreatic cholera. N Engl J Med 297:817–821, 1977.
105. Jensen RT, Gardener JD, Raufman JP, et al. Zollinger-Ellison syndrome. Current concepts and management. Ann Intern Med 8:59–75, 1983.
106. Johansson C, Kollberg B, Efendic S, Uvnas-Wallensten K. Effects of graded doses of somatostatin on gallbladder emptying and pancreatic enzyme output after oral glucose in man. Digestion 22:24–31, 1981.
107. Johansson C, Wisen O, Efendic S, Uvnas-Wallensten K. Effects of somatostatin on gastrointestinal propagation and absorption of oral glucose in man. Digestion 22:126–137, 1981.
108. Johnson JA, Fabri PJ, Lott JA. Serum gastrins in Zollinger-Ellison syndrome—Identification of localized disease. Clin Chem 26:867–870, 1980.
109. Kahan RS, Perez-Figaredo MRA, Neimanis A. Necrolytic migratory erythema. Distinctive dermatosis of the glucagonoma syndrome. Arch Dermatol 113:792–797, 1977.
110. Kahn CR, Levy AG, Gardner JD, et al. Pancreatic cholera: Beneficial effects of treatment with streptozotocin. N Engl J Med 292:941–945, 1975.
111. Katz R, Fischmann AVB, Galotta J, et al. Necrolytic migratory erythema, presenting as candidiasis, due to pancreatic glucagonoma. Cancer 44:558–563, 1979.
112. Kavlie H, White TT. Pancreatic islet beta-cell tumors and hyperplasia. Ann Surg 175:326–335, 1972.
113. Kent RB, van Heerden JA, Weiland LH. Nonfunctioning islet cell tumors. Ann Surg 193:185–190, 1981.
114. Kessinger A, Lemon HM, Foley JF. The glucagonoma syndrome and its management. J Surg Oncol 9:419–424, 1977.
115. Khandekar JD, Oyer D, Miller HJ, Vick NA. Neurologic involvement in glucagonoma syndrome. Response to combination chemotherapy with 5-fluorouracil and streptozotocin. Cancer 44:2014–2016, 1979.
116. Kimmel J, Pollack H, Hazelwood R. Isolation and characterization of chicken insulin. Endocrinology 83:1323, 1968.
117. Kitson HF, McCrossin RB, Jimenez M, Middleton A, Silink M. Somatostatin treatment of insulin excess due to B-cell adenoma in a neonate. J Pediatr 96:145–148, 1980.
118. Klee CB, Crouch TH, Richman PG: Calmodulin. Ann Rev Biochem 49:489, 1980.
119. Klein RF, Seino S, Sanz N, et al. High-performance liquid chromatography used to distinguish the autoimmune hypoglycemia syndrome from factitious hypoglycemia. J Clin Endocrinol Metab 61:571–574, 1985.
120. Konturek SJ, Kwiecien N, Obtuowicz W, et al. Effects of somatostatin-14 and somatostatin-28 on plasma hormonal and gastric secretory reponses to cephalic and gastrointestinal stimulation in man. Scand J Gastroenterol 20:31–38, 1985.
121. Korobkin MT, Palubinskas AJ, Glickman MG. Pitfalls in arteriography of cell tumors of the pancreas. Radiology 100:319–328, 1971.
122. Kothary PC, Fabri PJ, Gower W, et al. Evaluation of NH_2-terminus gastrins in gastrinoma syndrome. J Clin Endocrinol Metab 62:970–974, 1986.
123. Kothary PC, Vinik AI, Mahoney WC. Identification of gastrin molecular variants in gastrinoma syndrome. Regul Pept 17:71–84, 1987.
124. Kovaes K, Horvath E, Ezrin C, Sepp H, Elkan I. Immunoreactive somatostatin in pancreatic islet cell carcinoma accompanied by ectopic ACTH syndrome. Lancet 1:1365–1366, 1977.
125. Kraenzlin ME, Ching KC, Wood SM, Carr DH, Bloom SR. Long-term treatment of a VIPoma with somatostatin analogue resulting in remission of symptoms and possible shrinkage of metastases. Gastroenterology 88:185–187, 1985.

126. Krebs A, Teuscher A, Armagni C. Syndrome de glucagonome: Manifestations cutness. Ann Dermatol Venereol 105:637–639, 1978.
127. Krejs GJ, Orci L, Conlon M, et al. Somatostatinoma syndrome (biochemical, morphological, and clinical features). N Engl J Med 301:285–292, 1979.
127a. Krenning EP, Bakker WH, Breeman WAP, Koper JW, Kooij PP, Ausema L, Lameris JS, Reubi JC, Lamberts SWJ. Localisation of endocrine-related tumors with radioiodinated analogue of somatostatin. Lancet 1:242–244, 1989
128. Kvols LK. Metastatic carcinoid tumors and the carcinoid syndrome. A selective review of chemotherapy and hormonal therapy. Am J Med 81(suppl 6b):49–55, 1986.
129. Kvols LK, Buck M, Moertel CG, et al. Treatment of metastatic islet cell carcinoma with a somatostatin analogue (SMS 201-995). Ann Intern Med 107(2):162–168, 1987.
130. Kvols LK, Martin JK, Marsh HM, Moertel CG. Carcinoid crisis: Rapid reversal of the life threatening hypotension with a somatostatin analogue. N Engl J Med 313:1229–1230, 1985.
131. Kvols LK, Moertel CG, O'Connell MJ, et al. Treatment of the malignant carcinoid syndrome. Evaluation of a long-acting somatostatin analogue. N Engl J Med 315:663–666, 1986.
131a. Lamberts SWJ, Bakker WH, Reubi JC, Krenning EP. Treatment with Sandostatin and in vivo localization of tumors with radiolabeled somatostatin analogs. Metabolism 39 (supp2):152–155, 1990.
132. Lamers CB, Buis JT, Van Tongeren JH. Secretin-stimulated serum gastrin levels in hyperparathyroid patients from families with multiple endocrine adenomatosis-type I. Ann Intern Med 86:719–724, 1977.
133. Landor JH. Control of the Zollinger-Ellison syndrome by excision of primary and metastatic tumor. Am J Surg 147:406–409, 1984.
134. Larsson LI. Two distinct types of islet abnormalities associated with endocrine pancreatic tumors. Virchows Arch Pathol Anat 376:209–219, 1977.
135. Larsson LI. Gastrointestinal cells producing endocrine, neurocrine and paracine messengers. Clin Gastroenterol 9:485–615, 1989.
136. Larsson LI, Hirsch MA, Holst J, et al. Pancreatic somatostatinoma clinical features and physiologic implications. Lancet 1:666–668, 1977.
137. Larsson LI, Schwartz T, Lundquist G, et al. Pancreatic polypeptide in pancreatic endocrine tumors, possible implications in watery diarrhea syndrome. Am J Pathol 85:675–682, 1976.
138. Lefebvre J, Leievre G, Dalle-Furnari MA, et al. Glucagonoma avec acidocetose diabetique. Une observation. Diabete Metab 8:191, 1982.
139. Lennon JR, Sircus W, Bloom SR, et al. Investigation and treatment of recurrent VIPoma. Gut 16:821, 1975.
140. LeRoith D, Vinik AI, Epstein S, et al. Somatostatin and serum gastrin in normal subjects and in patients with pernicious anemia, chronic liver and renal diseases. S Afr Med J 49:1601–1605, 1975.
141. Levin G, Malmud L, Rock E, et al. Effects of somatostatin on gallbladder emptying in man. Clin Res 31:284A, 1983.
142. Lewis E, Tsai S, Vinik AI. The role of a long-acting somatostatin analogue (SMS 201-995) in the management of a patient with benign insulin secreting adenoma of the pancreas and a post-operative pancreatic fistula. Scand J Gastroenterol 21(suppl 119):217–222, 1986.
143. Lightman SL, Bloom SR. Cure of insulin-dependent diabetes mellitus by removal of a glucagonoma. Br Med J 1:367, 1974.
144. Linnestad P, Myrvang B, Ritland S, et al. Glucagonproduserende tumor i pancreas. Tidsskr Nor Laegeforen 103:1520–1522, 1983.
145. Long RG, Adrian TE, Barnes AJ, et al. Suppression of a pancreatic endocrine tumor secretion by long-acting somatostatin analogue. Lancet 2:764–767, 1979.
146. Loud FB, Holst JJ, Egense E, et al. Is somatostatin a humoral regulator of the endogenous pancreas and gastric acid secretion in man? Gut 26:445–449, 1985.

147. Lucas KG, Feldman JM. Flushing in the carcinoid syndrome and plasma kallikrein. Cancer 58:2290–2293, 1986.
148. Lunderquist A, Eriksson M, Ingemansson S, Larsson LI, Riechardt W. Selective pancreatic vein catheterization for hormone assay in endocrine tumors of the pancreas. Cardiovasc Radiol 1:117–124, 1987.
149. Lunderquist A, Tylen U. Phlebography of the pancreatic veins. Radiology 15:95–97, 1975.
150. Lundqist G, Krause U, Larsson LI, et al. A pancreatic-polypeptide-producing tumor associated with the WDMA syndrome. Scand J Gastroenterol 13:715–718, 1978.
151. Makhlouf G. Adenylate cyclase inhibitors. In: Janowitz HD, Sachar DB, eds. Frontiers of Knowledge in the Diarrheal Diseases. Upper Montclair, NJ, Projects in Health, 1979, p 337.
152. Malaisse-Lagae F, Stefan Y, Cox J, Perrelet A, Orci L. Identification of a lobe in the adult human pancreas rich in pancreatic polypeptide. Diabetologia 17:361–366, 1979.
153. Malagelada JR, Edis AJ, Adson MA, et al. Medical and surgical options in the management of patients with gastrinoma. Gastroenterology 84:1524–1532, 1983.
154. Manche A, Wood SM, Adrian TE, Welbourn RB, Bloom SR. Pancreatic polypeptide and calcitonin secretion from a pancreatic tumor—Clinical improvement after hepatic artery embolization. Postgrad Med J 59:313–314, 1983.
155. Mandarino L, Stenner D, Blanchard W, et al. Selective effects of somatostatin-14, -25 and -28 on in vitro insulin and glucagon secretion. Nature 291:76, 1981.
156. Marks V, Samols E. Diazoxide therapy of intractable hypoglycemia. Ann NY Acad Sci 150:442–454, 1968.
157. Marks V, Rose FC, Samols E. Hyperinsulinemia due to metastasizing insulinoma: Treatment with diazoxide. Proc R Soc Med 58:577–578, 1965.
158. Marks WH, Strodel WE, Lloyd RV, et al. Cervical metastases from small bowel carcinoid tumors. J Surg Oncol 24:135–141, 1983.
159. Maton PN, Camiller M, Griffin G, et al. The role of hepatic arterial embolization in the carcinoid syndrome. Br Med J 287:932–935, 1983.
160. Marynick SP, Fagadau WR, Duncan LA. Malignant glucagonoma syndrome: Response to chemotherapy. Ann Intern Med 93:453, 1980.
161. McArthur KE, Anderson SD, Durbin TE, et al. Clondine and Lidamidine to inhibit watery diarrhea in a patient with lung cancer. Ann Intern Med 96:323, 1982.
162. McCarthy DM. Report on the United States experience with cimetidine in Zollinger-Ellison syndrome and other hypersecretory states. Gastroenterology 74:453–458 1978.
163. McCarthy DM. The place of surgery in the Zollinger-Ellison syndrome. N Engl J Med 24:1344–1347, 1980.
164. McCarthy DM. The diagnosis and treatment of gastrinoma and Zollinger-Ellison syndrome. In: Santen RJ, Manni A, eds. Diagnosis and Management of Endocrine-Related Tumors. Boston, Martinus Nijhoff, 1984, pp 347–382.
165. McCarthy DM, Jensen RT. Zollinger-Ellison syndrome: Current Issues. In: Cohen S, Soloway R, eds. Hormone Producing Tumors of the Gastrointestinal Tract. Churchill Livingstone, 1985, p 25.
166. McCarthy DM, Weintraub B, Rosen S. Subunits of human chorionic gonadotropin in the Zollinger-Ellison syndrome. Gastroenterology 76:1198, 1979.
167. McGavran MH, Unger RH, Recant L, et al. A glucagon-secreting alpha cell carcinoma of the pancreas. N Engl J Med 274:1408–1413, 1966.
168. Megibow AJ, Bosniak MA, Ambos MA, Beranbaum ER. Thickening of the celiac axis and/or superior mesenteric artery: A sign of pancreatic carcinoma on computed tomography. Radiology 141:449–453, 1981.
169. Melmon KL, Sjoerdsma A, Oates JA, Laster L. Treatment of malabsorption and diarrhea of carcinoid syndrome with methysergide. Gastroenterology 48:18, 1965.
170. Mignon M, Ruszniewski P, Haffar S, et al. Current approach to the management of tumoral process in patients with gastrinoma. World J Surg 10:703–710, 1986.
171. Mignon M, Vallot T, Hervoir P, et al. Ranitidine versus cimetidine in the management of Zollinger-Ellison syndrome. In: Riley AJ, Salmon PR, eds. Ranitidine. Proceedings

of an International Symposium, World Congress of Gastroenterology, Stockholm, 1982. Amsterdam, Excerpta Medica, 1982, pp 169–177.
172. Miller DR. Functioning adenomas of pancreas with hyperinsulinism. Arch Surg 90:509–520, 1965.
173. Mitty HA, Efremidis S, Westkin MG, Dreiling DA, Rayfield EJ. Localization of insulinomas by radioimmunoassay of blood obtained by the transportal route. J Clin Endocrinol Metab 48:1035–1037, 1979.
174. Moertel CG. Treatment of the carcinoid tumor and the malignant carcinoid syndrome. J Clin Oncol 1:727–740, 1983.
175. Moertel CG, Hanley JA, Johnson LA. Streptozotocin alone compared with streptozotocin plus fluorouracil in the treatment of advanced islet cell carcinoma. N Engl J Med 303:1189–1194, 1980.
176. Molinie C, Naudan P, Daly JP, et al. Glucagonome: Survie de neuf années apres exerese. Nouv Presse Med 10:177, 1981.
177. Morowitz DA, Levine AE. Malignant Zollinger-Ellison syndrome: Remission of primary and metastatic pancreatic tumor after gastrectomy: Report of a case and review of the literature. Am J Gastroenterol 81:471–473, 1986.
178. Nankervis A, Proietto J, Ng KW, et al. The metabolic effects of chronic hyperglucagonemia. Clin Endocrinol 15:325, 1981.
179. Neri V, Bartorelli A, Faglia G. Effect of propranolol on the blood sugar, immunoreactive blood insulin in a patient with insulinoma. Acta Diabetol Lat 6:809–819, 1969.
180. Nobin A, Berg M, Ericsson MM, et al. Pancreatic polypeptide-producing tumors, report on two cases, Cancer 53:2688–2691, 1984.
181. Norton JA, Doppman JL, Collen MJ, et al. Prospective study of gastrinoma localization and resection in patients with Zollinger-Ellison Syndrome. Ann Surg 204:468–479, 1986.
182. Norton JA, Kahn CR, Schiebinger R, et al. Amino acid deficiency and the skin rash associated with glucagonoma syndrome. Ann Intern Med 91:213–215, 1979.
183. Noyes BE, Merarch M, Stein R, Agarwal KL. Detection and partial sequence analysis of gastrin mRNA by using an oligodeoxy-nucleotide probe. Proc Natl Acad Sci USA 76:1770–1774, 1979.
184. Oates JA, Pettinger WA, Doctor RB. Evidence for the release of bradykinin in the carcinoid syndrome. J Clin Invest 45:173–178, 1966.
185. Oberg K, Loof L, Bostrom H, et al. Hypersecretion of calcitonin in patients with the Verner-Morrison syndrome. Scand J Gastroenterol 16:135–144, 1981.
186. O'Dorisio TM, Vinik AI. Pancreatic polypeptide and mixed peptide-producing tumors of the gastrointestinal tract. In: Cohen S, Soloway RD, eds. Contemporary Issues in Gastroenterology. New York, Churchill Livingstone, 1985, p 117.
187. Orci L, Malaisse-Lagae F, Baeteus D, Penelet A: Pancreatic polypeptide-rich regions in human pancreas. Lancet 2:1200–1201, 1978.
188. Osei K, O'Dorisio TM. Malignant insulinoma: Effects of a somatostatin analogue (compound 201-995) on serum glucose, growth and gastroenteropancreatic hormones. Ann Intern Med 103:223–225, 1985.
189. Palmer JP, Werner PL, Benson JW, et al. Dominant inheritance of large molecular weight immunoreactive glucagon. J Clin Invest 61:763–769, 1978.
190. Pandol SJ, Korman LY, McCarthy DM, Gardner JD. Beneficial effects of oral lithium carbonate in the treatment of pancreatic cholera syndrome. N Engl J Med 302:1403–1404, 1980.
191. Passaro E. Localization of pancreatic endocrine tumors by selective portal vein catheterization and radioimmunoassay. Gastroenterology 77:806–807, 1979.
192. Passaro E, Gordon HE. Malignant gastrinoma following total gastrectomy. Arch Surg 108:444–448, 1974.
193. Pauwels S, Desmond H, Dimaline R, Dockray GJ. Identification of progastrin in gastrinomas, antrum, and duodenum by a novel radioimmunoassay. J Clin Invest 77:376–381, 1986.
194. Pedersen NB, Jonsson L, Holst JJ. Necrolytic migratory erythema and glucagon cell tumour of the pancreas: The glucagonoma syndrome. Acta Dermatovener (Stockholm) 56:391, 1976.

195. Pernow B, Waldenstrom J. Determination of 5-hydroxytryptamine, 5-hydroxy indoleacetic acid and histamine in 33 cases of carcinoid (argentaffinoma). Am J Med 23:16–25, 1957.
196. Pernow B, Waldenstrom J. Determination of 5-hydroxytryptamine, 5 hydroxyindolacetic acid and histamine in thirty three cases of carcinoid tumor (argentaffinoma). Am J Med 34:255–260, 1985.
197. Peters MN, Richardson CT, Feldman M, et al. Exploratory laparotomy, vagotomy and cimetidine for treatment of Zollinger-Ellison syndrome (ZES). Gastroenterology, 82:1149, 1982.
198. Pipeleers D, Couturier E, Gepts W, et al. Five cases of somatostatinoma: Clinical heterogeneity and diagnostic usefulness of basal and tolbutamide-induced hypersomatostatinemia. J Clin Endocrinol Metab 56:1236–1242, 1983.
199. Polak JM, Adrian TE, Bryant MG, et al. Pancreatic polypeptide in insulinomas, gastrinomas, vipomas, and glucagonomas. Lancet 1:328–330, 1976.
200. Prinz RA, Badrinath K, Banerji M, et al. Operative and chemotherapeutic management of malignant glucagon-producing tumors. Surgery 90:713, 1983.
201. Rao MB, O'Dorisio TM, George JM, et al. Angiotensin II and norepinephrine antagonize the effect of vasoactive intestinal peptide on rat ileum and colon. Peptides
201a. Reubi JC, Hacki WH, Lamberts SWJ. Hormone producing gastrointestinal tumors contain high density of somatostatin receptors. J Clin Endocrinol Metab 65:1127–1134, 1987.
201b. Reubi JC, Maurer R, von Werder K, Torhorst J, Klijn JG, Lamberts SWJ. Somatostatin receptors in human endocrine tumors. Cancer Res 47:551–558, 1987.
202. Richardson CT, Peters MN, Feldman M, et al. Treatment of Zollinger-Ellison syndrome with exploratory laparotomy, proximal gastric vagotomy, and H2-receptor antagonists: A prospective study. Gastroenterology 89:357–367, 1985.
203. Richter G, Stockmann F, Lembeke B, Conlon JM, Creutzfeldt W. Short-term administration of somatostatin analogue SMS 20-1995 in patients with carcinoid tumors. Scand J Gastroenterol 21(suppl 119):193–198, 1986.
204. Robins JM, Bookstein JJ, Oberman HA, Fajans SS. Selective arteriography in localizing islet cell tumors of the pancreas. Radiology 106:525–528, 1973.
205. Roche A, Raissonnier A, Gillon-Savouret MC. Pancreatic venous sampling and arteriography in the localizing insulinomas and gastrinomas: Procedure and results in 55 cases. Radiology 145:621–627, 1982.
206. Roti E, Ghinelli C, Bandini P, et al. Effects of somatostatin in a case of severe hypoglycemia due to nesidioblastosis. J Endocrinol Invest 4:209–212, 1981.
207. Said SI, Faloona GR. Elevated plasma and tissue levels of vasoactive intestinal polypeptide in the watery diarrhea syndrome due to pancreatic, bronchogenic and other tumors. N Engl J Med 293:155–160, 1975.
208. Samols E, Weir GC, Ramseur R, et al. Modulation of pancreatic somatostatin by adrenergic and cholinergic agonism and by hyper- and hypoglycemic sulfonamides. Metabolism 27(suppl 1):1219, 1978.
209. Sandler M, Karim SMM, William ED. Prostaglandin in amine-peptide-secreting tumors. Lancet 2:1053–1055, 1968.
210. Santangelo WC, O'Dorisio TM, Kim JG, Severino G, Krejs GJ. Pancreatic cholera syndrome—Effect of a synthetic somatostatin analogue on intestinal water and ion transport. Ann Intern Med 103:363–367, 1985.
211. Schally AV, Comaru-Schally AM, Redding TW. Antitumor effects of analogs of hypothalamic hormones in endocrine-dependent cancers. Proc Soc Exp Biol Med 175:259–281, 1985.
212. Schusdziarra V, Zyznar E, Rouiller D, et al. Splanchnic somatostatin. A hormonal regulator of nutrient homeostasis. Science 207:530, 1980.
213. Schwartz TW. Atropine suppression test for pancreatic polypeptide. Lancet 2:43, 1978.
214. Scuro LA, Lo Cascio V, Adami S, et al. Somatostatin inhibition of insulin secretion in insulin producing tumors. Metabolism 25:603–609, 1976.
215. Seal A, Yamada T, Debas H, et al. Somatostatin-14 and -28: Clearance and potency on gastric function in dogs. Am J Physiol 243:G97–G102, 1982.

216. Seino S, Fu ZZ, Marks W, et al. Characterization of circulating insulin in insulin autoimmune syndrome. J Clin Endocrinol Metab 62:64–69, 1986.
217. Seino S, Funakoshi A, Fu ZZ, Vinik AI. Identification of insulin variants in patients with hyperinsulinemia by reversed-phase high-performance liquid chromatography. Diabetes 34:1–7, 1985.
218. Shaklai M, Aderka D, Blum I. Suppression of hypoglycemia attacks and insulin release by propranolol in a patient with metastatic malignant insulinoma. Diabete Metab 3:155–158, 1977.
219. Sheppard M, Shapiro B, Pimstone B, et al. Metabolic clearance and plasma half disapperance time of exogenous somatostatin in man. J Clin Endocrinol Metab 48:50–53, 1979.
220. Shupack JL, Berczeller PH, Stevens DM. The glucagonoma syndrome. J Dermatol Surg Oncol 4:242–247, 1978.
221. Simpson S, Vinik AI, Marangos PJ, Lloyd RV. Immunohistochemical localization of neuron-specific enolase in gastroentero-pancreatic neuroendocrine tumors. Correlation with tissue and serum levels of neuron-specific enolase. Cancer 54:1364–1369, 1984.
222. Sircus W. Vagotomy in ZE syndrome. Gastroenterology 79:607–608, 1980.
223. Smith PL, Field M. In vitro antisecretory effects of trifluoroperazine and other neuroleptics in rabbit and human small intestine. Gastroenterology 78:1545–1553, 1980.
224. Solcia E, Capella C, Buffa R, et al. Morphological and functional classification of endocrine cells and related growths in the gastrointestinal tract. In: Glass GBJ, ed. Gastrointestinal Hormones. New York, Raven Press, 1980, pp 1–17.
225. Solt J, Kadas I, Polak JM, et al. A pancreatic-polypeptide-producing tumor of the stomach. Cancer 54:1101–1104, 1984.
226. Stabile BE, Passaro E Jr. Benign and malignant gastrinoma. Am J Surg 149:144–150, 1985.
227. Stabile BE, Morrow DJ, Passaro E Jr. The gastrinoma triangle: Operative implications. Am J Surg 147:25–31, 1984.
228. Stadil F, Stage G, Rehfeld JF, et al. Treatment of Zollinger-Ellison syndrome with streptozotocin. N Engl J Med 294:1440–1442, 1976.
229. Stark DD, Moss AA, Goldberg HI, Davis PL, Federle MP. Magnetic resonance and CT of the normal and diseased pancreas: A comparative study. Radiology 150:153–162, 1984.
230. Stark DD, Moss AA, Goldberg HI, Deveney CW, Way L. Computed tomography and nuclear magnetic resonance imaging of pancreatic islet cell tumors. Surgery 94:1024–1027, 1983.
231. Stark DD, Moss AA, Goldberg HI, Deveney CW. CT of pancreatic islet cell tumors. Radiology 150:491–494, 1984.
232. Stefanini P, Carboni M, Patrassi N, Basoli A. A Beta islet cell tumors of the pancreas: Results of a study on 1,067 cases. Surgery 75:597–609, 1974.
233. Stefanini P, Carboni M, Patrassi N, De Bernardinis NP, Blandamura V. The value of arteriography in the diagnosis and treatment of insulinomas. Am J Surg 131:352–356, 1976.
234. Stockmann F, Richter G, Lembcke B, Conlon JM, Creutzfeldt W. Scand J Gastroenterol 21(suppl 119):230–237, 1986.
235. Strauss GM, Weitzman SA, Aoki TT. Dimethyltriazenoimidazole carboxamide therapy of malignant glucagonoma. Ann Intern Med 90:57–58, 1979.
236. Strodel WE, Vinik AI, Jaffe BM, Eckhauser F, Thompson NW. Substance P in the localization of a carcinoid tumor. J Surg Oncol 27:106–111, 1984.
237. Strodel W, Vinik A, Lloyd RV, et al. Pancreatic polypeptide-producing tumors. Arch Surg 119:508, 1984.
238. Strodel W, Vinik A, Thompson NW, et al. Carcinoid tumors of the small intestine. In: Thompson NW, Vinik AI, eds. Endocrine Surgery Update. New York, Grune & Stratton, 1983, pp 293–320.
239. Swenson KH, Amon RB, Hanifin JM. The glucagonoma syndrome: A distinctive cutaneous marker of systemic disease. Arch. Dermatol 114:224–228, 1978.

240. Taniguch H, Murakami K, Morita S. Calcium antagonist (Diltiazem) for reversal of hypoglycemic symptoms in insulinoma. Lancet 2:501, 1977.
241. Teuscher A, Studer PP, Krebs A, et al. Diabetesverlauf und klinisches Bild bei Glucagonom. Schweiz Med Wochenschr 109:1273–1277, 1979.
242. Theodrosson-Norheim E, Norheism KO, Brodin E, et al. Neuropeptide K: A major tachykinin in plasma and tumor tissues from carcinoid patients. Biochem Biophys Res Commun 131:77–83, 1985.
243. Thompson NW, Eckhause FE. Malignant islet-cell tumors of the pancreas. World J Surg 8:940–951, 1984.
244. Thompson NW, Lloyd RV, Nishiyama RH, et al. MEN I pancreas: A histological and immunohistochemical study. World J Surg 8:561–574, 1984.
245. Thompson JC, Reeder DD, Villar HV, et al. Natural history and experience with diagnosis and treatment of the Zollinger-Ellinger syndrome. Surg Gynecol Obstet 140:721–739, 1975.
246. Thompson NW, Vinik AI, Eckhauser FE, Strodel WE: Extrapancreatic gastrinomas. Surgery 98:1113–1120, 1985.
247. Tomita T, Friesen SR, Kimmel JR. Pancreatic polypeptide cell hyperplasia with and without watery diarrhea syndrome. J Surg Oncol 16:11–20, 1980.
248. Tomita T, Friesen SR, Kimmel JR. Pancreatic polypeptide-secreting islet cell tumor. Cancer 57:129–133, 1986.
249. Tomita T, Friesen SR, Kimmel JR, Douli V, Pollock HG. Pancreatic polypeptide-secreting islet-cell tumors, a study of three cases. Am J Pathol 113:134–142, 1983.
250. Trenkner SW, Glazer GM. Techniques of endocrine organ imaging: Endocrine pancreas. In: Rankin S, ed. Strategies for Diagnostic Imaging: Endocrine System. London, Bailiere Tindall, in press.
251. Tsai ST, Eckhauser FE, Thompson NW, et al. Perioperative use of a long-acting somatostatin analogue (SMS 201-995) in patients with tumors of the gastroenteropancreatic axis. J Surg 100:788–795, 1986.
252. Tsai ST, Lewis E, Vinik AI. The use of a somatostatin analogue in the management of the flushing syndrome. Scand J Gastroenterol 21(suppl 119):267–274, 1985.
253. Turner RC, Lee ECG, Morris PJ, Harris EA, Dick R. Localization of insulinomas. Lancet 1:515–518, 1978.
254. Unger RH. Somatostinoma. N Engl J M 296:998–1000, 1977.
255. Vale W, Rivier C, Brown M. Regulatory peptides of the hypothalamus. Annu Rev Physiol 39:473–527, 1977.
256. Valverde I, Lemon HM, Kessinger A, Unver RH. Distribution of plasma glucagon immunoreactivity in a patient with suspected glucagonoma. J Clin Endocrinol Metab 42:804, 1976.
257. van Heerden JA, Smith SL, Miller LJ. The management of Zollinger-Ellison syndrome in patients with multiple endocrine neoplasm Type I, presented at Seventh Annual Meeting, American Association of Endocrine Surgeons, April 15, 1986.
258. Verner JV, Morrison AB. Islet cell tumor and a syndrome of refractory watery diarrhea and hypokalemia. Am J Med 25:374–380, 1958.
259. Verner JV, Morrison AB. Endocrine pancreatic islet disease with diarrhea: Report of a case due to a diffuse hyperplasia of non beta islet tissue with a review of 54 additional cases. Arch Intern Med 133:492–500, 1974.
260. Villar HV, Johnson DG, Lynch PJ, et al. Pattern of immunoreactive glucagon in portal, arterial and peripheral plasma before and after removal of glucagonoma. Am J Surg 141:148, 1981.
261. Vinik AI. Radioimmunoassay and bioassay of gastrin and somatostatin. J Clin Immunoassay 10(1):20–31, 1987.
262. Vinik AI, Glaser B. Pancreatic endocrine tumors. In: Dent TL, ed. Pancreatic Disease, Diagnosis and Therapy. New York, Grune & Stratton, 1981, pp 427–461.
263. Vinik AI, Thompson NW. Controversies in the management of Zollinger-Ellison syndrome. Ann Intern Med 105:956–959, 1986.
264. Vinik AI, Achem-Karam S, Owyang C. Gastrointestinal hormones in clinical medicine. In: Cohen MP, Foa PP, eds. Special Topics in Endocrinology and Metabolism. New York, Alan R Liss, 1983, vol 4, pp 93–138.

265. Vinik AI, Glowniak J, Glaser B, et al. Localization of gastroenteropancreatic (GEP) tumors. In: Johnson IDA, Thompson NW, eds. Surgery 2, Endocrine Surgery. London, Butterworth's International Medical Reviews, 1983, vol 6, pp 76–102.
266. Vinik AI, Levitt NS, Pimstone BL, Wagner L. Peripheral plasma somatostatin-like immunoreactive responses to insulin hypoglycemia and mixed meal in healthy subjects and in non-insulin-dependent maturity-onset diabetes. J Clin Endocrinol Metab 52(2):330–337, 1980.
267. Vinik AI, Seino S, Funakoshi A, et al. Familial hyperinsulinemia and insulin resistance associated with secretion of an abnormal insulin. J Clin Endocrinol Metab 62:645–652, 1986.
268. Vinik AI, Strodel WE, Cho KJ, Eckhauser FE, Thompson NW. Localization of hormonally active gastrointestinal tumors. In: Thompson NW, Vinik AI, eds. Endocrine Surgery Update. New York, Grune & Stratton, 1983, pp 195–218.
269. Vinik AI, Strodel WE, Eckhauser FE, Moattari R, Lloyd R. Somatostatinomas, PPomas, and neurotensionomas. Semin Oncol 14(3):263–281, 1987.
270. Vinik AI, Strodel WE, Lloyd RV, Thompson NW. Unusual gastroenteropancreatic (GEP) tumors and their hormones. In: Thompson NW, Vinik AI, eds. Endocrine Surgery Update. New York, Grune and Stratton, 1983, pp 293–320.
271. Vinik AI, Strodel WE, O'Dorisio TM. Endocrine tumors of the gastroenteropancreatic axis. In: Santen RJ, Manni A, eds. Diagnosis and Management of Endocrine-Related Tumors. Boston, Martinus Nijhoff, 1984, pp 305–329.
272. Vinik A, Tsai S, Moattari A, et al. Somatostatin analogue (SMS 201-995) in the management of gastroenteropancreatic tumors and diarrhea syndromes. Am J Med 81(suppl 6b):23–40, 1986.
273. Vinik AI, Tsai ST, Moattari AR, Cheung P. Somatostatin analogue (SMS 201-995) in patients with gastrinomas. Surgery 104(5):834–842, 1988.
274. Waldman DB, Gardner TD, Zfass AM, Makhlouf GM. Effects of vasoactive intestinal peptide, secretin, and related peptides on rat colonic transport and adenylate cyclase activity. Gastroenterology, 73:518–523, 1977.
275. Warner TFCS, Seo I, Madura JA, Polak JM, Pearse AGE. Pancreatic-polypeptide-producing apudoma of the liver. Cancer 46:1146, 1980.
276. Weil C. Gastroenteropancreatic endocrine tumors. Klivo 63:433–459, 1985.
277. Weir GC, Horton ES, Aoki TT, et al. Secretion by glucagonomas of a possible glucagon precursor. J Clin Invest 59:325–330, 1977.
278. Wesley JR, Vinik AI, O'Dorisio TM, Glaser B, Fink A. A new syndrome of symptomatic cutaneous mastocytoma producing vasoactive intestinal polypeptide (VIP). Gastroenterology 82:963–967, 1982.
279. Wilander E, Grimelius L, Portela-Gomes G et al. Substance P and enteroglucagon-like immunoreactivity in argentaffin and argyrophil mid gut carcinoid tumors. Scand J Gastroenterol 14(suppl):19–25, 1979.
280. Wolfe BM, Culebras JM, Sim AJW, et al. Substrate interaction in intravenous feeding: Comparative effects of carbohydrate and fat on amino acid utilization in fasting man. Ann Surg 186:518–540, 1977.
281. Wolfe MM, Alexander RW, McGuigan JE. Extrapancreatic, extraintestinal gastrinoma. N Engl J Med 306:1533–1536, 1982.
282. Wood SM, Kraenzlin ME, Adrian TE, Bloom SR. Treatment of patients with pancreatic endocrine tumors using a new long-acting somatostatin analogue: Symptomatic and peptide responses. Gut 26:438–444, 1985.
283. Wood SM, Kraenzlin ME, Adrian TE, et al. Treatment of patients with pancreatic endocrine tumours using a new long-acting somatostatin analogue. Symptomatic and peptide responses. Gut 26:438–444, 1985.
284. Young SW, Turner RJ, Castellino RA. A strategy for the contrast enhancement of malignant tumors using dynamic computed tomography and intravascular pharmacokinetics. Radiology 137:137–147, 1980.
285. Zollinger RM. Gastrinoma: Factors influencing prognosis. Surgery 97:49–54, 1985.
286. Zollinger RM, Ellison EH. Primary peptic ulceration of the jejunum associated with islet cell tumors of the pancreas. Ann Surg 142:709–723, 1955.
287. Zollinger RM, Martin EW, Carey LC, et al. Observations on the postoperative tumor growth behavior of certain islet cell tumors. Ann Surg 184:525–530, 1976.

CHAPTER

26

PANCREATIC ENDOCRINE TUMORS: SURGICAL ASPECTS

Neal E. Seymour and Dana K. Andersen

Thirty years after Langerhans's recognition of the pancreatic islets, Nicholls described an adenoma of islet cell origin as an autopsy finding in 1899.[56] The recognition of hypoglycemia and "dysinsulinism" in association with islet cell tumors followed the discovery of insulin in 1921, and in 1929 the first reported cure of the disease was achieved after the resection of an islet cell adenoma performed by Roscoe Graham.[24] Despite their relative rarity, these tumors have sparked a great deal of interest and represent a class of diseases for which a cure or marked clinical improvement is possible with operative treatment. It is now recognized that the endocrine cell tumors of the pancreas can exhibit a "pluripotential" ability to release multiple secretory products, and several characteristic clinical syndromes have been described that are associated with the secretion of biologically active peptide hormones. Pharmacologic agents have recently become available that alter the secretory behavior of pancreatic cells or the end-organ effects of their products, but there is little controversy surrounding the concept that, if feasible, surgical removal of the tumor should occur at an early point in every patient's management.

TUMOR LOCALIZATION

The technical aspects of the removal of pancreatic endocrine tumors are less dependent on histologic type per se and are more related to location, multicentricity, or the presence of metastasis. Frequently, small or ectopically located tumors are difficult to identify at operation. The value of precise localization is inestimable, and any information that is garnered preoperatively can potentially be of use to the surgeon. The circumstance of being unable to find a lesion at exploration is a consequence of the limitations of preoperative localization techniques, coupled with the frequent small size or multicentricity of these lesions.

Noninvasive radiologic imaging methods, while relatively free of morbid side effects, have not been as efficacious as selective arteriography in detecting very small tumors. Recently, computed tomographic (CT) scanning (Fig. 26-1) has achieved sensitivity in the range of 75% to 80%,[35,83] which is comparable to the best results reported with selective arteriography. Ultrasonographic methods have also improved greatly in recent years (Fig. 26-2), and while a sensitivity of roughly 50% does not rival that of arteriography, it is highly effective in the detection of hepatic metastases.[35] There remains a combined advantage in the performance of CT scanning, ultrasonography, and selective arteriography (Fig. 26-3) in the evaluation of each individual tumor.[83] Magnetic resonance imaging (MRI) is potentially of great use in the localization of even small endocrine tumors, but the published experience with MRI in this application is limited at the present time. Technical difficulties in pancreatic imaging are in the process of being overcome, and initial experience with islet cell tumors (Fig. 26-4) has yielded promising results.[44,61,82] New techniques of contrast enhancement, to improve the ability of MRI to visualize small, completely intrapancreatic tumors, are currently in development.

Transhepatic catheterization of the portal, superior mesenteric, and splenic veins for multiple hormone determinations has been used to localize most types of

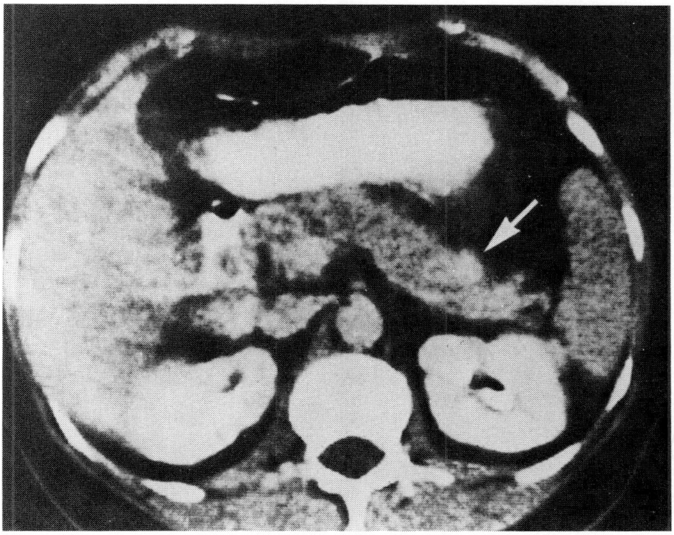

Figure 26-1. CT scan of a patient with Zollinger-Ellison syndrome. The CT scan with contrast material reveals within the pancreatic tail a 1-cm enhancing lesion (arrow) that was confirmed at surgery as a gastrinoma. (From Stark et al.[83] with permission.)

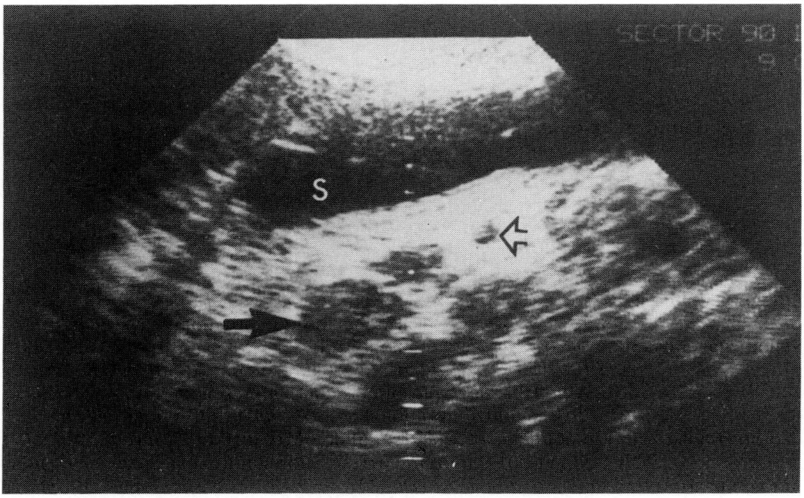

Figure 26-2. Transabdominal sonogram of a 14-year-old patient with insulinoma. The transverse sonogram demonstrates in the pancreatic head a 1.5-cm lesion (black arrow) that was confirmed at surgery as an insulinoma. S = fluid-filled stomach; open arrow = superior mesenteric artery. (From Telander et al.[86] with permission.)

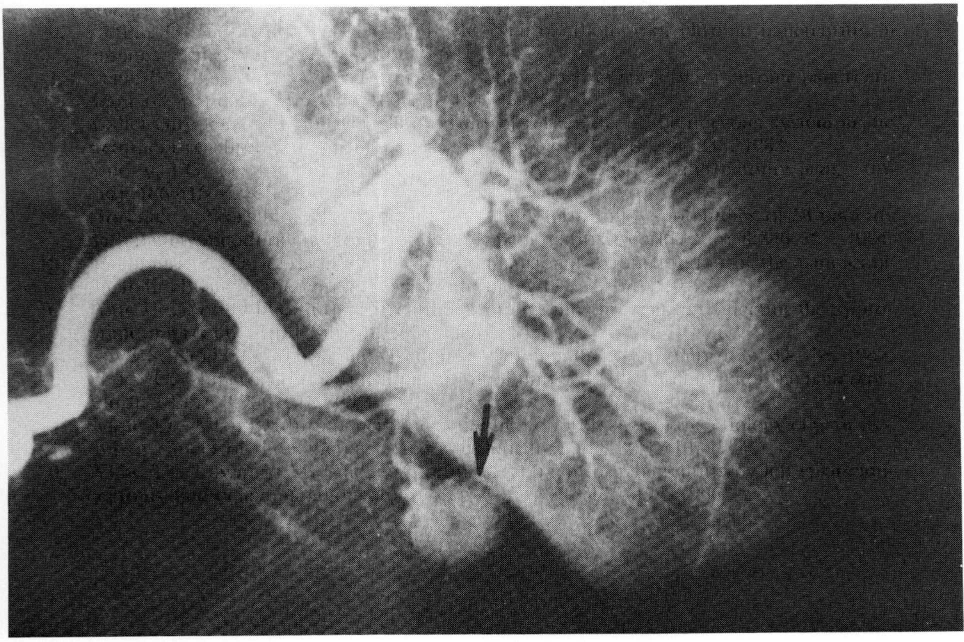

Figure 26-3. Selective splenic arteriogram in a 39-year-old patient with insulinoma. Contrast injection reveals in the pancreatic tail a 1-cm hypervascular lesion (arrow) that was confirmed at surgery as an insulinoma. (From Fraker and Norton[16] with permission.)

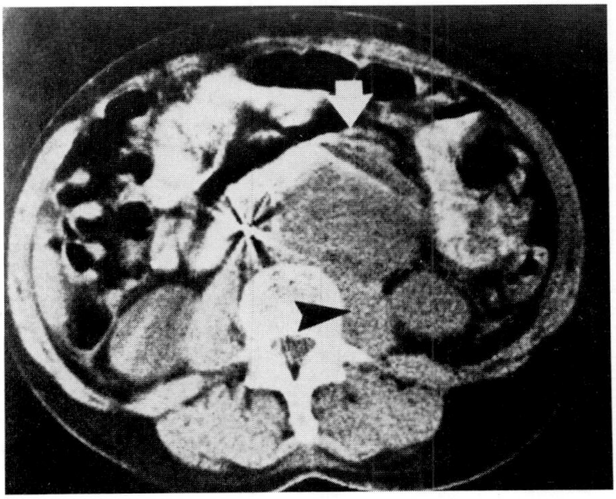

A

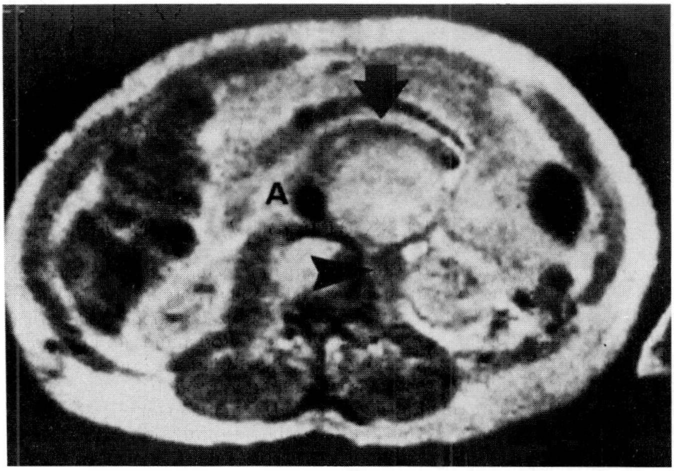

B

Figure 26-4. MRI of islet cell carcinoma. (A) A CT scan demonstrates a tumor (arrow) arising from the pancreatic tail. The tumor cannot be differentiated from psoas muscle (arrowhead). (B) MRI demonstrates an enhanced tumor mass (arrow) on T2 image, patency of the aorta (A), and differentiation of the tumor from the adjacent psoas muscle (arrowhead). (From Stark et al.[82] with permission.)

Site	IRI (μU/ml)			Glucose (mmol/l)
1. v port. centr.	• 29/19	v. hep. a. coel.	• 19/5 • 20/13	5.2
2. v. col.	• 18/13			
3. v. DP	• 25/14			
4. v DP	• 24/19			
5 v. ASPD	• 24/34			5.3
6. v. ileum.	• 15/10	v. hep. a. coel.	• 33/28 • 28/30	4.5
7. v. GCT	• 19/15			
8. v. GCT	• 19/19			
9. v. ASPD	• 13/17			3.3
10. v. lienal. dist.	• 14/17			
11. v. lienal.	• 16/18			
12. v. lienal.	• 25/27			
13. v. pancreat.	• 655/560			
14. v. pancreat.	• 6200/5200	a. coel. v. hep. dx.	• missed • 55/41	3.5
15. v. lienal.	• 21/26			
16. v. lienal.	• 179/308			
17. v. lienal.	• 86/116			3.7
18.-22. v. PSPD	• 10/14 13/17 13/18 11/13 12/15	a. coel. v. hep.	• 14/5 • 35/46	3.6

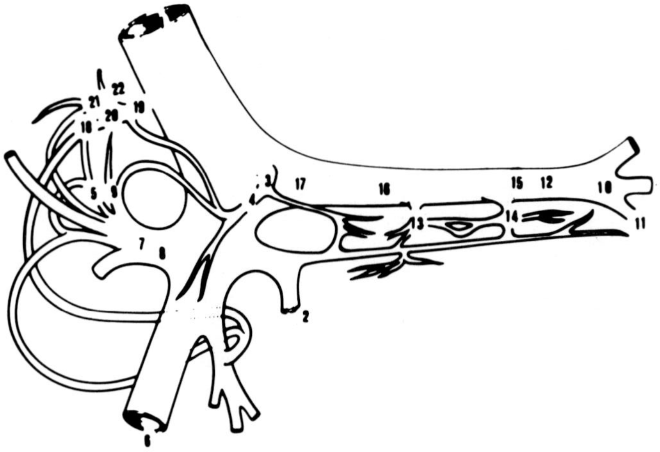

Figure 26-5. Results of immunoreactive insulin (IRI) determinations in a patient with insulinoma syndrome, negative ultrasonographic, and negative selective arteriographic results. Blood samples were obtained from 22 sites after percutaneous transhepatic portal venous catheterization, and from hepatic vein (v. hep.) and celiac artery (a. coel.). IRI results with two assay methods disclose large concentration (6200/5200 μU/mL) obtained from the pancreatic vein at site 14. Insulinoma of pancreatic tail was confirmed at surgery. (From Ingemansson et al.[26] with permission.)

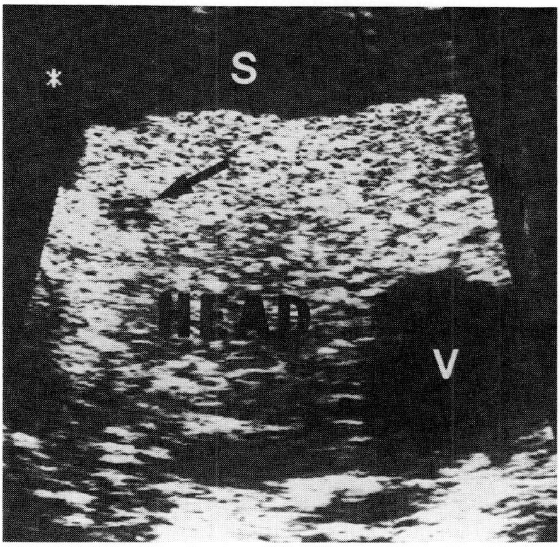

Figure 26-6. Intraoperative ultrasonography in a 12-year-old patient with multiple insulinomas and MEN-I syndrome. The intraoperative sonogram reveals a 0.3-cm hypoechoic mass (arrow) within the lateral portion of the pancreatic head, confirmed as insulinoma after subtotal resection performed for multiple lesions of the pancreas. S = saline in peritoneal cavity; V = superior mesenteric vein. (From Telander et al.[86] with permission.)

functional islet cell tumors. By selectively sampling venous effluent from small branches of these veins and then mapping concentration changes, one may localize a secretory source to a particular intra- or extrapancreatic area (Fig. 26-5). The vagaries of pancreatic venous drainage as well as the dilution of venous outflow from a tumor-bearing area with blood from non-tumor-bearing areas may each impair the precision achievable with this method. It has been described as an important technique in the localization of insulinomas, glucagonomas, and gastrinomas when CT scanning and selective arteriography fail to visualize the tumor.[25–27] Its usefulness when tumors are visualized by the more conventional means needs to be defined further.

Tumor localization may be aided further by the use of intraoperative realtime ultrasonography (Fig. 26-6).[36,39,75,76] This technique holds great promise in the precise localization of small tumors not palpable at operation, or tumors previously localized to a general region of the pancreas by selective venous sampling. It also may be of use in the assessment of the anatomic relationships between a tumor and surrounding structures, and in the possible detection of vascular invasion as well. Visualization of tumors as small as 3 mm has been reported with this technique, and initial controlled trials suggest that a significant number of small tumors that would otherwise remain undetected may be delineated with this intraoperative procedure.[57,86]

OPERATIVE CONSIDERATIONS

Operative exposure of the pancreas is best achieved with a transverse or Chevron upper abdominal incision. In the case of an individual with a narrow costal angle, a generous midline incision can provide adequate exposure.

Appropriate operative management of any pancreatic endocrine tumor requires mobilization of the entire pancreas. A Kocher maneuver provides exposure of the head and uncinate process; the anterior body and tail are exposed by opening the lesser sac in the avascular plane between the greater curvature of the stomach and the transverse colon. The tail of the pancreas is mobilized by incising the peritoneal attachments along the inferior border of the pancreas. The body and tail can be completely elevated by incising the parietal peritoneal attachments of the spleen and reflecting the spleen and distal pancreas medially. Manual examination of the mobilized pancreas by an experienced operator can reveal surprisingly small tumors, but the appreciation of small, deep-seated masses by palpation can be difficult.

The histologic diagnosis of malignancy in an endocrine tumor can be quite difficult to achieve; cellular pleomorphism and mitotic figures are unreliable indicators of malignancy. Therefore, at exploration, the liver and regional lymph nodes must be carefully inspected and any suspicious lesions or enlarged nodes biopsied. In the absence of obvious histologic findings of vascular or perineural invasion by the primary lesion, confirmed metastatic deposits are frequently the only evidence of a malignant neoplasm.

The actual removal of a pancreatic tumor can be accomplished by enucleation or regional resection. Large lesions of the pancreatic head may be amenable to removal only by pancreatoduodenectomy. Enucleation is preferred to resection for benign tumors and may be accomplished by dividing the pancreas over the mass and parallel to the main pancreatic duct, then "shelling out" the tumor using blunt dissection to avoid injury to the duct. This approach can be performed even for deep-seated tumors in the proximal pancreas when precise localization is available, and thus avoids pancreatoduodenectomy. The cavity left after this procedure should be left open and drained.[41] All sites of enucleation or margins of resection must be drained externally with either a sump or a closed drainage system.

Total pancreatectomy is rarely, if ever, indicated for islet cell tumors. Although it is used for diffuse processes such as nesidioblastosis or as the end result of serial "blind" pancreatic resections, advances in localization and medical treatment of functional tumors have largely obviated the need for its use even in these situations. In the management of patients with documented hypersecretion of hormones associated with generally benign, intrapancreatic tumors, and on the occasion of complete failure to detect the tumor after a thorough intraoperative search, a 75% distal pancreatectomy may be employed with subsequent careful evaluation of the resected specimen. It must be recalled that a 75% distal resection includes the anterior lobe of the pancreatic head. A resection margin at the level of the mesenteric artery and vein falls short of this goal.

CONTROVERSIES IN MANAGEMENT

Notwithstanding the general considerations regarding tumor localization and operative technique that apply to virtually all islet cell tumors, several aspects of the diagnosis, treatment, and general management of specific tumors continue to provoke debate and concern. Specific issues of controversy or special considerations are examined in detail in the sections that follow.

INSULINOMA

Clinical Features

Adenomas of the β cell are the most commonly reported pancreatic endocrine tumors, and much of what is applied in the localization and treatment of the other islet cell tumors has been derived from the management of insulinomas. The clinical manifestations of insulin-secreting tumors are well described, and "Whipple's triad" served as a criterion for exploration of patients suspected of having this disorder prior to the advent of routine insulin assays.[96]

The international series of 1067 cases compiled by Stefannini et al. provides the most complete picture currently available of the pathologic characteristics of insulinomas and their response to therapy.[84] Of the tumors in this series, 84% were found to be benign and the remaining 16% were malignant; 90% were single tumors. Distribution in the head, body, and tail was 32%, 30%, and 34%, respectively. And 53% were 1 to 5 cm; 34% were 5 to 10 cm. The histologic diagnosis of malignancy was frequently difficult, and the most reliable criteria were the presence of metastases, or demonstration of either vascular or perineural invasion. Metastatic spread was generally described as either hepatic or nodal.

Preoperative Studies and the Role of Transhepatic Hormone Sampling

Because of the small size and occasional multicentricity of insulinomas, and because of the possibility of being unable to palpate a tumor at the time of exploration, a concerted effort must be made to localize the tumor preoperatively. Ultrasonography and CT have been less efficacious in localizing tumors than selective angiography (Table 26-1). Fulton et al. reported successful preoperative angiographic detection of insulinomas in 90% of patients studied, using highly selective injections and digital subtraction methods.[19] The resolution of noninvasive imag-

TABLE 26-1. PREOPERATIVE AND INTRAOPERATIVE LOCALIZATION OF INSULINOMAS AT THE NATIONAL INSTITUTES OF HEALTH*

Localizing Study	Number	Detected (%)
Ultrasonography (preoperative)	3/12	(25)
CT scan	6/14	(43)
Selective angiography	16/19	(84)
Selective venous sampling	7/7	(100)
Intraoperative ultrasonography	6/7	(86)

* Modified from Fraker and Norton.[16]

ing studies has improved greatly in the past 10 years, however, and the most recent experience with CT has shown it to be almost equal in sensitivity to arteriography in the detection of insulinomas. The initial experience with MRI indicates that it should be a useful technique in the localization of insulinomas.[61,82] While technical difficulties remain to be resolved, MRI appears to have the potential to identify endocrine tumors less than 1.5 cm in diameter.[82] Although selective pancreatic venous catheterization with hormone sampling has been employed for insulinoma since 1978,[26] this diagnostic study is still not in widespread use, and some controversy exists regarding its precision.[35] Its use as an adjunct to other imaging techniques, palpation of pancreatic tissue, or intraoperative ultrasonography, has permitted localization of insulinomas that might not otherwise have been appreciated.[21,57,69] Furthermore, Glaser et al. reported the detection of insulinomas by selective venous catherization studies in six patients with fasting hypoglycemia in whom selective arteriography and CT scanning were negative.[21] The preoperative identification of a pancreatic region associated with hormone hypersecretion is clearly of value and may serve as a suitable indication for distal pancreatic resection. When hypersecretion appears to originate from the pancreatic head or portal regions, however, additional localization techniques are required before a suitable surgical course can be determined.

Operative Management Options

Enucleation is possible for most insulinomas because of their predominantly benign histologic condition and small size (Fig. 26-7). Pancreatic resection is performed for malignant insulinomas or when enucleation is technically difficult or dangerous. Since these tumors are evenly distributed throughout the pancreas,[84] there is a 25% chance that a 75% distal resection for an occult lesion will fail to control hyperinsulinism. Some authors advocate "blind" distal resection under these circumstances, however, with resection carried further to the right of this margin at repeat exploration if no clinical response occurs.[53] Careful attention to efforts to localize a tumor, including selective portal venous sampling and intraoperative ultrasonography, should obviate the need for repeated or subtotal resections.

Preoperative treatment with diazoxide has simplified the management of many patients with particularly severe hypoglycemia.[53] Preoperative hypoglycemia can also be avoided by taking steps to ensure that the patient has free access to food, and that oral intake is encouraged until the night before surgery, when an intravenous dextrose infusion is begun.

The clinical features of symptomatic hypoglycemia make its recognition straightforward in a patient with a diagnosed insulinoma. Its occurrence during surgery when clinical signs are masked by anesthesia can be catastrophic, however. Automatic glucose-monitoring devices with computerized insulin and glucose infusion systems for perioperative control of both hyper- and hypoglycemia are now in routine use.[73,74] These provide effective maintenance of euglycemia based on plasma glucose determinations performed at intervals as short as 1 minute. These systems permit monitoring of glucose concentrations for pertinent

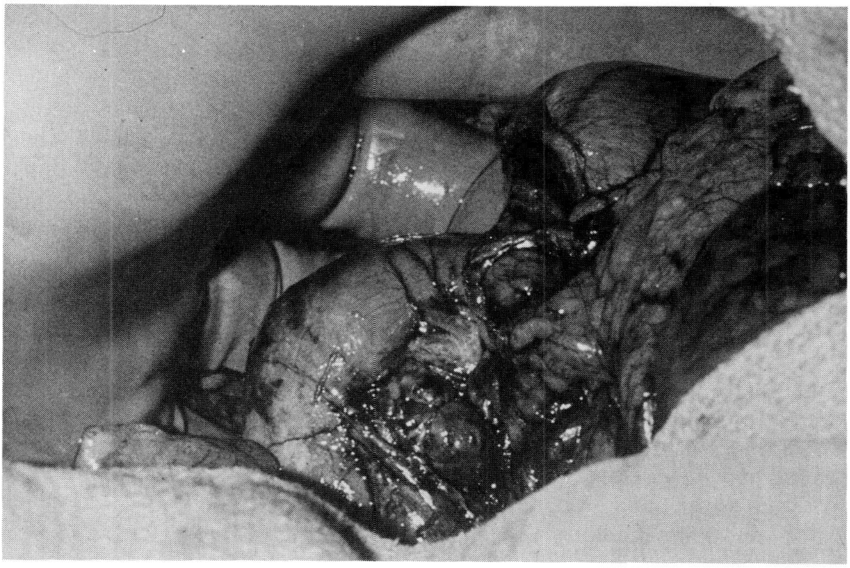

Figure 26-7. Insulinoma of pancreas. Operative appearance, after Kocher maneuver, of dark, well-encapsulated 1-cm lesion of pancreatic head. Lesion was enucleated with resolution of hypoglycemia.

intraoperative changes. The drawbacks of such a system, however, include their high cost and complexity. Alternatively, intraoperative glucose monitoring and prevention of hypoglycemia can be accomplished with simpler methods such as the use of a manual enzymatic glucose analyzer at frequent intervals intraoperatively, coupled with glucose administration as needed.[54] Intraoperative glucose should be maintained higher than 100 mg/dL. Failure to administer glucose on the grounds that it might mask rebound hyperglycemia after successful resection of a tumor can be hazardous. This rise is often delayed by up to 90 minutes when it does occur,[91] and both false-negative and false-positive interpretations of glucose values are possible.

GASTRINOMA

Evolution of Treatment Goals

The management of the Zollinger-Ellison syndrome (ZES) has been an area of unresolved controversy since the use of H_2-receptor antagonists first suggested that the end-organ sequelae of the syndrome could be controlled with a purely medical regimen. While the role of long-term medical therapy versus total gastrectomy has been hotly debated, the need for emergent surgical management of the complications of gastrinoma has declined, and attention has shifted toward efforts to surgically cure the underlying tumor.

Medical Versus Surgical Management of Acid Hypersecretion

Since Zollinger and Ellison reported the association of fulminant peptic ulceration and non-β islet cell tumors in 1955,[100] total gastrectomy has served as an extremely reliable means of controlling the peptic ulcer diathesis.[101] The first extensive trials with cimetidine in the treatment of ZES showed that the control of peptic ulceration achieved with medication alone could be comparable with the clinical results seen after total gastrectomy.[6,45,46] Both approaches to the control of acid hypersecretion are clearly effective. The continued support for the use of total gastrectomy in the management of ZES rests on the definitiveness of the procedure in halting acid production, the removal of patient compliance as a variable in antisecretory therapy, and the generally smooth postoperative response to total gastrectomy seen in ZES patients relative to other indications. If the insidious course of ZES cannot be altered by removal of the tumor, then the proven efficacy of total gastrectomy must be weighed against the requirement for a lifetime of strict adherence to a pharmacologic regimen. The choice of medical therapy commits the patient to follow-up acid output measurements to ensure adequate drug dose and meticulous compliance. For patients deemed unreliable or unwilling, this course may be unsuitable. Recurrent ulceration on high doses of cimetidine has occurred in up to 25% of those treated,[7,78] although the increased use of newer H_2-receptor blockers and omeprazole reduced this failure rate. Impressive results with medical therapy have been achieved at centers dedicated to providing specialized care of ZES patients.[43,58] No matter what the reason for failure of medical treatment, it must be recognized that an unfavorable response can result in the need for emergent surgical management of a peptic ulcer complication, with its attendant risk of morbidity and mortality. Even with the advent of more effective inhibitors of gastric acid secretion, the selected use of total gastrectomy in specific patients remains an important component of the management of gastrinoma.

Total gastrectomy could not be justified in the treatment of as indolent a condition as gastrinoma if the elective operative mortality rate were high. Mortality following total gastrectomy in 137 patients in the gastrinoma tumor registry prior to 1974 was 11 percent.[15] More recent reports indicate that with modern technique, postoperative mortality for total gastrectomy in ZES patients ranges from zero to five percent.[5,10,88] Unfavorable results generally occur only in patients operated on emergently, or in those with prior gastric surgery[5,11,50,89,97] (Table 26-2). Weight loss and nutritional deficiency are well-described complications which occur over the long-term after complete gastric resection performed for indications other than ZES. However, the postoperative nutritional status in ZES patients who have undergone total gastrectomy has been documented by Thompson et al. to be satisfactory based on multiple selected criteria.[88]

TABLE 26-2. MODERN SERIES (1978–1983) OF TOTAL GASTRECTOMY IN PATIENTS WITH ZES (OPERATIVE MORTALITY)*

Author (Ref)	No. of Patients	No. of Deaths
Bonfils et al.[5]	57	8†
Brennan et al.[7]	6	1
Deveney et al.[11]	38	1
Friesen[17]	16	0
Modlin et al.[50]	9	1‡
Stabile et al.[78]	10	0
Thompson et al.[88]	23	0
Thompson et al.[89]	14	0
Wilson[97]	16	0
Zollinger et al.[101]	34	1‡
TOTAL	223	12

Overall operative mortality: 5.4%
Operative mortality excluding
deaths after emergency gastrectomy: 2.8%

* Modified from Thompson et al.[88]
† Includes four with total gastrectomy done as an emergency, and four with previous gastric surgery.
‡ Total gastrectomy done as an emergency.

The use of H_2-receptor antagonists combined with vagotomy has recently been proposed to offer an advantage over medical management alone by reducing or occasionally eliminating the medication requirement, and Richardson et al. have advocated the use of proximal gastric vagotomy as an alternative to total gastrectomy when complete resection of tumor is judged impossible at laparotomy.[67,68] Since side effects of medical treatment do occur, and acid output must be monitored frequently on massive H_2-receptor blocker doses, significant reductions in medication requirements secondary to performance of a vagotomy is an attractive alternative to medical management alone. However, the requirement for long-term medical compliance remains, and clear cut evidence that vagotomy allows a permanent reduction in dosage of H_2-receptor antagonists relative to the duration of the disease, has not been demonstrated.

Tumor Resection Strategies

Improvement in survival through resection of the primary tumor has long been a goal in the management of gastrinoma. The misperception that the underlying disease is "controlled" if patients are maintained ulcer-free, can result in failure to definitively treat that population of patients who may have resectable tumors. In 40 cases accumulated over 30 years by Zollinger, 71% of the 21 deaths in the series were related to tumor progression.[101] However, 5-year survival with complete tumor resection was 76% compared with 21% following incomplete resection. The Mayo Clinic experience with 44 patients undergoing exploration for gastrinoma indicates that the potential for complete cure of the ZES exists in a small but not insignificant percentage of patients.[43] Tumor resection resulted in recurrence-free follow-up in 16% of patients, while exclusion of patients with MEN-I or metastatic disease at the time of surgery increased the apparent cure rate to 20%, or 7 out of 35 patients. ''Cured'' patients required no further medical or surgical treatment for acid hypersecretion. Multifocality of tumors was not found to preclude curative resection if all detectable tumor was removed. Norton and co-workers at the National Institutes of Health have shown that with careful imaging techniques and preoperative identification of patients with MEN-I and metastatic disease, up to 30% of gastrinomas may be surgically curable.[58] Friesen achieved long-term eugastrinemia in 43% of patients who underwent aggressive resection of pancreatic and extrapancreatic gastrinomas.[17] Therefore, if a tumor is amenable to resection, total gastrectomy may not be required, provided the patient is followed carefully for evidence of recurrence. At exploration, those patients who have residual tumor or unresectable disease can be treated definitively for acid hypersecretion by total gastrectomy,[10,17,88] although the urgency or even necessity of this procedure has been debated. Extrapancreatic gastrinomas appear to offer a higher probability of cure after removal that do tumors within the pancreas, as the majority of favorable results have been achieved following excision of duodenal submucosal tumors[5,43,62,88] (Fig. 26-8). Single gastrinomas re-

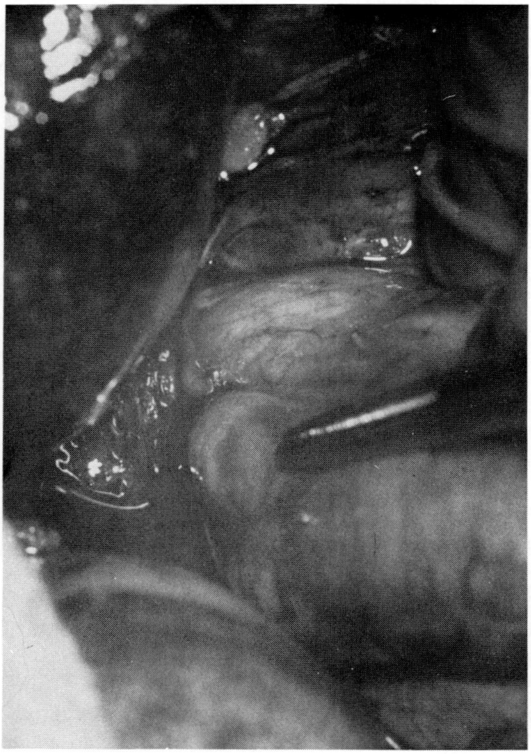

Figure 26-8. Duodenal gastrinoma. Operative appearance of 1-cm intramural gastrinoma on lateral surface of duodenal C loop. Lesion was resected without cure of hypergastrinemia. (From Andersen[2] with permission.)

sected from the liver, small bowel mesentery, and lymph nodes[79,98] all have been associated with long-term survival and eugastrinemia (Table 26-3). It is unclear whether gastrinomas, particularly those found in abdominal lymph nodes, arise de novo in these locations. Since many patients with anomalously located tumors have undergone prior ulcer operations, it has been suggested that some primary tumors might have been fortuitously removed.[10]

Patients with gastrin-secreting tumors in the setting of MEN-I rarely benefit from attempts at resection, probably as a consequence of the diffuse nature of their intrapancreatic disease.[43] Familial tumors are less frequently metastatic at the time of diagnosis than sporadic gastrinomas and have been associated with 10-year survivals as high as 71% to 89%.[88,99] The expected benefit of surgical exploration in patients with familial tumors, however, is a matter of debate. With the possibility of curative excision excluded, the only indication for surgery is total gastrectomy or vagotomy. The current trend is therefore toward increased use of omeprazole or H_2-receptor antagonist therapy alone, at least as the initial form of treatment, in MEN-I patients.

Historically, a large percentage of gastrinomas have eluded localization both preoperatively and at exploration. With the recognition that cure is possible with identification and removal of isolated tumors, preoperative localization has become as critical a priority as with other islet cell tumors. A prospective analysis of detection techniques showed arteriography to be the most sensitive method (60%) followed by CT (40%).[58] Others have found selective arteriography to be much less successful for gastrinoma than for insulinoma.[88] Variable results have been achieved with portal venous sampling for gastrin. A significant benefit in locating tumors not otherwise detectable at laparotomy has been shown at some institutions,[8,69] while others have reported that information obtained with this technique was not felt to be of use at surgery.[9,48,90] The recent prospective NIH series found a preponderance of gastrin gradients localized to the pancreatic head, whether or not a tumor was located at surgery. This raises the question of whether a patient without a demonstrable tumor might benefit from pancreatoduodenectomy performed solely on the basis of positive venous sampling. Although a limited number of successful resections in this situation have been reported,[81] the risks of a radical procedure must be weighed against the comparatively favorable prognosis of patients without discrete, identifiable tumors who are treated with alternative therapy. Intraoperative ultrasonography may increase the possibility of visualizing tumors within regions of the pancreas suggested by venous sampling and may therefore permit enucleation or more limited resection.

The principal cause of late death in patients with gastrinoma is the progression of hepatic metastases.[67,107] This has proved to be an exceedingly difficult problem to treat, and the prognosis becomes dismal in this setting. Some limited benefit has been demonstrated with 5-fluorouracil and streptozotocin treatment.[51] A recent report of selected patients with metastatic disease undergoing aggressive resection of all identifiable tumor, followed by adjuvant chemotherapy, showed some survival benefit compared with a nonsurgically treated cohort.[60] Only a small number of patients, however, prove to have metastatic disease that is amenable to resection. Increasingly, an aggressive surgical approach to the gastrinoma patient has been advocated, and it now appears appropriate to explore all

TABLE 26-3. COLLECTED RATES OF "CURE" FOLLOWING RESECTION OF GASTRINOMAS*

Author (Ref)	Year	Number of Patients	Length of Follow-up (yrs)	Number of Cures	Pancreatic Tumor	Duodenal Tumor	Extrapancreatic or Extraintestinal
Rawson et al.[66]	1960	1	16	1	1		
Parrish and Rawlins[63]	1965	1	6	1	1		
Zollinger and Moore[102]	1968	25	20	1	1		
Zollinger et al.[101]	1980	15†	4–10	1		1	
Bonfils et al.[5]	1981	92	1–6	5		5	
Wilson[97]	1982	28	3–21	5	1		4
Friesen[17]	1982	23	3–10	10	6	2	2
Wolfe et al.[98]	1982	18	3–11	5		1	4
Barreras et al.[2]	1982	1	7	1	1		
Malagelada et al.[43]	1983	53	3–10	7	1	5	1
Deveney et al.[10]	1983	52	1–10	6	6		
Thompson et al.[88]	1983	27	1–4	3		1	2
Landor[38]	1984	1	2	1		1	
Stabile and Passaro[77]	1985	65	1.5–10	6	3	2	1
Miyata et al.[49]	1986	1	1	1			1
Norton et al.[60]	1986	52	0.5–4	7	2	1	4
Ellison et al.[12]	1987	20†	2–6	8	3	3	2
Total (percent)		475		69(15)	26	22	21

* Modified from Ellison et al.[12]
† Additional patients.

patients with sporadic gastrinoma to assess resectability and to attempt surgical removal of the neoplasm in patients in whom removal is feasible.

GLUCAGONOMA

Suspicion and Detection of the Tumor

The glucagonoma syndrome, elucidated clearly by McGavran et al. in 1966,[47] called attention to the peculiar spectrum of findings associated with glucagon hypersecretion and probably contributed to the increased number of cases described after 1970. It is now widely recognized that any suspicious migratory skin lesions in a diabetic patient should prompt the appropriate diagnostic tests for glucagonoma. If immunoreactive glucagon levels are found to be significantly elevated, the presence of a tumor should be investigated.

In a review of 47 patients with the glucagonoma syndrome, 57% had metastases at the time of initial exploration, while 32% had disease localized to a particular region of the pancreas, without evidence of extension of their disease.[23] Three of these patients went on to develop recurrent tumor after resection of the pancreatic primary. Of the 34 pancreatic tumors identified, 30 were to the left of the superior mesenteric vessels, probably as a consequence of the general localization of α cells to the dorsal region of the pancreas. Because the majority of tumors in this series were distal and larger on average than insulinomas, surgical treatment consisted generally of distal pancreatic resection. Tumors that were identified with concurrent metastases were not resected, nor were hepatic metastases.

Glucagonomas do not ordinarily represent as difficult a localization problem as insulinomas often do, since it is the exception to find single tumors smaller than 3 cm.[23] Ultrasonography, CT scan, and selective arteriography have been used effectively in localizing pancreatic glucagonomas. Ingemansson et al.[25] and Vinik et al.[94] have reported the successful use of transhepatic pancreatic venous sampling in locating glucagonomas in the pancreas. The effectiveness of this technique in identifying and localizing glucagon-secreting tumors when other localization techniques are negative remains to be demonstrated, but the initial experience is promising.

Perioperative Management

Control of diabetes and nutritional support should be preoperative priorities in patients with glucagonoma. The fairly constant finding of weight loss even in the absence of malignant or metastatic disease is probably due to the catabolic effects of glucagon. Weight loss can be accompanied by hypoaminoacidemia and hypoproteinemia to varying degrees. A course of preoperative parenteral alimentation may be indicated in those patients with significantly impaired nutrition. There is evidence to suggest that the characteristic migratory rash seen with glucagonoma may be related to hypoaminoacidemia. After serum proteins returned to normal with total parenteral nutrition, improvement in the cutaneous manifestations of the tumor was reported by Norton et al.[59] The causes of the thrombotic phenomena associated with glucagonomas have not been adequately explained, but clearly these patients are at increased risk of deep venous thrombosis and pulmonary embolism.[70] If deep venous thrombosis is suspected, heparinization should be started immediately. Some surgeons have recommended prophylactic preoperative heparinization for all patients with glucagonoma.[31]

Operative Strategies

At operation, distal resection can be curative for truly intrapancreatic lesions. Since glucagonomas may be slow-growing, debulking of widespread disease often provides palliation from the diabetes, weight loss, skin rash, and miscellaneous manifestations of the tumor. Significant improvement in symptoms was achieved in 13 of 17 patients who underwent palliative resection for proven metastatic glucagonoma.[52] The mean response, however, was less than 1 year, and mean survival was less than 2 years. Disease-free survival 6 years after subtotal distal pancreatectomy for a glucagonoma of the pancreatic neck with resection of nodal metastatic spread has recently been reported.[22]

It has been hoped that with increasing awareness of the physical findings in patients with glucagonoma, some improvement in the management of these tumors would result from earlier recognition. This has not yet been borne out, and recent reports of glucagonomas[80] would suggest that the actual incidence of malignant disease at the time of diagnosis is higher than that reported previously. Unfortunately, glucagonomas frequently remain unsuspected, and therefore undetected, until metastatic disease indicates their presence. Only widespread acceptance of routine measurement of glucagon levels in diabetic patients will result in an increased survival of patients with this potentially curable tumor.

VIPOMA

Diagnostic Considerations

The syndrome of watery diarrhea, hypokalemia, and achlorhydria (WDHA) in association with a non-β islet cell tumor was first described by Verner and Morrison in 1958.[92] Various hormonal products have been implicated in the metabolic derangements seen in the WDHA syndrome, but vasoactive intestinal peptide is felt to be the most prevalent symptom-causing humoral product of these tumors.[3,71] In the evaluation of patients with the hallmark of this disease, profuse (3 L/day or more) watery diarrhea, plasma immunoreactive vasoactive intestinal polypeptide (VIP) levels often aid in the establishment of the diagnosis. Pancreatic polypeptide levels are often elevated concurrently, and it has been suggested by Polak et al. that this may be a marker for a pancreatic as opposed to an extrapancreatic hormone source.[64]

Surgical Treatment

Resection of the tumor currently offers the only possibility of cure and the best possibility of long-term remission in the symptoms for both benign and malignant disease. Even resection of a recurrent metastatic vipoma may result in significant clinical improvement.[55] Cumulative experience with vipoma indicates that multicentricity is a rare finding[80] but that 40% of tumors are malignant and 30% metastatic at the time of diagnosis.[42] There is also a 10% incidence of extrapancreatic tumors of primarily sympathetic neural origin.

Perioperative Management

Because these patients usually present with a prolonged history of diarrhea, metabolic and nutritional disorders are frequently encountered and must be corrected prior to surgery.[93] Hypokalemia, hypomagnesemia, and other electrolyte or acid–base abnormalities can be difficult to treat in the presence of ongoing gastrointestinal fluid losses. Unfortunately, the massive secretory diarrhea of the Verner-Morrison syndrome can be extremely refractory to treatment. The successful use of a long-acting somatostatin analog to decrease the stool output in patients with vipoma has now been established,[13,95] and appears to offer an important form of therapy in the preoperative stabilization of these patients (Fig. 26-9). Metastatic or irresectable tumors associated with the WDHA syndrome may also respond to prolonged somatostatin analog therapy as well.

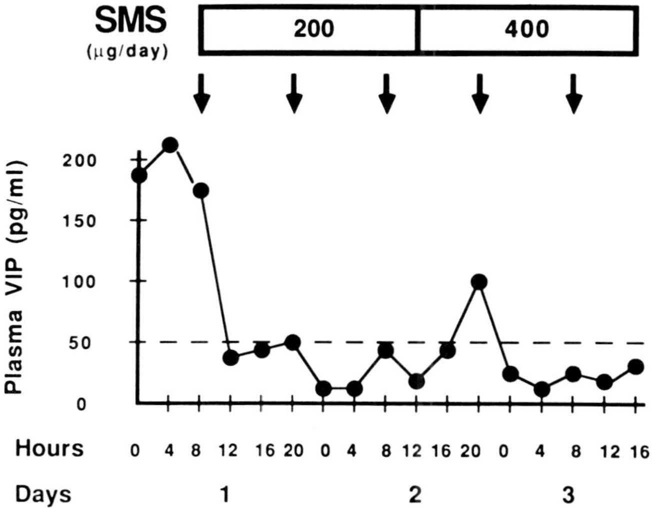

Figure 26-9. Effect of somatostatin analog octreotide on VIP levels in a patient with metastatic vipoma. The decline in VIP levels coincided with a disappearance of diarrhea. (From Vinik et al.[95] with permission.)

OTHER TUMORS

Somatostatinoma

Other rarer hormonally active tumors arising from endocrine tissue of the pancreas have been described and surgically treated. Nonfunctioning islet cell adenomas and carcinomas are also detected with increasing frequency[33,87] and require resection as well.

The precise incidence of somatostatinoma is unknown, and extensive surgical experience with this tumor is lacking. Although rarely encountered, it may be an underdiagnosed disease since the principal components of the somatostatinoma syndrome, cholelithiasis and mild diabetes mellitus, are ubiquitous problems.[34] Some of the reported cases were, in fact, discovered incidentally at the time of exploration for cholecystectomy. The combined presence of mild diabetes, pathologic biliary lesions, and steatorrhea should alert the clinician to the possibility of a somatostatin-secreting tumor and the need for appropriate investigations including the ascertaining of somatostatin levels. No prospective evaluations of localization techniques have been undertaken, but CT, ultrasonography, and selective angiography have been employed. Most reported cases of somatostatinoma have demonstrated intrapancreatic tumors,[20,40] but extrapancreatic tumors have also been described.[29,30] Reviews of cases of somatostatinomas have revealed most of these tumors to be malignant at the time of diagnosis with up to an 83% incidence of hepatic metastases.[72] Prolonged survival is possible with resection, even for malignant disease,[32,72] but often requires radical procedures. Earlier recognition of the clinical signs of the disease and aggressive and early surgical intervention may result in an improvement in the operative results with this tumor.

PPoma

Pancreatic polypeptide (PP) levels have been found to be elevated alone and concurrently with other hormones from a variety of islet cell tumors.[4] It has been suggested as a serum marker for islet cell tumors in general,[65] and by Friesen et al. as a marker for MEN-I.[18] The clinical presentations of tumors secreting only PP (PPoma) do not clearly indicate a particular spectrum of complaints, and they have been described as *silent lesions,*[85] although abdominal pain, weight loss, and other nonspecific complaints are frequently noted. The usefulness of PP as a general marker for the presence of islet cell tumors makes it a particularly useful screening test in patients with suspected familial endocrinopathies, or for patients with suspected pancreatic masses, or for patients with the most common manifestation of an MEN syndrome, hyperparathyroidism.

Carcinoid Tumors

Carcinoid tumors are relatively common lesions, although fewer than 10% are extraintestinal, and pancreatic carcinoids represent a particularly unusual manifestation of the disease. These lesions may present with the classic symptoms of flushing and diarrhea; these vasodilatory and gastrointestinal manifestations are dependent on the relative effects of substance P and serotonin released from the tumor. Measurement of levels of serotonin, or serotonin metabolites such as urinary 5-hydroxyindoleacetic acid, forms the most reliable diagnostic maneuver,[14] although provocative testing may be required for definitive diagnosis. Recently, the value of pentagastrin as a simple and reliable stimulant has been demonstrated, with flushing, elevations in serotonin levels, or both, elicited after bolus intravenous infusion.[1]

The surgical management of pancreatic carcinoids is frequently complicated by the presence of metastatic disease, and therapy must therefore be directed toward effective palliation of what are frequently disabling symptoms. Resection of metastatic tumor is advisable when feasible,[28] for relief of symptoms and prolongation of survival. Widespread hepatic metastases may require pharmacologic therapy for symptom relief, and the serotonin receptor antagonist ketanserin[1] as well as a long-acting somatostatin analog[37] have proved useful in this regard. Antineoplastic therapy is frequently unsuccessful in metastatic carcinoid, although combination chemotherapy with addition of streptozotocin may result in a beneficial response in as many as 40% of patients.[37] While the long-term prognosis is poor in patients with metastatic disease, an aggressive approach to "debulking" the tumor mass carries significant benefit for these islet cell tumor patients in particular.

REFERENCES

1. Ahlman H, Dahlstrom A, Gronstad K, et al. The pentagastrin test in the diagnosis of the carcinoid syndrome. Ann Surg 201:81–86, 1985.
2. Andersen, DK. Current diagnosis and management of Zollinger-Ellison syndrome. Ann Surg 210:685–703, 1989.
3. Bloom SR, Polak JM. The role of VIP in pancreatic cholera. In: Thompson JC, ed. Gastrointestinal Hormones. Austin, University of Texas Press, 1975, pp 635–642.
4. Bloom SR, Polak JM. Hormone profiles. In: Bloom SR, Polak JM, eds. Gut Hormones. New York, Churchill Livingstone, 1981, pp 555–560.
5. Bonfils S, Landor JH, Mignon M, Hervoir P. Results of surgical management in 92 consecutive patients with Zollinger-Ellison syndrome. Ann Surg 194:692–697, 1981.
6. Bonfils S, Mignon M, Gratton J. Cimetidine treatment of acute and chronic Zollinger-Ellison syndrome. World J Surg 3:597–604, 1979.
7. Brennan MF, Jensen RT, Wesley RA, et al. The role of surgery in patients with Zollinger-Ellison syndrome (ZES) managed medically. Ann Surg 196:239–245, 1982.
8. Burchurth F, Stage JG, Stadil F, et al. Localization of gastrinomas by transhepatic portal catheterization and gastrin assay. Gastroenterology 77:444–450, 1979.
9. Cherner JA, Doppman JL, Norton JA, et al. Selective venous sampling for gastrin to localize gastrinomas. A prospective assessment. Ann Intern Med 105:841–847, 1986.
10. Deveney CW, Deveney KE, Stark D, et al. Resection of gastrinomas. Ann Surg 198:546–553, 1983.
11. Deveney CW, Deveney K, Way LW. The Zollinger-Ellison syndrome—23 years later. Ann Surg 188:384–393, 1978.
12. Ellison EC, Carey LC, Sparks J, et al. Early surgical treatment of gastrinoma. Am J Med 82(suppl 5B):17–24, 1987.
13. Ellison EC, O'Dorisio TM, Benson GD. Modulation of functional gastrointestinal tumors by endogenous and exogenous somatostatin. Am J Surg 151:668–675, 1986.

14. Feldman JM, O'Dorisio TM. Role of neuropeptides and serotonin in the diagnosis of carcinoid tumors. Am J Med 81 (suppl 6B):41–48, 1986.
15. Fox PA, Hofmann JW, Wilson SD, DeCosse JJ. Surgical management of the Zollinger-Ellision syndrome. Surg Clin North Am 54:395–407, 1974.
16. Fraker DL, Norton JA. Localization of insulinomas and gastrinomas. JAMA 259:3601–3605, 1988.
17. Friesen SR. Treatment of the Zollinger-Ellison syndrome: A 25 year assessment. Am J Surg 143:331–338, 1982.
18. Friesen SR, Tomita T, Kimmel JR: Pancreatic polypeptide update: Its roles in detection of the trait for multiple endocrine adenopathy syndrome, type I and pancreatic polypeptide-secreting tumors. Surgery 94:1028–1037, 1983.
19. Fulton RE, Sheedy PF II, McIlrath DC, et al. Preoperative angiographic localization of insulin-producing tumors of the pancreas. Am J Roentgenol 123:367–377, 1975.
20. Ganda OP, Weir GC, Soeldner JS, et al. "Somatostatinoma": A somatostatin-containing tumor of the endocrine pancreas. N Engl J Med 296:963–967, 1977.
21. Glaser B, Valtysson G, Fajans SS, et al. Gastrointestinal/pancreatic hormone concentrations in the portal venous system of nine patients with organic hyperinsulinism. Metabolism 30:1001–1010, 1981.
22. Hendry WS, Munro A. Pancreatic glucagonoma with lymph node metastases: Disease-free survival six years after resection. J R Coll Surg Edinb 31:115–116, 1986.
23. Higgins GA, Recant L, Fischman AB. The glucagonoma syndrome: Surgically curable diabetes. Am J Surg 137:142–148, 1979.
24. Howland G, Campbell WR, Maltby EJ, Robinson WL: Dysinsulinism: Convulsions and coma due to islet cell tumor of the pancreas with operation and cure. JAMA 93:674–679, 1929.
25. Ingemansson S, Holst J, Larsson L, Lunderquist A. Localization of glucagonomas by catheterization of the pancreatic veins and with glucagon assay. Surg Gynecol Obstet 145:509–516, 1977.
26. Ingemansson S, Kuhl C, Larsson L, et al. Localization of insulinomas and islet cell hyperplasia by pancreatic vein catheterization and insulin assay. Surg Gynecol Obstet 146:725–734, 1978.
27. Ingemansson S, Larsson L, Lunderquist A, Stadil F. Pancreatic vein catheterization with gastrin assay in normal patients and in patients with Zollinger-Ellison syndrome. Am J Surg 134:558–563, 1977.
28. Jaffe BM. Surgery for gut hormone–producing tumors. Am J Med 82(suppl 5B):68–76, 1987.
29. Jensen SL, Christiansen LA, Oxholm A, Holst JJ. Duodenal somatostatinoma. Br J Surg 71:159, 1984.
30. Kaneko H, Yanaihara N, Ito S, et al. Somatostatinoma of the duodenum. Cancer 44:2273–2279, 1979.
31. Kaplan EL, Michelassi F. Endocrine tumors of the pancreas and their clinical syndromes. Surg Annu 18:181–223, 1986.
32. Kelly TR. Pancreatic somatostatinoma. Am J Surg 146:671–673, 1983.
33. Kent RB III, Van Heerden JA, Weiland LH. Non-functioning islet cell tumors. Ann Surg 193:185–190, 1981.
34. Krejs GH, Orci L, Conlon JM, et al. Somatostatinoma syndrome: Biochemical, morphologic and clinical features. N Engl J Med 30 1:285–292, 1978.
35. Krudy AG, Doppman JL, Jensen RT, et al. Localization of islet cell tumors by dynamic CT: Comparison with plain CT, arteriography, sonography, and venous sampling. Am J Radiol 143:585–589, 1984.
36. Kuhn FP, Gunther R, Ruckert K, Beyer J. Ultrasonic demonstration of small pancreatic islet cell tumors. J Clin Ultrasound 10:173–175, 1982.
37. Kvols LK, Buck M. Chemotherapy of metastatic carcinoid and islet cell tumors. Am J Med 82(suppl 5B):77–83, 1987.
38. Landor JH. Control of the Zollinger-Ellison syndrome by excision of primary and metastatic tumor. Am J Surg 147:406–409, 1984.

39. Lane RJ, Coupland GAE. Operative ultrasonic features of insulinomas. Am J Surg 144:558–587, 1982.
40. Larsson LI, Hirsch MA, Holst JJ, et al. Pancreatic somatostatinoma—Clinical features and physiologic implications. Lancet 1:666–668, 1977.
41. Linnquist S. Insulinoma of the pancreatic head: Results from two surgical strategies. Acta Chir Scand 152:217–221, 1986.
42. Long RG, Bryant MG, Mitchell SJ, et al. Clinicopathological study of pancreatic and ganglioneuroblastoma tumors secreting vasoactive intestinal polypeptide (vipomas). Br Med J 282:1767–1771, 1981.
43. Malagelada JR, Edis AJ, Adson MA, et al. Medical and surgical options in the management of patients with gastrinoma. Gastroenterology 84:1524–1532, 1983.
44. May G, Gardiner R. Clinical Imaging of the Pancreas. New York, Raven Press, 1987, pp 146–149.
45. McCarthy DM. Report on the United States experience with cimetidine in Zollinger-Ellison syndrome and other hypersecretary states. Gastroenterology 74:453–458, 1978.
46. McCarthy DM: The place of surgery in the Zollinger-Ellison syndrome. N Engl J Med 302:1344–1347, 1980.
47. McGavran MH, Unger RH, Recant L, et al. A glucagon-secreting alpha-cell carcinoma of the pancreas. N Engl J Med 274:1408–1413, 1966.
48. Mignon M, Ruszniewski P, Haffar S, et al. Current approach to the management of tumoral process in patients with gastrinoma. World J Surg 10:793–810, 1986.
49. Miyata M, Nakao K, Sakamoto T, et al. Removal of metastatic gastrinoma: A case report. Surgery 99:245–248, 1986.
50. Modlin IM, Jaffe BM, Sank A, Albert D. The early diagnosis of gastrinoma. Ann Surg 196:512–577, 1982.
51. Moertel CG, Hanley JA, Johnson LA. Streptozotocin alone compared with streptozotocin plus fluorouracil in the treatment of advanced islet cell carcinoma. N Engl J Med 303:1189–1194, 1980.
52. Montenegro F, Lawrence GD, Macon W, Pass C. Metastatic glucagonoma. Improvement after surgical debulking. Am J Surg 139:424–427, 1980.
53. Moss NH, Kaplan EL. Insulinoma and nesidioblastosis. In Surgical Diseases of the Pancreas. Howard JM, Jordan GL, Reber HA (eds). Philadelphia, Lea & Febiger, pp 814–828, 1987.
54. Muir JJ, Endres SM, Offord K, et al. Glucose management in patients undergoing operation for insulinoma removal. Anesthesiology 59:371–375, 1983.
55. Nargorney DM, Bloom SR, Polak JM, Blumgart LH. Resolution of Verner-Morrison syndrome by resection of metastatic vipoma. Surgery 93:238–253, 1983.
56. Nicholls AG. Simple adenoma of the pancreas arising from an island of Langerhans. J Med Res 8:385–395, 1902.
57. Norton JA, Cromack DT, Shawker TM, et al. Intraoperative ultrasonic localization of islet cell tumors. A prospective comparison to palpation. Ann Surg 207:160–168, 1988.
58. Norton JA, Doppman JL, Collen MJ, et al. Prospective study of gastrinoma localization and resection in patients with Zollinger-Ellison syndrome. Ann Surg 204:468–479, 1986.
59. Norton JA, Kahn CT, Schiebinger R, et al. Amino acid deficiency and the skin rash associated with glucagonoma. Ann Intern Med 91:213–215, 1979.
60. Norton JA, Sugarbaker PH, Doppman JL. Aggressive resection of metastatic disease in selected patients with malignant gastrinoma. Ann Surg 203:352–359, 1986.
61. Ohtomo K, et al. MRI of islet cell tumors of the pancreas: Preliminary results. Rinsho Hoshasen 31:551–553, 1986.
62. Oberhelman HA Jr. Excisional therapy for ulcerogenic tumors of the duodenum: Long term results. Arch Surg 104:447–453, 1972.
63. Parrish JA, Rawlins DC. Intestinal mucosa in the Zollinger-Ellison syndrome. Gut 6:286–289, 1965.

64. Polak JM, Bloom SR, Adrian TE, et al. Pancreatic polypeptide in insulinomas, gastrinomas, VIPomas and glucagonomas. Lancet 1:328–330, 1976.
65. Prinz RA, Bermes EW, Kimmel JR, Marangos PJ. Serum markers for pancreatic islet cell and intestinal carcinoid tumors: A comparison of neuron-specific enolase, beta-human chronic gonadotropin and pancreatic polypeptide. Surgery 94:1019–1023, 1983.
66. Rawson AB, England MT, Gillan CG, et al. Zollinger-Ellison syndrome with diarrhea and malabsorption. Observations on a patient before and after pancreatic islet cell tumor removal without resort to gastric surgery. Lancet 2:131–134, 1960.
67. Richardson CT, Feldman M, McClelland RN, et al. Effect of vagotomy in Zollinger-Ellison syndrome. Gastroenterology 77:682–686, 1979.
68. Richardson CT, Peters MN, Feldman M, et al: Treatment of Zollinger-Ellison syndrome with exploratory laparotomy, proximal gastric vagotomy, and H2-receptor antagonists. A prospective study. Gastroenterology 89:357–367, 1985.
69. Roche A, Raisonnier A, Gillon-Savouret M-C. Pancreatic venous sampling and arteriography in localizing insulinomas and gastrinomas: Procedures and results in 55 cases. Radiology 145:621–627, 1982.
70. Roggli VI, Judge DM, McGavran MH. Duodenal glucagonoma: A case report. Hum Pathol 10:350–356, 1979.
71. Said SI, Faloona GR. Elevated plasma tissue levels of vasoactive intestinal polypeptide in the watery diarrhea syndrome due to pancreatic, bronchogenic and other tumors. N Engl J Med 293:155–160, 1975.
72. Sakazaki S, Umeyama K, Nakagawa H, et al. Pancreatic somatostatinoma. Am J Surg 146:674–679, 1983.
73. Schwartz SS, Horwitz DL, Zehfus B, et al. Use of a glucose controlled insulin infusion system (artificial beta cell) to control diabetes during surgery. Diabetologia 16:157–164, 1979.
74. Schwartz SS, Horowitz DL, Zehfus B, et al. Continuous monitoring and control of plasma glucose during operation for removal of insulinomas. Surgery 85:702–707, 1979.
75. Sigel B, Duarte B, Coelho JCU, et al. Localization of insulinomas of the pancreas at operation by real-time ultrasound scanning. Surg Gynecol Obstet 156:145–147, 1983.
76. Sigel B, Machi J, Ramos J, et al. The role of imaging ultrasound during pancreatic surgery. Ann Surg 200:486–493, 1984.
77. Stabile BE, Passaro E. Benign and malignant gastrinoma. Am J Surg 149:144–150, 1985.
78. Stabile BE, Ippoliti AF, Walsh JH, Passaro E Jr. Failure of H2 blockers in the treatment of gastrinomas. Am J Surg 145:17–23, 1983.
79. Stabile BE, Morrow DJ, Passaro E Jr. The gastrinoma triangle: Operative implications. Am J Surg 147:25–31, 1984.
80. Stacpoole PW. The glucagonoma syndrome: Clinical features, diagnosis and treatment. Endocr Rev 2:347–361, 1981.
81. Stadil F, Stage JG. The Zollinger-Ellison syndrome. Clinics on Endocrinology and Metabolism 8:433–446, 1979.
82. Stark DD, Moss AA, Goldberg HI, et al. Magnetic resonance and CT of the normal and diseased pancreas: A comparative study. Radiology 150:153–162, 1984.
83. Stark DD, Moss AA, Goldberg HI, Deveney CW. CT of pancreatic islet cell tumors. Radiology 150:491–494, 1984.
84. Stefannini P, Carboni M, Patrassi N, Basoli A. Beta-islet cell tumors of the pancreas: Results of a study on 1067 cases. Surgery 75:597–609, 1974.
85. Strodel WE, Vinik AI, Lloyd RV, et al. Pancreatic polypeptide-producing tumors. Silent lesions of the pancreas? Arch Surg 119:508–514, 1984.
86. Telander RL, Charboneau JW, Haymond MW. Intraoperative ultrasonography of the pancreas in children. J Pediatr Surg 21:262–266, 1986.
87. Thompson GB, Van Heerden JA, Grant CS, et al. Islet cell carcinomas of the pancreas: A twenty year experience. Surgery 104:1011–1017, 1988.

88. Thompson JC, Lewis BG, Wiener I, Townsend CM. The role of surgery in the Zollinger-Ellison syndrome. Ann Surg 197:594–607, 1983.
89. Thompson JC, Way LW, Hallenbeck GA, Jones RS. Zollinger-Ellison syndrome (symposium). Contemp Surg 14:77–122, 1979.
90. Thompson NE, Vinik AL, Eckhauser FE, Strodel WE. Extrapancreatic gastrinomas. Surgery 98:113–120, 1985.
91. Tutt GO, Edis AJ, Service FJ, Van Heerden JA. Plasma glucose monitoring during operations for insulinoma. A critical reappraisal. Surgery 88:351–356, 1980.
92. Verner JV, Morrison AB. Islet cell tumor and a syndrome of refractory watery diarrhea and hypokalemia. Am J Med 25:374–380, 1958.
93. Verner JV, Morrison AB. Endocrine pancreatic islet cell disease with diarrhea: Report of a case due to diffuse hyperplasia of non-beta islet tissue with a review of 54 additional cases. Arch Intern Med 133:492–500, 1974.
94. Vinik AI, Strodel WE, Cho KJ, et al. Localization of hormonally active gastrointestinal tumors. In: Thompson NW, Vinik AI, eds. Endocrine Surgery Update. New York, Grune & Stratton, 1983, pp 195–218.
95. Vinik AI, Tsai ST, Cheung P, et al. Somatostatin analog (SMS 201-995) in the management of gastroenteropancreatic tumors and diarrhea syndromes. Am J Med 81(suppl 6B):23–40, 1986.
96. Whipple AO, Frantz VK. Adenoma of the islet cells with hyperinsulinism: A review. Ann Surg 101:1299–1335, 1935.
97. Wilson SD. The role of surgery in children with Zollinger-Ellison syndrome. Surgery 92:682–692, 1982.
98. Wolfe MM, Alexander RW, McGuigan JE. Extrapancreatic, extraintestinal gastrinoma: Effective treatment by surgery. N Engl J Med 306:1533–1536, 1982.
99. Zollinger RM. Gastrinoma: Factors influencing prognosis. Surgery 97:49–54, 1985.
100. Zollinger RM, Ellison EH. Primary peptic ulcerations of the jejunum associated with islet cell tumors of the pancreas. Ann Surg 142:709–723, 1955.
101. Zollinger RM, Ellison EC, Fabri PJ, et al. Primary peptic ulcerations of the jejunum associated with islet cell tumors. Twenty-five year appraisal. Ann Surg 192:422–430, 1980.
102. Zollinger RM, Moore FT. Zollinger-Ellison syndrome comes of age. JAMA 204:361–365, 1968.

CHAPTER

27

CANCER OF THE PANCREAS: THE STATUS OF RADIATION AND CHEMOTHERAPY

Marc L. Citron, Frederick P. Smith, and Philip Vigneri

EDITORIAL COMMENT

The Gastrointestinal Tumor Study Group trial of adjuvant radiation therapy and fluorouracil after curative pancreatic resection showed a clear survival advantage at 2 and 5 years. We agree with the authors that this is an important advance and look for further confirmation of these results. The treatment can be accomplished with only mild to moderate toxicity. For unresectable locally advanced disease, the combination of chemotherapy, usually fluorouracil, and radiation has produced only modest increases in survival of 8 versus 5 months. Because of the toxicity and the lack of a clear demonstration of improvement in quality of life, treatment should be thoroughly discussed with the individual patient so that he or she can participate in the decision regarding treatment. For widespread metastatic disease, with a median survival of approximately 3 months, multiple drug chemotherapy and radiation continues to be used in clinical trials, and patients should probably receive treatment only within such trials.

CONTROVERSY

The poor results of surgical resection alone have led to increased interest in adjuvant therapy. Is there any improvement and is it worthwhile? In patients with unresectable disease and very limited life expectancy, do chemotherapy and/or radiation increase the length of survival, and perhaps more important, do they improve the quality of life?

The value of chemotherapy in the management of patients with adenocarcinoma of the pancreas has been brought into question because of its limited impact on survival. Further, the risk–benefit ratio for patients receiving chemotherapy has not been well addressed in the literature even though the toxicities of this treatment have been commonly recognized by both clinicians and patients.

Patients with adenocarcinoma of the pancreas can be grouped into three categories at presentation: those resected with curative intent, those with locally unresectable disease, and those with metastatic disease well beyond the confines of the organ.[15] For the purpose of discussing the controversies in management, we will use this classification of disease manifestation.

TUMOR RESECTABLE WITH CURATIVE INTENT

Surgery still represents the only modality with curative potential for this disease. In spite of advances in imaging, however, less than 15% of patients are resectable.[30] Even when resected, the median survival is 12 months, and less than 10% of patients survive 5 years.[6] Elsewhere in this text the merits of different surgical techniques are described, and the reader is referred to those sections to review the controversies surrounding different surgical approaches (Chapters 23 and 24). Our premise will be that if surgical resection is feasible, the tumor should be resected. Surgery may also provide the potential for palliation with bypass of the stomach, of which the outlet may be compromised, and biliary diversion in the jaundiced patient. We will not debate the alternative merits of percutaneous stents since these are detailed elsewhere.

Until recently, curative surgery had been the sole treatment for patients with resectable lesions. However, a prospective randomized trial by the Gastrointestinal Tumor Study Group (GITSG) evaluated the role of adjuvant chemotherapy and radiation therapy versus observation alone (controls) following curative resection of the pancreas.[14,18] In the first phase of this trial, there were 22 control patients; another 21 evaluable patients received 5-fluorouracil (5-FU) mg/m^2 by intravenous bolus for the first 3 days of two 2000- rad segments given in a split-course manner. Beginning 1 month after completion of radiation, 5-FU was given weekly for 2 years. Median survival in the group randomized to no adjuvant treatment was 10.9 months, compared with 21 months for those receiving adjuvant therapy. None of the control group but four of the treatment group (19%) were survivors beyond 5 years.

Since the control arm had an inferior survival and accrual to the trial was exceedingly slow (the number of authors almost approximated the number of patients in each arm), GITSG discontinued the control arm but continued to accrue patients to the treatment group. The median survival for this new cohort of 32 patients assigned to the same adjuvant regimen, but not part of the randomized trial, was about 21 months, similar to that of the treatment group in the randomized study.

What conclusions can be drawn from this trial? First, combined chemotherapy and radiation confers a modest but real survival benefit in the adjuvant setting. Second, 2 years of chemotherapy, as used in this trial, is excessive in view of the fact that over 50% of the patients are dead by 21 months. Conversely, it is not clear whether chemotherapy should be limited merely to the time of radiation. It is appealing to speculate that chemotherapy is acting as a radiosensitizer and thus exerting its maximal effect in preventing local recurrence, but there is no evidence to support that contention. Despite chemotherapy's lack of activity in patients with metastatic disease, it may have some biological effects on microscopic distant disease in ambulatory patients who have undergone prior pancreatic resection. Support for this idea comes from recent data regarding a variety of malignancies, including non-small lung cancer, a tumor that is resistant to chemotherapy in the presence of high tumor load but is more sensitive in its earlier stages of disease.[8]

Since there is an improvement in survival for patients receiving adjuvant therapy, the single most important issue is whether this survival advantage outweighs the attendant morbidity and possible mortality in such treatment. A large experience upon which to base an answer does not exist. Generally, myelosuppression is not a major problem in combined-modality programs in which 5-FU is given as an infusion or bolus with or without other agents.[5,10,19,29]

Short-term radiation effects of nausea, appetite suppression, and vomiting may be more severe, but a significant difference from radiation alone cannot be demonstrated from the reported series. Alternatively, many patients have been treated with combined modalities and have experienced only minimal side effects. Long-term effects of chronic gastritis, ulceration, or bowel obstruction have not been a problem due to the poor survival beyond 18 months.

In the absence of other data to determine the risk–benefit ratio of adjuvant therapy, the decision to use this must be based on the GITSG trial and the bias of the clinician's own experience. It is our opinion that adjuvant therapy can be delivered in most cases with mild-to-moderate toxicity that reverses after the completion of treatment.

UNRESECTABLE DISEASE

Locally advanced disease describes tumor that, while confined to the organ, proves unresectable by virtue of contiguous involvement of the celiac plexus, inferior vena cava, and/or adjacent viscera. For locally advanced pancreatic cancer, the median survival in the untreated patient is approximately 5 months.[31] With radiation alone, little survival advantage seems to exist.[7] Palliation of pain and biliary obstruction may be feasible with such therapy, however.[16] In 1969, Moertel et al. appeared to ascribe for the first time survival advantage to the addition of 5-FU to irradiation in this state of disease.[25] This produced a mean survival of 10 months in contrast to 4 months without 5-FU. Subsequent reports have established the merit of this combined modality of therapy for locally advanced carcinoma of the pancreas.

The GITSG compared high-dose radiation alone (6000 rad) with that same dose combined with 5-FU, and with a moderate radiation dose (4000 rad) plus 5-FU. Of 225 patients entered in this study, 194 were evaluable for survival. Forty percent of patients treated with 5-FU and radiation were alive at 1 year, compared with 10% of patients treated with radiation alone. A median survival of 40 weeks was found for both 5-FU–radiation groups; in contrast, radiation alone produced a median survival of 23 weeks. Toxicity was comparable for all three groups.

Mild-to-moderate nausea and vomiting occurred in 28% to 48% of patients. Myelosuppression was common, but severe leukopenia was rarely encountered. There were no treatment-related deaths.

Therefore, for locally advanced pancreatic cancer, there appears to be convincing, reproducible evidence that supports the merit of adding chemotherapy. The survival advantage of such treatment, although resulting in almost doubling the expected life span, is small, and virtually all patients succumb from disease within 2 years of diagnosis.

There have been attempts to improve these results employing alternative modalities of delivering irradiation. These include higher dosage[12] and intraoperative,[34] interstitial,[32] neutron,[28] and helium radiation sources. To date, however, there is little advantage demonstrated for these methods of treating locally advanced carcinoma of the pancreas over the combined-modality approach described above. For this stage of disease, therefore, it is the authors' opinion that 5-FU plus irradiation represents the standard of comparison. However, the average survival in most series with this approach is about 8 months, and similar results have been described by some[20] but not others[13a] with chemotherapy alone.

The acute toxicity of combined chemotherapy and radiation can be considerable but is usually reversible and rarely life-threatening. More severe toxicity has been produced by raising the dose of 5-FU. The effect of treatment on the quality of life has not been studied. Although combined chemotherapy and irradiation is said to relieve pain, this conclusion is based usually on the subjective report by the physician rather than the standard end points used in analgesic studies. The added financial cost of approximately $5000 at some institutions is an important consideration, especially for patients with limited resources.

METASTATIC DISEASE

Metastatic carcinoma, extending well beyond the pancreas, has had a dismal prognosis, with median survivals measuring from a few weeks to 3 months. Metastases occur frequently in the liver and occasionally in the lung, bone, and peritoneum. By the time the diagnosis is established, patients are often debilitated from malnutrition secondary to profound anorexia and subsequent cachexia. Many patients are jaundiced and poor candidates for any management beyond palliative, symptomatic support. This has perpetuated the existing pessimism shared by most professionals dealing with this disease.

Chemotherapy has been the treatment pursued in the majority of published reports on the management of metastatic disease. On single drugs used, 5-FU, streptozotocin, mitomycin, and doxorubicin, among others, have been reported to produce responses in varying proportions of patients treated.[4,26] Ranges of response from 0% to 30% can be found in the literature.[4,26] It is important to recognize that the definition of response may vary greatly. In the authors' estimation, response should mean a volumetric shrinkage of tumor of at least 50% either attended by symptomatic improvement in pain or nutritional status or at least without any clinical deterioration. The duration of response should be at least 2 months. When these criteria are brought to bear on single-drug therapy of metastatic pancreatic cancer, the response rates rarely approach 20%, and the vast majority of these tend to be short-lived.

Combination chemotherapy of pancreatic carcinoma was initially encouraging. Kovach and co-workers—in a randomized study using 5-FU alone, bischloroethylnitrosourea (BCNU) alone, and the combination—reported 16%, 0%, and 33% response rates, respectively.[21] The median duration of survival for all patients was 6 months. The benefit of the combination seemed to be confirmed in an independent trial by Lokich and Skarin.[23]

Wiggins and co-workers initiated a trial of 5-FU with streptozotocin and mitomycin C (SMF) and in 10 of 23 patients reported responses with the survival advantage to responders of 10 months, in contrast to 3 months for nonresponders.[33] Bukowski and his associates reported similar results with their studies of an SMF combination.[3] Five of 16 (31%) responded to treatment. This seemed to be further corroborated by a large group trial; the Southwest Oncology Group reported a 40% response rate to the SMF program in metastatic pancreatic cancer.[2]

Smith subsequently reported on the treatment of 25 patients with a program incorporating 5-FU with doxorubicin and mitomycin C (FAM).[27] Ten of the 25 patients appeared to have objective tumor regressions as noted above, with survival in these "responders" averaging 9 months in contrast to 3 months for the nonresponders. Furthermore, it was found that the survival for responding patients in relapse was 3 months, equivalent to that of nonresponders or the natural "expected" survival of a patient with metastatic pancreatic carcinoma. Bitran and his colleagues reported similar results with their FAM program.[1]

These results unfortunately have not been reproducible in larger cooperative trials. The GITSG, comparing SMF with FAM, obtained response rates of approximately 12% with a slight advantage in survival for SMF-treated patients but only averaging 12 weeks or 3 months—the natural life expectancy of the patient with metastatic pancreatic cancer.[13]

Many explanations may be offered for these apparent discrepancies in results, including lack of homogeneity of patient populations, slight differences in treatments, parameters used to gauge tumor response, and investigator bias. The parameter used to measure response may be the most critical factor. It has been our observation that bulky tumor masses in the pancreas may never reflect a response noted in the same individual's liver metastases. This is drawn not only from our observations in the above-cited studies[3,21,23,33] but also from reexploring two patients with persistent, unchanged tumor masses in the pancreas only to find fibrotic masses with microscopic residual carcinoma.[28]

It is also important to note that there appear to be survival benefits in "responders." A great deal of controversy exists in this observation. Perhaps these individuals would do equally well with supportive care only. We will not pursue this controversy here but establish that this observation tends to be universal; responders, by definition, do better than those patients who do not achieve tumor reduction with therapy. It should be further emphasized that the ultimate benefit of any intervention lies in its favorable comparison with a different or nonintervention (control) group. In this country, such trials are difficult to accomplish with our educated patient population usually biased toward one or the other.

In a pilot study based on results from a nude mouse–human pancreatic tumor xenograft model,[22] Hudis et al. tested the combination of cisplatin, cytarabine, and caffeine (CAC) in patients with advanced pancreatic cancer; a 39% partial remission rate was found in patients with measurable tumor.[17] Those same workers recently completed a randomized phase III trial in 80 patients comparing CAC with a standard SMF regimen. Preliminary analysis of this study shows response rates of about 10% in both arms. Median survival was 3.5 months and 5.3 months in the CAC and SMF arms, respectively.[9]

A randomized controlled trial has been reported from the United Kingdom. Mallinson and co-workers, using a combination of chemotherapy, compared treatment with control in patients with advanced pancreatic cancer.[24] A marked survival advantage was found in 21 treated patients when compared with 19 untreated controls. Median survival was 44 weeks in the treatment arm and only 9 weeks in the control group. This difference in survival cannot be easily explained. By virtue of more frequent physician visits, it is possible that the treatment group received better supportive care that factored into their longer survival. Likewise, it is possible that patients in the no-treatment group may have not received follow-up care in physicians' offices but were treated at home or in a hospice. It is also likely that the idea of receiving treatment was a motivating force for patients to live, whereas the idea of receiving no treatment had the opposite effect on the control group. These are important considerations because there were no objective responses to chemotherapy in the treatment group. There are other problems with this report that might affect its conclusions: (1) patients without histologic confirmation of cancer were included, and (2) the arms were not balanced for performance status as well as other important prognostic factors.

In summary, chemotherapy is widely employed for treating patients with metastatic pancreatic cancer. None of the chemotherapy regimens has shown significant survival advantage. Routine application of chemotherapy in this setting, therefore, needs examination because of its associated toxicity. It appears that patients who experience tumor shrinkage may benefit from prolongation of life with symptomatic relief; however, there is no evidence to date that they have experienced an objective improvement in their quality of life.

Since there is no established therapy for patients with metastatic disease, these patients are best treated on clinical trial. For nonprotocol patients, chemotherapy should be reserved for ambulatory patients with no prior chemotherapy treatment. If there is no objective or subjective improvement within 8 weeks, it would be reasonable to discontinue treatment.

REFERENCES

1. Bitran J, Desser R, Kosloff M, et al. Treatment of metastatic pancreatic and gastric adenocarcinoma with 5-fluorouracil, adriamycin, and mitomycin-C (FAM). Cancer Treat Rep 63:2049–2051, 1979.
2. Bukowski R, Abderholden R, Hewlett J, et al. Phase II trial of streptozotocin, mitomycin-C, and 5-fluorouracil (SMF) in adenocarcinoma of the pancreas. Cancer Clin Trials 3:321–324, 1980.

3. Bukowski R, Schacter LS, et al. Phase II trial of 5-FU, Adriamycin, mitomycin-C, and streptozotocin in pancreatic adenocarcinoma. Cancer 50:197–200, 1982.
4. Carter SK. The integration of chemotherapy into a combined modality approach for cancer treatment, VI: Pancreatic adenocarcinoma. Cancer Treat Rev 2:193–214, 1975.
5. Cola LR, Engstrom PF, Paul A. Nonsurgical management of esophageal cancer: Report of a study of combined radiotherapy and chemotherapy. J Clin Oncol 5:1783–1790, 1987.
6. Cooperman AM, Herter FP, Marboe CA, et al. Pancreatoduodenal resection and total pancreatectomy—An institutional review. Surgery 90:705–718, 1981.
7. Dobelbower RR, Borgelt BB, et al. Precision radiotherapy for cancer of pancreas. Int J Radiat Oncol Biol Phys 6:1121–1133, 1980.
8. Dillman RO, Seagren SL, Propert K, et al. Protochemotherapy improves survival in regional non-small cell lung cancer (NSCLC). Proc Am Soc Clin Oncol 7:195, 1988. Abstract.
9. Dougherty JB, Kelsen D, Kemeny N, et al. Advanced pancreatic cancer: A phase I-II trial of cisplatin, high-dose cytarabine, and caffeine. JNCI 81:1735–1738, 1989.
10. Douglas HO, Subramanian H. Survival of patients with locally unresectable but not widely metastatic pancreatic adenocarcinoma. Proc Am Assoc Cancer Res 21:150, 1980. Abstract 598.
11. The Gastrointestinal Tumor Study Group. A multi-institutional comparative trial of radiation therapy alone and in combination with 5-fluorouracil for locally unresectable pancreatic carcinoma. Ann Surg 189:205–208, 1979.
12. The Gastrointestinal Tumor Study Group. Therapy of locally unresectable pancreatic carcinoma: A randomized comparison of high dose (6000 rads) radiation alone, moderate dose radiation (4000 rads) + 5-fluorouracil, and high dose radiation + 5-fluorouracil. Cancer 48:1705–1710, 1981.
13. The Gastrointestinal Tumor Study Group. Phase II studies of drug combinations in advanced pancreatic carcinoma: Fluorouracil plus doxorubicin plus mitomycin-C and two regimens of streptozotocin plus mitomycin-C plus fluorouracil. J Clin Oncol 4:1794–1798, 1986.
13a. The Gastrointestinal Tumor Study Group. Treatment of locally unresectable carcinoma of the pancreas: comparison of combined-modality therapy (chemotherapy plus radiotherapy) to chemotherapy alone. J Natl Cancer Inst 80:751–755, 1988.
14. Gastrointestinal Tumor Study Group. Further evidence of effective adjuvant combined radiation and chemotherapy following curative resection of pancreatic cancer. Cancer 59:2006–2010, 1987.
15. Gullo J, Citron M, Smith F, et al. Gastric and pancreatic cancer. In: Advances in Cancer Treatment. The Hague, Martinus-Mijhoff Press, 1980, pp 125–147.
16. Haslam JB, Cavanaugh PJ, Stroup SL. Radiation therapy in the treatment of irresectable adenocarcinoma of the pancreas. Cancer 32:1341–1345, 1973.
17. Hudis C, Kelsen D, Dougherty J, et al. A randomized trial of streptozotocin (S), mitomycin (M), and 5-fluorouracil (F) (SMF) vs. cisplatin (C), Ara-C (A), and caffeine (C) (CAC) in advanced pancreas cancer (PC). Abstract, Proc of ASCO, Vol., p. 107, March 1990.
18. Kaiser MH, Ellenberg SS. Pancreatic cancer: Adjuvant combined radiation following curative resection. Arch Surg 120:899–903, 1985.
19. Kalra J, Cortes E, Chen S, et al. Effective multimodality treatment for advanced epidermoid carcinoma of the female genital tract. J Clin Oncol 1:413–415, 1983.
20. Klaasen DJ, MacIntyre GE, Cotton PF, et al. Treatment of locally unresectable cancer of the stomach and pancreas: A randomized comparison of 5-fluorouracil alone with radiation plus concurrent and maintenance 5-fluorouracil, an Eastern Cooperative Oncology Group study. J Clin Oncol 3:373–378, 1985.
21. Kovach JS, Moertel LG, Schutt AJ. A controlled study of combined 1,3-bis(2-chloroethyl)-1-nitrosourea and 5-fluorouracil therapy for advanced gastric and pancreatic cancer. Cancer 33:563–567, 1974.
22. Kyriazis AP, Kyriazis AA, Yagoda A. Enhanced therapeutic effect of *cis*-diamminedichloroplatinum (II) against nude mouse–grown human pancreatic adenocarcinoma

when combined with I-D-arabinofuranosyl-cytosine and caffeine. Cancer Res 45:6083–6087, 1985.

23. Lokich J, Skarin A. Combination therapy with 5-fluorouracil (5-FU) and 1,3-bis(2-chloroethyl)-1-nitrosourea (BCNU) for disseminated gastrointestinal carcinoma. Cancer Chemo Rep 56:653–657, 1972.
24. Mallinson CN, Rake MO, Cocking JB, et al. Chemotherapy in pancreatic cancer: Results of a controlled, prospective, randomised, multicentre trial. Br Med J 281:1589–1591, 1980.
25. Moertel CG, Childs DS, Reitemeir RJ, et al. Combined 5-fluorouracil and supervoltage radiation therapy of locally unresectable gastrointestinal cancer. Lancet 2:865, 1967.
26. Smith F, Schein P. Chemotherapy of pancreatic cancer. Semin Oncol 6:368–377, 1979.
27. Smith F, Hoth D, Levin B, et al. 5-Fluorouracil, Adriamycin, and mitomycin-C (FAM): Chemotherapy for advanced adenocarcinoma of the pancreas. Cancer 46:2014–2018, 1980.
28. Smith FP, Schein PS, MacDonald JS, et al. Fast neutron irradiation for locally advanced pancreatic cancer. Int J Radiat Oncol Biol Phys 7:1527, 1981.
29. Taylor SG IV, Murthy AK, Showel JL, et al. Improved control in advanced head and neck cancer with simultaneous radiation and cisplatin/5-FU chemotherapy. Cancer Treat Rep 69:933–939, 1985.
30. Trade M. The surgical treatment of pancreatic cancer. Surgery 28:35, 1985.
31. Whittington R, Dobelbower RR, Mohiuddin M, et al. Radiotherapy of unresectable pancreatic carcinoma: A six year experience with 104 patients. Int J Radiat Oncol Biol Phys 7:1639–1644, 1981.
32. Whittington R, Solin L, Mohiuddin M, et al. Multimodality therapy of localized unresectable pancreatic adenocarcinoma. Cancer 54:1991, 1984.
33. Wiggans G, Wolley PV, et al. Phase II trial of streptozotocin, mitomycin-C, and 5-fluorouracil (SMF) in the treatment of advanced pancreatic cancer. Cancer 41:387–391, 1978.
34. Wood W, Shipley WU, Gunderson LL, et al. Intraoperative irradiation for unresectable pancreatic carcinoma. Cancer 49:1272, 1982.

Index